ESSENTIALS

of

OBSTETRICS

and

GYNECOLOGY

NEVILLE F. HACKER, M.B.B.S. (Qld), MRCOG, MRACOG, FACOG, FACS

Director of Gynecologic Oncology;
Associate Professor of Obstetrics and Gynecology

J. GEORGE MOORE, M.D., FACOG, FACS

Professor and Chairman, Department of Obstetrics and Gynecology

University of California, Los Angeles School of Medicine, Los Angeles, California

1986

W. B. SAUNDERS COMPANY

Philadelphia / London / Toronto / Mexico City / Rio de Janeiro / Sydney / Tokyo / Hong Kong

W. B. Saunders Company: West Washington Square
Philadelphia, PA 19105

Library of Congress Cataloging-in-Publication Data

Main entry under title:

Essentials of obstetrics and gynecology.

1. Gynecology.   2. Obstetrics.
   I. Hacker, Neville.   II. Moore, J. George, 1917-
   [DNLM: 1. Gynecology. 2. Obstetrics. WQ 100 E783]

RG101.E87 1986   618.1   85–19658

ISBN 0–7216–1227–X

Editor: Dana Dreibelbis

Production Manager: Frank Polizzano

Page Layout Artist: Joan Sinclair

Essentials of Obstetrics and Gynecology   ISBN 0–7216–1227–X

Last digit is the print number: 9   8   7   6   5   4   3

To our dear wives,
Estelle and Mary Lou,
without whose patience and understanding
this book would not have been possible,
and for Geoff, Graeme, Sharon,
Barbara and Terence

CONTRIBUTORS

EDITORS

NEVILLE F. HACKER, M.B.B.S. (Qld), MRCOG, MRACOG, FACOG, FACS
Associate Professor of Obstetrics and Gynecology and Director of Gynecologic Oncology, UCLA School of Medicine.
Breast Disease: A Gynecologic Perspective; Principles of Cancer Therapy; Vulvar and Vaginal Cancer

J. GEORGE MOORE, M.D., FACOG, FACS
Professor and Chairman of Obstetrics and Gynecology, UCLA School of Medicine.
Female Reproductive Anatomy; Obstetric and Gynecologic Evaluation; Benign Diseases of the Uterus; Benign Tumors of the Ovaries and Fallopian Tubes; Endometriosis and Adenomyosis

SECTION EDITORS

CALVIN J. HOBEL, M.D.
Professor of Obstetrics and Gynecology and Pediatrics, UCLA School of Medicine; Director of Maternal-Fetal Medicine and Associate Director of Obstetrics and Gynecology, Cedars-Sinai Medical Center.
Prenatal Care; Normal Labor, Delivery, and the Puerperium; Resuscitation of the Newborn; Operative Obstetrics

JONATHAN S. BEREK, M.D.
Associate Professor of Obstetrics and Gynecology, UCLA School of Medicine.
Ovarian Cancer; Gestational Trophoblastic Neoplasia

JOHN MARSHALL, M.D.
Professor of Obstetrics and Gynecology, UCLA School of Medicine; Chairman of Obstetrics and Gynecology, Harbor/UCLA Medical Center.
Amenorrhea and Abnormal Uterine Bleeding

OTHER CONTRIBUTORS

JUAN J. ARCE, M.D.
Associate Professor of Obstetrics and Gynecology, Charles R. Drew Postgraduate Medical School; Chief, Division of Obstetrics, Martin Luther King, Jr. General Hospital.
Antepartum Hemorrhage

A. DAVID BARNES, M.D.
Attending Obstetrician and Gynecologist, Kern County Medical Center, Bakersfield, California.
Ovulation, Fertilization, and Implantation

RICHARD A. BASHORE, M.D.
Professor of Obstetrics and Gynecology, UCLA School of Medicine.
Dystocia

NARENDER N. BHATIA, M.D.
Assistant Professor of Obstetrics nad Gynecology, UCLA School of Medicine; Director of Gynecologic Urology, Harbor/UCLA Medical Center and Cedars-Sinai Medical Center.
Pelvic Relaxation and Urinary Problems

CLIFFORD BOCHNER, M.D.
Fellow in Maternal-Fetal Medicine, Department of Obstetrics and Gynecology, Cedars-Sinai Medical Center.
Anatomic Characteristics of the Fetal Head and Maternal Pelvis

J. ROBERT BRAGONIER, M.D., Ph.D.
Adjunct Professor of Obstetrics and Gynecology, UCLA School of Medicine; Chairman of Obstetrics and Gynecology, CIGNA Medical Center.
Human Sexuality; Sexual Assault

CHARLES R. BRINKMAN III, M.D.
Professor of Obstetrics and Gynecology and Chief, Division of Obstetrics, UCLA School of Medicine.
Obstetric and Gynecologic Evaluation; Hypertensive Disorders of Pregnancy

JOHN E. BUSTER, M.D.
Professor of Obstetrics and Gynecology, UCLA School of Medicine; Chief, Division of Reproductive Endocrinology, Harbor/UCLA Medical Center.
Dysmenorrhea and the Premenstrual Syndrome

MARIA BUSTILLO, M.D.
Assistant Professor of Obstetrics and Gynecology, UCLA School of Medicine; Attending Obstetrician and Gynecologist, Harbor/UCLA Medical Center.
Puberty and Precocious Puberty

MARY E. CARSTEN, Ph.D.
Professor of Obstetrics, Gynecology and Anesthesiology, UCLA School of Medicine.
Endocrinology of Pregnancy and Parturition

R. JEFFREY CHANG, M.D.
Associate Professor of Obstetrics and Gynecology, UCLA School of Medicine.
Virilism and Hirsutism

GAUTAM CHAUDHURI, M.D., Ph.D.
Assistant Professor of Obstetrics and Gynecology, UCLA School of Medicine.
Abortion

KENNETH A. CONKLIN, M.D., Ph.D.
Associate Professor of Anesthesiology and Director of Obstetric Anesthesia, UCLA School of Medicine.
Obstetric Analgesia and Anesthesia

IRVIN M. CUSHNER, M.D., M.P.H.
Professor of Obstetrics and Gynecology and Chief, Division of Women's Health, UCLA School of Medicine.
Contraception and Sterilization

WILLIAM J. DIGNAM, M.D.
Professor of Obstetrics and Gynecology and Chief, Division of Gynecology, UCLA School of Medicine.
Conditions Requiring Surgery During Pregnancy; Ectopic Pregnancy

LARRY C. FORD, M.D.
Assistant Professor of Obstetrics and Gynecology, UCLA School of Medicine.
Pelvic Inflammatory Disease

MICHELLE FOX, M.S.
Genetic Counselor and Genetic Clinic Coordinator, UCLA School of Medicine.
Genetic Counseling and Prenatal Diagnosis

ANN GARBER, Dr.P.H.
Assistant Clinical Professor of Obstetrics and Gynecology, UCLA School of Medicine; Director, Genetic Counseling, Cedars-Sinai Medical Center.
Teratology

ANNE D. M. GRAHAM, M.D.
Assistant Professor of Obstetrics and Gynecology, UCLA School of Medicine.
Preterm Labor and Premature Rupture of Membranes

WILLIAM A. GROWDON, M.D.
Assistant Professor of Obstetrics and Gynecology, UCLA School of Medicine.
Embryology and Congenital Anomalies of the Female Genital System

JOHN GUNNING, M.D.
Adjunct Associate Professor of Obstetrics and Gynecology, UCLA School of Medicine; Chief, Division of Gynecology, Harbor/UCLA Medical Center.
Vaginal and Vulvar Infections

LEWIS A. HAMILTON, Jr., M.D.
Associate Professor of Obstetrics and Gynecology and Director of Medical Education in Obstetrics and Gynecology, Charles R. Drew Postgraduate Medical School.
Intrauterine Growth Retardation, Intrauterine Fetal Demise, and Post-term Pregnancy

HUNTER A. HAMMILL, M.D.
Assistant Professor of Obstetrics and Gynecology, Case Western Reserve University, Cleveland, Ohio.
Pelvic Inflammatory Disease

GEORGE S. HARRIS, M.D.
Emeritus Clinical Professor of Obstetrics and Gynecology, University of Southern California School of Medicine; Director of Clinical Research in Obstetrics and Gynecology, Cedars-Sinai Medical Center.
Gynecologic Operative Techniques

ROBERT H. HAYASHI, M.D.
Professor of Obstetrics and Gynecology and Director of Maternal-Fetal Medicine, University of Michigan, Ann Arbor, Michigan.
Postpartum Hemorrhage and Puerperal Sepsis

HOWARD L. JUDD, M.D.
Professor of Obstetrics and Gynecology and Chief, Division of Reproductive Endocrinology, UCLA School of Medicine.
Menopause

THOMAS B. LEBHERZ, M.D.
Professor of Obstetrics and Gynecology, UCLA School of Medicine.
Benign Lesions of the Vulva, Vagina, and Cervix

RONALD S. LEUCHTER, M.D.
Assistant Clinical Professor of Obstetrics and Gynecology, UCLA School of Medicine.
Gynecologic Operative Techniques; Uterine Corpus Cancer

JOHN K. H. LU, Ph.D.
Associate Professor of Obstetrics and Gynecology and Anatomy, UCLA School of Medicine.
Physiology and Biochemistry of the Normal Reproductive Cycle

ARNOLD L. MEDEARIS, M.D.
Assistant Professor of Obstetrics and Gynecology, UCLA School of Medicine; Director of Antenatal Testing, Cedars-Sinai Medical Center.
Immunology of Pregnancy; Fetal Malpresentations; Multiple Gestation

DAVID R. MELDRUM, M.D.
Associate Professor of Obstetrics and Gynecology and Director of Infertility, UCLA School of Medicine.
Infertility

ROBERT MONOSON, M.D.
Adjunct Assistant Professor of Obstetrics and Gynecology, UCLA School of Medicine.
Rhesus Isoimmunization

JOHN MORRIS, M.D. (Deceased)
Former Associate Professor of Obstetrics and Gynecology, Charles R. Drew Postgraduate Medical School; Former Chief, Division of Reproductive Sciences, Martin Luther King, Jr. General Hospital
Antepartum Hemorrhage

SUHA H. N. MURAD, M.D.
Associate Professor of Anesthesiology, UCLA School of Medicine; Director of Obstetric Anesthesia, Harbor/UCLA Medical Center.
Normal Labor, Delivery, and the Puerperium

JOHN NEWNHAM, M.B.B.S., FRACOG
Fellow, Division of Maternal-Fetal Medicine, Department of Obstetrics and Gynecology, Cedars-Sinai Medical Center.
Operative Obstetrics

BAHIJ NUWAYHID, M.D.
Professor of Obstetrics and Gynecology, McGill University; Director of Maternal-Fetal Medicine, Women's Pavilion, Royal Victoria Hospital, Montreal, Canada.
Medical Complications of Pregnancy

GARY OAKES, M.D.
Adjunct Associate Professor of Obstetrics and Gynecology, UCLA School of Medicine; Director of Perinatal Outreach, Cedars-Sinai Medical Center.
Infections in Pregnancy

ANDREA J. RAPKIN, M.D.
Assistant Professor of Obstetrics and Gynecology, UCLA School of Medicine.
Chronic Pelvic Pain

ANTHONY E. READING, Ph.D.
Assistant Professor of Psychiatry and Biobehavioral Science, Neuropsychiatric Institute, UCLA Medical Center.
Human Sexuality; Sexual Assault

MICHAEL G. ROSS, M.D., Ph.D.
Assistant Professor of Obstetrics and Gynecology, UCLA School of Medicine; Attending Obstetrician and Gynecologist, Harbor/UCLA Medical Center.
Normal Labor, Delivery, and the Puerperium

EDWARD W. SAVAGE, Jr., M.D.
Adjunct Associate Professor of Obstetrics and Gynecology, UCLA School of Medicine; Professor of Obstetrics and Gynecology, Charles R. Drew Postgraduate Medical School; Chief, Division of Gynecology, Martin Luther King, Jr. General Hospital.
Cervical Dysplasia and Cancer

JAMES R. SHIELDS, M.D.
Consultant Perinatologist, Medical Center of Tarzana, Tarzana, California.
Fetal Malpresentations; Multiple Gestation

KLAUS J. STAISCH, M.D.
Associate Professor of Obstetrics and Gynecology, University of Minnesota Medical School; Director of Obstetrics, Hennepin County Medical Center, Minneapolis, Minnesota.
Identification and Management of Fetal Distress During Labor

KHALIL TABSH, M.D.
Associate Clinical Professor of Obstetrics and Gynecology, UCLA School of Medicine; Director, Maternal-Fetal Medicine, Northridge Hospital Medical Center, Northridge, California.
Genetic Counseling and Prenatal Diagnosis; Rhesus Isoimmunization

PAUL J. TOOT, M.D.
Chairman of Obstetrics and Gynecology, Kern County Medical Center, Bakersfield, California.
Ovulation, Fertilization, and Implantation

MACLYN E. WADE, M.D.
Professor of Obstetrics and Gynecology, UCLA School of Medicine; Chairman of Obstetrics and Gynecology, Cedars-Sinai Medical Center.
Uterine Corpus Cancer

NATHAN WASSERSTRUM, M.D., Ph.D.
Assistant Professor of Obstetrics and Gynecology, Baylor College of Medicine, Houston, Texas.
Maternal Physiology

PREFACE

A generation ago most schools of medicine in the United States presented courses in theoretical obstetrics and gynecology extending over a period of 18 months, supplemented by practical clerkships of 8 to 16 weeks in the third and fourth years. Most students procured as source textbooks a fairly complete compendium of obstetrics and another in gynecology. These texts not only served the students in medical school but were of great value during their housestaff training and were added to their reference library as they entered practice.

During the decade of the 1960's, theoretical obstetrics and gynecology in many institutions was condensed into a general course known as "An Introduction to Clinical Medicine" or "The Pathophysiology of Disease." Practical work in the clinics and wards was condensed into core clerkships, and in obstetrics and gynecology the "core" was generally restricted to six or eight weeks with electives available in subspecialty areas (high-risk obstetrics, gynecologic oncology, reproductive endocrinology, acting internships, and outpatient gynecology). This condensation of experience into the "core" of obstetrics and gynecology during the clinical years left students with a difficult choice in selecting a textbook that would not overwhelm them with information yet would still stimulate their interest in the subject. Understandably it became increasingly difficult to hold the student responsible for a critical body of knowledge.

Textbooks prescribed for the core clerkships often do not have sufficient depth and sometimes do not possess key references or practical information. On the other hand, the classic texts of obstetrics and gynecology or gynecologic surgery are generally considered by students to be too expensive or too comprehensive for them to absorb during the clerkship. This book is a response to their dilemma. The chapters have all been written by members of the Obstetrics and Gynecology Faculty at the University of California, Los Angeles (UCLA) Medical Center and its affiliated hospitals—Harbor (LA County) General Hospital, Cedars-Sinai Medical Center, Martin Luther King, Jr. General Hospital, and Kern County Medical Center. Some authors have changed their institutional affiliation prior to the publication of the book. It is hoped that the book will serve the needs of the student, be useful during housestaff training, and be a helpful text in the medical practitioner's library. Fundamental principles and practice of obstetrics and gynecology are presented succinctly, but we have endeavored to cover all important aspects of the subject in sufficient detail to allow a reasonable understanding of the pathophysiology and a safe approach to clinical management.

The text is divided into five sections: an introductory section, obstetrics, reproductive endocrinology, gynecology, and gynecologic oncology. Special emphasis is given to family planning and important aspects of women's health. The basic operations of obstetrics and gynecology are included to allow a reasonable understanding of the technical procedures. Drs. Neville F. Hacker and J. George Moore have been responsible for the overall organization of the book. The most difficult tasks have been to maintain uniformity of style and to keep the text within 550 pages without sacrificing essential information. Drs. Calvin Hobel, John Marshall, J. George Moore, and Jonathan Berek have organized their particular sections. Dr. Hacker has been largely responsible for the final editing of all the sections.

This book would not have been possible without the special help of the following individuals to whom we are most grateful: Gwynne Gloege, the very talented principal medical illustrator at UCLA, who was responsible for the overall uniformity and high quality of the illustrations; Yao-shi Fu, M.D., and Roberta Nieberg, M.D., from the Department of Pathology, who provided illustrations and advice regarding gynecologic pathology; Norman Chang, who was responsible for the photography; and Linda Olt, who provided invaluable editorial assistance and also prepared the index. At W. B. Saunders, we are particularly grateful to Dana Dreibelbis, the Executive Editor who provided the initial inspiration and subsequent guidance for this project. Finally, this project would never have been completed without the untiring efforts, skill, and ever cheerful countenance of Cheri Buonaguidi, the Obstetrics and Gynecology student coordinator at UCLA. She carefully read and accurately typed each version of the manuscript and worked with each of the contributors until all chapters were completed.

J. GEORGE MOORE, M.D.
NEVILLE F. HACKER, M.D.

CONTENTS

III GYNECOLOGY
    J. George Moore—Subeditor

IV REPRODUCTIVE ENDOCRINOLOGY
John Marshall—Subeditor

V GYNECOLOGIC ONCOLOGY
Jonathan S. Berek—Subeditor

I

INTRODUCTION

FEMALE REPRODUCTIVE ANATOMY

J. GEORGE MOORE

The scope of obstetrics and gynecology assumes a reasonable background in reproductive anatomy, physiology, and endocrinology. A physician cannot effectively practice obstetrics and gynecology without understanding the physiologic processes that transpire in a woman's life as she passes through infancy, adolescence, reproductive maturity, and the menopause. As the various clinical problems are addressed, it is important to consider those anatomic and physiologic changes that normally take place at key points in a woman's life cycle. Virtually all organ systems are involved, and much of gynecology involves monitoring normal physiologic changes.

Most of this text deals with the disruptive deviations from normal female anatomy and physiology, whether they be congenital, functional, traumatic, inflammatory, neoplastic, or even iatrogenic. As the etiology and pathogenesis of clinical problems are considered, each must be studied in the context of normal anatomy and physiology. This chapter discusses those aspects of female reproductive anatomy that are essential to obstetrics and gynecology.

PERINEUM

The perineum represents the inferior boundary of the pelvis. It is bounded superiorly by the levator ani muscles and inferiorly by the skin between the thighs (Fig. 1–

1). Anteriorly, the perineum extends to the symphysis pubis and the inferior borders of the pubic bones. Posteriorly, it is limited by the ischial tuberosities, the sacrotuberous ligaments, and the coccyx. The superficial and deep transverse perineal muscles cross the pelvic outlet between the two ischial tuberosities and divide the space into the urogenital triangle anteriorly and the anal triangle posteriorly.

The urogenital diaphragm is a fibromuscular sheet that stretches across the pubic arch. It is pierced by the vagina, urethra, the artery of the bulb, the internal pudendal vessels, and the dorsal nerve of the clitoris. Its inferior surface is covered by the crura of the clitoris, the vestibular bulbs, the greater vestibular (Bartholin's) glands, and the superficial perineal muscles. The Bartholin's glands are situated just posterior to the vestibular bulbs, and their ducts empty into the introitus just below the labia minora. They are often the site of gonococcal infections and painful abscesses.

EXTERNAL GENITALIA

The external genitalia are referred to collectively as the vulva. As shown in Figure 1–2, the vulva includes the mons veneris, labia majora, labia minora, clitoris, vulvovaginal (Bartholin's) glands, fourchette, and perineum. The most prominent features of the vulva, the labia majora, are large, hair-cov-

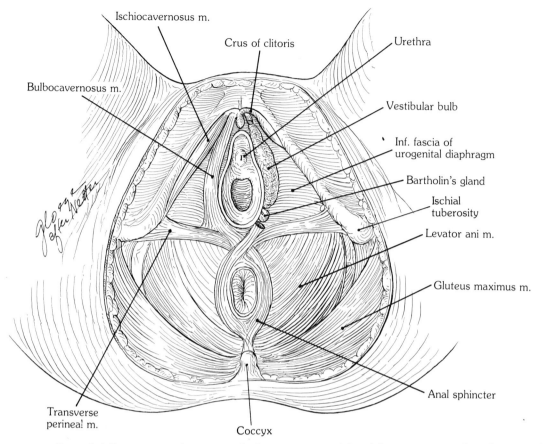

Ischiocavernosus m.

Crus of clitoris

Urethra

Bulbocavernosus m.

Vestibular bulb

Inf. fascia of
urogenital diaphragm

Bartholin's gland

Ischial
tuberosity

Levator ani m.

Gluteus maximus m.

Anal sphincter

Transverse
perineal m.

Coccyx

Figure 1–1 The perineum, showing superficial structures on the left and deep structures on the right.

ered folds of skin that contain sebaceous glands and lie on either side of the introitus. The labia minora lie medially and contain no hair but have a rich supply of venous sinuses, sebaceous glands, and nerves. The labia minora may vary from scarcely noticeable structures to leaf-like flaps measuring up to 3 cm in length. Anteriorly, each splits into two folds. The posterior pair of folds attach to the inferior surface of the clitoris where they unite to form the frenulum of the clitoris. The anterior pair unite like a hood over the clitoris, forming the prepuce. Posteriorly, the labia minora extend almost to the fourchette.

The clitoris lies just in front of the urethra and consists of the glans, the body, and the crura. Only the glans of the clitoris is visible externally. The body, composed of a pair of corpora cavernosa, extends superiorly for a distance of several centimeters and divides into two crura, which are attached to the undersurface of either pubic ramus. Each crus is covered by the corresponding ischio-

cavernosus muscle. The vestibular bulbs (equivalent to the corpus spongiosum of the penis) extend posteriorly from the glans on either side of the lower vagina. Each bulb is attached to the inferior surface of the perineal membrane and covered by the bulbocavernosus muscle. These muscles aid in constricting the venous supply to the erectile vestibular bulbs and also act as the sphincter vaginae.

As the labia minora are spread, the vaginal introitus, guarded by the hymenal ring, is seen. Usually, the hymen is represented only by a circle of carunculae myrtiformes around the vaginal introitus. However, the hymen may take many forms, such as a cribriform plate with many small openings or a completely imperforate diaphragm.

The vestibule of the vagina is that portion of the introitus extending inferiorly from the hymenal ring between the labia minora; the fourchette represents the posterior portion of the vestibule just above the perineal body.

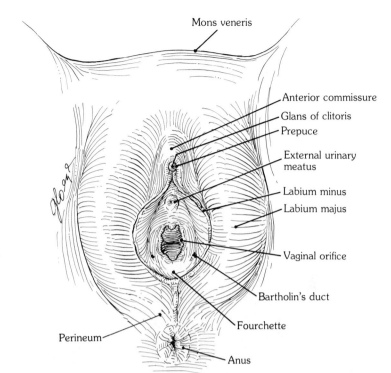

Figure 1–2 Female external genitalia.

Mons veneris

Anterior commissure
Glans of clitoris
Prepuce
External urinary meatus
Labium minus
Labium majus
Vaginal orifice
Bartholin's duct
Fourchette
Perineum
Anus

Most of the vulva is innervated by the branches of the pudendal nerve. Anterior to the urethra, the vulva is innervated by the ilioinguinal and genitofemoral nerves.

VAGINA

The vagina is a flattened tube extending from the hymenal ring at the introitus up to the fornices that surround the cervix (Fig. 1–3). Its epithelium is stratified squamous in type, normally devoid of mucous glands and hair follicles, and nonkeratinized. Deep to the vaginal epithelium are the muscular coats of the vagina, which consist of an inner circular and an outer longitudinal smooth muscle layer. Remnants of the mesonephric ducts may sometimes be demonstrated along the vaginal wall in the subepithelial layers and may give rise to Gartner's duct cysts. The vagina averages about 8 cm in length, although its size will vary considerably with age, parity, and the status of ovarian function. An important anatomical feature is the immediate proximity of the posterior fornix of the vagina to the pouch of Douglas, which allows easy access to the peritoneal cavity from the vagina, either by culdocentesis or colpotomy.

UTERUS

The uterus consists of the cervix and the uterine corpus, which are joined by the isthmus (Fig. 1–4). The latter represents a transitional area wherein the endocervical epithelium gradually changes into the endometrial lining. In late pregnancy, this area elongates and is referred to as the lower uterine segment.

The cervix is generally 2 to 3 cm in length. The portion that protrudes into the vagina and is surrounded by the fornices is covered with a nonkeratinizing squamous epithelium. At about the external cervical os, the squamous epithelium changes to a simple columnar epithelium, the site of transition being referred to as the squamocolumnar junction. The cervical canal is lined by an irregular, arborized, simple columnar epithelium, which extends into the stroma as cervical "glands" or crypts.

The uterine corpus is a thick, pear-shaped organ, somewhat flattened anteroposteriorly, that consists of interlacing, smooth muscle fibers. The endometrial lining may vary from 2 to 10 mm in thickness, depending on the stage of the menstrual cycle. Most of the surface of the uterus is covered by the peritoneal mesothelium.

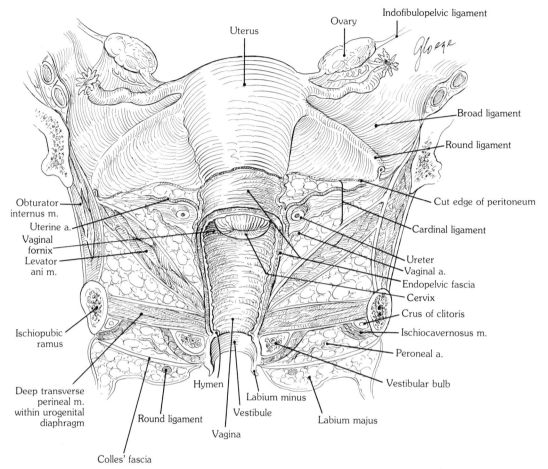

Figure 1–3 Coronal section of the pelvis at the level of the uterine isthmus and ischial spines, showing the ligaments supporting the uterus.

Four paired sets of ligaments are attached to the uterus. Each *round ligament* inserts on the anterior surface of the uterus just in front of the fallopian tube, passes to the pelvic side wall in a fold of the broad ligament, traverses the inguinal canal, and ends in the labium majus. The round ligaments are of little supportive value but help to keep the uterus anteverted. The *uterosacral ligaments* are condensations of the endopelvic fascia that arise from the sacral fascia and insert into the posterior inferior portion of the uterus at about the level of the isthmus. These ligaments contain sympathetic and parasympathetic nerve fibers that supply the uterus. They provide important support for the uterus and are also important in precluding the development of an enterocele. The *cardinal ligaments* (Mackenrodt's) are the other important supporting structures of the uterus that prevent prolapse. They extend from the pelvic fascia on the lateral pelvic walls and

insert into the lateral portion of the cervix and vagina, reaching superiorly to the level of the isthmus. The *pubocervical ligaments* pass anteriorly around the bladder to the posterior surface of the pubic symphysis.

In addition, there are four peritoneal folds. Anteriorly, the *vesicouterine fold* is reflected from the level of the isthmus onto the bladder. Posteriorly, the *rectouterine fold* passes from the posterior wall of the uterus, to the upper fourth of the vagina, and thence onto the rectum. It forms a cul-de-sac called the pouch of Douglas. Laterally, the two *broad ligaments* each pass from the side of the uterus to the lateral wall of the pelvis. Between the two leaves of each broad ligament are contained the fallopian tube, the round ligament, the ovary, and the ovarian ligament, in addition to nerves, blood vessels, and lymphatics. The fold of broad ligament containing the fallopian tube is called the mesosalpinx. Between the end of the tube

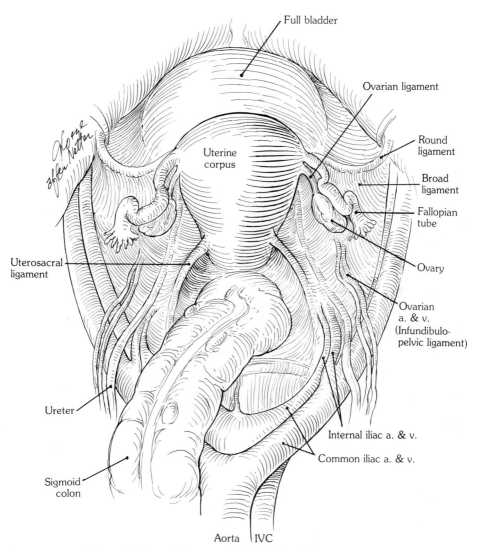

Figure 1–4 View of the organs in the female pelvis.

and the pelvic side wall, adjacent to the common iliac vessels, is the *infundibulopelvic ligament,* which contains the vessels and nerves for the ovary.

FALLOPIAN TUBES

The oviducts are bilateral muscular tubes (about 10 cm in length) with lumina that connect the uterine cavity with the peritoneal cavity. They are enclosed in the medial four fifths of the superior aspect of the broad ligament. The tubes are lined by a ciliated, columnar epithelium that is thrown into branching folds. That segment of the tube within the wall of the uterus is referred to as the *interstitial portion.* The medial portion of each tube is superior to the round ligament, anterior to the ovarian ligament, and relatively fixed in position. This nonmobile portion of the tube has a fairly narrow lumen and is referred to as the *isthmus.* As the tube proceeds laterally, it is located anterior to the ovary, then passes around the lateral portion of the ovary and down towards the cul-de-sac. The *ampullary* and *fimbriated* portions of the tube are suspended from the broad ligament by the mesosalpinx and are quite mobile. The mobility of the fimbriated end of the tube plays an important role in fertility.

OVARIES

The ovaries are oval, flattened, compressible organs, approximately 3 by 2 cm in size. They are situated on the superior surface of the broad ligament and are suspended between the ovarian ligament medially and the suspensory ligament of the ovary or infundibulopelvic ligament laterally and superiorly. Each occupies a position in the ovarian fossa (of Waldeyer), which is a shallow depression on the lateral pelvic wall just posterior to the external iliac vessels and anterior to the ureter and hypogastric vessels. In endometriosis and salpingo-oophoritis, the ovaries may be densely adherent to the ureter. Generally, the serosal covering and the tunica albuginea of the ovary are quite thin, and developing follicles and corpora lutea are readily visible.

The blood supply to the ovaries is provided by the long ovarian arteries that arise from the abdominal aorta immediately below the renal arteries. These vessels course downward and cross laterally over the ureter at the level of the pelvic brim, passing branches to the ureter and the fallopian tube. The ovary also receives substantial blood supply from the uterine artery. The venous drainage from the right ovary is directly into the inferior vena cava, while that of the left ovary is into the left renal vein (Fig. 1–5).

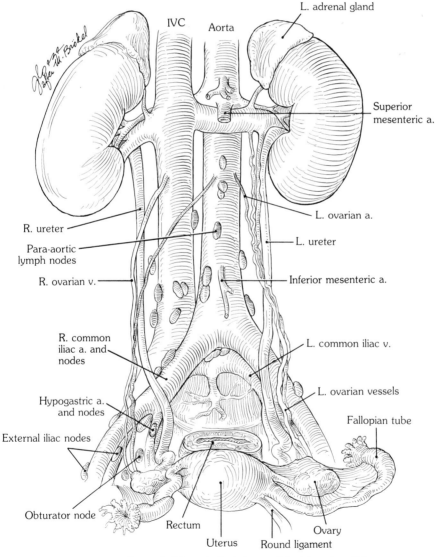

Figure 1–5 Lymphatic drainage of the internal genital organs.

URETERS

The ureters extend 25 to 30 cm from the renal pelves to their insertion into the bladder at the trigone. Each descends immediately under the peritoneum, crossing the pelvic brim beneath the ovarian vessels just anterior to the bifurcation of the common iliac artery. In the true pelvis, the ureter initially courses inferiorly, just anterior to the hypogastric vessels, and stays closely attached to the peritoneum. It then passes forward along the side of the cervix and beneath the uterine artery toward the trigone of the bladder.

LYMPHATIC DRAINAGE

The lymphatic drainage of the vulva and lower vagina is principally to the inguino-femoral lymph nodes and then to the external iliac chains (see Fig. 55–3). The lymphatic drainage of the cervix takes place through the parametria (cardinal ligaments) to the pelvic nodes (the hypogastric, obturator, and external iliac groups) and then to the com-mon iliac and para-aortic chains. The lym-phatic drainage from the endometrium is through the broad ligament and infundibu-lopelvic ligament to the pelvic and para-aortic chains. The lymphatics of the ovaries pass via the infundibulopelvic ligaments to the pelvic and para-aortic nodes (Fig. 1–5).

LOWER ABDOMINAL WALL

Since most intra-abdominal gynecologic operations are performed through lower ab-dominal incisions, it is important to review the anatomy of the lower abdominal wall with special reference to the muscles and fasciae. After transecting the skin, subcuta-neous fat, superficial fascia (of Camper), and deep fascia (of Scarpa), the anterior rectus sheath is encountered (Fig. 1–6). The rectus sheath is a strong fibrous compartment formed by the aponeuroses of the three lat-eral abdominal wall muscles. The aponeu-roses meet in the midline to form the linea alba and partially encase the two rectus ab-dominis muscles. The composition of the

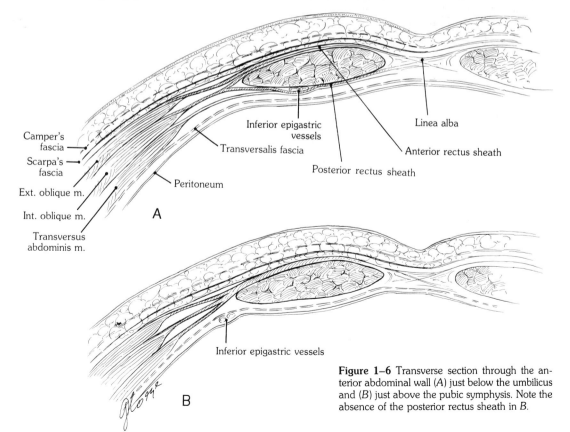

Camper's fascia
Scarpa's fascia
Ext. oblique m.
Int. oblique m.
Transversus abdominis m.
Transversalis fascia
Peritoneum
Inferior epigastric vessels
Posterior rectus sheath
Anterior rectus sheath
Linea alba
A

Inferior epigastric vessels
B

Figure 1–6 Transverse section through the an-terior abdominal wall (A) just below the umbilicus and (B) just above the pubic symphysis. Note the absence of the posterior rectus sheath in B.

rectus sheath differs in its upper and lower portions. Above the midpoint between the umbilicus and the symphysis pubis, the rectus muscle is encased anteriorly by the aponeurosis of the external oblique and the anterior lamina of the internal oblique aponeurosis; posteriorly by the aponeurosis of the transversus abdominis and the posterior lamina of the internal oblique aponeurosis. In the lower fourth of the abdomen, the posterior aponeurotic layer of the sheath terminates in a free crescentic margin, the semilunar fold of Douglas.

Each rectus abdominis muscle, encased in the rectus sheath on either side of the midline, extends from the superior aspect of the symphysis pubis to the anterior surface of the fifth, sixth, and seventh costal cartilages. A varying number of tendinous intersections (three to five) cross each muscle at irregular intervals, and a transverse rectus surgical incision forms a new fibrous intersection during healing. The muscle is not attached to the posterior sheath, and, following separation from the anterior sheath, can be retracted laterally, as in the Pfannenstiel incision. Each rectus muscle has a firm aponeurosis at its attachment to the symphysis pubis, and this tendinous aponeurosis can be transected if necessary to improve exposure, as in the Cherny incision, and resutured securely during closure of the abdominal wall.

The inferior epigastric arteries arise from the external iliac arteries and proceed superiorly just lateral to the rectus muscles between the transversalis fascia and the peritoneum. They enter the rectus sheaths at the level of the semilunar line and continue their course superiorly just posterior to the rectus muscles. In a transverse rectus muscle-cutting incision, the epigastric arteries can be retracted laterally or ligated to allow a wide peritoneal incision.

ABDOMINAL WALL INCISIONS

The most commonly used lower abdominal incision in gynecologic surgery is the Pfannenstiel incision (Fig. 1–7). Although it does not always give sufficient exposure for extensive operations, it has cosmetic advantages in

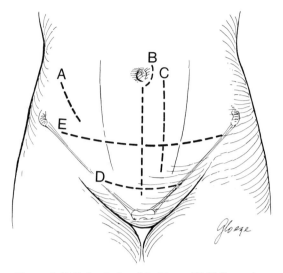

Figure 1–7 Abdominal wall incisions: (A) McBurney's, (B) lower midline, (C) left lower paramedian, (D) Pfannenstiel or Cherny, and (E) transverse.

that it is generally 2 cm above the symphysis pubis, and the scar is later covered by the pubic hair. Because the rectus abdominis muscles are not cut, eviscerations and wound hernias are extremely uncommon. For extensive pelvic procedures (e.g., radical hysterectomy and pelvic lymphadenectomy), a transverse muscle cutting incision (Maylard) at a slightly higher level in the lower abdomen gives sufficient exposure. In addition, the skin incision falls within lines of Langer, so a good cosmetic result can be expected. When it is anticipated that upper abdominal exploration will be necessary, such as in a patient with suspected ovarian cancer, a midline incision through the linea alba or a paramedian vertical incision is indicated.

SUGGESTED READING

Clemente CD: Regional Atlas of the Human Body. Philadelphia, Lea and Febiger, 1975.

Grant JCB: An Atlas of Human Anatomy. 7th ed. Baltimore, Williams and Wilkins Co, 1978.

Maylard EA: Directions of abdominal incisions. Br J Med 2:895, 1907.

Smout CFV, Jacoby F, Lillie EW: Gynecological and Obstetrical Anatomy. Baltimore, Williams and Wilkins Co, 1969.

Ulfelder H: Mechanism of pelvic support in women. Am J Obstet Gynecol 72:856, 1956.

Chapter Two

OBSTETRIC AND GYNECOLOGIC EVALUATION

CHARLES R. BRINKMAN III and J. GEORGE MOORE

As in most areas of medicine, a careful history and physical examination form the basis for patient evaluation and clinical management in obstetrics and gynecology. This chapter outlines the essential details of the clinical evaluation of the obstetric and gynecologic patient and also discusses some pertinent ethical considerations and obstetric statistics.

OBSTETRIC HISTORY

A complete history must be recorded at the time of the prepregnancy evaluation or at the initial antenatal visit. Several detailed standardized forms are available for recording the pertinent aspects of the antenatal history, but this does not negate the need for a detailed history taken personally by the physician who will be caring for the patient throughout pregnancy. During the history-taking, major opportunities arise to provide counseling and explanations that serve to establish close rapport and to allay apprehensions.

Previous Pregnancies

Each prior pregnancy should be reviewed in chronological order and the following information recorded:

1. *Date of delivery* (or pregnancy termination).

2. *Location of delivery* (or pregnancy termination). Recording the city, name of hos-

pital, and name of the attending physician may become important if further details are required.

3. *Duration of gestation* (recorded in weeks). When correlated with birth weight, this information allows an assessment of fetal growth patterns. The gestational age of any spontaneous abortion is of etiologic significance.

4. *Type of delivery* (or method of terminating pregnancy). This information is important for planning the method of delivery in the present pregnancy. A difficult forceps delivery or a cesarean section may require a personal review of the labor and delivery records.

5. *Duration of labor* (recorded in hours). This may alert the physician to the possibility of an unusually long or short labor.

6. *Type of anesthesia.* Any complications of anesthesia should be noted.

7. *Maternal complications.* Urinary tract infections, vaginal bleeding, hypertension, and postpartum complications may be repetitive; such knowledge is helpful in anticipating problems with the present pregnancy.

8. *Newborn weight* (in grams or pounds and ounces). This information may give indications of gestational diabetes, fetal growth problems, or cephalopelvic discordance.

9. *Newborn gender.* This may provide insight into patient and family expectations and may indicate certain genetic risk factors.

10. *Fetal and neonatal complications.* Certain questions may be asked to elicit any problems and to determine the need to obtain

11

further information. Inquiry should be made as to whether or not the baby had any problems after it was born, whether or not the baby breathed and cried right away, and whether or not the baby left the hospital with the mother. In addition to providing an assessment of risks, answers to questions such as these may allow insight into the mother's attitude during this pregnancy.

Menstrual History

A good menstrual history is essential, since it is the determinant for establishing the expected date of confinement (EDC). Nägele's rule for establishing the EDC is to subtract three months and add seven days to the first day of the last normal menstrual period (LMP). For example:

LMP—July 20, 1985 (7/20/85)
EDC—April 27, 1986 (4/27/86)

This calculation depends upon a normal 28-day cycle, and adjustments must be made for longer or shorter cycles. Any bleeding or spotting since the last normal menstrual period should be reviewed in detail. Many abnormalities may be associated with bleeding in the first and second trimester, such as threatened abortion, ectopic pregnancy, placenta previa, and cervical neoplasia.

Contraceptive History

This information is important for risk assessment. Oral contraceptives taken during early pregnancy have been associated with birth defects, and retained intrauterine devices can cause early pregnancy loss and premature delivery. Discussion of contraception also allows the physician to gain insight into whether or not the pregnancy was planned and desired.

Medical History

The importance of a good medical history cannot be overemphasized. In addition to common disorders such as diabetes mellitus, hypertension, and renal disease, all serious conditions should be recorded. An episode of hepatitis would dictate laboratory evaluation for a carrier state. An unexplained period of proteinuria would require investigations to rule out undiagnosed renal disease or a collagen vascular disease such as systemic lupus erythematosus.

Surgical History

Each surgical procedure should be recorded chronologically, including age, hospital, surgeon, and complications. Trauma must also be listed, since a fractured pelvis may result in diminished pelvic capacity.

Social History

The social history not only plays a role in risk assessment, but provides insight into the patient's personal qualities. Habits such as smoking or alcohol and drug abuse are important factors that must be recorded and managed appropriately. The patient's contact or exposure to domesticated animals, particularly cats, with their associated risk of toxoplasmosis, is an important item to uncover.

The patient's type of work and lifestyle may affect the pregnancy. A woman who does heavy manual labor may not be able to continue working throughout the entire pregnancy, while one with a more sedentary position may continue to work until the onset of labor.

OBSTETRIC PHYSICAL EXAMINATION

General Physical Examination

This procedure must be thorough and performed as early as possible in the prenatal period. A cursory or perfunctory examination is not sufficient, since this may be the first complete examination the woman has had since childhood. A complete physical examination provides an opportunity to detect previously unrecognized abnormalities. Normal baseline levels must also be established, particularly those of weight, blood pressure, funduscopic appearance, and cardiac status.

Pelvic Examination

The initial pelvic examination should be done early in the prenatal period and should include (1) inspection of the external genitalia, vagina, and cervix, (2) collection of cytologic specimens from the ectocervix and endocervical canal, and (3) palpation of the cervix, uterus, and adnexa.

Palpation of the uterus is important. Uterine abnormalities may be detected, and the approximate duration of gestation determined. The estimate of gestational age by uterine size becomes less accurate as pregnancy progresses. Rectal and rectovaginal examinations are also important aspects of this initial pelvic evaluation.

Clinical Pelvimetry

This assessment is carried out following the bimanual pelvic examination and before the rectal examination. It is important that clinical pelvimetry be carried out systematically. The details of clinical pelvimetry are described in Chapter 9.

DIAGNOSIS OF PREGNANCY

The diagnosis of pregnancy and its location may be quite challenging during the early weeks of amenorrhea. For the most part, pregnancy is diagnosed on clinical grounds without the necessity of resorting to laboratory or imaging methods. Indeed, unless there is some specific clinical or social reason that makes early diagnosis desirable, cost-effective practice would dictate a purely clinical diagnosis.

Symptoms of Pregnancy

The most common symptoms in the early months of pregnancy are amenorrhea, urinary frequency, breast engorgement, nausea, tiredness, and easy fatigability. Amenorrhea in a previously normally menstruating, sexually active woman should be considered to be caused by pregnancy until proven otherwise. Urinary frequency is most likely caused by the pressure of the enlarged uterus upon the bladder. Morning urgency upon awakening is common in early pregnancy. Breast engorgement, which many women are aware of in the luteal phase, continues and becomes exaggerated in early pregnancy. The cause of nausea during early pregnancy has not been fully explained.

Signs of Pregnancy

The signs of pregnancy may be divided into those that are presumptive, those that are probable, and those that are positive.

The *presumptive signs* are primarily those associated with skin and mucous membrane changes. Discoloration and cyanosis of the vulva, vagina, and cervix are related to the generalized engorgement of the pelvic organs and are, therefore, nonspecific. The dark discoloration of the vulva and vaginal walls is known as Chadwick's sign. Pigmentation of the skin and abdominal striae are nonspecific and unreliable signs. The most common sites for pigmentation are the midline of the lower abdomen and over the bridge of the nose and under the eyes. The former is called the linea nigra, while the latter sites are called chloasma or the mask of pregnancy. Chloasma is also a fairly uncommon side effect of oral contraceptives.

The *probable signs* of pregnancy are those mainly related to the detectable physical changes in the uterus. During early pregnancy, the uterus changes its size, shape, and consistency. Early uterine enlargement tends to be in the anteroposterior diameter so that the uterus becomes globular. Uterine consistency becomes softer, and it may not be possible to palpate the connection between the cervix and fundus. This change is referred to as Hegar's sign. The cervix also begins to soften early in pregnancy. Later, ballottement of the fetus or a fetal part and mapping of a fetal outline by palpation are also probable signs of pregnancy. Finally, the palpatory presence of uterine contractions is a probable sign of pregnancy, although other causes of uterine enlargement can result in uterine contractions.

The *positive signs* of pregnancy include the detection of a fetal heart beat and the recognition of fetal movements. Modern Doppler techniques for detecting the fetal heart beat may be successful as early as 10 weeks and are nearly always positive by 12 weeks. Fetal heart tones can usually be detected with a stethoscope between 16 and 20 weeks. The multiparous woman generally recognizes fetal movements between 16 and 18 weeks, while the primigravida usually does not recognize fetal movements until 18 to 20 weeks. An experienced observer may palpate fetal movements with increasing reliability after 20 to 24 weeks.

Laboratory Tests for Pregnancy

Pregnancy Tests. Tests to detect pregnancy have revolutionized early diagnosis. Although they are considered a probable sign of pregnancy, the accuracy of these tests is good. All commonly used methods depend upon the detection of chorionic gonadotropin or its beta subunit. Depending upon the specific sensitivity of the test, pregnancy may be suspected even prior to a missed period. The available tests and their sensitivities are discussed in Chapter 37.

Diagnostic Ultrasound. The imaging technique of ultrasound has made a significant contribution to the diagnosis and evaluation of pregnancy. Using real-time ultrasound, a fetal image can be detected by 6 to 7 weeks and a beating heart shortly thereafter. Radiographic imaging depends upon detection of the fetal skeleton, which is usually not seen until 16 weeks.

GYNECOLOGIC HISTORY

A full history is equally as important in evaluating the gynecologic patient as in evaluating a patient in general medicine or surgery. The history-taking must be systematic to avoid omissions, and it should be conducted with sensitivity and without haste.

Following the introductory amenities, recording the referral source, age, place of birth, education, and present occupation conveniently sets the tone for a friendly and nonadversarial interview.

Present Illness

The patient is asked to state her main complaint and to relate her present illness sequentially in her own words. Pertinent negative accounts should be recorded, and, as far as possible, questions should be reserved until after the patient has described the course of her illness. Generally, the history provides substantial clues to the diagnosis, so it is important to fully evaluate the more common symptoms encountered in gynecologic patients.

Abnormal Vaginal Bleeding. Vaginal bleeding before the age of 10 and after the age of 52 is cause for concern and requires investigation. These are the limits of normal menstruation, and although the occasional woman may menstruate regularly and normally up to the age of 57 or 58 years, it is important to ensure that she is not bleeding from uterine cancer or from exogenous estro-

gens. Prolongation of menses beyond seven days or bleeding between menses, except for a brief *"kleine regnung"* at ovulation, may connote abnormal ovarian function, uterine myomata, or endometriosis.

Abdominal Pain. Many gynecologic problems are associated with abdominal pain. The common gynecologic causes of acute lower abdominal pain are salpingo-oophoritis with peritoneal inflammation, torsion and infarction of an ovarian cyst, or rupture of an ectopic pregnancy. Chronic lower abdominal pain is generally associated with endometriosis, chronic pelvic inflammatory disease, or large pelvic tumors.

Amenorrhea. The most common causes of amenorrhea are pregnancy and the normal menopause. It is abnormal for a young woman to reach the age of 17 without menstruating (primary amenorrhea). Pregnancy should be suspected in a woman between 15 and 45 years of age who fails to menstruate within 35 days from the first day of her last menstruation. In a patient with amenorrhea who is not pregnant, enquiry should be made about menopausal or climacteric symptoms such as hot flashes, vaginal dryness, or depression.

Other pertinent symptoms of concern in a gynecologic patient's present illness include dysmenorrhea, premenstrual tension, fluid retention, leukorrhea, constipation, dyschezia, dyspareunia, and abdominal distension. Lower back and sacral pain may indicate uterine prolapse, enterocele, or rectocele.

Menstrual History

The menstrual history should include the age at menarche (average is 12 to 13 years), interval between periods (21 to 35 days with a median of 28 days), duration of menses (average is 5 days), and character of the flow (scant, normal, heavy, with or without clots). Any intermenstrual bleeding (metrorrhagia) should be noted. The date of onset of the last menstrual period (LMP), as well as the date of the previous menstrual period (PMP), should be recorded. Enquiry should be made regarding menstrual cramps (dysmenorrhea), and, if present, the age of onset, severity, and character of the cramps should be recorded, together with an estimate of the disability incurred. Midcycle pain (*mittelschmerz*) and a midcycle increase in vaginal secretions are indicative of ovulatory cycles.

Contraceptive History

The type and duration of each contraceptive method must be recorded, along with any attendant complications. These may include amenorrhea or thromboembolic disease with oral contraceptives; dysmenorrhea, heavy bleeding (menorrhagia), or pelvic infection with the intrauterine device; or contraceptive failure with the diaphragm.

Obstetric History

Each pregnancy, delivery, and any associated complications are listed.

Marital History

The date and duration of each marriage should be recorded, along with the purported reason for termination. The health and relationship of the husband or consort(s) may provide insight into the present complaints. Enquiry should be made regarding any pain (dyspareunia), bleeding, or dysuria associated with sexual intercourse. Sexual satisfaction must be tactfully evaluated.

Past History

As in the obstetric history, any significant past medical or surgical history should be recorded, as should the patient's family history.

Systemic Review

A review of all other organ systems should be undertaken. Habits (tobacco, alcohol, drug abuse), medications, usual weight with recent changes, and loss of height (osteoporosis) are important parts of the system review.

GYNECOLOGIC PHYSICAL EXAMINATION

General Physical Examination

A complete physical examination must be performed on each new patient and repeated at least annually. The initial examination should include the patient's height, weight, and arm span (in adolescent patients or those with endocrine problems) and should be carried out with the patient completely disrobed but suitably draped. The examination should be systematic and should include the points that follow.

Vital Signs. Temperature, pulse rate, respiratory rate, and blood pressure should be recorded.

General Appearance. The patient's body build, posture, state of nutrition, demeanor, and state of well-being should be recorded. A well-described general appearance should allow the patient to be identified on the ward after the description in the chart has been read.

Head and Neck. The evaluation should include the ears, throat, tonsils, cervical lymph nodes, thyroid gland, and fundi. Evidence of supraclavicular lymphadenopathy, oral lesions, webbing of the neck, or goiter may be pertinent to the gynecologic assessment.

Breasts. The breast examination, discussed in Chapter 39, is particularly important in gynecologic patients.

Heart and Lungs. A complete examination of the heart and lungs is of importance, particularly in a patient requiring surgery. The presence of a pleural effusion may be indicative of a disseminated malignancy, particularly ovarian cancer.

Abdomen. Examination of the abdomen is critical in the evaluation of the gynecologic patient. The contour, whether flat, scaphoid, or protuberant, should be noted. The latter appearance may suggest ascites. The presence and distribution of hair, especially in the area of the escutcheon, should be recorded, as should the presence of striae or operative scars.

Abdominal tenderness must be determined by placing one hand flat against the abdomen in the nonpainful areas initially, then gently and gradually exerting pressure with the fingers of the other hand (Fig. 2–1). Rebound tenderness (a sign of peritoneal irritation), muscle guarding, and abdominal rigidity should be gently elicited, again first in the nontender areas. A "doughy" abdomen in which the guarding increases gradually as the pressure of palpation is increased is often seen with a hematoperitoneum.

It is important to palpate any abdominal mass. The size should be specifically noted. However, other characteristics may be even more important in suggesting the diagnosis,

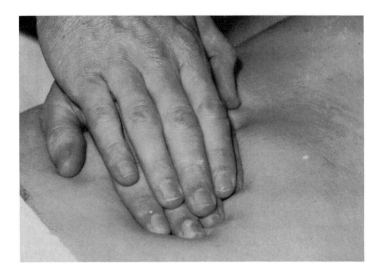

Figure 2–1 Palpation of the abdomen by placing the left palm flat against the abdominal wall and then gently exerting pressure with the fingers of the right hand.

such as whether the mass is cystic or solid, smooth or nodular, fixed or mobile, and whether or not it is associated with ascites. In determining the reason for abdominal distension (tumor, ascites, or distended bowel), it is important to percuss carefully the areas of tympany (gaseous distension) and dullness. A large tumor is generally dull on top with loops of bowel displaced to the flanks. Dullness that shifts as the patient turns onto her side (shifting dullness) is suggestive of ascites.

The presence and character of the peristaltic waves are important. High-pitched, tinkling bowel sounds suggest the recent onset of a bowel obstruction, while the absence of peristalsis may connote peritonitis or a long-standing bowel obstruction.

Back. Abnormal curvature of the vertebral column (dorsal kyphosis or scoliosis) is an important observation in evaluating osteoporosis in a postmenopausal woman. Costovertebral angle tenderness suggests pyelonephritis, while psoas muscle spasm may occur with gynecologic infections. A sciatic radiation of pain may suggest orthopedic problems or a recurrent pelvic malignancy impinging on the sciatic nerve.

Extremities. The presence or absence of varicosities, edema, pedal pulsations, and cutaneous lesions are important in evaluating and managing the gynecologic patient.

Pelvic Examination

In a gynecologic patient, pelvic examination may represent the most important part of the assessment. It must be conducted sys-

tematically and with careful sensitivity, especially if it is the patient's first such examination. The procedure should be unhurried, performed with smooth and gentle movements, and accompanied by reasonable explanations.

Vulva. The character and distribution of hair, the degree of development or atrophy of the labia, and the character of the hymen (imperforate or cribriform) and introitus (virginal, nulliparous, or multiparous) should be noted. Any clitoromegaly should be noted, as should cysts, tumors, or inflammation of the Bartholin's gland. The urethra and Skene's glands should be inspected for any purulent exudates. The labia should be inspected for any inflammatory, dystrophic, or neoplastic lesions, as described in Chapters 29 and 55. Perineal relaxation and scarring should be noted, as they may cause dyspareunia and defects in rectal sphincter tone.

Speculum Examination. The vagina and cervix are inspected with an appropriately sized bivalve speculum (Fig. 2–2), which should be warmed under the tap and lubricated only with warm water so as not to interfere with the examination of cervical cytology or any vaginal exudate (see Chapter 33). After gently spreading the labia to expose the introitus, the speculum should be inserted with the blades entering the introitus transversely, then directed posteriorly along the vagina with pressure exerted against the relatively insensitive perineum to avoid contacting the sensitive urethra. As the anterior blade reaches the cervix, the speculum is opened to bring the cervix into view. As the

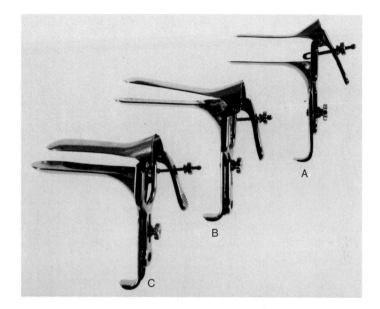

Figure 2–2 *A*, Pediatric speculum; *B*, Pederson speculum; and *C*, Graves speculum. The Pederson speculum is narrower and more appropriate for examining a nulliparous patient.

vaginal epithelium is inspected, it is important to rotate the speculum through 90 degrees, so that lesions on the anterior or posterior walls of the vagina ordinarily covered by the blades of the speculum will not be overlooked. Vaginal wall relaxation should be sought using either a Sims' speculum or the posterior blade of a bivalve speculum (see Chapter 35). The patient is asked to bear down (Valsalva's maneuver) or to cough in order to demonstrate any stress incontinence. If the patient's complaint involves urinary stress or urgency, this portion of the examination should be carried out before emptying the bladder.

The cervix should be inspected to determine its size, shape, and color. The nulliparous patient generally has a conical, unscarred cervix with a circular, centrally placed os; the multiparous cervix is generally bulbous with a transverse configuration of the os (Fig. 2–3). Any purulent cervical discharge should be cultured. Plugged, distended cervical glands (nabothian follicles) may be seen on the ectocervix. In premenopausal women, the squamocolumnar junction of the cervix is usually visible around the cervical os, particularly in patients of low parity. Postmenopausally, the junction is invariably retracted within the endocervical canal.

Bimanual Examination. The bimanual pelvic examination provides information about the uterus and adnexa (fallopian tubes and ovaries). During this portion of the examination, the urinary bladder should be emp-

tied; if it is not, the internal genitalia will be difficult to delineate, and the procedure is apt to be uncomfortable for the patient. Occasionally, because of pain-evoked guarding, the bimanual examination must be carried out under anesthesia. The labia are separated, and the gloved, lubricated index finger is inserted into the vagina, avoiding the sensitive urethral meatus. Pressure is exerted posteriorly against the perineum and puborectalis muscle, which causes the introitus to gape somewhat, thereby allowing the middle finger to be inserted as well. Intromission of the two fingers into the depth of the vagina may be facilitated by having the patient bear down slightly.

The cervix is palpated for consistency, contour, size, and tenderness to motion. If the

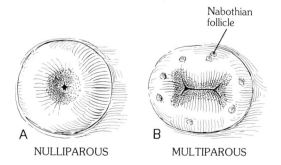

Figure 2–3 *A*, Cervix of a nulliparous patient and *B*, cervix of a multiparous patient. Note the circular os in the nulliparous cervix and the transverse os, due to lacerations at childbirth, in the multiparous cervix.

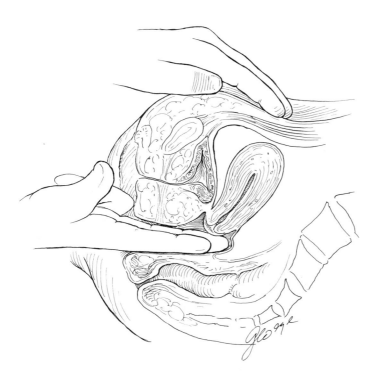

Figure 2–4 Bimanual evaluation of the uterus by gently pressing the uterus with the vaginal fingers against the abdominal hand.

vaginal fornices are absent, as may occur in postmenopausal women, it is not possible to appreciate the size of the cervix on bimanual examination. This can only be determined on rectovaginal or rectal examination.

The uterus is evaluated by placing the abdominal hand flat on the abdomen with the fingers pressing gently just above the symphysis pubis. With the vaginal fingers supinated in either the anterior or posterior vaginal fornix, the uterine corpus is pressed gently against the abdominal hand (Fig. 2–4). As the uterus is felt between the examining fingers of both hands, the size, configuration, consistency, and mobility of the organ are appreciated. If the muscles of the abdominal wall are not compliant, or if the uterus is retroverted, the outline, consistency, and mobility must be determined by ballottement with the vaginal fingers in the fornices; however, in these circumstances, it is impossible to discern uterine size accurately.

By shifting the abdominal hand to either side of the midline and gently elevating the lateral fornix up to the abdominal hand, it may be possible to outline an adnexal mass (Fig. 2–5). The left adnexa are best appreciated with the fingers of the left hand in the vagina (Fig. 2–6). The examiner should stand sideways, facing the patient's left, with the left hip maintaining pressure against the left elbow, thereby providing better tactile sensation because of the relaxed musculature in the forearm and examining hand. The pouch of Douglas is also carefully assessed for nodularity or tenderness, as may occur with endometriosis, pelvic inflammatory disease, or metastatic carcinoma.

It is usually impossible to feel the normal tube, and conditions must be optimal to appreciate the normal ovary. The ovary has the size and consistency of a shelled oyster and may be felt with the vaginal fingers as they are passed across the under surface of the abdominal hand. The ovaries are very tender to compression, and the patient is uncomfortably aware of any ovarian compression or movement during the examination.

It may be impossible to differentiate between an ovarian or tubal mass or even a lateral uterine mass. Generally, left adnexal masses are more difficult to evaluate than those on the right because of the position of the sigmoid colon on the left side of the pelvis.

Rectal Examination

The anus should be inspected for lesions, hemorrhoids, or inflammation. Rectal sphincter tone should be recorded and any mucosal

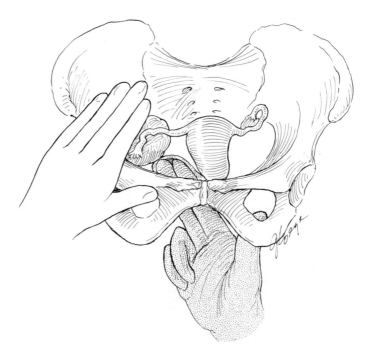

Figure 2–5 Bimanual examination of the right adnexa.

lesions noted. A guaiac test should be performed to determine the presence of occult blood.

A rectovaginal examination is helpful in evaluating masses in the cul-de-sac, the rectovaginal septum, or adnexa. It is essential in evaluating the parametrium in patients with cervical cancer (Fig. 2–7). Following hysterectomy, or in postmenopausal patients with obliteration of the vaginal fornices, rec-

tal examination is very helpful in evaluating the adnexa. Rectal examination may also be essential in differentiating between a rectocele and an enterocele. The rectovaginal bimanual examination may be necessary in a virginal or nulliparous patient in whom two fingers cannot be accommodated adequately in the vagina. In an infant or child, the bimanual evaluation is done with the rectal finger pressed against the suprapubic fingers.

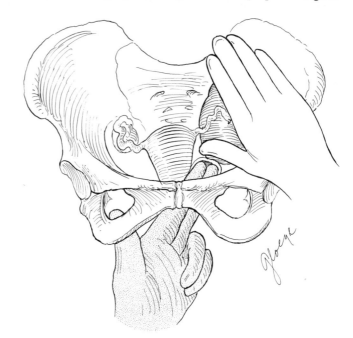

Figure 2–6 Bimanual examination of the left adnexa. Note that the fingers of the left hand are in the vagina.

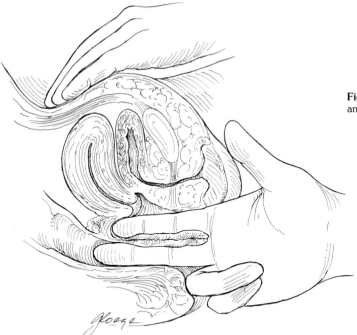

Figure 2–7 Rectovaginal bimanual examination.

Laboratory Evaluation

Following the history and physical examination, appropriate laboratory tests should be ordered. Tests normally include a urinalysis, complete blood count, erythrocyte sedimentation rate, and blood chemistry. Special tests, such as tumor markers and hormone assays, are obtained when indicated.

Assessment

A reasonable differential diagnosis should be possible with the information gleaned from the history, physical examination, and laboratory tests. The plan of management should aim toward a chemical or histologic confirmation of the definitive diagnosis, and the appropriate therapeutic options, along with the rationale for each option, should be listed.

ETHICAL CONSIDERATIONS

In few areas of medicine is it necessary to be more sensitive to the emotional and psychological needs of the patient than in the fields of obstetrics and gynecology. By their very nature, the history and physical exami-

nation may cause embarrassment to some patients. The members of the medical care team are individually and collectively responsible for ensuring that each patient's privacy and modesty are respected while providing the highest level of medical care. This objective is particularly challenging, but not impossible, on a teaching service.

The clinician should strive to meet the highest expectations of the patients in dress, manner, and attitude. While a casual and familiar approach may be acceptable to many younger patients, it may offend others and be quite inappropriate for a great many older patients. Different circumstances with the same patient may dictate different levels of formality. Cleanliness and good grooming are mandatory when dealing with patients in the outpatient or hospital setting. The manner of dress should avoid extremes and should at all times be neat and clean.

Patients should be addressed courteously and respectfully. Great care must be taken in discussing medical conditions, since the discussions are easily misinterpreted by the patient, and the emotional impact can be devastating. A bedside discussion with the patient must be carried out with more care and sensitivity than coffee room repartee with medical colleagues. Medical slang must be avoided. No matter how trivial the problem, it is important to the patient, and there is no place for a casual approach or frivolous attitude on the part of the physician.

Entrance to the patient's room should be announced by a knock and spoken identification. An appropriate salutation using the patient's surname and a personal introduction with the stated reason for the visit are minimal requirements before any questions are asked or an examination is begun. It is advisable that the general physical and pelvic examinations be carried out in the presence of a chaperone.

OBSTETRIC STATISTICS

Vital statistics are provided by the National Center for Health Statistics. Despite the approximate three-year delay in compiling yearly birth and death reports, the statistics facilitate an understanding of the impact of human reproduction on a population.

Births

The *birth rate* is the number of live births per 1000 population. It is frequently used as an index of the need for obstetric services. During 1982, 3,680,537 live births were registered in the United States. This figure represents a small increase (1 percent) over the 3,629,238 births registered in 1981. Provisional data for 1983 indicate a decline of about 2 percent from the final total for 1982. The birth rate was 15.9 live births per 1000 population in 1982, 1 percent higher than the 1981 rate of 15.8. Provisional statistics for 1983 indicate a decline of about 3 percent in the birth rate.

The birth rate for women aged 15 to 17 increased by 1 percent, while rates for women aged 18 to 19, 20 to 24, and 25 to 29 years declined by 1 percent or less. In contrast, rates for women aged 30 to 34 and 35 to 39 years increased by 5 and 6 percent, respectively, and the rate for women aged 40 to 44 years increased by 3 percent. These trends continue the pattern generally observed for the last decade, namely the marked shift in childbearing to later ages. For example, the proportion of all births occurring in teenagers fell from 19 percent in 1975 to 14 percent in 1982, while the proportion of births occurring to mothers aged 30 years and older increased from 17 to 22 percent during this period.

The *fertility rate* is the number of live births per 1000 females in the population between the ages of 15 and 44 years. The number of women of childbearing age (15 to 44) increased 2 percent between 1979 and 1980, with the largest increases found in women aged 30 to 34 and 35 to 39. The fertility rate was 67.3 live births per 1000 women aged 15 to 44 years, less than 1 percent below the rate in 1981 of 67.4. A decline of about 3 percent in the fertility rate is indicated for 1983 according to provisional data.

The *sex ratio* at birth in 1982 was 1051 male births per 1000 female births. This ratio has ranged between 1051 and 1055 since 1968.

Maternal Mortality

A *maternal death* is one attributed to complications of pregnancy, childbirth, and the puerperium. The *maternal mortality rate* is the number of maternal deaths per 100,000 live births. In 1982, 292 women died of maternal causes, and the maternal mortality rate was 7.9 deaths per 100,000 live births. Black women were three times as likely as white women to die of causes associated with pregnancy, childbirth, and the puerperium. The maternal mortality rate has decreased dramatically during the past 30 years, having been 83.3 deaths per 100,000 live births in 1950. The main reason for this decline is the improvement in medical care. The most important improvements have been in obstetric training and in the implementation of continuing educational programs that have helped improve the standard of care to a wider section of the population.

The major causes of maternal mortality, which account for more than half of all maternal deaths, remain the same: hemorrhage, hypertension, and infection.

The *perinatal mortality rate* is the number of stillbirths and neonatal deaths per 1000 live births. As with maternal mortality, the perinatal mortality rate has dropped dramatically over the past 30 years from 39.7 per 1000 live births in 1950 to 17 per 1000 live births in 1981. The drop in mortality has been most dramatic in the past 15 years, the result, it is thought, of improvements in obstetric care and neonatal intensive care. The major cause of perinatal mortality is prematurity, and improvements in prenatal care are progressively reducing the incidence of this occurrence.

GLOSSARY

The following is a listing of some frequently used terms in obstetrics.

Gravidity   The total number of pregnancies in a given patient.

Parity   The number of pregnancies a patient has carried to viability (20 weeks or more). It should be noted that both gravidity and parity refer to the number of *pregnancies,* not fetuses or infants delivered. A multiple gestation is counted as one pregnancy. Therefore, a woman who is currently pregnant and has had one previous singleton pregnancy and one previous twin gestation would be G_3P_2. A woman who is currently pregnant and has had one abortion and one ectopic pregnancy would be G_3P_0.

A system used to express more information involves including under parity the number of term pregnancies, premature deliveries, abortions, and living children. Using this system, a woman who is G_5P_{2112} would be currently pregnant for the fifth time, and have had 2 term pregnancies, 1 premature delivery, and 1 abortion. She would currently have two living children.

Premature delivery   Delivery of an infant weighing between 500 and 2500 gm after 20 weeks' and prior to 37 weeks' gestation.

Abortus   Fetus or embryo weighing less than 500 gm (400 gm in California), delivered before 20 weeks' gestation. The fetus should not have a crown-rump length of more than 16.5 cm.

Fetal death   Death occurring *in utero* prior to birth and after 20 weeks' gestation. It is synonymous with stillbirth.

Neonatal death   An infant death occurring after delivery and prior to 29 days of age.

Perinatal death   Fetal or infant death occurring after 20 weeks' gestation and before 29 neonatal days.

Fetal death (stillbirth) rate   The number of fetal deaths per 1000 births.

Neonatal death rate   The number of neonatal deaths per 1000 live births.

Infant death rate   The number of infant deaths per 1000 live births up to the first year of life.

SUGGESTED READING

Guidelines for Perinatal Care. Elk Grove Village, IL, American Academy of Pediatrics, and Washington, DC, American College of Obstetricians and Gynecologists, 1983.

National Center for Health Statistics. Monthly Vital Statistics Report: Advance Report of Final Mortality Statistics, 1982. Vol 33, No 9 (Suppl), Sept 28, 1984.

National Center for Health Statistics. Monthly Vital Statistics Report: Advance Report of Final Mortality Statistics, 1982. Vol 33, No 9 (Suppl), Dec 20, 1984.

O'Sullivan JB, Mahan CM, Charles D, Dandrow RV: Screening criteria for high-risk gestational diabetic patients. Am J Obstet Gynecol 116:895, 1973.

Sachs BP, Layde PM, Rubin GL, et al: Reproductive mortality in the United States. JAMA 247(20):2789, 1982.

II

MATERNAL-FETAL MEDICINE

Calvin J. Hobel — SUBEDITOR

OVULATION, FERTILIZATION, AND IMPLANTATION

A. DAVID BARNES and PAUL J. TOOT

Reproduction is affected by a complex series of physiologic processes. In this chapter, ovulation, fertilization, and implantation are described. Amniotic fluid, which protects the fetus during intrauterine life, is also discussed.

FOLLICULAR DEVELOPMENT

Primordial follicles undergo sequential development, differentiation, and maturation until a mature graafian follicle is produced. The follicle then ruptures, releasing the ovum. Subsequent luteinization of the ruptured follicle produces the corpus luteum.

In response to gonadotropins and ovarian steroids, the follicle cells become cuboidal, and stromal cells around the follicle become prominent. The ovum enlarges and develops a prominent nucleolus. A clear gelatinous material surrounds the ovum forming the *zona pellucida*, which contains microscopic canals. The surrounding granulosa cells multiply rapidly, and the innermost three or four layers become cuboidal and adherent to the ovum, forming the *cumulus oophorus*. A fluid-filled antrum forms among the granulosa cells. As the liquor continues to accumulate, the antrum enlarges and the centrally located primary oocyte comes to be against the wall of the follicle.

Follicle-stimulating hormone (FSH) receptors are present in granulosa cells. Under FSH stimulation, the granulosa cells proliferate, and the number of FSH receptors per follicle increases markedly. Thus, the growing primary follicle becomes increasingly more sensitive to stimulation by FSH. Subsequently, both estradiol and testosterone receptors also appear in the granulosa cells. Surrounding the granulosa cells is a thin basement membrane. Outside this membrane the connective tissue cells organize themselves into two coats, the *theca interna and externa*. (Theca is the Greek word for "sheath.")

Differentiation of Secondary Follicles

Secondary follicles are larger, contain more granulosa and theca interna cells, and have a central antrum. The antrum progressively enlarges with antral or follicular fluid, which contains both pituitary and ovarian steroid hormones. Secondary follicles possess aromatase enzyme systems in granulosa cells and luteinizing hormone (LH) receptors in both granulosa and theca interna cells. Thus, they aromatize androgens into estrogens and respond to LH stimulation with steroidogenesis.

Maturation of Graafian Follicles

The further maturation of secondary follicles into mature graafian follicles requires the sequential development of receptor molecules for FSH, estradiol, testosterone, and luteinizing hormone (LH) and of aromatase enzymes. LH stimulation increases the synthesis of androgens by theca interna cells. Androgens are aromatized into estrogens, either within the theca interna cells (one-cell theory) or after diffusion into the granulosa cells (two-cell theory). Estrogens, particularly estradiol, enhance the induction of FSH receptors and act synergistically with FSH to increase LH receptors. In growing follicles, the presence of sufficient numbers of LH receptors not only enhances androgen synthesis and estrogen formation, but also ensures follicular maturation and ovulation. The granulosa cells of the cumulus oophorus, which are in close contact with the zona pellucida, become elongated and form the *corona radiata*. The latter is shed with the oocyte at ovulation.

Follicular Atresia

During each cycle, a cohort of follicles is selected for development into primary, secondary, and graafian follicles. Among these many developing follicles, usually only one continues its differentiation and maturation into a graafian follicle that ovulates. The remaining follicles undergo atresia. On the basis of antral fluid steroid levels, growing follicles can be identified as either estrogen- or androgen-predominant. Follicles greater than 8 mm in diameter are usually estrogen-predominant, while smaller follicles are usually androgen-predominant. Furthermore, in larger estrogen-predominant follicles, antral fluid FSH concentrations continue to rise while blood FSH levels are declining. In contrast, in smaller androgen-predominant follicles, antral fluid FSH values decrease as blood FSH levels decline; thus, the intrafollicular steroid milieu appears to play an important role in determining whether a follicle undergoes maturation or atresia.

Ovulation

During the late follicular phase, the maturing follicle secretes large amounts of estrogen, and the rapidly increasing blood estradiol levels stimulate the hypothalamus and the pituitary to initiate both the LH and FSH midcycle surges. The preovulatory LH surge initiates a sequence of structural and biochemical changes that culminate in ovulation. Prior to ovulation, there is general dissolution of the entire follicular wall and localized disintegration of that portion of the wall that

is on the surface of the ovary, both presumably due to proteolytic enzymes. With degeneration of the cells on the surface, a stigma forms, and the follicular basement membrane finally bulges through the stigma. When this ruptures, the oocyte and corona radiata are expelled into the peritoneal cavity and ovulation occurs.

Ovulation is now known from ultrasound studies to be a gradual phenomenon, with the collapse of the follicle taking from several minutes to as long as an hour or more. The oocyte adheres to the surface of the ovary, allowing an extended period during which the muscular contractions of the tube may bring it in contact with the tubal epithelium. Probably both muscular contractions and tubal ciliary movement contribute to the transportation of the oocyte into and along the tube. Ciliary activity is not essential, since at least some women with immotile cilia become pregnant.

At birth, primary oocytes are in the prophase of the first meiotic division. They continue in this phase until the next maturation division occurs in conjunction with ovulation. A few hours preceding ovulation, the chromatin is resolved into distinct chromosomes, and meiotic division takes place with unequal distribution of the cytoplasm to form a *secondary oocyte* and the *first polar body*. Each element contains 23 chromosomes, each in the form of two monads. The second maturation spindle forms immediately and remains at the surface. No further development takes place until after ovulation and fertilization have occurred. At that time, and prior to the union of the male and female pronuclei, another division occurs to reduce the chromosomal component of the egg pronucleus to 23 single chromosomes (22 + X), each composed of one monad. The *ovum* and a *second polar body* are thus formed. The first polar body may also divide.

Luteinization and Corpus Luteum Function

After ovulation and under the influence of LH, the granulosa cells of the ruptured follicle undergo luteinization. These luteinized granulosa cells, plus the surrounding theca cells, capillaries and connective tissue, form the corpus luteum, which produces copious amounts of progesterone and some estradiol. The normal functional life span of the corpus

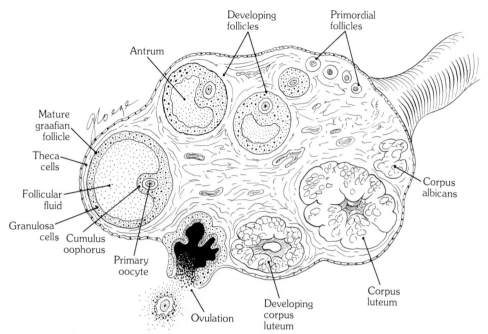

Figure 3–1 Schematic representation of the sequence of events occurring in the ovary during a complete follicular cycle. Adapted with permission from Yen SC, Jaffe R (eds): Reproductive Endocrinology. Philadelphia, W. B. Saunders, 1978, p. 64.

luteum is about 14 days. After this time, it regresses, unless pregnancy occurs, and is gradually replaced by an avascular scar called a corpus albicans. The events occurring in the ovary during a complete cycle are shown in Figure 3–1.

SPERMATOGENESIS, SPERM CAPACITATION, AND FERTILIZATION

Fertilization, or conception, is the union of male and female pronuclear elements. Conception takes place in the fallopian tube, after which the fertilized ovum continues to the uterus where implantation occurs and development begins.

Spermatogenesis requires about 74 days. Together with transportation, a total of about three months elapses before sperm are ejaculated. The sperm achieve motility during their transport through the epididymis, but sperm capacitation, which renders them capable of fertilization, does not occur until they are removed from the seminal plasma after ejaculation.

Estrogen levels are high at the time of ovulation, resulting in an increased amount, decreased viscosity, and changed electrolyte content of the cervical mucus. These are the most favorable characteristics for sperm penetration. The average ejaculate contains 2 to 5 ml of semen; 200 to 300 million sperm may be deposited in the vagina, 60 to 90 percent of which are morphologically normal. Less than 200 sperm achieve proximity to the egg. Only one sperm fertilizes the single egg released at ovulation.

The major loss of sperm occurs in the vagina following coitus, with expulsion of semen from the introitus playing an important role. In addition, there is digestion of sperm by vaginal enzymes, destruction of some by the vaginal acidity, phagocytosis of sperm along the reproductive tract, and some further loss from passage through the fallopian tube into the peritoneal cavity.

Those sperm that do migrate from the alkaline environment of the semen to the alkaline environment of the cervical mucus exuding from the cervical os are directed along channels of lower viscosity mucus into the cervical crypts where they are stored for later ascent. Two waves of passage to the tubes may occur. Uterine contractions, probably facilitated by prostaglandins in the seminal plasma, propel sperm to the tubes within five minutes. Some evidence indicates that these sperm may not be as capable of fertilization as those that arrive later largely under their own power. It is of interest, however, that the seminal concentrations of prostaglandins have been found to be lower in males of infertile couples. Sperm may be found within the peritoneal cavity for long periods, but it is conjectural whether or not they are capable of fertilization. Ova are usually fertilized within 12 hours of ovulation.

Capacitation is the physiologic change sperm must undergo in the female reproductive tract prior to fertilization. Human sperm can acquire the ability to fertilize after a short incubation in defined media without residence in the female reproductive tract. Therefore, *in vitro* fertilization is possible.

The *acrosome reaction* is one of the principal components of capacitation. The acrosome, a modified lysosome, lies over the sperm head as a kind of "chemical drill-bit" designed to enable the sperm to burrow its way to the oocyte (Fig. 3–2). The overlying plasma membrane and the outer acrosomal membrane become unstable and eventually break down, releasing hyaluronidase, a neuraminidase, and corona-dispersing enzyme. Acrosin, bound to the remaining inner acrosomal membrane, may play a role in the final penetration of the zona pellucida. The latter contains species-specific receptors for the plasma membrane. After traversing the zona, the postacrosomal region of the sperm head fuses with the oocyte membrane, and the sperm nucleus is incorporated into the ooplasm. This process triggers release of the contents of the cortical granules that lie at the periphery of the oocyte. This cortical reaction results in changes in the oocyte membrane and zona pellucida that prevent the entrance of further sperm into the oocyte.

The process of capacitation may be inhibited by a factor in the semen, thus preserving maximum enzyme release to allow effective penetration of the corona and zona pellucida surrounding the oocyte. The cellular investments of the oocyte may further activate the sperm, thus facilitating penetration to the oocyte membrane. The corona is not required for normal fertilization to occur, however, since its removal has no effect on the rate or quality of fertilization *in vitro*. The major function of these surrounding granulosa cells and their intercellular matrix may be to serve as a sticky mass that causes adherence to the ovarian surface and the mucosa of the tubal epithelium.

Following penetration of the oocyte, the sperm nucleus decondenses to form the male pronucleus, which approaches and finally fuses with the female pronucleus at syngamy to form the *zygote*. Fertilization restores the diploid number of chromosomes and determines the sex of the zygote.

CLEAVAGE, MORULA, BLASTOCYST

Following fertilization, cleavage occurs. This consists of a rapid succession of mitotic divisions that produces a mulberry-like mass known as a morula. Fluid is secreted by the outer cells of the morula, and a single fluid-filled cavity develops, known as the blastocyst cavity. An inner-cell mass can be defined, attached eccentrically to the outer layer of flattened cells; the latter becomes the trophoblast. The embryo at this stage of development is called a blastocyst, and the zona pellucida disappears at about this time.

IMPLANTATION

The fertilized ovum reaches the endometrial cavity about three days after ovulation. Hormones influence egg transport. Estro-

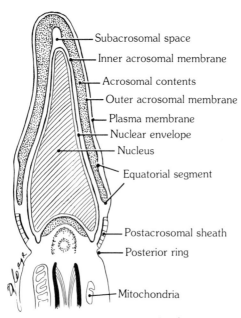

Subacrosomal space
Inner acrosomal membrane
Acrosomal contents
Outer acrosomal membrane
Plasma membrane
Nuclear envelope
Nucleus
Equatorial segment
Postacrosomal sheath
Posterior ring
Mitochondria

Figure 3–2 The sperm head.

gen causes "locking" of the egg in the tube, and progesterone reverses this action. Prostaglandins (PGs) have diverse effects. PGE relaxes the tubal isthmus, while PGF stimulates tubal motility. It is unknown whether or not abnormalities of egg transport play a role in infertility, but in animal studies, acceleration of ovum transport will cause a failure of implantation.

Upon reaching the uterine cavity, the embryo undergoes further development for two to three days before implanting. The zona is shed and the blastocyst then adheres to the endometrium, a process probably dependent on changes in the surface characteristics of the embryo, such as electrical charge and glycoprotein content. A variety of proteolytic enzymes may play a role in separating the endometrial cells and digesting the intercellular matrix.

Initially, the wall of the blastocyst facing the uterine lumen consists of a single layer of flattened cells. The thicker opposite wall has two zones, the trophoblast and the inner cell mass (embryonic disc). The latter differentiates at 7.5 days into a thick plate of primitive "dorsal" ectoderm and an underlying layer of "ventral" endoderm. Between the embryonic disc and trophoblast appear

small cells that enclose a space that becomes the amniotic cavity.

Under the influence of progesterone, decidual changes occur in the endometrium of the pregnant uterus. The endometrial stromal cells enlarge and form polygonal or round decidual cells. The nuclei become round and vesicular and the cytoplasm becomes clear, slightly basophilic, and surrounded by a translucent membrane. During pregnancy, the decidua thickens to a depth of 5 to 10 mm. The *decidua basalis* is the decidua directly beneath the site of implantation. The *decidua capsularis* is the portion overlying the developing ovum and separating it from the rest of the uterine cavity. *Decidua vera* (parietalis) is the remaining lining of the uterine cavity (Fig. 3–3). The space between the decidua capsularis and decidua vera is obliterated by the fourth month with fusion of the capsularis and vera.

The decidua basalis enters into the formation of the basal plate of the placenta. The spongy zone of the decidua basalis consists mainly of arteries and dilated veins. The decidua basalis is invaded extensively by trophoblastic giant cells that first appear as early as the time of implantation. *Nitabuch's layer* is a zone of fibrinoid degeneration where the

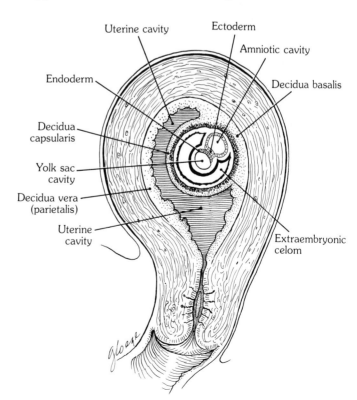

Figure 3–3 Early stage of implantation.

trophoblast meets the decidua. When the decidua is defective, as in placenta accreta, Nitabuch's layer is absent.

When the free blastocyst contacts the endometrium after four to six days, the syncytiotrophoblast, a syncytium of cells, differentiates from the cytotrophoblast. At about 9 days, lacunae, irregular fluid-filled spaces, appear within the thickened trophoblastic syncytium. This is soon followed by the appearance of maternal blood within the lacunae, as maternal tissue is destroyed, and the walls of the mother's capillaries are eroded. As the blastocyst burrows deeper into the endometrium, the trophoblastic strands branch to form the solid, primitive villi traversing the lacunae. The villi, which are first distinguished about the twelfth day after fertilization, are the essential structures of the definitive placenta. Located originally over the entire surface of the ovum, the villi later disappear, except over the most deeply implanted portion, the future placental site.

Embryonic mesenchyme first appears as isolated cells within the cavity of the blastocyst. When the cavity is completely lined with mesoderm, it is termed the *extraembryonic celom*. Its membrane, the chorion, is composed of trophoblasts and mesenchyme. When the solid trophoblast is invaded by a mesenchymal core, presumably derived from cytotrophoblast, secondary villi are formed.

Maternal venous sinuses are tapped about 15 days after fertilization. By the seventeenth day, both fetal and maternal blood vessels are functional, and a placental circulation is established. The fetal circulation is completed when the blood vessels of the embryo are connected with chorionic blood vessels that are formed from cytotrophoblast. Proliferation of cellular trophoblasts at the tips of the villi produces cytotrophoblastic columns that progressively extend through the peripheral syncytium. Cytotrophoblastic extensions from columns of adjacent villi join together to form the cytotrophoblastic shell, which attaches the villi to the decidua. By the nineteenth day of development, the cytotrophoblastic shell is thick. Villi contain a central core of chorionic mesoderm, where blood vessels are developing, and an external covering of syncytiotrophoblasts or syncytium.

By three weeks, the relationship of the chorion to the decidua is evident. The greater part of the chorion, denuded of villi, is designated the smooth chorion or "chorion laeve." Until near the end of the third month, the chorion laeve remains separated from the amnion by the extraembryonic celomic cavity. Thereafter, amnion and chorion are in intimate contact. The villi adjacent to the decidua basalis enlarge and branch (chorion frondosum) and progressively assume the form of the fully developed human placenta (Fig. 3–4). By 4.5 months, the chorion laeve contacts and fuses with the decidua vera, thus obliterating most of the uterine cavity.

VARIATIONS IN THE PLACENTA

Placental implantation variations include *bipartite* or *tripartite placentas,* where vessels cross between incompletely divided lobes; *duplex* or *triplex placentas*, where blood vessels do not cross between the completely divided lobes; and *placenta succenturiate*, where blood vessels course through the membranes to connect the distant accessory lobe(s) to the main placenta. Eccentric insertion of the umbilical cord results in a *battledore placenta,* which is of no clinical significance. With *velamentous insertion* of the cord, blood vessels course unprotected for long distances through the membranes to insert into the margin of the placenta. In both placenta succenturiate and velamentous insertion, the blood vessels course through the membranes and may pass over the internal cervical os, where they are in a position to be compressed by the presenting fetal part or torn at the time of membrane rupture. Either of these events may be a disaster for the fetus.

In *placenta circumvallata* (Fig. 3–5), there is a large central circular depression on the fetal surface of the placenta surrounded by an elevated ridge. Amnion and chorion are folded back on themselves, forming a double layer of fetal membranes at this site. It is believed that the regression of villi, which originally surrounded the whole chorion, went too far, and the placental plate became too small. Secondary proliferation of villi had to occur after the membranes became attached to the edge of the original placenta. The incidence of abortion in early pregnancy and bleeding in late pregnancy is increased with placenta circumvallata.

Placenta membranacea results from persistence of the villi of the chorion laeve as well

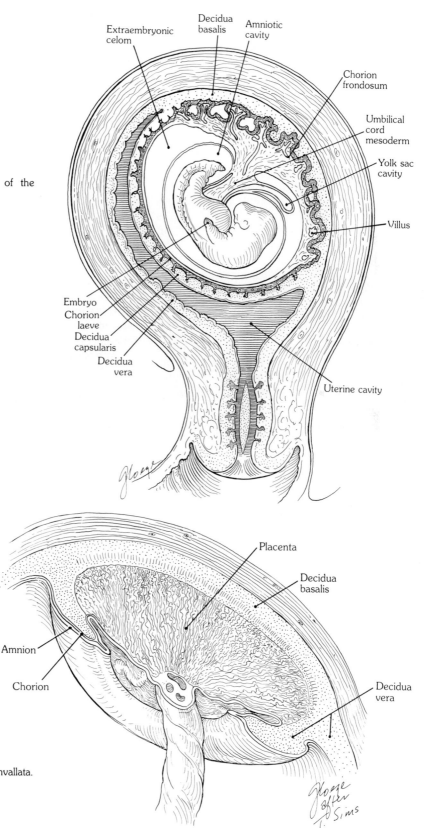

Figure 3–4 Relationship of the chorion to the placenta.

Extraembryonic celom

Decidua basalis

Amniotic cavity

Chorion frondosum

Umbilical cord mesoderm

Yolk sac cavity

Villus

Uterine cavity

Embryo

Chorion laeve

Decidua capsularis

Decidua vera

Figure 3–5 Placenta circumvallata.

Placenta

Decidua basalis

Decidua vera

Amnion

Chorion

as the chorion frondosum, producing a large, thin placenta that entirely surrounds the fetal membranes. Separation and expulsion may be incomplete during the third stage of labor, increasing the incidence of postpartum hemorrhage.

AMNIOTIC FLUID

Throughout normal pregnancy, the amniotic fluid compartment allows the fetus room for growth, movement, and development. Without amniotic fluid, the uterus would contract and compress the fetus. In cases of leakage of amniotic fluid early in the first trimester, the fetus may develop structural abnormalities including facial distortion, limb reduction, and abdominal wall defects secondary to the uterine compression.

Toward midpregnancy (20 weeks), the amniotic fluid becomes increasingly important for fetal pulmonary development. The latter requires a fluid-filled respiratory tract and the ability of the fetus to "breathe" *in utero,* moving amniotic fluid in and out of the lungs. The absence of adequate amniotic fluid during midpregnancy is associated with pulmonary hypoplasia at birth, often incompatible with life.

The amniotic fluid also has a protective role for the fetus. It contains antibacterial activity and acts to inhibit the growth of potentially pathogenic bacteria. During labor and delivery, the amniotic fluid continues to serve as a protective medium for the fetus, aiding dilatation of the cervix. The premature infant with its fragile head may benefit most from delivery with the amniotic membranes intact (en caul). In addition, the amniotic fluid may serve as a means of communication for the fetus. Fetal maturity and readiness for delivery may be signaled to the maternal uterus via fetal urinary hormones excreted into the amniotic fluid.

Volume and Composition

Amniotic fluid volume and composition are regulated by a complex system of fluid exchange between maternal and fetal fluid compartments. The amniotic fluid may represent an extension of the fetal extracellular fluid compartment. During the first trimester of pregnancy, the volume of the amniotic fluid is minimal (5 to 25 ml), arising from transudation of fetal plasma through the nonkeratinized fetal skin or umbilical cord, or of maternal plasma through the vascularized uterine decidua. This fluid is iso-osmotic with fetal and maternal plasma, although essentially devoid of protein. Beginning in the second trimester, the amniotic fluid becomes a dynamic model of fluid exchange. The human fetus at term is estimated to excrete 600 to 700 ml per day of hypotonic urine into the amniotic cavity, accounting for the hypo-osmolality of the amniotic fluid. The fetal respiratory tract actively secretes up to 250 ml per day into the amniotic fluid. Fetal swallowing at term removes 500 ml per day of fluid, and the remainder is resorbed by a flow of water across the chorioamnion in response to the osmotic gradient created by the hypo-osmotic amniotic fluid and the iso-osmotic maternal plasma. Consequently, the volume of amniotic fluid at term (700 to 1000 ml) is continually exchanged every 24 hours.

Abnormalities of the amniotic fluid may thus occur as a result of changes in fetal renal function, swallowing, lung fluid production, or transchorionic water flow. The fetus may autonomously regulate the fetal sites of amniotic fluid secretion and resorption through hormones including vasopressin, cortisol, and catecholamines.

Oligohydramnios

Oligohydramnios refers to a marked deficiency in the volume of amniotic fluid. A diminished volume of amniotic fluid may produce fetal hypoxia as a result of umbilical cord compression secondary to fetal movements or uterine contractions. Furthermore, the passage of fetal meconium into a reduced volume of amniotic fluid results in a thick, particulate suspension that may cause fetal respiratory compromise.

It is essential to classify oligohydramnios according to its etiology. Oligohydramnios is associated with intrauterine growth retardation in 60 percent of cases. When associated with ultrasonic evidence of asymmetric growth retardation, fetal compromise is highly likely. Those cases secondary to spontaneous rupture of fetal membranes may not be associated with prior fetal distress. Oligohydramnios may occur as a result of fetal stress *in utero*; the secretion of fetal stress hormones (catecholamines, vasopressin) may inhibit lung fluid secretion and urine production, while perhaps promoting fluid resorption via fetal swallowing. Finally, there are cases associated with a variety of fetal malformations, such as Potter's syndrome (renal agenesis), in which detailed ultrasonic and genetic evaluations are necessary.

Polyhydramnios

Polyhydramnios refers to an excessive amount of amniotic fluid, usually exceeding two liters. The fluid usually accumulates slowly, although acute hydramnios may occasionally occur, particularly with a twin gestation. The complications of polyhydramnios include an increased risk of premature labor (due to hyperdistension of the uterus), maternal respiratory discomfort, umbilical cord prolapse at the time of rupture of the membranes, and fetal malpresentation.

The etiologies of polyhydramnios may be discussed in terms of sites of fluid secretion and resorption. Fetal anomalies in which decreased swallowing or gastrointestinal absorption occurs (anencephaly, duodenal atresia, tracheoesophageal fistula) are often associated with polyhydramnios. Occasional anomalies of the pulmonary system (cystic adenomatoid malformation of the lung) may be associated with increased fluid production. Abnormalities of transchorionic water flow may result in the accumulation of excess fluid, as sometimes occurs in diabetic pregnancies. In addition, polyhydramnios occurs in most pregnancies marked by immune or nonimmune hydrops. The fetus and placenta become edematous in this condition, as a result of fetal congestive heart failure, hypoproteinemia, or severe anemia. Transudation of placental fluid, as well as increased fetal production of fluid, may account for the polyhydramnios.

If polyhydramnios is suspected, a definitive diagnosis may be made by ultrasound. A complete ultrasonic fetal evaluation should be performed to exclude hydrops or malformations. Maternal testing should include screening for diabetes, a Rhesus antibody titer, glucose-6-phosphate dehydrogenase determination, hemoglobin electrophoresis, and viral titers when appropriate.

Although it is possible to drain the excessive amniotic fluid via amniocentesis, the reaccumulation of up to one liter per day limits this approach. Beta-agonist tocolytic agents to decrease uterine activity may be of value, and the patient should be advised to rest as much as possible. In the acute form, induction of labor may be necessary to relieve severe maternal distress.

SUGGESTED READING

Boyd JD: The Human Placenta. Cambridge, Heffer and Sons Ltd, 1970.

McNatty NP, Makris A, DeGrazier C, et al: The production of progesterone, androgens, and estrogens by granulosa cells, thecal tissue, and stromal tissue from human ovaries in vitro. J Clin Endocrinol Metab 49:678, 1979.

Pitkin RM: Acute polyhydramnios recurrent in successive pregnancies: Management with multiple amniocenteses. Obstet Gynecol 48 (Suppl):42s, 1976.

Queenan JT, Gadow EC: Polyhydramnios: Chronic versus acute. Am J Obstet Gynecol 108:349, 1970.

Queenan JT, Thompson W, Whitfield CR, et al: Amniotic fluid volumes in normal pregnancies. Am J Obstet Gynecol 114:34, 1972.

Seeds AE: Current concepts of amniotic fluid dynamics. Am J Obstet Gynecol 138:575, 1980.

Speroff L, Glass RH, Kase NG: Clinical Gynecologic Endocrinology and Fertility. 3rd ed. Baltimore, Williams and Wilkins, 1983.

Chapter Four

MATERNAL PHYSIOLOGY

NATHAN WASSERSTRUM

Maternal adjustments in pregnancy are designed to support the requirements of fetal homeostasis and growth without unduly jeopardizing maternal well-being. This is accomplished by adapting maternal systems to deliver energy and growth substrates to the fetus and to remove inappropriate heat and waste products. In addition, the sheer physical presence of the enlarging uterus impinges on diverse maternal functions, including circulation, respiration, and renal function. The limits of the fetal role in maintaining fetal homeostasis are clear. Although breathing movements and urine production occur *in utero,* the fetal lung and kidney appear to play no role in fetal respiration and excretion. However, the fetus is capable of redistributing its cardiac output and oxygen delivery among different organs in response to physiologic demands.

NORMAL VALUES IN PREGNANCY

The normal values for several hematologic, biochemical, and physiologic indices during pregnancy differ markedly from the nonpregnant range and may also vary according to the duration of the pregnancy. These alterations are shown in Table 4–1.

CARDIOVASCULAR SYSTEM

Cardiac Output

The hemodynamic changes associated with pregnancy are summarized in Table 4–2. The plasma volume rises as early as the sixth week of pregnancy and plateaus at approximately 50 percent above nonpregnant levels by about 32 to 34 weeks' gestation, after which there is little further change. The red blood cell mass appears to continue to rise throughout pregnancy. Hence, if iron stores are adequate, the hematocrit tends to rise from the second to the third trimester. Cardiac output rises by the tenth week of gestation; it reaches about 40 percent above nonpregnant levels by 20 to 24 weeks, after which there is little change. Cardiac output reaches its peak while blood volume is still rising and reflects increases in both stroke volume and heart rate.

Intravascular Pressures

Systolic pressure falls only slightly during pregnancy, while diastolic pressure decreases more markedly, beginning in the first trimester, reaching its nadir in midpregnancy, then returning toward nonpregnant levels by term. These changes reflect the elevated cardiac output and reduced peripheral resistance that characterize pregnancy; toward the end of pregnancy, vasoconstrictor tone normally increases, and with it the blood pressure. The normal rise of blood pressure toward prepregnant levels as term approaches must be recognized, and the implications for the diagnosis of pre-eclampsia appreciated (see Chapter 14).

Blood pressure, as measured with a sphygmomanometer cuff around the brachial artery, varies with posture. In late pregnancy, it is probably highest when the gravida is sitting, somewhat lower when she is lying

TABLE 4–1 COMMON LABORATORY VALUES IN PREGNANCY

TEST	NORMAL RANGE (NONPREGNANT)	CHANGE IN PREGNANCY	TIMING
Serum Chemistries			
Albumin	3.5–4.8 gm/dl	↓ 1 gm/dl	Most by 20 wk, then gradual
Calcium (total)	9–10.3 mg/dl	↓ 10%	Gradual fall
Chloride	95–105 mEq/L	No significant change	Gradual rise
Creatinine (female)	0.6–1.1 mg/dl	↓ 0.3 mg/dl	Most by 20 wk
Fibrinogen	1.5–3.6 gm/L	↑ 1–2 gm/L	Progressive
Glucose, fasting (plasma)	65–105 mg/dl	↓ 10%	Gradual fall
Potassium (plasma)	3.5–4.5 mEq/L	↓ 0.2–0.3 mEq/L	By 20 wk
Protein (total)	6.5–8.5 gm/dl	↓ 1 gm/dl	By 20 wk, then stable
Sodium	135–145 mEq/L	↓ 2–4 mEq/L	By 20 wk, then stable
Urea nitrogen	12–30 mg/dl	↓ 50%	First trimester
Uric acid	3.5–8 mg/dl	↓ 33%	First trimester, rise at term
Urinary Chemistries			
Creatinine	15–25 mg/kg/day (1–1.4 gm/day)	No significant change	
Protein	Up to 150 mg/day	Up to 250–300 mg/day	By 20 wk
Creatinine clearance	90–130 ml/min per 1.73 m^2	↑ 40–50%	By 16 wk
Serum Enzymatic Activities			
Amylase	23–84 IU/L	↑ 50–100%	Controversial
Transaminase			
Glutamic pyruvic (SGPT)	5–35 mU/ml	No significant change	
Glutamic oxaloacetic (SGOT)	5–40 mU/ml	No significant change	
Hematocrit (female)	36–46%	↓ 4–7%	Bottoms at 30–34 wk
Hemoglobin (female)	12–16 gm/dl	↓ 1.5–2 gm/dl	Bottoms at 30–34 wk
Leukocyte count	4.8–10.8 × 10^3/mm^3	↑ 3.5 × 10^3/mm^3	Gradual
Platelet count	150–400 × 10^3/mm^3	Slight decrease	
Serum Hormone Values			
Cortisol (plasma)	8–21 µg/dl	↑ 20 µg/dl	
Prolactin (female)	25 ng/ml	↑ 50–400 ng/ml	Gradual, peaks at term
Thyroxine, total (T$_4$)	5–11 gm/dl	↑ 5 mg/dl	Early sustained
Triiodothyronine, total (T$_3$)	125–245 ng/dl	↑ 50%	Early sustained

Adapted and reproduced with permission from Main DM, Main EK: Obstetrics and Gynecology, A Pocket Reference. Chicago, Year Book Medical Publishers, Inc., 1984, p 7.

down (a minority show a dramatic fall due to vena caval compression), and lower still when she lies on one side.

When elevations in blood pressure are clin- ically detected during pregnancy, it is custom- ary to repeat the measurement with the pa- tient on her side. This practice usually introduces a systematic error. In the lateral

TABLE 4–2 CARDIOVASCULAR CHANGES IN PREGNANCY

PARAMETER	AMOUNT OF CHANGE	TIMING
Arterial blood pressures		
Systolic	↓ 4–6 mm Hg	All bottom at 20–24 wks, then rise gradu-
Diastolic	↓ 8–15 mm Hg	ally to prepregnancy values at term
Mean	↓ 6–10 mm Hg	
Heart rate	↑ 12–18 BPM	Early 2nd trimester, then stable
Stroke volume	↑ 10–30%	Early 2nd trimester, then stable
Cardiac output	↑ 33–45%	Peaks in early 2nd trimester, then stable until term

Adapted and reproduced with permission from Main DM, Main EK: Obstetrics and Gynecology, A Pocket Reference. Chicago, Year Book Medical Publishers, Inc., 1984, p 18.

position, the blood pressure cuff around the brachial artery is raised about 10 cm above the heart. This leads to a hydrostatic fall in measured pressure, yielding a reading about 7 mm Hg lower than if the cuff was at heart level, as occurs during sitting or supine measurements.

Mechanical Circulatory Effects of the Gravid Uterus

As pregnancy progresses, the enlarging uterus displaces and compresses various abdominal structures, including the iliac veins and inferior vena cava (and probably also the aorta) with marked effects. The supine position accentuates this venous compression, producing a fall in venous return, and hence cardiac output. In most gravidas, a compensatory rise in peripheral resistance minimizes the fall in blood pressure. However, in up to 10 percent of gravidas, there is a significant fall in blood pressure accompanied by symptoms of nausea, dizziness, and even syncope. This "supine hypotensive syndrome" is relieved by changing position to the side. It is noteworthy (and of some diagnostic value) that the expected baroreflexive tachycardia, which normally occurs in response to other maneuvers that reduce cardiac output and blood pressure, does not accompany caval compression. In fact, bradycardia is often associated with the syndrome.

The venous compression by the gravid uterus elevates pressure in veins draining the legs and pelvic organs, thereby exacerbating varicose veins in the legs and vulva and causing hemorrhoids. As expected, venous pressure is unaltered in the arm, where drainage is not compromised by the uterus. The rise in venous pressure is the major cause of the lower extremity edema that characterizes pregnancy. The hypoalbuminemia associated with pregnancy also shifts the balance of the other major factor in the Starling equation—colloid osmotic pressure—in favor of fluid transfer from the intravascular to the extracellular space. Because of venous compression, the rate of blood flow in the lower veins is also markedly reduced, predisposing to thrombosis. The various effects of caval compression are somewhat mitigated by the development of a paravertebral collateral circulation that permits blood from the lower body to bypass the occluded inferior vena cava.

During late pregnancy, the uterus can also partially compress the aorta and its branches; this is thought to account for the observation in some patients of lower pressure in the femoral artery compared with the brachial artery. This aortic compression can be accentuated during uterine contractions and may be a cause of fetal distress when a patient is in the supine position. This phenomenon has been referred to as the *"Poseiro effect."* Clinically, it can be suspected when the femoral pulse is not palpable.

Regional Blood Flow

Blood flow to most regions of the body increases and plateaus relatively early in pregnancy. Notable exceptions occur in the uterus, kidney, and skin, in each of which blood flow increases with gestational age. Two of the major increases (those to the kidney and to the skin) serve purposes of elimination—the kidneys of waste material, the skin of heat. Both processes require plasma rather than whole blood, which gives point to the disproportionate increase of plasma over red blood cells in the blood expansion.

Control of Cardiovascular Changes

The precise mechanisms accounting for the cardiovascular changes in pregnancy remain to be proven. It has been suggested that the rise in cardiac output and fall in peripheral resistance during pregnancy might be explained in terms of the circulatory response to an arteriovenous shunt, represented by the uteroplacental circulation. However, the elevations in cardiac output and uterine blood flow follow different time courses in pregnancy, the former reaching its maximum in the second trimester, the latter increasing to term.

Oxygen-Carrying Capacity of Blood

As indicated above, plasma volume expands proportionately more than red blood cell volume, leading to a fall in hematocrit. The optimum hematocrit is 35 for the white gravida and 33 for the black gravida. Hematocrits below 27 to 29, or above 39 to 41, are associated with progressively less favorable outcomes. In spite of the relatively low "optimal" hematocrit, the arteriovenous oxygen difference in pregnancy is below nonpregnant levels. This supports the concept that the hemoglobin concentration in pregnancy is more than sufficient to meet oxygen-carrying requirements.

Although the epidemiologic data are inadequate, it appears that a high proportion of women in the reproductive age group enter pregnancy without sufficient stores of iron to meet the increased needs of pregnancy.

RESPIRATORY SYSTEM

The major respiratory changes in pregnancy are due to three factors: the mechanical effects of the enlarging uterus, the increased total body oxygen consumption, and the respiratory stimulant effects of progesterone.

Respiratory Mechanics in Pregnancy

The changes in lung volume and capacities associated with pregnancy are detailed in Table 4–3. As pregnancy progresses, the enlarging uterus elevates the resting position of the diaphragm. This results in a less negative intrathoracic pressure and a decreased resting lung volume, that is, a decreased functional residual capacity (FRC). The enlarging

uterus produces no impairment in diaphragmatic or thoracic muscle motion. Hence, the vital capacity (VC) remains unchanged. These characteristics—reduced FRC with unimpaired VC—are analogous to those seen in pneumoperitoneum and contrast with those seen in severe obesity or abdominal binding in which the elevated diaphragm is accompanied by decreased excursions of the respiratory muscles. Reductions in both the expiratory reserve volume and residual volume contribute to the reduced FRC.

Oxygen Consumption and Ventilation

Total body oxygen consumption increases about 15 to 20 percent in pregnancy. Approximately half of this increase is accounted for by the uterus and its contents. The remainder is accounted for mainly by increased maternal renal and cardiac work; smaller increments are due to work of the respiratory muscles and the breasts.

In general, a rise in oxygen consumption is accompanied by cardiorespiratory responses that facilitate oxygen delivery (i.e., by increases in cardiac output and alveolar ventilation). To the extent that elevations in cardiac output and alveolar ventilation keep pace with the rise in oxygen consumption, the arteriovenous oxygen difference and the arterial partial pressure of carbon dioxide

TABLE 4–3   LUNG VOLUMES AND CAPACITIES IN PREGNANCY

TEST	DEFINITION	CHANGE IN PREGNANCY
Respiratory rate	—	No significant change
Tidal volume	The volume of air inspired and expired at each breath	Progressive rise throughout pregnancy of 0.1–0.2 L
Expiratory reserve volume	The maximum volume of air that can be additionally expired after a normal expiration	Lowered by about 15% (0.55 L in late pregnancy compared with 0.65 L postpartum)
Residual volume	The volume of air remaining in the lungs after a maximum expiration	Falls considerably (0.77 L in late pregnancy compared with 0.96 L postpartum)
Vital capacity	The maximum volume of air that can be forcibly inspired after a maximum expiration	Unchanged, except for possibly a small terminal diminution
Inspiratory capacity	The maximum volume of air that can be inspired from resting expiratory level	Increased by about 5%
Functional residual capacity	The volume of air in lungs at resting expiratory level	Lowered by about 18%
Minute ventilation	The volume of air inspired or expired in one minute	Increased by about 40% as a result of the increased tidal volume and unchanged respiratory rate

Adapted and reproduced with permission from Main DM, Main EK: Obstetrics and Gynecology, A Pocket Reference. Chicago, Year Book Medical Publishers, Inc., 1984, p 14.

(PCO_2), respectively, remain unchanged. In pregnancy, the elevations in both cardiac output and alveolar ventilation are greater than those required to meet the increased oxygen consumption. Hence, despite the rise in total body oxygen consumption, the arteriovenous oxygen difference and arterial PCO_2 both fall. The fall in PCO_2, by definition, indicates hyperventilation.

The rise in minute ventilation reflects an approximate 40 percent increase in tidal volume at term; the respiratory rate does not change during pregnancy.

When injected into normal nonpregnant subjects, progesterone increases ventilation. The respiratory center becomes more sensitive to CO_2 (i.e., the curve describing the ventilatory response to increasing CO_2 has a steeper slope). Such increased respiratory center sensitivity to CO_2 characterizes pregnancy and probably accounts for the hyperventilation of pregnancy.

Alveolar Arterial Gradient and Arterial Blood Gases

As noted above, pregnancy is characterized by hyperventilation (the arterial PCO_2 falls to a level of 27 to 32 mm Hg) and its associated respiratory alkalosis. Renal compensatory bicarbonate excretion leads to a final pH between 7.40 and 7.45. During labor (without conduction anesthesia), the hyperventilation associated with each contraction produces a further transient fall in PCO_2. By the end of the first stage of labor, when cervical dilation is complete, a decrease in arterial PCO_2 persists, even between contractions.

In general, when alveolar PCO_2 falls during hyperventilation, alveolar PO_2 shows a corresponding rise, leading to a rise in arterial PO_2. This occurs in pregnancy, and in the first trimester, the mean arterial PO_2 may be 106 to 108 mm Hg. There is a slight downward trend in arterial PO_2 as gestation proceeds. This reflects, at least in part, an increased alveolar arterial gradient, possibly resulting from the decrease in FRC discussed previously, which leads to ventilation-perfusion mismatch.

Dyspnea of Pregnancy

In general, airway resistance is unchanged or even decreased in pregnancy. Despite this absence of obstructive or restrictive effects, dyspnea is a common symptom in pregnancy. Gravida with dyspnea of pregnancy show no changes in pulmonary function tests, compared to those without the symptom. However, these women tend to demonstrate a relatively higher nonpregnant PCO_2. It has therefore been suggested that with pregnancy, the marked change in PCO_2 to unusually low levels results in the sensation of dyspnea.

RENAL PHYSIOLOGY

Anatomic Changes in the Urinary Tract

The urinary collecting system, including the calyces, renal pelves, and ureters, undergoes marked dilatation in pregnancy, as is readily seen on intravenous urograms. The dilatation is generally more prominent on the right side, begins in the first trimester, is present in 90 percent of women at term, and may persist until the twelfth to sixteenth postpartum week. This occurrence probably reflects the influence of both humoral and physical factors. Progesterone appears to produce smooth muscle relaxation in various organs, including the ureter. As the uterus enlarges, partial obstruction of the ureter occurs at the pelvic brim in both the supine and upright positions. Because of the relatively greater effect on the right side, a role has been ascribed to the dilated ovarian venous plexus. Ovarian venous drainage is asymmetric, with the right vein emptying into the inferior vena cava and the left into the ipsilateral renal vein.

Although it was previously thought that in pregnancy dilatation is accompanied by decreased ureteral peristalsis, more recent studies suggest that this is not the case. The gestational hypertrophy of ureteral smooth muscle and hyperplasia of their connective tissue are also evinced against the common notion of "floppy" ureters in pregnancy.

Renal Blood Flow and Glomerular Filtration Rate

Renal plasma flow and the glomerular filtration rate (GFR) increase early in pregnancy, plateauing at about 40 percent above nonpregnant levels by midgestation, then remaining unchanged to term. The mechanism of these increases is unclear. A facile explanation based on the marked volume expansion associated with pregnancy is insufficient. As was true for cardiac output, renal blood flow and GFR (clinically measured as the creatinine clearance) reach their peak relatively early in pregnancy, before the greatest increase in intravascular and extracellular volume occur. The elevated GFR is reflected in lower serum levels of creatinine and urea nitrogen, as noted in Table 4–1.

Fluid Volumes

The maternal extracellular volume, which consists of intravascular and interstitial components, increases throughout pregnancy, leading in effect to a state of physiologic extracellular hypervolemia. The intravascular volume, which consists of plasma and red cell components, increases approximately 50 percent during pregnancy. The plasma component increases approximately twice as much as the red cell mass (leading to a fall in hematocrit beginning early in pregnancy), and the two components follow different time courses, as discussed earlier. Maternal interstitial volume shows its greatest increase in the last trimester.

The magnitude of the rise in maternal plasma volume correlates with the size of the fetus; it is particularly marked in multiple gestation. Multipara with poor reproductive histories show smaller increments in plasma volume and GFR, when compared with those with a history of normal pregnancies and normal-sized babies.

While the changes in volume of the different body compartments and in the various humoral and physical factors known to affect volume can be described, volume regulation in pregnancy is poorly understood. Several physiologic factors involved in the renal handling of sodium, and hence in extracellular fluid volume regulation, undergo dramatic changes during pregnancy. These are summarized in Table 4–4.

Renin-Angiotensin System in Pregnancy

The elements of the renin-angiotensin system are markedly altered in pregnancy. Plasma concentrations of renin, renin substrate, angiotensin I, and angiotensin II are increased. Renin levels remain elevated throughout pregnancy. It is possible that at least a portion of the elevated renin measured in the peripheral blood of pregnant women may represent a different, high-molecular-weight form or an inactive form of the enzyme.

The uterus, like the kidney, can produce renin, and extremely high concentrations of renin occur in the amniotic fluid. The role played by this renin is not yet clear.

HOMEOSTASIS OF MATERNAL ENERGY SUBSTRATES

The metabolic regulation of energy substrates, including glucose, amino acids, fatty acids, and ketone bodies, is complex and interrelated.

TABLE 4–4   FACTORS INFLUENCING URINARY SODIUM EXCRETION DURING PREGNANCY

FACTORS INCREASING SODIUM EXCRETION	FACTORS DECREASING SODIUM EXCRETION

Marked increase in glomerular filtration rate
Increased progesterone production
Natriuretic hormones (argininevasopressin, vasodilatory prostaglandins, neurophysins, melanocyte-stimulating hormone)
Physical factors:
   Decreased plasma albumin, which produces a decreased postglomerular oncotic pressure
	Elevated plasma aldosterone concentration
	Increased concentration of other potentially salt-retaining hormones (desoxycorticosterone, estrogen, cortisol, placental lactogen, prolactin)
	Physical factors:
	   Increased filtration fraction producing an increased postglomerular oncotic pressure
	   Uteroplacental vasculature may simulate arteriovenous shunt
	   Increased ureteral pressure

Adapted with permission from Lindheimer MD, Katz AI: The renal response to pregnancy. In Brenner BM, Rector FC Jr (eds): The Kidney. 2nd ed. Philadelphia, WB Saunders Co, 1981, p 1774.

Insulin Effects and Glucose Metabolism

In pregnancy, the insulin response to glucose stimulation is augmented. By the tenth week of normal pregnancy and continuing to term, fasting concentrations of insulin are elevated and those of glucose reduced. Until midgestation, these changes are accompanied by improved intravenous glucose tolerance (although oral glucose tolerance remains unchanged). Glycogen synthesis and storage by the liver increases, and gluconeogenesis is inhibited. Thus, during the first half of pregnancy, the anabolic actions of insulin are potentiated.

After early pregnancy, insulin resistance emerges, so glucose tolerance is impaired. The fall in serum glucose for a given dose of insulin is reduced, compared with earlier pregnancy. There is prolonged elevation of circulating glucose after meals, although fasting glucose remains reduced, as in early pregnancy.

A variety of humoral factors have been suggested to account for the anti-insulin environment of the latter part of pregnancy. Perhaps the most important is human placental lactogen (hPL), which antagonizes the peripheral effects of insulin. It is secreted by the placenta into the maternal circulation in amounts parallel to placental growth. Free levels of cortisol are also increased. In addition, progesterone may exert some anti-insulin effects.

Other potential diabetogenic factors that probably do not play important roles in producing glucose intolerance in pregnancy should be considered. Although basal levels of glucagon are elevated in pregnancy, secretion of glucagon is suppressed normally by a glucose challenge. Growth hormone is not elevated, and the pituitary response to hypoglycemia is diminished. Finally, the half-life of intravenous insulin is unchanged during pregnancy; therefore, accelerated metabolic degradation probably does not play a role in glucose intolerance.

Lipid Metabolism

The potentiated anabolic effects of insulin that characterize early pregnancy lead to the inhibition of lipolysis. During the second half of pregnancy, however, probably as a result of rising hPL, lipolysis is augmented, and the plasma concentration of free fatty acids after an overnight fast is elevated. Teleologically, the free fatty acids act as substrates for maternal energy metabolism, while glucose and amino acids cross the placenta to the fetus. In the humoral milieu of the second half of the pregnancy, the increased free fatty acids lead to ketone body (beta-hydroxybutyrate and acetoacetate) formation. Pregnancy is thus associated with an increased risk of ketoacidosis, especially after prolonged fasting.

In the context of maternal lipid metabolism, mention must be made of the most dramatic lipid change in pregnancy, the rise in fasting triglyceride concentration.

PLACENTAL TRANSFER OF NUTRIENTS

The transfer of substances across the placenta occurs by several mechanisms, including simple diffusion, facilitated diffusion, and active transport. Several physiochemical factors, such as molecular size, degree of ionization, and lipid solubility, affect the rate of diffusion. Substances with molecular weights greater than 1000, such as polypeptides and proteins, cross the placenta slowly, if at all.

Amino acids are actively transported across the placenta, making fetal levels higher than maternal. Glucose is transported by facilitated diffusion, leading to rapid equilibrium with only a small maternal-fetal gradient. Free fatty acids diffuse passively across the placenta, and fetal levels are lower than maternal levels. Glucose is the main energy substrate of the fetus. However, recent studies suggest that amino acids and lactate may contribute up to 25 percent of fetal oxygen consumption. The degree and mechanism of placental transfer of these and other substances are summarized in Table 4–5.

OTHER ENDOCRINE CHANGES

Thyroid

The thyroid gland normally shows moderate enlargement during pregnancy. This is not due to elevation of thyroid-stimulating hormone, which remains unchanged.

Circulating thyroid hormone exists in two

TABLE 4–5 MATERNAL-FETAL TRANSFER DURING PREGNANCY

FUNCTION	SUBSTANCE	PLACENTAL TRANSFER
Glucose homeostasis	Glucose	Excellent—"facilitated diffusion"
	Amino acids	Excellent—active transport
	Free fatty acids (FFA)	Very limited—essential FFA only
	Ketones	Excellent—diffusion
	Insulin	No transfer
	Glucagon	No transfer
Thyroid function	Thyroxine (T_4)	Very poor—diffusion
	Triiodothyronine (T_3)	Poor—diffusion
	Thyrotropin-releasing hormone (TRH)	Good
	Long-acting thyroid stimulatory hormone (LATS)	Good
	Thyroid-stimulating hormone (TSH)	Negligible transfer
	Propylthiouracil	Excellent
Adrenal hormones	Cortisol	Excellent transfer and active placental conversion of cortisol to cortisone
	ACTH	No transfer
Parathyroid function	Calcium	Active transfer against gradient
	Magnesium	Active transfer against gradient
	Phosphorus	Active transfer against gradient
	Parathyroid hormone	Not transferred
Immunoglobulins	IgA	Minimal passive transfer
	IgG	Good—both passive and active transport from seven weeks' gestation
	IgM	No transfer

Adapted and reproduced with permission from Main DM, Main EK: Obstetrics and Gynecology, A Pocket Reference. Chicago, Year Book Medical Publishers, Inc., 1984, p 37.

primary active forms: *thyroxine* (T_4) and *triiodothyronine* (T_3). The former circulates in higher concentrations, is more highly protein-bound, and is less metabolically potent than T_3, for which it may serve as a prohormone. Circulating T_4 is bound to carrier proteins, approximately 85 percent to *thyroxine-binding globulin* (TBG), and most of the remainder to another protein, *thyroxine-binding prealbumin*. It is believed that only the unbound fraction of the circulating hormone is biologically active. TBG is increased during pregnancy because the high estrogen levels induce increased hepatic synthesis. The body responds by raising total circulating levels of T_4 and T_3. The net effect is that the free, biologically active concentration of each hormone is unchanged from the nonpregnant state. Therefore, clinically, the free T_4 index, which corrects the total circulating T_4 for the amount of binding protein, is an appropriate measure of thyroid function, with the same normal range as in the nonpregnant state. Thyroid hormones do not cross the placenta.

Adrenal

Adrenocorticotrophic hormone (ACTH) and plasma cortisol are both elevated from three months' gestation to delivery. Although less so than thyroid hormones, circulating cortisol is also bound, primarily by a specific plasma protein, *corticosteroid-binding globulin* (CBG) or *transcortin*. Unlike the thyroid hormones, the mean unbound level of cortisol is elevated in pregnancy; there is also some loss of the diurnal variation that characterizes its concentration in nonpregnant women. It is not clear to what extent this elevated cortisol is responsible for some of the "pseudo-Cushingoid" features of pregnancy, such as striae gravidarum and impaired glucose tolerance.

WEIGHT GAIN IN PREGNANCY

The average weight gain in pregnancy uncomplicated by generalized edema is 12.5 kg

TABLE 4–6 ANALYSIS OF WEIGHT GAIN IN PREGNANCY

TISSUES AND FLUIDS	INCREASE IN WEIGHT (gm) UP TO:			
	10 weeks	20 weeks	30 weeks	40 weeks
Fetus	5	300	1500	3400
Placenta	20	170	430	650
Amniotic fluid	30	350	750	800
Uterus	140	320	600	970
Mammary gland	45	180	360	405
Blood	100	600	1300	1250
Interstitial fluid (no edema or leg edema)	0	30	80	1680
Maternal stores	310	2050	3480	3345
Total weight gained	650	4000	8500	12,500

Adapted with permission from Hytten F, Chamberlain G (eds): Clinical Physiology in Obstetrics. Oxford, Blackwell Scientific Publications, 1980, p 221.

(28 lb). The components of this weight gain are indicated in Table 4–6. The products of conception comprise only about 40 percent of the total maternal weight gain.

PLACENTAL TRANSFER OF OXYGEN AND CARBON DIOXIDE

Fetal Oxygenation

The uteroplacental circulation subserves fetal gas exchange. Figure 4–1 demonstrates the normal blood gases on the maternal and fetal sides of the placenta. The umbilical vein of the fetus, like the pulmonary vein of the adult, carries the circulation's most highly oxygenated blood. The umbilical venous Po_2 of about 28 mm Hg is relatively low by adult standards. The fetus normally lives at these low oxygen tensions. The delivery system produces a large fall in oxygen tension from the uterine artery to the umbilical vein—analogous in the adult to the fall in oxygen tension from inspired air (Pio_2 = 150) to the pulmonary veins (Po_2 = 100). This relatively low fetal tension is essential for survival *in utero,* because a high Po_2 initiates adjustments, such as closure of the ductus arteriosus, which normally occur in the neonate but would be harmful *in utero.*

The placenta receives 60 percent of the combined ventricular output, while the postnatal lung receives 100 percent of the cardiac output. Unlike the lung, which consumes insignificant amounts of the oxygen it transfers, more than 20 percent of the oxygen derived from maternal blood at term is consumed by placental tissue. The degree of functional and anatomic shunting of placental blood past exchange sites is approximately 20 percent, some tenfold greater than in the lung. The cause of this functional shunting is probably a mismatch between maternal and fetal blood flow at the exchange sites, analogous to the ventilation perfusion inequalities that may occur in the lung.

Fetal and Maternal Hemoglobin Dissociation Curves

Most of the oxygen in blood is carried by hemoglobin in red blood cells. The maximum amount of oxygen carried per gram of hemoglobin, that is, the amount carried at 100 percent saturation, is fixed at 1.34 ml. However, the affinity of hemoglobin for oxygen, which is the percent saturation at a given oxygen tension, depends on chemical conditions. As is illustrated in Figure 4–2, when compared with nonpregnant adults, the binding of oxygen by hemoglobin is much greater in the fetus. In contrast, maternal affinity is lower. The shape of the fetal oxygen dissociation curve permits larger amounts of oxygen to be transported per unit of blood at relatively low oxygen tensions. Furthermore, the difference between maternal and fetal hemoglobin dissociation curves permits transplacental transfer of large volumes of oxygen. Thus, transplacental equilibration of maternal blood with a Po_2 of 30 mm Hg and saturation of 55 percent, will result in fetal blood with a Po_2 of 30 mm Hg but a saturation of almost 80 percent.

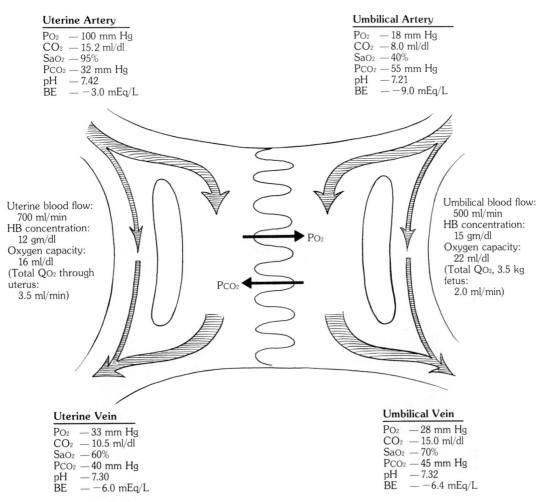

Uterine Artery

Po₂ — 100 mm Hg
CO₂ — 15.2 ml/dl
SaO₂ — 95%
Pco₂ — 32 mm Hg
pH — 7.42
BE — −3.0 mEq/L

Umbilical Artery

Po₂ — 18 mm Hg
CO₂ — 8.0 ml/dl
SaO₂ — 40%
Pco₂ — 55 mm Hg
pH — 7.21
BE — −9.0 mEq/L

Uterine blood flow:
700 ml/min
HB concentration:
12 gm/dl
Oxygen capacity:
16 ml/dl
(Total QO₂ through
uterus:
3.5 ml/min)

Po₂

Pco₂

Umbilical blood flow:
500 ml/min
HB concentration:
15 gm/dl
Oxygen capacity:
22 ml/dl
(Total QO₂, 3.5 kg
fetus:
2.0 ml/min)

Uterine Vein

Po₂ — 33 mm Hg
CO₂ — 10.5 ml/dl
SaO₂ — 60%
Pco₂ — 40 mm Hg
pH — 7.30
BE — −6.0 mEq/L

Umbilical Vein

Po₂ — 28 mm Hg
CO₂ — 15.0 ml/dl
SaO₂ — 70%
Pco₂ — 45 mm Hg
pH — 7.32
BE — −6.4 mEq/L

Figure 4–1 Placental transfer of oxygen and carbon dioxide. (Adapted from Bonica JJ: Obstetric Analgesia and Anesthesia, 2nd ed. Amsterdam, World Federation of Societies of Anesthesiologists, 1980, p. 29. Used with permission.)

Figure 4–2 The oxygen dissociation curve of fetal blood compared with maternal blood. The central continuous curve is of normal adult blood. A vertical line at an oxygen pressure of 30 mm Hg divides the curves. The fetal curve normally operates below that level, and the maternal curve above it. (Reproduced with permission from Hytten F, Chamberlain G (eds): Clinical Physiology in Obstetrics. Oxford, Blackwell Scientific Publications, 1980, p 472.)

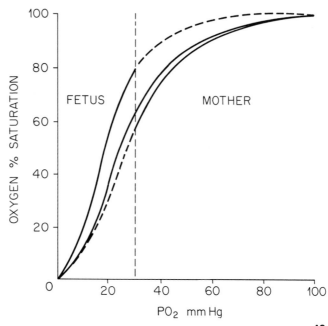

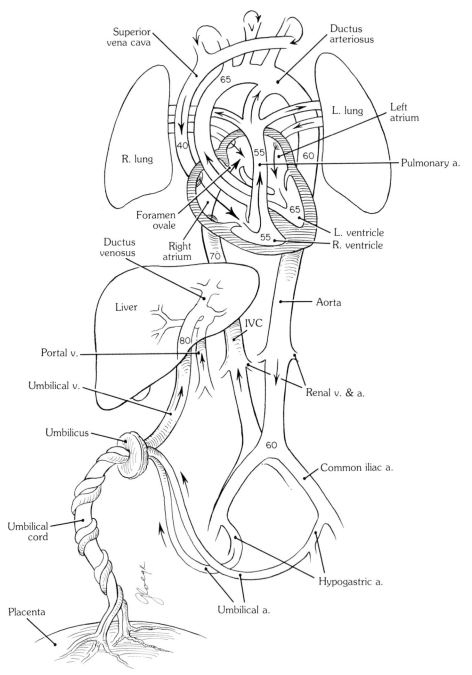

Figure 4–3 The fetal circulation. Numbers represent approximate values of per cent saturation of blood with oxygen *in utero*. (Adapted with permission from Parer JJ: Fetal circulation. *In* Sciarra JJ (ed): Obstetrics and Gynecology. Vol 3, Maternal and Fetal Medicine. Hagerstown, MD, Harper and Row, 1984, p 2.)

The decrease in the affinity of hemoglobin for oxygen produced by a fall in pH is referred to as the Bohr effect. Because of the unique situation in the placenta, a double Bohr effect facilitates oxygen transfer from mother to fetus. When CO_2 and fixed acids are transferred from fetus to mother, the associated rise in fetal pH increases the fetal red blood cell affinity for oxygen uptake; the concomitant reduced maternal blood pH decreases oxygen affinity and promotes its unloading from maternal red cells.

FETAL CIRCULATION

Several anatomic and physiologic factors must be noted in considering the fetal circulation (Fig. 4–3 and Table 4–7).

The normal adult circulation is a series circuit. The blood circulates serially through the right heart, to the lungs, then through the left heart, to the systemic circulation, finally returning to the right heart. In the fetus, such a series circulation does not exist. Instead, output of the right ventricle is about double that of the left ventricle, blood from both ventricles circulates to the lower body, and only a small fraction of right ventricular output goes to the lungs.

The fetal circulation is characterized by channels (ductus venosus, foramen ovale, and ductus arteriosus) and preferential streaming, which function to maximize the delivery of more highly oxygenated blood to the upper body and brain, less highly oxygenated blood to the lower body, and very low blood flow to the nonfunctional lungs. The umbilical vein, carrying oxygenated (80 percent saturated) blood from the placenta to the fetal body, enters the portal system. A portion of this umbilical-portal blood passes through the hepatic microcirculation, where oxygen is extracted, and thence through the hepatic veins into the inferior vena cava. The remainder enters the ductus venosus, which bypasses the liver and directly enters the inferior vena cava. The inferior vena cava also receives the unsaturated (25 percent saturated) venous return from the lower body. As it enters the heart, the inferior vena cava carries the most highly oxygenated blood (70 percent saturated) to reach the heart.

Before it mixes with the unsaturated blood returning via the superior vena cava (25 percent saturated), approximately one third of inferior vena caval blood preferentially streams across the foramen ovale into the left atrium. There, it mixes with the relatively meager pulmonary venous return, goes to the left ventricle, and thence to the aorta. The proximal aorta, carrying the most highly saturated blood leaving the heart (65 percent saturated) gives off branches that supply the brain and upper body. In its descending portion, the aorta is joined by the ductus arteriosus branch of the pulmonary artery, carrying relatively less saturated blood (55 percent saturated). The saturation of the descending aortic blood supplying the lower body (60 percent saturated) is thus lower than that supplying the brain and upper body.

The role of the ductus arteriosus must be emphasized. As noted above, one third of the highly saturated inferior caval blood flows through the foramen ovale directly into the left atrium. The remaining two thirds enters the right atrium and right ventricle. Unsaturated superior vena caval blood is directed toward the tricuspid valve, leading to a relatively lower saturation of right compared with left ventricular blood; in normal fetuses, essentially no superior vena caval blood traverses the foramen ovale into the left atrium. Right ventricular output enters the pulmo-

TABLE 4–7 COMPONENTS OF THE FETAL CIRCULATION

FETAL STRUCTURE	FROM/TO	ADULT REMNANT
1. Umbilical vein	Umbilicus/ductus venosus	Ligamentum teres hepatis
2. Ductus venosus	Umbilical vein/inferior vena cava (bypasses liver)	Ligamentum venosum
3. Foramen ovale	Right atrium/left atrium	Closed atrial wall
4. Ductus arteriosus	Pulmonary artery/descending aorta	Ligamentum arteriosum
5. Umbilical artery	Common iliac artery/umbilicus	1. Superior vesical arteries 2. Lateral vesicoumbilical ligaments

Adapted and reproduced with permission from Main DM, Main EK: Obstetrics and Gynecology, A Pocket Reference. Chicago, Year Book Medical Publishers, Inc., 1984, p 34.

nary trunk, from which its major portion bypasses the lungs by flowing through the ductus arteriosus to the descending aorta. Although the descending aorta supplies branches to the lower fetal body, the major portion of descending aortic flow goes to the umbilical arteries, which return deoxygenated blood to the placenta.

SUGGESTED READING

Bieniarz J, Grottogini JJ, Curuchet E, et al: Aortocaval compression by the uterus in late human pregnancy. II. An arteriographic study. Am J Obstet Gynecol 100:203, 1968.

Bieniarz J, Maqueda E, Caldeyro-Barcia R: Compression of aorta by the uterus in late human pregnancy. I. Variation between femoral and brachial artery pressure with changes from hypertension to hypotension. Am J Obstet Gynecol 95:795, 1966.

Elkayam R, Gleicher N: Cardiovascular physiology of pregnancy. In Elkayam R, Gleicher N (eds): Cardiac Problems in Pregnancy: Diagnosis and Management of Maternal and Fetal Disease. New York, Alan R Liss, 1982, p 5.

Garn SM, Ridella SA, Petzold AS, et al: Maternal hematologic levels and pregnancy outcomes. Semin Perinatol 5:155, 1981.

Heymann MA: Fetal cardiovascular physiology. In Creasy RK, Resnick R (eds): Maternal-Fetal Medicine. Philadelphia, WB Saunders Co, 1984, p 259. .

Hytten FR, Chamberlain G (eds): Clinical Physiology in Obstetrics. Oxford, Blackwell Scientific Publications, 1980.

Lindheimer MD, Katz AI: The renal response to pregnancy. In Brenner BM, Rector FC Jr (eds): The Kidney. 2nd ed. Philadelphia, WB Saunders Co, 1981.

Longo LL: Some physiological implications of altered uteroplacental blood flow. In Moawad AH, Lindheimer MD (eds): Uterine and Placental Blood Flow. New York, Masson Publishing USA, 1982, p 93.

Prowse CM, Gaensler EA: Respiratory and acid base changes during pregnancy. Anesthesiology 26:381, 1965.

Tulchinsky D, Ryan KJ: Maternal-Fetal Endocrinology. Philadelphia, WB Saunders Co, 1980.

Chapter Five

IMMUNOLOGY OF PREGNANCY

ARNOLD L. MEDEARIS

Pregnancy represents one of the most significant areas of study for the immunobiologist. The reasons for the success of gestation in both normal and abnormal pregnancies remain unclear because the fetus is antigenically dissimilar to the mother. The immunologic response of the mother to her fetus is an area of increasing interest.

The importance of immunology to obstetrics is often not appreciated. The identification of the Rhesus factor, and the development of a preventive program utilizing immunosuppression of the maternal response to fetal cell leakage at the time of delivery, are two of the first major successes in the field of perinatology.

Briefly addressed in this chapter are four areas in which an initial understanding of immunology is important. These are (1) the immunobiology of the maternal-fetal interaction, (2) the immunologic response during normal pregnancy, (3) the role of immunology in pregnancy-associated conditions, and (4) the maternal and fetal effects of autoimmune diseases in pregnancy.

IMMUNOBIOLOGY OF THE MATERNAL-FETAL INTERACTION

The maintenance of the antigenically dissimilar fetus in the uterus of the mother is of primary importance in obstetrics. Most of the recent attention in this field has come from the study of organ transplantation. The presence of the fetus is analogous to the grafting of tissues or organs between two individuals of the same species who are genetically dissimilar. Since all humans (except identical twins) are considered to be genetically dissimilar (allogeneic), such transplants are referred to as allografts. There are a number of mechanisms that have been proposed to account for the tolerance and subsequent success of the fetal allograft.

The primary sites of modulation of the maternal response to the fetus are the uterus, regional lymphatics, and the placental surface. The uterus has been considered to be an immunologically privileged site, similar to the anterior chamber of the eye, the adrenal gland, and the cheek pouch of the hamster. These sites appear to have decreased or altered afferent lymphatic systems that allow them to modify the host response to an allograft, and it appears that a similar mechanism may apply in the uterus during pregnancy. The T cells, which primarily mediate the cellular response to foreign tissue by acting to either help or suppress the immune response, are also locally altered in pregnancy. Pregnancy-related suppressor T cells capable of decreasing the maternal lymphocyte response have been described. These cells, in conjunction with placental interventions, can lead to an altered local immunologic environment.

The separate vascular compartments found in the hemomonochorial placentation of the human effectively remove the fetus from direct contact with the maternal immunologic defense system. This allows the placenta to function as an interface between two distinct systems. Tight trophoblastic intercellular junctions and a fibrinous covering of the trophoblast lead to control of the cellular and molecular fetomaternal transport. In addition, the placenta lacks the major histocompatibility (HLA) antigens that are necessary for the maternal lymphocytes to initiate an effective immunologic response.

The placenta produces a number of pregnancy-associated plasma proteins and steroids that may alter the maternal immune response. These include pregnancy-specific beta-1 glycoprotein (SP1), human placental lactogen (hPL), and human chorionic gonadotropin (hCG), as well as the sex steroids estrogen and progesterone. All of these substances have been shown to nonspecifically suppress the local immune response in pregnancy.

In addition, the placenta functions as an immunoabsorbent to decrease the response against the fetus. Antibodies that are generated by the maternal immune response against paternal antigens in the placental surface (masking antibodies) and local immune complexes (blocking antibodies) may be trapped in the placenta. These complexes can modify and/or block the immune response by facilitating enhancing antibodies and cellular suppression.

These mechanisms, which are summarized in Table 5–1, are thought to account for the maternal tolerance and the lack of host rejection seen in the majority of pregnancies.

IMMUNOLOGIC RESPONSE DURING NORMAL PREGNANCY

The mother's immunologic defense system remains intact during pregnancy. While allowing the fetal allograft to exist, the mother must still be able to protect herself and her fetus from infection and antigenically foreign substances. The nonspecific mechanisms of the immunologic system (including phagocytosis and the inflammatory response) are not affected by pregnancy. The specific mechanisms of the immune response (humoral and cellular) are also not significantly affected. There is no significant change in the leukocyte count. The percentage of B or T lymphocytes is not altered, nor is there any consistent alteration in their performance during pregnancy.

Immunoglobulin levels do not change in pregnancy. The levels of specific maternal IgG antibodies are of particular importance because of their ability to cross the placenta. Maternal IgG is the major component of the fetal immunoglobulin *in utero* and the early neonatal period. IgG is the only immuno-

TABLE 5–1 PROPOSED MECHANISMS FOR THE SUCCESS OF THE FETAL ALLOGRAFT

| MATERNAL | | FETAL | |
Systemic	Uterus and Local Lymphatic System	Placenta	Systemic
None (Normal cell mediated immunity)	1. Privileged immunologic site 2. Localized, nonspecific suppression induces tolerance and generates suppressor T cells	1. Separation of the maternal-fetal circulations, including tight local barriers 2. Lack of expression of the major histocompatibility antigen (HLA) at the maternal-fetal interface 3. Nonspecific local immunosuppression through placental proteins and hormones 4. Immunoabsorbent effect of placental proteins and hormones 5. Production of masking and blocking antibodies 6. Generation of immune cell blockage	Unidentified humoral and cellular immunosuppressive elements

globulin that is transported across the placenta. Significant passive immunity can be transferred in this manner to the fetus and aids in protecting it from infection during the perinatal period. IgM, because of its larger molecular size, is unable to cross the placenta. The other immunoglobulins—IgA, IgD, and IgE—are also confined to the maternal compartment and do not present any direct harm or benefit to the fetus.

The fetal immune system develops early. Lymphocytes are present by the seventh week and antigen recognition is demonstrable by the twelfth week. All of the immunoglobulin classes except IgA have fetal components present by week twelve. Production of the various immunoglobulins is progressive throughout gestation. The newborn fetus at term has developed a sufficient defense system to combat bacterial and viral challenges.

ROLE OF IMMUNOLOGY IN PREGNANCY-ASSOCIATED CONDITIONS

The major pregnancy-associated immunologic disease process is hemolytic disease of the newborn. Rhesus factor incompatibility, which is the most important of these conditions, is discussed in Chapter 25.

Hemolytic disease secondary to non-Rhesus sensitization and the destruction of lymphocytes or platelets secondary to sensitization against specific surface antigens all have the same pathogenesis. Fetal cellular antigens leak into the maternal circulation, primarily at birth, and initiate an immune response. The reaction to these foreign antigens is by the humoral component (B cells) of the immune system. Antibody production is initiated and IgM and/or IgG immunoglobulins are produced. Many times, no response or only a weak response can be measured. IgG, if present in low concentration, does not cause any appreciable fetal compromise. However, high levels of IgG can lead to a destructive response if the fetal antigen against which it is directed is present in the current or a subsequent pregnancy. Antibodies to white cells and platelets are not routinely evaluated. Fetal lymphopenia or thrombocytopenia may occur secondary to maternal sensitization, but these are diagnosed infrequently.

An exception to the above mechanism is found in ABO incompatibility, where naturally occurring antibodies can be found prior to any fetal cellular leakage. These antibodies are generally IgM and not clinically significant. However, in group O individuals, both IgG and IgM antibodies may occur naturally, and the IgG antibodies may cross the placenta. ABO incompatibility occurs largely in mothers of blood group O with infants of blood group A or B. The hemolytic disease is less severe than Rhesus hemolytic disease, and hydrops fetalis does not occur.

Blood transfusions can also sensitize the mother to fetal red cell antigens. If the patient has a history of receiving a red cell transfusion and is sensitized to one of the irregular antigens, it is important to confirm the antigen status of the father, if possible, to determine whether or not the fetus is at risk for hemolytic disease. For example, if the patient has antibodies to Kell and the father is Kell-negative, the fetus could not inherit the Kell antigen and would therefore not be at risk.

It has been postulated that pre-eclampsia has an immunologic basis. However, no consistent abnormality has been demonstrated in the immune system of pre-eclamptic patients studied by current techniques. While pre-eclampsia may represent a form of late fetal rejection, the evidence is not yet compelling.

AUTOIMMUNE DISEASE IN PREGNANCY

An autoimmune disease is one in which antibodies are developed against the host's own tissues. A number of autoimmune diseases can significantly affect either the maternal or fetal outcome in pregnancy. These include rheumatoid arthritis, systemic lupus erythematosus (SLE), idiopathic thrombocytopenic purpura, isoimmune thrombocytopenia, Graves' disease, and myasthenia gravis. A summary of the interactions of primary immunologic disorders and pregnancy is shown in Table 5–2. In general, the severity of maternal disease depends on the end organ primarily involved. The fetus is affected if an IgG antibody is produced against a vital organ.

Rheumatoid Arthritis

Rheumatoid arthritis is a chronic systemic disease that affects individuals between the

TABLE 5–2 AUTOIMMUNE DISEASE IN PREGNANCY

DISEASE	EFFECT OF DISEASE ON THE PREGNANCY		EFFECT OF PREGNANCY ON THE DISEASE	ANTIBODIES THAT CROSS THE PLACENTA
	Mother	Fetus		
Rheumatoid arthritis	No significant effect	No significant effect Teratogenic effects of medication	Improved commonly	None
Idiopathic thrombocytopenic purpura	Ante-, intra-, and postpartum hemorrhage	Fetal hemorrhage (particularly intracranial bleeding)	None	Platelet antibodies
Thrombotic thrombocytopenic purpura	No significant effect	Similar to ITP	None	Platelet antibodies
Graves' disease	No significant effect	Intrauterine growth retardation Neonatal thyrotoxicosis	Improved during pregnancy Exacerbation postpartum	Long-acting thyroid stimulator (LATS)
Myasthenia gravis	No significant effect	Transient neonatal myasthenia	Variable during pregnancy Moderate exacerbation postpartum	Anti-acetylcholinesterase
Systemic lupus erythematosus	Increased incidence of uterine infection Increased incidence of pre-eclampsia	Abortion (spontaneous) Prematurity Intrauterine growth retardation Stillbirth Congenital heart block Endomyocardial fibrosis	Exacerbation of the disease Deterioration of renal condition Anemia, leukopenia, and thrombocytopenia	Various tissues and membranes

ages of 20 and 60 years, most commonly females. It is manifested primarily in the joints, but extra-articular manifestations may also be present, including subcutaneous nodules on the extensor surfaces of the forearms and involvement of the cardiac, pulmonary, ocular, nervous, and lymphatic systems. Due to the deposition of immune complexes in the blood vessels, vasculitis may be present. The kidneys are usually spared.

Investigations. Laboratory findings include a normocytic, normochromic anemia; leukopenia; elevated platelet count; high sedimentation rate; and hypergammaglobulinemia. The rheumatoid factor may be present in about 80 percent of affected individuals, while the antinuclear antibody test is positive in about 20 percent.

Treatment. Drug treatment is recommended for those individuals who are symptomatic or in whom the clinical picture worsens.

SALICYLATES. Salicylates are the mainstay of drug treatment in rheumatoid arthritis. They interfere with platelet aggregation, although bleeding is rare. The drugs have been used during pregnancy and are known to cross the placental barrier. Maternal side effects include prolonged gestation and greater blood loss during delivery and in the immediate postpartum period. Reports of fetal and neonatal side effects are mainly related to clotting defects. As prostaglandin inhibitors, they pose the potential risks of affecting premature closure of the ductus arteriosus in the fetus and causing pulmonary hypertension in the neonate. Although parents should be aware of the potential maternal and fetal-neonatal risks, clinical experience suggests that salicylates are relatively safe when taken during pregnancy.

NONSTEROIDAL ANTI-INFLAMMATORY AGENTS. These drugs are used when salicylates fail to relieve the inflammatory response. Several preparations are available, among which are indomethacin, ibuprofen, and naproxen. None of these drugs has been studied in depth during pregnancy, although it is known that they cross the placenta and reach the fetus. As antiprostaglandins, they pose risks to the fetus and neonate similar to those of salicylates.

DISEASE SUPPRESSIVE MEDICATIONS. Such agents include gold, antimalarials, and penicillamine. *Gold* toxicity includes skin rashes, bone marrow suppression, and nephro- and hepatotoxicity. Gold is protein-bound, crosses the placenta very poorly, and has no reported fetal and neonatal side effects. *Antimalarials* compare favorably with gold. Side effects are mainly gastrointestinal and ocular. Since they cross the placenta readily, they are not recommended during pregnancy. *Penicillamine* is one of the newer drugs. It compares favorably with gold and has the same drug toxicity problems as gold salts. Since it crosses the placenta, the potential risks to the fetus are enormous. It should not be used during pregnancy.

CYTOTOXIC AGENTS. Cyclophosphamide and azathioprine have been used in several controlled trials in patients with rheumatoid arthritis. Their main side effect is bone marrow toxicity. They should be avoided during pregnancy.

STEROIDS. Although steroids are the best available anti-inflammatory agents, their use should be limited to severe cases in which other drug regimens have failed. Aside from their maternal and fetal side effects, systemic steroids may mask the inflammatory response to the joints and allow bone destruction to proceed unabated. Intra-articular steroids are useful, have limited systemic side effects, and may even be used in pregnant women with minimal concern about fetal and neonatal well-being.

Prognosis. Prognosis during pregnancy is usually good, with the majority of the patients (75 percent) showing improvement.

Systemic Lupus Erythematosus

Systemic lupus erythematosus (SLE) is a chronic connective tissue disease that is characterized by multiple system involvement. The disease tends to affect young women in the second to fourth decade, although it may occur at any age. The incidence of SLE has increased dramatically over the past two decades, the present estimate being one case per 1000 population.

Manifestations. The clinical and laboratory manifestations are variable. This prompted the American Rheumatism Association to list 14 criteria that include the most common findings in SLE patients (Table 5–3). The presence of any four of these manifestations correlates very highly with the clinical presence of lupus.

Once the diagnosis of SLE is made, it is

TABLE 5–3 AMERICAN RHEUMATISM ASSOCIATION CRITERIA FOR SYSTEMIC LUPUS ERYTHEMATOSUS

1. Facial erythema (butterfly rash)
2. Discoid lupus
3. Raynaud's phenomenon
4. Alopecia
5. Photosensitivity
6. Oral and nasopharyngeal ulceration
7. Arthritis without deformity
8. Positive LE preparation
9. Chronic false-positive test for syphilis (VDRL)
10. Profuse proteinuria (greater than 3.5 gm/day)
11. Cellular casts
12. Pleurisy or pericarditis
13. Psychosis or convulsions
14. Hemolytic anemia, leukopenia, or thrombocytopenia

imperative to follow the disease activity. The hallmark of this connective tissue disorder is the presence of various circulating antibodies, including anti-DNA, anti-RNA, antiplatelet, and many others. The presence of anti-DNA and depressed complement levels (C3) are frequently connected with disease activity and specifically with lupus nephritis. In a small number of patients (most probably those who are free of lupus nephritis), there is no correlation between these serologic findings and the activity of the disease.

Association with Pregnancy. Patients with SLE should be counseled against pregnancy during the active phase of the disease. Additionally, they should be informed about the potential maternal, fetal, and neonatal complications. Pregnancy counseling should cover the areas discussed below.

FLARE-UPS. In patients with mild disease or those who enter the pregnancy with the disease quiescent, no major flare-ups are encountered during pregnancy or the postpartum period.

GENETIC PENETRANCE. First-degree relatives of patients with SLE have about a 12 percent incidence of the disease, compared with an incidence of 0.001 percent in the general population.

PREGNANCY OUTCOME. Although fertility rates are not affected in patients with SLE, the abortion and stillbirth rates are much higher than normal. Arteriolitis (decidual vasculitis) affecting the uterine vessels has been implicated. Even if the pregnancy continues, the poor blood supply to the utero-placental circulation may result in a growth-retarded fetus. Recent studies suggest a good fetal outcome if renal functions are preserved.

NEONATAL STATUS. A number of offspring have been found with congenital heart block, endomyocardial fibrosis, skin rashes, and circulating antibodies. The association between maternal SLE and fetal-neonatal cardiac conditions is strong, and it is felt that the presence of maternal antibodies to the fetal heart may play a role in their development.

Treatment. The management of SLE in pregnancy does not differ from accepted management practices in the nonpregnant individual. The presence of anti-DNA antibodies and depressed complement levels are suggestive of active disease or impending flare-up. Systemic steroids are the mainstay of treatment, and the daily dose should be adjusted according to the individual needs. Cytotoxic or antimalarial drugs that pose great risk to the fetus should be avoided. If circulating lupus anticoagulant is present, low-dose steroids might be of some help. Fetal studies (non-stress test, contraction stress test, obstetric sonograms) are indicated after fetal viability has been reached.

The management of labor and delivery follows obstetric indications. Mothers who are using systemic steroids or who have received such medications for a period of several months are at risk of manifesting adrenal insufficiency and should receive intravenous hydrocortisone sodium succinate (Solu-Cortef), 100 mg every 8 hours, or an equivalent dose of corticosteroids, during labor and for 48 to 72 hours postdelivery. Patients who were receiving steroids during pregnancy can then revert to their previous dose, while if the patient was not on systemic steroids during pregnancy, the steroids commenced during labor may be tapered gradually over a period of several weeks. Breast feeding is not contraindicated during the period of steroid treatment.

Contraceptive Counseling. Contraceptive counseling is essential for patients with SLE. Oral contraceptives are known to induce lupus-like manifestations in healthy women and might worsen the symptoms in patients with SLE. Intrauterine devices may lead to recurrent pelvic infections, especially if steroids or cytotoxic agents are in use by the patient. The risk of heavy vaginal bleeding is increased if thrombocytopenia or a circulating anticoagulant is present. For the above reasons, oral contraceptives or intrauterine devices should be avoided. Barrier methods are the safest, although the risk of pregnancy is higher. In patients who have completed their family or in whom the disease is far-advanced or debilitating, permanent sterilization is recommended.

Idiopathic Thrombocytopenic Purpura (ITP)

Although the exact etiology is not known, this entity is associated with systemic lupus erythematosus, lymphoma, viral infection, and thyroid disease. Available information suggests that platelet production is normal or increased, but peripheral platelet destruction exceeds bone marrow production. An IgG immunoglobulin has been isolated from the plasma of these patients. When this immunoglobulin attaches itself to the platelets, it causes structural damage. Subsequently, these platelets are sequestered in the reticuloendothelial system.

Treatment. Every effort should be made to uncover the underlying etiologic factors and to treat them accordingly. Low platelet counts *per se* should not be treated. Only when associated petechiae and hemorrhages are present is treatment recommended. Corticosteroids, in a dose equivalent to 60 to 80 mg per day of prednisone, are given initially, maintained for two to three weeks, then tapered slowly. Within two weeks of commencing corticosteroid treatment, the platelet count increases, although it may remain below control levels. Even in the absence of changes in the platelet level, hemostasis is improved. Splenectomy should be considered for patients who fail to respond to corticosteroid treatment. Platelet transfusions are not recommended, except in life-threatening situations, since they are destroyed quickly in the peripheral circulation.

The treatment of ITP during pregnancy follows the same guidelines outlined above. Since the platelet-associated IgG immunoglobulin crosses the placenta, fetal thrombocytopenia might develop. About 50 percent of fetal mortality in ITP patients is attributed to hemorrhage. There is poor correlation between maternal and fetal platelet counts, and a decision to perform a cesarean section should not be based solely on maternal platelet levels. Serious neonatal hemorrhage is unlikely to occur if the neonatal platelet count exceeds 50,000/cu mm.

Two approaches might be utilized for management of labor and delivery in the pregnant patient with ITP.

1. Cesarean section may be performed at or near term and prior to the onset of labor.

2. The onset of spontaneous labor may be awaited. When cervical dilatation allows fetal blood sampling, a fetal platelet count is obtained. If the count is less than 50,000/cu mm, a cesarean section is done; otherwise, vaginal delivery is allowed.

Thrombotic Thrombocytopenic Purpura (TTP)

TTP is a syndrome that includes thrombocytopenic purpura, hemolysis, fragmentation of red blood cells, fever, and neurologic and renal manifestations. The maternal mortality rate is about 60 to 70 percent.

In the treatment of TTP, splenectomy for maternal indications has been recommended, although newer therapeutic approaches have significantly reduced maternal mortality. Recent advances include exchange transfusions, infusion of fresh frozen plasma, and administration of antiplatelet medication.

Miscellaneous Disorders

The immunologic disorders caused by receptor antibodies, Graves' disease, and myasthenia gravis have primary fetal effects. *Graves' disease,* which is discussed in Chapter 16, can cause neonatal thyrotoxicosis due to the transplacental passage of long-acting thyroid stimulator (LATS). The fetus of the mother with *myasthenia gravis* can experience transient symptoms of muscle weakness during the neonatal period similar to those ex-

perienced by the mother. Both of these conditions are exacerbated postpartum.

Recently, subclinical autoimmune disease and circulating lupus-like anticoagulants have been implicated as a cause of *recurrent abortion, early fetal loss,* and severe *intrauterine growth retardation.* When these conditions are present and unexplained in a patient, it may be helpful to obtain an antinuclear antibody titer, although patients with immunologic problems represent a small proportion of the total number of patients with these pregnancy complications. No therapy has been shown to consistently improve outcome in this group.

SUGGESTED READING

Adelsberg BR: Immunology of pregnancy. Mt Sinai J Med 52:5, 1985.

Beer AE, Billingham RE: The Immunobiology of Mammalian Reproduction. Englewood Cliffs, New Jersey, Prentice-Hall Inc, 1976.

Bernales R, Bellanti J: Fetal and neonatal immunology. In Quilligan EJ, Kretchmer N (eds): Fetal and Maternal Medicine. New York, John Wiley and Sons, 1980, p 267.

Cauchi M: Obstetric and Perinatal Immunology. London, Edward Arnold Publishers, 1981.

Dhindsa DS, Schumacher GFB: Immunological Aspects of Infertility and Fertility Regulation. Amsterdam, Elsevier North Holland Inc, 1980.

Jones WR: Immunological aspects of reproduction. Clin Obstet Gynecol 6(3):383, 1979.

Jones WR, Storey B, Norton G, et al: Pregnancy complicated by acute idiopathic thrombocytopenic purpura. J Obstet Gynaecol Br Commonwealth 81:330, 1974.

Lockshin MD, Gibofsky A, Peebles CL, et al: Neonatal lupus erythematosus with heart block: Family study of a patient with anti SS-A and SS-B antibodies. Arthritis Rheum 26:210, 1983.

Oliver TK, Kirschbaum TH, Scott JR (eds): Immunology of Reproduction. In Seminars in Perinatology. New York, Grune and Stratton, Vol 1, No 2, April 1977.

Scott JS, Maddison PG, Taylor PV, et al: Connective tissue disease, antibodies in ribonucleoprotein, and congenital heart block. N Engl J Med 309:209, 1983.

Wegmann TG, Gill TJ: Immunology of Reproduction. London, Oxford University Press, 1983.

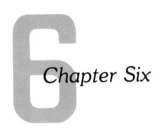

Chapter Six

PRENATAL CARE

CALVIN J. HOBEL

The objective of prenatal care is to assure that every wanted pregnancy is given the maximal chance to culminate in the delivery of a healthy baby, without impairing the health of the mother. It is known that prenatal care is associated with improved reproductive outcome, but it is not certain which components of the total process are responsible. The purpose of this chapter is to describe the components of modern prenatal care.

PREPREGNANCY HEALTH CARE

The concept of prepregnancy health care has been established, and ideally, prenatal care should be a continuation of such a physician-supervised program for women. For example, prepregnancy counseling provides the woman and her husband or the future father of the child with information about the potential risks of a pregnancy (see Chapter 7). Prepregnancy management of the diabetic to assure optimal control of blood glucose levels during the early weeks of pregnancy has the potential of preventing birth defects.

SPECIFIC OBJECTIVES OF PRENATAL CARE

The precise content of prenatal care has been defined by the American College of Obstetricians and Gynecologists. The specific objectives are to prevent and manage those conditions that cause poor pregnancy outcomes. These conditions include premature labor and delivery, intrauterine growth retardation, birth defects, hypertension, diabetes mellitus, perinatal infections, and post-term pregnancy.

COMPONENTS OF PRENATAL CARE

Access to prenatal care is very important. Community education is important for reaching patients who choose not to seek prenatal care. The majority of prenatal care services are provided outside the hospital setting. Established links among the private doctor's office, the community clinic, and the hospital are important to allow access to ancillary services for high-risk patients.

The First Visit

At the first prenatal visit, a thorough history must be taken and physical examination performed, as outlined in Chapter 2. A complete assessment of risk must also be undertaken. This may be done in an organized fashion using a standardized form. One such system is the Problem Oriented Prenatal Risk Assessment System (POPRAS).

In assessing risk at the first and subsequent visits, historic facts must be considered (subjective information), together with the findings on physical examination and the results of laboratory and other special tests (objective information). In some centers, weighted scores are assigned to each problem to allow a more precise assessment of risk to be made. Once problems are identified, a specific plan of action should be established for each problem.

ROUTINE TESTS DURING PREGNANCY

In ordering laboratory tests, it is appropriate to strike a balance between the benefits of the information obtained and the cost of the test. Certain laboratory evaluations, which have either become traditional or are legislatively mandated, may be questioned from the standpoint of cost-effectiveness. Therefore, appropriate individualization should be exercised for each prenatal patient. Table 6–1 lists the commonly performed evaluations.

Cervical Cytology

This test should be carried out on every newly pregnant woman unless a normal Papanicolaou smear has been obtained within the past six months.

Blood Count

Hematologic investigations can, for all practical purposes, be restricted to the determination of either the hemoglobin concentration or the packed red cell volume (hematocrit). A white cell count and differential are not cost-effective but may identify the rare

TABLE 6–1 PRENATAL LABORATORY TESTS AND INVESTIGATIONS

ROUTINE
1. Cervical cytology
2. Complete blood count (CBC)
3. Urinalysis (UA) and screen for bacilluria
4. Blood group, Rh factor, and antibody screen
5. Serology test for syphilis
6. Rubella antibody titer

COMMONLY PERFORMED
7. Blood glucose screen
8. Serum alpha-fetoprotein (AFP)
9. Ultrasound
10. Tuberculin skin testing

OTHER TESTS
11. Cervical culture for *Neisseria gonorrhoeae* and group B streptococci
12. Toxoplasmosis antibody test
13. Hepatitis B surface antigen (HBsAg) titer
14. Sickle cell preparation or hemoglobin electrophoresis in all previously unscreened black women

case of leukemia that occurs during pregnancy if there is any clinical suspicion. All black women who have not previously been screened for the sickle trait should be screened with either a sickle-cell preparation or a hemoglobin electrophoresis. Anemic women of Mediterranean extraction should be evaluated with a hemoglobin electrophoresis to detect thalassemia.

Urinalysis

A "clean-catch" midstream urine specimen should be obtained and subjected to the following tests: (1) analysis for the presence of glucose, ketones, and protein; (2) microscopic examination of the sediment; and (3) either quantitative culture or a biochemical screen for the presence of bacilluria. This latter evaluation is probably cost-effective when balanced against the incidence and associated morbidity of urinary tract infections in pregnancy.

Blood Group, Rhesus Factor, and Antibody Screen

Every pregnant woman should have a blood group, Rhesus (Rh) factor, and antibody screen performed at the first prenatal visit. If alerted by a positive screen, the antibody present can be identified and the patient appropriately managed (see Chapter 25).

Test for Syphilis

A serologic test for syphilis is mandated by law in virtually all states. Early diagnosis and treatment of syphilis reduce perinatal morbidity.

Rubella Antibody Screen

A rubella antibody screen should be done on each prenatal patient who is known to be susceptible (nonimmune) or whose status is unknown. Following delivery, nonimmune women should be offered the rubella vaccine.

Glucose Screen

Glucose screening for gestational diabetes is best carried out between 24 and 28 weeks, when insulin requirements are maximal. Sev-

TABLE 6–2 SCREENING TESTS FOR
DIABETES MELLITUS

TEST	NORMAL PLASMA GLUCOSE
Fasting	<100 mg/dl
1 hour after 50 gm glucose load	<135 mg/dl
2 hours after 100 gm glucose load	<140 mg/dl

eral screening methods are acceptable, as outlined in Table 6–2. Any patient 25 years of age or older should be screened. Risk factors for diabetes mellitus are shown in Table 6–3.

Serum Alpha-fetoprotein Test

Each pregnant woman should be counseled regarding the availability of the maternal serum alpha-fetoprotein test. This test, which may predict an open neural tube defect, is best carried out between 16 and 20 weeks. Further evaluation of patients with elevated levels is discussed in Chapter 7.

Ultrasound

Ultrasonic dating of the pregnancy and an ultrasonic fetal survey to detect gross abnormalities have been recommended in some clinics as a routine part of early prenatal care. Routine ultrasonography will be most cost-effective in patients in whom the date of the last menstrual period is uncertain and in patients with a family history of congenital anomalies. Considerable individualization should be exercised in making the decision to order this evaluation. If ultrasound is performed, it is most informative between 16 and 20 weeks.

Tuberculin Skin Testing

All prenatal patients who have no history of tuberculosis should be skin-tested with 0.1

TABLE 6–3 RISK FACTORS FOR
DIABETES MELLITUS

1. Age 25 years or older
2. Obesity
3. Family history of diabetes mellitus
4. Previous infant weighing greater than 4000 gm
5. Previous stillborn infant
6. Previous congenitally deformed infant
7. Previous polyhydramnios
8. History of recurrent abortions

ml of purified protein derivative (PPD) containing 5 tuberculin units. If the test is negative, no further work-up is necessary. If the test is positive and the patient asymptomatic, a chest x-ray should be obtained. If negative, no further work-up is necessary and no treatment should be given antepartum. If active disease is suspected, the patient should be hospitalized and have her sputum, gastric aspirates, and morning urine cultured and tested with acid-fast stains. Chemotherapy should then be commenced.

Other Tests

Some clinics routinely culture the cervix and urethra for gonorrhea; others obtain the culture only in a high-risk patient. A cervical culture identifying group B streptococci and treatment near term may be very helpful in reducing the risk of neonatal infection. A *toxoplasmosis antibody test* for all cat owners is appropriate. Nonimmune patients should be advised to avoid contact with cats and, particularly, cat excrement. A *hepatitis B surface antigen (HBsAg) titer* to detect the carrier state should be obtained in all patients giving a history of type B hepatitis or hepatitis of unknown type.

SUBSEQUENT PRENATAL CARE

Careful surveillance of the obstetric patient is directed toward the identification of developing problems that may affect the fetus adversely.

Weight Gain

The pregnant patient should be weighed at each visit. A total weight gain of 26 to 28 pounds is ideal for most pregnancies. Excessive weight gain is not harmful, although it may be associated with gestational diabetes. Sudden weight gain in the third trimester is a warning sign of impending pre-eclampsia. Inadequate weight gain or weight gain of less than 10 pounds at 28 weeks is associated with the risk of premature labor or intrauterine fetal growth retardation. Deviation from normal may require counseling or referral to a dietitian.

Urinalysis

At each visit, a urine sample should be checked for sugar and protein. Urine samples obtained in the clinic are usually two to three hours postprandial and, therefore, may contain sugar. If glycosuria is identified, a repeat sample should be obtained in the fasting state to rule out glycosuria, which is a possible first sign of diabetes. Proteinuria may be a sign of renal disease or pre-eclampsia.

Blood Pressure

Blood pressure should be monitored at each visit to allow early detection of pre-eclampsia. Both the systolic and diastolic pressures are normally lowest at the end of the second and the beginning of the third trimester.

Gestational Age Estimate and Fundal Height Measurements

At each visit, the gestational age must be assessed and recorded. From 22 weeks until term, the fundal height, measured in centimeters (cm) from the symphysis pubis to the top of the fundus, is equivalent to the gestational age in weeks. A discrepancy of greater than 2 to 3 cm suggests a size/dates problem. This may be the first indication of a multiple gestation (size at least 3 cm more than dates) or of intrauterine growth retardation (size at least 3 cm less than dates). An ultrasonic examination is indicated for further evaluation of a size/dates discrepancy.

Examination of the Abdomen

Beginning at 28 weeks, systematic examination of the abdomen is carried out to identify the attitude, lie, presentation, and position of the fetus. The fetal heart should also be auscultated.

The *attitude* refers to the relationship of parts of the fetus to each other. Normally, the fetus conforms to the shape of the uterus and the attitude is one of complete flexion. The fetus is folded, with its back convex, head flexed, and thighs over the abdomen. The arms are crossed over the thorax leaving a protected space for the umbilical cord between the face and the knees. With a deflexed attitude, as in a brow presentation, the head is extended and the spinal curvature reduced.

The *lie* of the fetus is the relationship of the long axis of the fetus to the long axis of the mother. The lie can be either longitudinal, transverse, or oblique.

The *presenting part* is the portion of the fetus that descends first through the birth canal. When the lie is longitudinal, the presenting part is either the head (cephalic presentation) or breech (breech presentation). When the lie is transverse, the presenting part can be the shoulder.

The *position* refers to the relationship of some definite part of the fetus (the denominator) to the maternal pelvis. For example, in vertex presentations, the denominator is the occiput, while in breech presentations, the denominator is the sacrum.

Leopold Maneuvers. The fetal location within the uterus is determined by the maneuvers of Leopold. The *first maneuver* is carried out with the physician facing the patient's head and standing to one side as she lies supine on the examining table. The examiner's hands palpate the fundal area and distinguish which part of the fetus occupies the fundus. The head is round and hard, while the breech is irregular and soft.

The *second maneuver* is accomplished when the hands are placed on either side of the abdomen to determine on which side the fetal back lies. The back is linear and firm, while the extremities have multiple parts. The location of the back can help determine the position of the fetus.

The *third maneuver* is done with a single examining hand placed just above the symphysis to determine the presenting part. The presenting part is grasped between the thumb and third finger. The unengaged vertex is round, firm, and ballotable, while the breech is irregular and nodular.

The *fourth maneuver* is done with the examiner facing the patient's feet and placing both hands on either side of the lower abdomen just above the inlet. This maneuver determines head flexion or extension. When pressure is executed in the direction of the inlet, one hand usually descends further than the other. When the head is flexed, the cephalic prominence (brow) preventing descent of one hand is on the same side as the small parts, while when the head is extended, the occiput is felt prominently on the same side as the back.

The Leopold maneuvers should be carried out at each visit during the third trimester to identify an abnormal lie, presentation, or position of the fetus.

SPECIAL CONCERNS DURING PREGNANCY

Exercise

Exercise is a very important part of maintaining health. Exercise is beneficial during pregnancy because it helps to maintain a feeling of well-being. The amount of exercise should be maintained at approximately the same level as before pregnancy. A patient who does not exercise should not be advised to begin an aggressive program during pregnancy. However, a mild exercise program designed to improve strength and flexibility of muscles should be encouraged. Muscle strength and flexibility are thought to improve posture and muscle tone and reduce common discomforts of pregnancy. Aggressive exercise, such as prolonged jogging and skiing, should be avoided because posture changes brought about by the developing fetus can affect balance.

Work

Limiting the amount of work during pregnancy is recommended to avoid fatigue. Heavy forms of housework or heavy employment outside the home should be discouraged. For women who do work, rest periods are recommended to reduce the likelihood of fatigue. Stressful work during pregnancy is associated with a greater risk of preterm delivery and poor fetal growth.

Travel and Change in Residence

In general, travel by car, train, or airplane is not harmful during pregnancy. However, fatigue must be avoided by taking frequent rest periods. Of greatest concern is the stress associated with travel or a change in residence, which is thought to be associated with preterm labor.

Sexual Intercourse

Sexual intercourse may continue throughout pregnancy, except in patients at risk for abortion or premature labor or in patients with placenta previa. Labor may follow coitus near term, probably because of the effect of prostaglandins in seminal fluid.

Bathing

Tub bathing or showers are permitted during pregnancy. Care must be taken to avoid slipping on the wet surface of the bath or shower because of the mother's altered center of gravity.

ASSESSMENT OF FETAL WELL-BEING

The assessment of fetal health is challenging, since the fetus is not easily seen or heard. During the past 15 years, electronic advances have provided new technology that has made the fetus more accessible and allowed visualization of the fetus and the recording of intrauterine fetal events. A combination of the nonstress test, contraction stress test, and real-time ultrasonic assessment is used to assess fetal well-being.

Figure 6–1 presents an algorithm that may be used to follow a high-risk pregnancy. Table 6–4 indicates the recommended frequency for biophysical profile testing for various high-risk conditions.

TABLE 6–4 RECOMMENDED FREQUENCY FOR BIOPHYSICAL PROFILE TESTING

HIGH-RISK CONDITION	FREQUENCY
Intrauterine growth retardation (IUGR),	
Mild	Weekly
Moderate*	Twice weekly
Diabetes mellitus	
Class A	Weekly, 37 to 40 weeks
	Twice weekly, beyond 40 weeks
Class B and worse	Twice weekly, beginning at 34 weeks
Post-term pregnancy	Twice weekly, beginning at 42 weeks
Other	
Maternal or physician concern	Weekly
Decreased fetal movements	Weekly
Other high-risk conditions	Weekly

*For severe IUGR, delivery is usually indicated.

ANTENATAL TESTING GUIDELINES

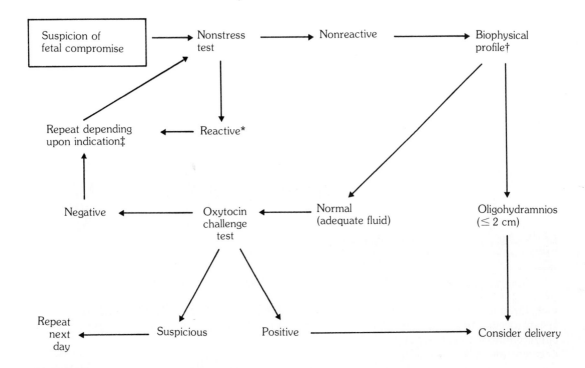

*All pregnancies complicated by IUGR or postdatism should have a complete biophysical profile that includes an ultrasonic evaluation.

†Ultrasonic assessment: (A) fetal movements, 3 per 10 minutes; (B) fetal breathing, 30 per 10 minutes; (C) amniotic fluid, > 2 cm in vertical dimension.

‡See Table 6-4.

Figure 6–1 Algorithm for the antenatal evaluation of a high-risk pregnancy.

Nonstress Test

The first assessment of fetal well-being is the nonstress test. With the mother resting in the lateral supine position, a continuous fetal heart rate tracing is obtained using external Doppler equipment. The mother reports each fetal movement, and the effects of the fetal movements on heart rate are determined. A normal fetus responds to fetal movement with an acceleration in fetal heart rate of 15 beats or more per minute above the baseline for at least 15 seconds (Fig. 6–2). If at least two such accelerations occur in a 20-minute interval, the fetus is regarded as being healthy, and the test is said to be reactive. A nonreactive nonstress test is shown in Figure 6–3.

Ultrasonic Assessment

The next step in prenatal assessment is to determine the adequacy of amniotic fluid volume by real-time ultrasound. Reduced fluid (oligohydramnios) suggests fetal compromise. In addition, when there is reduced amniotic fluid, the fetus is more likely to become compromised due to umbilical cord compression. *Fetal breathing* (chest wall movements) and *fetal movements* (stretching and rotational movements) are also used to assess the fetus. A fetus who has at least 30 breathing movements in 10 minutes or three body movements in 10 minutes is considered healthy. A combination of a reactive nonstress test, adequate amniotic fluid, and adequate fetal breathing and fetal movement is frequently referred to as a *"normal biophysical profile."*

Contraction Stress Test

The contraction stress test is a test for uteroplacental dysfunction, a common condition in the high-risk pregnancy. A dilute infusion of oxytocin is given to establish at

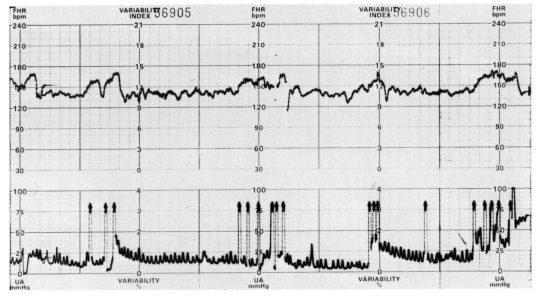

Figure 6–2 Reactive nonstress test. Note the fetal heart rate accelerations with fetal movements.

least three uterine contractions in 10 minutes. If late decelerations are observed with each contraction, the test is positive. If only one deceleration is observed, the test is suspicious. When the test is positive, the patient should usually be delivered.

SPECIAL PROGRAMS FOR HIGH-RISK PREGNANCIES

For any high-risk pregnancy, it is essential to establish gestational age as early as possible, preferably during the first trimester. If

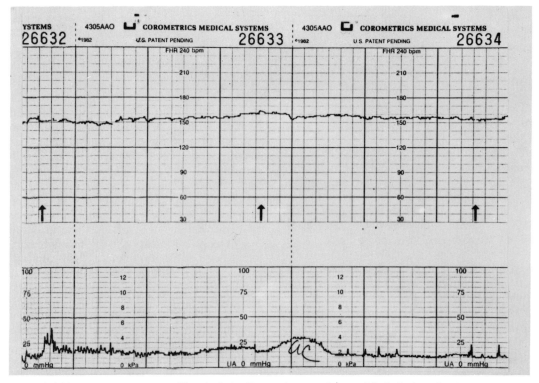

Figure 6–3 Nonreactive nonstress test. Note the lack of beat-to-beat variability and the lack of acceleration of the fetal heart rate with fetal movements (arrows).

gestational age is questionable according to either the history or physical examination, an ultrasound should be obtained for measurement of the biparietal diameter, head and abdominal circumferences, and femur length. These measurements will establish gestational age as accurately as possible and provide baseline values for future comparison.

For the purpose of illustration, four special problems will be discussed that lend themselves to identification, assessment, intervention, and prevention of perinatal morbidity or mortality. These are preterm labor, intrauterine growth retardation, diabetes mellitus, and post-term pregnancy.

Low Birth Weight Infants

In modern obstetrics, low birth weight is the leading cause of poor pregnancy outcome. Low birth weight infants can be either preterm (less than 37 weeks' gestational age) or growth retarded (small for gestational age). Table 6–5 lists those factors that identify patients at risk for preterm labor and intrauterine growth retardation. Following identification of patients at risk, a special prenatal care program should be instituted to reduce the incidence of the problem.

Preterm Labor. Patients at risk for preterm labor need additional assessments at each prenatal visit. Uterine activity, which is always abnormal prior to 30 weeks, should be monitored, and a pelvic examination performed to identify early effacement and/or cervical dilatation. In addition, these patients should be taught the symptoms and signs of preterm labor and advised to go to the hospital immediately should labor start. They should also be advised to avoid manual labor, sexual intercourse, long trips, and smoking, and to rest in bed as much as possible. Patients with evidence of uterine activity and/or early cervical changes may require more extensive interventions, such as prolonged bed rest, work leave, and/or oral tocolytics (uterine relaxants).

Intrauterine Growth Retardation (IUGR). One of the first clinical signs suggesting an abnormality of fetal growth is a discrepancy

TABLE 6–5 PRENATAL IDENTIFICATION OF HIGH-RISK PREGNANCIES

PRENATAL RISK CONDITIONS	HISTORIC RISK FACTORS	DEVELOPING RISK FACTORS
Preterm labor	Previous history of induced abortion, preterm delivery, or neonatal death Habitual abortion Uterine/cervix anomaly History of genitourinary infections Renal disease Smoking Psychiatric hospitalization Low socioeconomic status Maternal age <20 or >35 Single parent Heavy work Long travel	Size/dates discrepancy Severe anemia Threatened abortion Incompetent cervix Surgery Multiple pregnancy Bleeding after 20 weeks Pre-eclampsia Polyhydramnios Urinary tract infection Preterm effacement and/or dilatation of the cervix Engagement of fetal head before 36 wks
Intrauterine growth retardation	Previous low birth weight infant Race (black) Height ≤62 inches Weight ≤100 pounds Narcotic abuse Cigarettes ≥ 1 pack/day Chronic hypertension	Pregnancy-induced hypertension Threatened abortion Congenital malformations
Diabetes mellitus	Age greater than 25 years Previous macrosomic infant Previous perinatal death Family history of diabetes	Size greater than dates Abnormal screen or glucose tolerance test Multiple pregnancy Polyhydramnios Glycosuria
Post-term	Patient under 19 years Previous post-term pregnancy	Threatened abortion Congenital malformations

TABLE 6–6 PRENATAL INTERVENTIONS FOR SELECTED HIGH-RISK CONDITIONS

PRENATAL RISK CONDITION	SELECTED ASSESSMENT	SELECTED INTERVENTIONS
Preterm labor	Uterine activity Cervical length and dilatation	Patient education Bed rest (3 times daily) Work leave Oral tocolytics
Intrauterine growth retardation	Uterine activity Fetal assessment	Patient education Bed rest Early management of medical problems Nutritional counseling Stop smoking
Diabetes mellitus	Home glucose monitoring Fetal assessment	Patient education Dietary management Insulin

Post-term	Fetal assessment	Induction of labor if abnormal
		  fetal assessment profile
		  or ripe cervix

between uterine size and gestational age as determined by the last menstrual period (size/dates discrepancy). When the fundus fails to increase in size, an ultrasound should be obtained to facilitate the diagnosis of IUGR. One of the earliest sonographic findings of poor fetal growth is an abdominal circumference below the tenth percentile. When IUGR is diagnosed, serial testing for fetal well-being is indicated (Table 6–4). Implementation of the interventions listed in Table 6–6 is known to help improve fetal growth, and the abdominal circumference may return to normal (fiftieth percentile). In cases of severe IUGR, all fetal measurements (abdomen, head, and femur) can be reduced. Oligohydramnios (amniotic fluid pocket 2 cm × 2 cm or less on ultrasound) indicates fetal compromise and warrants induction of labor.

Diabetes

Greater attention is being placed on the early recognition of patients at risk for glucose intolerance (Table 6–3). Once diagnosed special interventions are necessary (Table 6–6) and later in pregnancy antenatal testing is required (Table 6–4). Early in pregnancy, the fetus is at increased risk for malformations and poor fetal growth, while late in pregnancy the fetus is at risk for excessive growth and sudden intrauterine fetal death.

Post-Term Pregnancy

The post-term pregnancy (greater than 42 weeks) has been the most common late preg-

nancy problem associated with fetal and newborn morbidity and mortality. There are limited prenatal historic and developing problems for early identification of this problem (Table 6–5). To prevent poor outcome, a systematic approach should be undertaken for the assessment of fetal well-being using a combination of fetal heart rate monitoring, real-time ultrasonic assessment of amniotic fluid volume, fetal breathing patterns, and fetal movements (see Chapter 23). The post-term pregnancy requiring this special assessment is usually one without other medical problems and with a cervix not favorable for induction of labor.

PREVENTIVE HEALTH CARE

Management during pregnancy presents an opportunity for patient education and the practice of preventive medicine. Most women do not have regular contact with a team of health care professionals at any other time in their lives. Childbirth preparation classes for both the patient and her husband are very educational, particularly during the first pregnancy. The presence and encouragement of the baby's father can be most helpful during labor and delivery. These classes provide an important opportunity for both parents to enhance bonding to the infant prior to birth.

While prenatal and obstetric information is of primary importance, other topics that may have lifelong relevance can be introduced and emphasized during prenatal care. The pregnancy itself is frequently a strong motivator for women to eliminate potentially harmful habits or dietary patterns and to become more aware of their general health. Therefore, a systematic approach to the dissemination of preventive health care information will generally be well-received by the pregnant woman at this time.

SUGGESTED READING

Bragonier JR, Cushner IM, Hobel CJ: Social and personal factors in the etiology of preterm birth. In Fuchs F, Stubblefield PG (eds): Preterm Birth, Causes, Prevention, and Management. New York, Macmillan Publishing Co, 1984, p 64.

Chamberlain G: The pregnancy clinic. Br Med J 11:29, 1980.

Collings CA, Curet LB, Mullin JP: Maternal and fetal responses to a maternal aerobic exercise program. Am J Obstet Gynecol 145:702, 1983.

Evertson LR, Paul RH: Antepartum fetal heart rate testing: The nonstress test. Obstet Gynecol 132:895, 1978.

Freeman RK, Anderson G, Dorchester W: A prospective multi-institutional study of antepartum fetal heart rate monitoring. II. Contraction stress test versus nonstress test for primary surveillance. Am J Obstet Gynecol 143:778, 1982.

Fuhrmann K, Reiher H, Semmler K, et al: Prevention of congenital malformations in infants of insulin-dependent diabetic mothers. Diabetes Care 6:219, 1983.

Herron MA, Katz M, Creasy RK: Evaluation of a preterm birth prevention program: Preliminary report. Obstet Gynecol 59:452, 1982.

Hobel CJ: Routine antenatal laboratory tests. In Queenan J, Hobbins J (eds): Protocols for High-Risk Pregnancies. Oradell, NJ, Medical Economics Co Inc, 1982, p 19.

Hobel CJ: Identification of the patient at high-risk. In Bolognese RJ, Schwarz RH (eds): Perinatal Medicine: Management of the High-Risk Fetus and Neonate. Chapter 1. Baltimore, Williams and Wilkins Co, 1978.

Manning FA, Platt LA, Sipo L: Antepartum fetal evaluation: Development of a fetal biophysical profile. Am J Obstet Gynecol 136:787, 1980.

Standards for Obstetrics/Gynecology Services, 5th ed. The American College of Obstetricians and Gynecologists, Washington DC, 1982, p 9.

Tafari N, Naeye RL, Cobezie A: Effects of maternal undernutrition and heavy physical work during pregnancy on birth weight. Br J Obstet Gynaecol 87:222, 1980.

7 Chapter Seven

GENETIC COUNSELING AND PRENATAL DIAGNOSIS

KHALIL TABSH and MICHELLE FOX

Expanding knowledge of human genetics and technical advances in prenatal diagnosis have had a significant impact on the practice of obstetrics. Physicians must be cognizant of genetic screening procedures in order to identify patients suitable for genetic counseling, carrier detection, and prenatal diagnosis. This chapter includes information on the screening of patients for genetic counseling, as well as the indications and techniques employed for prenatal diagnosis. In addition, the most common genetic disorders and their patterns of inheritance are discussed.

PATIENTS REQUIRING GENETIC COUNSELING AND PRENATAL DIAGNOSIS

The most important screening tool available to every physician is the personal and family history. Ideally, couples should be questioned about their health history before they decide to have children.

The major reason couples are referred for prenatal diagnosis is age. Women over 34 years of age have an increased risk of giving birth to children with chromosomal abnormalities. Controversy exists as to whether or not men over 50 years of age have an increased risk of fathering children with chromosomal abnormalities.

Other major indications for prenatal diagnosis include a history of (1) a previous stillborn child with birth defects; (2) a pre-

vious child born with mental retardation, chromosomal abnormality, or known genetic disorder; (3) multiple fetal losses; or (4) a baby who has died in the neonatal period. It is crucial to establish an accurate diagnosis of the affected family member by obtaining medical records, autopsy reports, and laboratory data, or by having the family member examined by a geneticist.

Individuals of various ethnic or racial backgrounds should be screened for genetic diseases that are more prevalent in that particular group. The common genetic diseases for which screening is advisable on ethnic grounds are Tay-Sachs disease in the Ashkenazi Jewish population of Eastern European background (carrier frequency 1 in 27), sickle-cell anemia in black Americans (carrier frequency 1 in 10), and thalassemia in Mediterranean populations (carrier frequency believed to be 1 in 30 among Italian-Americans.) There is no reason to wait until a patient becomes pregnant to initiate screening for these disorders, since the possibility of their occurrence can be determined beforehand. Prenatal diagnosis by amniocentesis is advisable for Tay-Sachs disease, sickle-cell anemia, and many of the thalassemias when both partners have been identified as carriers.

Until recently, identification of the "at-risk pregnancy" has depended on maternal age or the prior birth of a child already affected by a genetic disorder. With the advent of maternal serum alpha-fetoprotein (AFP) testing, screening is now available to identify the woman at risk of having a child with a neural tube defect. Maternal screening may help a very large population of women who would not take advantage of amniocentesis because of the risk of miscarriage, but would undergo a simple blood test during pregnancy.

Although not directly affecting the obstetrician, specific screening programs in most states identify newborns with biochemical genetic disorders, such as phenylketonuria and galactosemia. Infants identified as having these diseases are placed on special dietary regimens and escape the mental retardation and physical problems that have characterized the untreated cases.

DIAGNOSTIC PROCEDURES

The procedures noted below can be carried out either singly or in combination to facilitate the diagnosis of genetic disorders (Table 7–1).

Amniocentesis

Amniocentesis, the withdrawal of amniotic fluid from the amniotic sac, is the most widely utilized prenatal diagnostic test. It was originally used in the 1950s to analyze amniotic fluid for evidence of Rh sensitization during the third trimester of pregnancy. Techniques for culturing amniotic cells became available in the 1960s and led to the first prenatal diagnosis of Down's syndrome in 1967. The

TABLE 7–1 TECHNIQUES FOR THE PRENATAL DIAGNOSIS OF GENETIC DISEASES IN THE FETUS

Midtrimester amniocentesis
Maternal blood screening
  Serum alpha-fetoprotein
  Rhesus factor determination
Fetal ultrasonography
Fetoscopy
  Visualization
  Fetal tissue sampling
  Fetal blood sampling
  Fetal liver biopsy
Chorionic villus sampling
Fetal blood sampling under ultrasonic
  direction by needling
  (a) fetal heart
  (b) cord insertion into placenta

majority of patients undergoing amniocentesis are referred because of advanced maternal age.

Counseling. An important part of this diagnostic technique is counseling. Patients must be informed of the risks and benefits of amniocentesis before making a decision regarding its advisability. The increased risk of miscarriage associated with amniocentesis is about 0.5 percent. Follow-up studies of infants in amniocentesis and control groups have revealed no statistically significant differences with respect to infant deaths, illnesses, frequency of physical abnormalities, or psychomotor or language development.

Patients should be informed about two types of fetal abnormalities that can be screened for with this technique: chromosomal problems and neural tube defects. Amniotic fluid AFP values are done routinely, even though the problem of neural tube defects is not an age-related one. Counseling must include the fact that other chromosomal abnormalities in addition to Down's syndrome can be diagnosed by this procedure. Many couples have been faced with difficult decisions regarding the diagnosis of Turner's syndrome (45, XO) or Klinefelter's syndrome (47, XXY), both of which are caused by abnormalities occurring in sex chromosomes and are characterized by growth, activity, and learning problems.

Patients must be reminded that an amniocentesis is not a guarantee of a normal, healthy baby. Every female undertaking a pregnancy has a 2 to 3 percent risk of delivering a baby with structural congenital anomalies. The incidence of structural anomalies does not increase with maternal age, and prenatal diagnostic tests do not lower the incidence. Patients often ask to be "tested for everything." At the present time, approximately 80 to 100 specific genetic disorders can be diagnosed by amniocentesis in addition to chromosomal abnormalities and neural tube defects. Some of these genetic disorders are exceedingly rare, and testing is offered only to families who have already had an affected child. It is impractical in terms of cost-effectiveness, and the amount of fluid that would be required for testing procedures, to consider screening any one individual for all known entities.

Technique. Amniocentesis is an outpatient procedure performed 16 to 20 weeks after the first day of the last menstrual period. It is recommended that the procedure not be carried out earlier than 16 weeks because there is an insufficient number of fetal squamous cells in the fluid. Guided by ultrasound, a 20- or 21-gauge needle with a stylet is introduced through the abdominal wall under sterile conditions, with the aid of local anesthesia. The stylet is removed and 20 ml of amniotic fluid is aspirated. The initial 2 ml of amniotic fluid may be discarded to lessen the chance of maternal contamination. The aspirated amniotic fluid is then taken to the laboratory for cell culturing, karyotyping, and biochemical analysis. Chromosomal analysis of cultured amniotic cells takes approximately two weeks. Most reports indicate a 99 to 99.6 percent accuracy for chromosomal results.

Maternal Serum Alpha-Fetoprotein (AFP) Screening

Shortly after elevated amniotic fluid AFP levels were shown to be associated with open neural tube defects, it was discovered that AFP was also elevated in blood samples of the women carrying affected fetuses. Maternal serum AFP screening takes place optimally in the sixteenth to eighteenth week of gestation. If the initial serum sample shows an elevated AFP level, a second sample is obtained. If the second sample remains elevated, an ultrasound is done to rule out multiple gestation, fetal demise, or inaccurate gestational age (all of which can give false-positive results). If none of these factors contributes to the elevated serum AFP level, an amniocentesis is recommended for a more definitive diagnosis.

Maternal serum AFP screening is a controversial issue for several reasons. One of the primary concerns is the large number of false-positive results obtained at the time of the initial blood test, which causes increased maternal anxiety. This problem can be lessened by adopting a higher cutoff level, but then the sensitivity decreases. Normal serum AFP levels do not guarantee a normal baby, as closed neural tube defects may not produce elevated AFP. Another problem facing the maternal serum AFP screening program is that of timing. Many patients do not schedule their first prenatal visit until after 20 weeks of pregnancy.

Ultrasonography

Level II ultrasound* is becoming extremely useful as a diagnostic procedure to identify structural abnormalities of the fetus. The use of this level of ultrasound to identify birth defects should be conducted at a tertiary medical center by an experienced ultrasonographer.

Structural defects that have been diagnosed with this technique include craniospinal abnormalities (anencephaly, hydrocephaly, spina bifida, microcephaly), gastrointestinal anomalies (omphalocele, gastroschisis), excretory system anomalies (renal agenesis, renal dysplasia, urinary obstruction), skeletal dysplasias, and congenital heart defects.

Diabetic women have an increased risk of delivering children with birth defects, such as congenital heart defects. Echocardiograms of the fetus are now being used to delineate congenital heart defects in diabetic women and in women who have had a previously affected child or who themselves have a congenital heart defect.

Recently, fetal blood samples have been obtained by needling the heart and umbilical cord at its placental insertion site under ultrasonic direction. The risks of this procedure are not known, but it may be useful in patients with hematologic disorders such as hemophilia and beta-thalassemia.

Fetoscopy

Fetoscopy is a prenatal diagnostic procedure that makes it possible to visualize the fetus, sample fetal blood, or obtain a fetal skin biopsy. It has been useful in the diagnosis of hematologic disorders, such as hemophilia and beta-thalassemia, and potentially fatal skin disorders. The procedure has also been used to perform fetal liver biopsy for the prenatal diagnosis of ornithine transcarbamylase deficiency. The first positive diagnosis based on an anatomical finding at the time of fetoscopy was that of Ellis-van-Creveld syndrome, an autosomal recessive dwarfing syndrome with postaxial polydactyly. Measurement of the limb lengths by ultrasound suggested the diagnosis, and fe-

---

*Level I ultrasound is used to establish gestational age, localize the placenta, and identify the presentation of the fetus.

toscopy identified the extra digits on each hand.

Fetoscopy is an outpatient procedure monitored by ultrasonography and usually performed between 18 and 20 weeks' gestation. The fetoscope is a 15- to 20-cm-long endoscopic instrument containing fiberoptic illumination housed in a cannula. It provides the physician with a two- to fivefold magnification of the fetus. Fetal blood sampling by fetoscopy is successful in approximately 90 percent of cases. The risk of spontaneous abortion following fetoscopy is currently 3 to 5 percent.

Until recently, carrier females for hemophilia A were faced with the same situation as a carrier female for Duchenne's muscular dystrophy. Identification of fetal sex could be made by amniocentesis, but the male fetus is normal 50 percent of the time. Currently, an accurate prenatal diagnosis of hemophilia A can be made by fetoscopy. The ratio of factor VIII procoagulant antigen to factor VIII-released antigen can be measured by fetal blood sampling. An affected fetus has an abnormally reduced ratio (less than 0.20).

The application of fetoscopy is less than optimal. Only a limited portion of the fetus can be visualized. Fetal blood sampling for hemoglobinopathies is already obsolete in some cases, such as alpha-thalassemia, because of advances in restriction endonuclease DNA analysis. Also, ultrasonic techniques are improving so rapidly that their accuracy may approach that of direct visualization of the fetus.

CONGENITAL AND HEREDITARY DISORDERS

Chromosomal Disorders

Chromosomal abnormalities occur in 0.5 percent of live births, but the incidence associated with spontaneous abortions is much higher and estimated to be approximately 50 percent. The most common chromosomal abnormalities among liveborn infants are sex chromosomal aneuploidies (i.e., Turner's syndrome, Klinefelter's syndrome), balanced Robertsonian translocations (translocations between groups D and D or D and G), and autosomal trisomies such as Down's syndrome.

Women over 34 years of age are at increased risk of giving birth to children with autosomal trisomies (i.e., trisomy 21, 13, or 18; Fig. 7–1) or some sex chromosomal abnormalities (i.e., Turner's syndrome, 45, XO; Klinefelter's syndrome, 47, XXY; Fig. 7–2). The overall risk of Down's syndrome is 1 per 800 live births. It increases to about 1 per 300 live births for women who are 35 to 39 years of age and to about 1 in 80 for those 40 to 45 years of age (Table 7–2). The incidence of Down's syndrome diagnosed at the time of amniocentesis is considerably higher. In women 35 to 39 years of age, the rate is

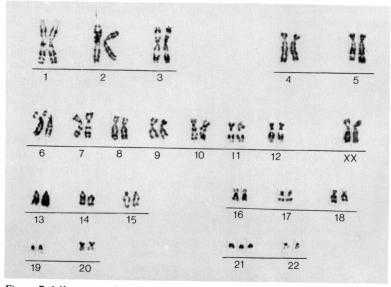

Figure 7–1 Karyotype of a patient with Down's syndrome (47,XX + 21).

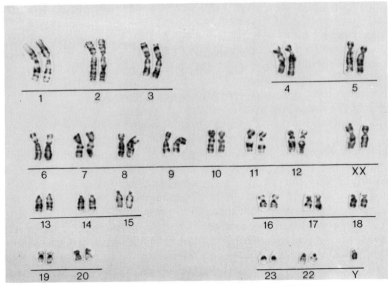

Figure 7–2 Karyotype of a patient with Klinefelter's syndrome (47,XXY).

about 1 in 125; in those 40 to 45, it is about 1 in 20. The discrepancy between the rate of occurrence at delivery and that at amniocen-

TABLE 7–2   RISK OF HAVING AN INFANT
             WITH DOWN'S SYNDROME BY
             MATERNAL AGE

MATERNAL AGE (years)	FREQUENCY OF DOWN'S SYNDROME
30	1/885
31	1/826
32	1/725
33	1/592
34	1/465
35	1/365
36	1/287
37	1/225
38	1/176
39	1/139
40	1/109
41	1/85
42	1/67
43	1/53
44	1/41
45	1/32
46	1/25
47	1/20
48	1/16
49	1/12

Reproduced with permission from Hook EB, Chambers GM: Estimated rates of Down's syndrome in live births by one year maternal age intervals in a New York State study—Implications of the risk figures for genetic counselling and cost-benefit analysis of prenatal diagnosis programs. Birth Defects: Orig Art Ser 13(3A):123, 1977.

tesis is believed to be due in part to fetal loss in the late second and third trimester.

Ninety-five percent of cases of Down's syndrome are nondisjunctional events leading to 47 chromosomes with an extra number 21 autosome, while 4 percent have a karyotype of translocation Down's syndrome with 46 chromosomes and the extra number 21 chromosome attached to an autosome. Parents of a child with Down's syndrome should be karyotyped to exclude the possibility of a familial balanced translocation. The most common translocation involving the 21 chromosome is an attachment to a 14 or 15 chromosome, and less commonly a 21 or 22 chromosome. The remaining 1 percent of individuals with Down's syndrome are mosaics, having two populations of cells, one with 46 chromosomes (a normal karyotype) and one with 47 chromosomes.

A couple who has had a previous child with trisomy 21 (Down's syndrome) or another meiotic nondisjunctional type of chromosomal abnormality is believed to be at a small increased risk (about 1 percent) of giving birth to another child with a chromosomal abnormality and should be referred for amniocentesis.

Approximately 1 in 500 individuals carries a balanced translocation. Fetuses receiving unbalanced chromosomal material have a 50 percent chance of being affected.

Blood chromosomal studies should be performed on a couple following three or more spontaneous abortions because in approximately 3 to 5 percent of such couples, one member is a balanced translocation carrier. Depending on the type of translocation found, the recurrence risk for spontaneous abortions and/or defective offspring can be estimated. These couples should be alerted to the advisability of having an amniocentesis because of their increased risk.

Single Gene Disorders

Single gene disorders are uncommon (occurring in about 1 percent of live births), but they can result in a great medical and psychosocial burden.

Autosomal Recessive Disorders. With autosomal recessive disorders, two affected genes must be present for manifestation of the disease. Usually there is no family history of another affected individual. If there is a family history, siblings of either sex are equally as likely to be affected. Depending on the rarity of the disorder, the parents, who are obligate carriers, may be cosanguineous (blood relatives). A couple who has had one child with an autosomal recessive disorder has a 25 percent chance of giving birth to another abnormal child.

Many autosomal recessive disorders may be diagnosed prenatally by amniocentesis. Tay-Sachs disease, sickle-cell anemia, alphathalassemia, and many inborn errors of metabolism can be detected by studying amniotic fluid and/or cultured amniotic cells.

The most common autosomal recessive disorder affecting Caucasian offspring is *cystic fibrosis,* which, at the present time, cannot be diagnosed prenatally. In addition, it is not yet possible to detect a carrier. Even though 1 in 20 Caucasians carries the gene for cystic fibrosis, it is only after individuals have had an affected child that they learn they are carriers. Measurement of alkaline phosphatase from the amniotic fluid of mothers at risk for cystic fibrosis shows some promise for prenatal diagnosis.

With the exception of Tay-Sachs disease, heterozygote detection is not available for biochemical genetic disorders, so it is usually only after the birth of an affected child that a couple knows that each of them is a carrier. The majority of the biochemical genetic disorders are associated with early death or serious medical consequences, most often profound mental retardation. Parents faced

with a known prenatal diagnosis of an affected fetus usually elect to terminate the pregnancy. To date, two biochemical genetic disorders, vitamin B_{12}-responsive and biotin-responsive multiple carboxylase deficiencies, have been treated successfully *in utero.*

PRENATAL DIAGNOSIS. The prenatal diagnosis of sickle-cell anemia and some forms of thalassemia is now possible using amniotic fluid fibroblasts and specific restriction endonucleases. The first step in this procedure is the isolation of DNA from the nuclei of the amniotic fluid fibroblasts. The DNA is then digested by bacterial enzymes, restriction endonucleases, that cleave DNA at specific sites, producing fragments of reproducible size. In the case of sickle cell anemia, a single change in base-pairing (mutation) is identified by a specific restriction endonuclease. After digestion, the DNA fragments are separated by size with electrophoresis and transferred to a nitrocellulose filter. The filter-bound DNA fragments are hybridized to ^{32}P-labeled known DNA sequences. Unhybridized DNA fragments are washed away, and the filter is autoradiographed. Depending on the specific banding pattern found, a diagnosis of sickle cell carrier status, noncarrier status, or affected sickle-cell fetus can be made.

Autosomal Dominant Disorders. In autosomal dominant disorders, only one abnormal gene is necessary for disease manifestation. The affected individual has a 50 percent chance of passing the gene and the disorder on to offspring. Unaffected offspring cannot pass on the gene or the disorder. The occurrence and transmission of the genes are not influenced by gender; male and females are equally affected.

In cases in which the parents of an affected individual are clinically normal, the disorder has resulted from a spontaneous mutation of genetic material. The hallmark of autosomal dominant diseases is their variable expressivity. It is often an important issue in a genetics clinic to decide whether a child is affected by a spontaneous mutation or is the product of a parent with minimal expression of the same gene. A careful history and physical examination of family members, in addition to possible biochemical, radiologic, or histologic testing, may have to be carried out to determine the parents' carrier or noncarrier status.

Some of the common autosomal dominant disorders include tuberous sclerosis, neurofibromatosis, achondroplasia, craniofacial synostosis, adult-form polycystic kidney disease, and several types of muscular dystrophy. Prenatal diagnosis by amniocentesis has not been successful in screening for the majority of autosomal dominant disorders.

PRENATAL DIAGNOSIS BY LINKAGE ANALYSIS. Linked genes are those with loci present on the same chromosome. Genes are arranged in a linear array on the chromosomes. Two genes that are situated near each other on the same chromosome tend to be transmitted as a unit. In other words, the principle of independent assortment does not apply to linked genes. When gene coding for a single gene disorder is closely linked to a polymorphic marker gene, the frequency of transmission of a particular trait can be studied. For a linkage to be informative, the linkage must be a close one, and the polymorphic marker must have multiple alleles.

MYOTONIC DYSTROPHY. This type of muscular dystrophy is characterized by myotonia (muscle weakness and wasting), gonadal dysfunction, cataracts, and mental retardation. There is no definitive marker for the prenatal diagnosis of myotonic dystrophy, but there is a known linkage between myotonic dystrophy and the ABH secretory locus. Prenatal diagnosis can be carried out by determination of the secretor status of the amniotic fluid of the "at-risk fetus." The secretor status of the fluid reflects the secretor genotype of the fetus. Unfortunately, only 5 to 10 percent of families have informative genotypes.

Sex-Linked Disorders. Sex-linked disorders are due to recessive genes located on the X chromosome. X-linked genes primarily affect males, while females are the unaffected (or mildly affected) carriers of the gene. There is no male-to-male transmission of X-linked disorders.

X-linked disorders can occur because of new mutations of genetic material as a sporadic event, or from the inheritance of the X-linked recessive gene from the carrier mother. In some cases, it may be difficult to distinguish between the two situations. Female carriers of X-linked disorders have a 50 percent chance of giving birth to affected sons. They also have a 50 percent chance of passing the carrier status on to their daughters. The most common sex-linked disorders are *Duchenne's muscular dystrophy* (DMD), and *fragile-X mental retardation*.

PRENATAL DIAGNOSIS. Women at risk of giving birth to a son with DMD, by virtue of previously having had a son with the disorder or of having a family history of its occurrence (affected brother or maternal uncle), may elect to undergo an amniocentesis to determine fetal sex. Many attempts have been made to identify affected males prenatally, but none have been successful. The patient who is a carrier for DMD is then faced with the choice of aborting any male fetus (half will be normal) or carrying it to term in the hope that it will not be affected.

Fragile-X mental retardation may account for 4 percent of mentally retarded males. Prenatal diagnosis of this disorder has been reported and may become more important as increasing numbers of males are identified with the fragile-X chromosome.

Multifactorial Disorders

In each disorder previously discussed, there is a known and predictable pattern of inheritance. However, the majority of birth defects are inherited in a multifactorial fashion, which means that both genes and the environment play a role. The common multifactorial disorders are cleft lip and/or palate, neural tube defects (spina bifida or anencephaly), congenital heart defects, and pyloric stenosis.

Neural tube defects occur in about 1 per 1000 births in the United States. In Northern Ireland, Wales, and Scotland, the incidence of neural tube defects is 6 to 8 per 1000 births. Although the etiology is unknown, recent data have suggested that the mothers may be folic acid–deficient, and periconceptional vitamin supplementation has been recommended.

Both *anencephaly* (congenital absence of the forebrain) (Fig. 7–3) and *spina bifida* (open spine) are believed to occur prior to 30 days' gestation because of failure of the neural tube to close. Newborns with anencephaly are stillborn or die within the first few days of life. Newborns with spina bifida have a variable course, depending on the site of the lesion and whether or not it is a *meningocele* (herniation of the meninges through an open spinal defect with the cord remaining in its usual position) or a *myelocele* (herniation of the spinal cord). Infants with a myelocele are at risk for muscle paralysis

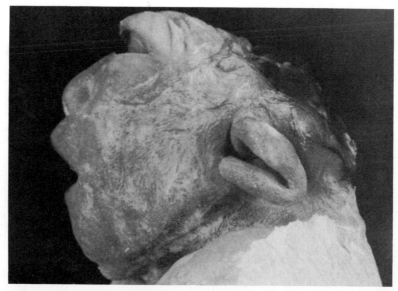

Figure 7–3 Infant with anencephaly. Note the absence of development of the vault of the skull caused by congenital absence of the forebrain.

or weakness below the level of the lesion and incontinence of bowel and bladder. In approximately 75 percent of cases, hydrocephalus is also present.

In multifactorial disorders in general, and in neural tube defects in particular, the couple who has given birth to one affected child has an increased risk of approximately 3 percent of giving birth to another. Sisters of women who have had an affected child are also at an increased risk.

In 85 percent of cases of spina bifida, the neural tube defect is "open" with the fetal central nervous system in direct communication with the amniotic fluid. Amniotic fluid alpha-fetoprotein (AFP) levels are elevated when the fetus has an open neural tube defect. AFP is produced primarily by the fetal liver during the second trimester of pregnancy and normally enters the amniotic fluid via the fetal urine. Elevated alpha-fetoprotein levels in the amniotic fluid represent a specific biochemical marker for open neural tube defect and other congenital malformations, including omphalocele and gastroschisis. It is assumed that the amniotic fluid levels of alpha-fetoprotein are elevated because of leakage through exposed vessels. The accuracy of amniotic AFP determination in the prenatal diagnosis of neural tube defects is approximately 95 percent.

FUTURE OF PRENATAL DIAGNOSIS

The field of prenatal diagnosis is expanding rapidly, and existing techniques are being refined. The most promising new prenatal diagnostic technique is chorionic villus biopsy. By sampling the chorion, the prenatal diagnosis of chromosomal abnormalities and some biochemical genetic defects can be made in the first trimester. The chorionic biopsy is accomplished by introducing a catheter through the cervix. Direct study of the dividing cells can identify a chromosomal abnormality in 48 hours at 10 weeks' gestation. Although the psychological advantages of early prenatal diagnosis are clear, this technique is still experimental, and the risks associated with it are presently unknown.

Until recently, prenatal diagnosis of an affected fetus has led to a decision to either terminate the pregnancy or start preparing for the birth of an affected child. Fetal surgery may provide the choice of *in utero* treatment for specific structural abnormalities, such as hydrocephalus or diaphragmatic hernia, or it may prevent kidney damage by treating posterior urethral valve obstruction.

Recombinant DNA is a challenging new technology that will have a great impact on the field of biochemical genetics and prenatal diagnosis. Using the restriction endonucleases previously described in this chapter, segments of human DNA may be inserted into plasmid or bacteriophage vectors and then amplified during proliferation of a host bacterium. If human DNA from a single chromosome is treated with appropriate restriction endonucleases, inserted into the plasmid and then cloned, it is possible to obtain clones of cells containing a single gene-length segment of human DNA. If enough clones are selected, a "library" of DNA segments representing all the genes of the human chromosome can be obtained. Radioactive probes can then be used to hybridize to specific DNA segments. By utilizing recombinant DNA technology and chorionic villus biopsy, many single gene disorders may be prenatally diagnosable during the first trimester of pregnancy in the near future.

SUGGESTED READING

Antonarakis SE, Phillips JA, Kazazian HH: Genetic diseases: Diagnosis by restriction endonuclease analysis. J Pediatr 100:845, 1982.

Crandall BF, Kasla W, Matsumoto M: Prenatal diagnosis of neural tube defects (NTD): Experience with acetylcholinesterase gel electrophoresis. Am J Med Genet 12:361, 1982.

Crandall BF, Lebherz TB, Rubinstein B, et al: Follow-up of 2000 second trimester amniocenteses. Obstet Gynecol 56:625, 1980.

Crandall BF, Lebherz TB, Rubinstein B, et al: Chromosome findings in 2500 second trimester amniocenteses. Am J Med Genet 5:345, 1980.

Gerbie AB, Elias S: Technique for midtrimester amniocentesis for prenatal diagnosis. Semin Perinatol 4:159, 1980.

Goossens M, Dumez Y, Kaplan L, et al: Prenatal diagnosis of sickle-cell anemia in the first trimester of pregnancy. N Engl J Med 309:831, 1983.

Hobbins JC, Grannum P, Berkowitz RL, et al: Ultrasound in the diagnosis of congenital anomalies. Am J Obstet Gynecol 134:331, 1979.

Hook EB: Rates of chromosome abnormalities at different maternal ages. Obstet Gynecol 58:282, 1981.

Kaback MM, Greenwald S, Brossman R: Carrier detection and prenatal diagnosis in Tay-Sachs disease: Summary experience in the first decade. Pediatr Res 15:1138A, 1981.

Macri JN, Baker DA, Baim RS: Diagnosis of neural tube defects by evaluation of amniotic fluid. Clin Obstet Gynecol 24:1081, 1981.

NICHD National Registry for Amniocentesis Study Group: Midtrimester amniocentesis for prenatal diagnosis: Safety and accuracy. JAMA 236:1471, 1976.

Rodeck CH, Nicolaides KH: The use of fetoscopy for prenatal diagnosis and treatment. Semin Perinatol 7:118, 1983.

Simoni G, Brambati B, Danesino C, et al: Efficient direct chromosome analyses and enzyme determinations from chorionic villi samples in the first trimester of pregnancy. Hum Genet 63:349, 1983.

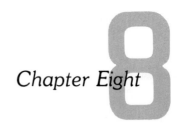

Chapter Eight

TERATOLOGY

ANN GARBER

A teratogen is any agent or factor that can cause abnormalities of form or function (birth defects) in an exposed fetus. Such abnormalities include fetal wastage and intrauterine fetal growth retardation, malformations due to abnormal growth and morphogenesis, and abnormal central nervous system performance.

It was not until the teratogenic effects of rubella infection were demonstrated in 1941 that any notable consideration was given to environmental factors and their potential deleterious effects on human pregnancy. In the succeeding decades, the susceptibility of the fetus to many environmental factors has been appreciated.

Probably the best known teratogen is thalidomide, which was shown to cause phocomelia and other malformations in the offspring of mothers who had been given the drug during pregnancy. Thalidomide is unique in that it is the only example of a teratogen that when introduced to the pregnant population led to a dramatic epidemic of a specific malformation; withdrawal of the drug led to a virtual disappearance of the malformation. The thalidomide experience provided compelling evidence that, unless proven otherwise, chemical and physical agents must be seriously regarded as having a potential for adverse effects on the human fetus. In 1962, drug law amendments were enacted that led to regulations requiring that new drugs not be administered to pregnant women until preliminary studies indicated reasonable evidence of the drug's safety and effectiveness in animals, and subsequently in men and nonpregnant women.

Although drugs are the most obvious source for teratogenic exposure, clinicians must also take measures to protect the pregnant patient from the potential hazards associated with today's technology and lifestyle. Chemical waste disposals, alcohol, tobacco, cosmetics, and occupational agents are substances that individuals are exposed to daily. Some of these agents are known teratogens, while the fetal effects of others are not known.

EXPOSURE

Several studies indicate that pregnant women are being exposed to a large number of potential teratogens. Results of the Collaborative Perinatal Project indicate that during the first trimester alone, as many as 32 percent of pregnant women are exposed to analgesics (mostly aspirin), 18 percent to immunizing agents, 16 percent to antimicrobial and antiparasitic agents, and 6 percent to sedatives, tranquilizers, and antidepressants. Although some teratogenic exposures are unavoidable, the great majority of agents, including radiation and drugs, are readily avoidable.

PATHOGENIC MECHANISMS

Teratogens may affect embryogenesis by the disturbance of one or more developmental processes. They may produce hypoplasia or hyperplasia of developing tissues, failure of cellular differentiation or interaction, or mechanical disruption of a cell. Often, the end result of teratogenic action is an organ with too few cells. Subsequently, the organ system may fail to fully develop because of lack of a critical mass required for cellular differentiation.

Cell growth, differentiation, interaction, and migration are basic characteristics of embryological development. Thus, environmental insults frequently affect more than one tissue or organ system. Cellular disturbances can occur as a result of many different teratogenic agents, and, conversely, the effect of a particular teratogen is influenced by a number of important factors (Table 8–1). In addition, congenital anomalies frequently caused by teratogenic agents also occur in fetuses not exposed to teratogens. Although teratogenicity is difficult to prove in humans, evidence of one or more of the observations listed in Table 8–2 provides support for a teratogenic insult.

PRINCIPLES OF TERATOLOGY

Fetal Susceptibility

The efficacy of a particular teratogen is, in part, dependent on the genetic makeup of both mother and fetus, as well as on a number of factors related to the maternal-fetal environment. For instance, many congenital abnormalities, such as oral clefts, congenital heart disease, and neural tube defects, are inherited through multifactorial inheritance. These types of birth defects are thought to be due to a combination of several genes and environmental insults. The recurrence risk for a similar abnormality in subsequent pregnancies is small, but increased compared with the risk in the overall population. Thus, some fetuses are predisposed to certain malformations because of their genetic makeup; such fetuses would be particularly susceptible to

TABLE 8–1 FACTORS THAT INFLUENCE THE EFFECT OF TERATOGENIC AGENTS

1. Nature and dose of the agent
2. Stage of embryonic development
3. Fetal susceptibility
4. Interaction with other environmental factors

TABLE 8–2 INDICATORS OF POTENTIAL TERATOGENICITY IN HUMANS

1. Case-control studies demonstrate a relationship between exposure to the agent and a particular anomaly.
2. The timing of exposure is consistent with the embryological development of the malformed organs.
3. The incidence of an anomaly rises upon introduction of a new drug.
4. Animal studies confirm the relationship between a particular agent and a specific malformation.

teratogens that raise the risk for that malformation.

Fetal vulnerability may also be influenced by maternal variability in the ability to metabolize a teratogen, maternal variability in the rate of placental transfer, or differences in fetal metabolism.

Dose

Depending on the particular teratogen, there may be (1) no apparent effect at a low dose; (2) an organ-specific malformation at an intermediate dose; or (3) a spontaneous abortion at a high dose. Additionally, smaller doses administered over several days may produce a different effect from a single large dose.

Timing

Three stages of teratogenic susceptibility may be identified based on gestational age (Figure 8–1). Prior to implantation (one week in humans), there is no demonstrable teratogenic effect. During the subsequent two weeks, the fetus is relatively resistant to teratogenic insult. The most vulnerable stage is between 3 and 8 weeks during the period of organogenesis. The timing determines which organ system or systems are affected. Unfortunately, most women do not realize they are pregnant until this critical period of development is well underway.

From about the fourth month of pregnancy to the end of gestation, embryonic development consists primarily of increasing organ size. With the exception of a limited number of tissues (brain and gonads), teratogenic exposure after the fourth month usually causes decreased growth without malformation.

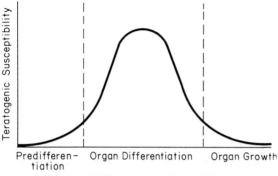

Teratogenic Susceptibility

Predifferen-   Organ Differentiation   Organ Growth
tiation

PERIOD OF GESTATION

Figure 8–1 Schematic representation of embryonic periods of differential susceptibility to a teratogen. During the first weeks of embryogenesis, a teratogen can be lethal, but if the embryo survives, it will not necessarily be malformed. Following the period of maximum susceptibility, a teratogen can interfere with growth but will not directly affect organogenesis. Secondary effects (e.g., vascular occlusion) could still produce anomalies. (Reprinted with permission from Simpson JL: Disorders of Sexual Differentiation. Etiology and Clinical Delineation. New York, Academic Press, 1976, p 46.)

Nature of the Teratogenic Agents

Although few agents are known to cause serious malformations in a large proportion of exposed individuals, there are probably hundreds of potentially teratogenic agents, given the right set of circumstances (susceptible fetus, embryologically vulnerable period, large teratogenic dose). Furthermore, certain drugs combined with other drugs may be capable of producing malformations, although neither agent would be teratogenic when taken alone.

TERATOGENIC AGENTS

Teratogens may be categorized into three broad categories: (1) drugs and chemical agents, (2) infectious agents, and (3) radiation. The list that follows is far from exhaustive.

Drugs and Chemical Agents

Alcohol. Since ethanol is one of the most abused substances in this country, it is perhaps surprising that the adverse effects of ethyl alcohol on fetal development were not fully realized until recently. The frequency of the *fetal alcohol syndrome* (FAS) runs as high as 0.2 percent, and an additional 0.4 percent of newborns show less severe features of the disorder.

The spectrum of anomalies caused by prenatal ingestion of ethanol is wide, and the frequency and severity appear to be dose-related. As little as one ounce of absolute alcohol twice per week appears to increase the risk of spontaneous abortion two- to fourfold. One ounce of absolute alcohol daily (two drinks) may be enough to produce mild features of FAS, such as low birth weight.

The clinical features of FAS are summarized in Table 8–3. The most consistent findings in babies with this disorder include (1) prenatal growth deficiency for weight, height, and head circumference; (2) distinct craniofacial features; and (3) mild to moderate mental retardation. The average IQ among FAS individuals is 65, but may range from 16 to 105. Hypotonia is a frequent finding, along with poor motor coordination.

It is of utmost importance that alcoholic women of reproductive age be aware of the serious risks posed by prenatal alcohol consumption. It is not possible to state the safe level of ethanol intake. Even moderate exposure to the fetus has been associated with partial features of FAS. Until more detailed risk information becomes available, the safest advice is to avoid alcohol consumption during pregnancy.

TABLE 8–3   CLINICAL FEATURES OF THE FETAL ALCOHOL SYNDROME

Craniofacial
 Eyes: Short palpebral fissures, ptosis, strabismus, epicanthic folds, myopia, microphthalmia
 Ears: Poorly formed concha, posterior rotation
 Nose: Short, hypoplastic philtrum
 Mouth: Prominent lateral palatine ridges, micrognathia, cleft lip or palate, faulty enamel
 Maxilla: Hypoplastic
Cardiac
 Murmurs, atrial septal defect, ventricular septal defect, tetralogy of Fallot
Central Nervous System
 Mild to moderate mental retardation, microcephaly, poor coordination, hypotonia
Growth
 Prenatal onset growth deficiency
Muscular
 Hernias of diaphragm, umbilicus, or groin
Skeletal
 Pectus excavatum, abnormal palmar creases, nail hypoplasia, scoliosis

Antianxiety Agents. This class of drugs is of special interest because it contains the now well-described teratogen thalidomide. Typical features of thalidomide exposure included phocomelia, ear anomalies, cardiac malformations, esophageal or duodenal atresia, and renal agenesis.

Antianxiety agents are currently used by a significant number of pregnant women. Data regarding their teratogenicity are conflicting, although exposure to meprobamate or chlordiazepoxide has been associated with a greater than fourfold increase in severe congenital anomalies. No specific pattern of anomalies is apparent.

Diazepam (Valium) crosses the placenta and accumulates in the fetal circulation. Pregnant women exposed to diazepam during the first trimester should be counseled as to the possible increased risk of oral clefts, although the incidence is probably well below 1 percent.

Antineoplastic Agents. Aminopterin and methotrexate, both of which are folic acid antagonists, have been clearly established as teratogens. Exposure prior to 40 days' gestation is lethal to the embryo; later exposure during the first trimester produces fetal effects, including intrauterine growth retardation, craniofacial anomalies, abnormal positioning of extremities, mental retardation, early miscarriage, stillbirth, and neonatal death.

Alkylating agents have been associated with fetal anomalies, including severe intrauterine growth retardation, fetal death, cleft palate, microphthalmia, limb reduction anomalies, and poorly developed external genitalia. The first trimester is a particularly dangerous time for use of these drugs.

Antibiotics. The majority of studies on the teratogenicity of antibiotics have failed to reveal an increased risk to the fetus. A few, however, appear to pose potential harm.

Although no consistent reports of fetal abnormalities have been associated with tetracycline exposure in the first trimester, fetal exposure beyond the fourth month of pregnancy has been shown to result in deciduous teeth that appear yellow with hypoplasia of the enamel. There is also an increased susceptibility to caries.

About 10 to 15 percent of fetuses exposed to streptomycin and closely related compounds, such as dihydrostreptomycin, will develop serious eighth nerve damage with subsequent hearing loss.

Anticoagulants

COUMARIN DERIVATIVES. Use of coumarin during the first trimester is associated with an increased risk of spontaneous abortion, intrauterine growth retardation, central nervous system defects, stillbirth, and a characteristic syndrome of craniofacial features known as the *fetal warfarin syndrome*. Embryologically, the most vulnerable time appears to be between six and nine weeks after conception. As many as 30 percent of exposed fetuses suffer pregnancy loss or serious teratogenic consequences.

HEPARIN. Heparin has major advantages over coumarin anticoagulants during pregnancy because it does not cross the placenta. Therefore, it should be used routinely for anticoagulation during the first trimester and after 36 weeks' gestation.

Anticonvulsants. Approximately 1 of every 200 pregnant women is epileptic and faces an increased risk for significant fetal abnormalities. It is not clear whether the major proportion of this risk is due to anticonvulsant therapy or to a potential teratogenic effect of the underlying convulsive disorder. However, the specific patterns of fetal malformations associated with different anticonvulsant agents support the concept that the drugs contribute significantly to the pathogenesis of congenital malformations.

DIPHENYLHYDANTOIN (DILANTIN). A specific syndrome, known as the *fetal hydantoin syndrome* (FHS), has been described, the clinical features of which include craniofacial abnormalities, limb reduction defects, prenatal onset growth deficiency, mental retardation, and cardiovascular anomalies. Overall, approximately 10 percent of exposed fetuses demonstrate FHS, while an additional 30 percent may have isolated features of the syndrome. Furthermore, recent investigations suggest that hydantoins may have a prenatal carcinogenic effect in that several exposed infants with signs of FHS have subsequently developed neuroblastomas.

Pregnant epileptic women should be counseled as to the risks of these agents and be advised to either discontinue their use or take the lowest dose capable of controlling seizures.

OXAZOLIDINEDIONE ANTICONVULSANTS.

Trimethadione (Tridione) and paramethadione (Paradione), used to treat petit mal epilepsy, have been associated with a characteristic malformation syndrome in exposed fetuses. The clinical features include craniofacial abnormalities, prenatal onset growth deficiency, and an increased frequency of mental retardation and cardiovascular abnormalities. Additionally, exposure to these agents has been associated with an increased risk of fetal loss. Taken together, women using trimethadione or paramethadione face an 85 percent risk for pregnancy loss or major congenital anomalies. Because of this serious teratogenic potential, and since petit mal epilepsy is rare during reproductive years, oxazolidinedione anticonvulsants are contraindicated during pregnancy.

VALPROIC ACID. *In utero* exposure to valproic acid (Depakene), a relatively new anticonvulsant, produces congenital malformations similar to those found in the fetal hydantoin syndrome. Although normal births associated with prenatal valproic acid exposure have been reported, this drug should be avoided during pregnancy.

PHENOBARBITAL. Phenobarbital is considered to be the antiepileptic drug of choice during pregnancy. The true teratogenicity of phenobarbital is difficult to assess because other drugs are usually taken in combination with this agent, but the risk appears to be very low. Other potential complications of phenobarbital include neonatal withdrawal symptoms and neonatal hemorrhage. Fetal addiction should not be a complication at the dosage levels required for seizure control.

Hormones

PROGESTINS AND ESTROGEN/PROGESTIN COMBINATIONS. A large number of pregnant women are exposed to progestins or progestin/estrogen combinations for the management of threatened abortion or because they continue taking birth control pills unaware that they are pregnant. The most consistent abnormality associated with the use of progestins during pregnancy is masculinization of the external genitalia in female fetuses. The magnitude of this risk appears to be between 1 and 2 percent.

The teratogenicity of estrogen and progestin combinations is more difficult to assess. Potential problems include congenital heart defects, nervous system defects, limb reduction malformations, and modified development of sexual organs. Except for the latter category, no firm evidence for a causal relationship exists.

CLOMIPHENE. Clomiphene is used to induce ovulation but should not be used after conception has occurred. This agent has been associated with an increased risk of neural tube defects and Down's syndrome. It is not clear whether the malformations are due to a drug effect or are related to the underlying subfertility state. Until further information is available, women exposed to clomiphene after conception should be counseled as to the potentially increased risks. Maternal serum alpha-fetoprotein screening and amniocentesis should be made available to such patients.

Miscellaneous Agents

DIURETICS. Although there is evidence of diuretic teratogenicity in rodents, teratogenicity has not been clearly demonstrated in humans.

VITAMIN A. Vitamin A analogues, such as isotretinoin (Accutane), have been marketed in the United States since 1982 for treatment of severe acne. Since 1982, a number of reports suggesting the teratogenicity of these drugs have been published. Affected infants demonstrate craniofacial malformations, psychomotor retardation, congenital heart defects, and central nervous system malformations. The exact risk for serious defects following exposure during the first trimester has not yet been established, but it appears to be substantial. Thus, physicians have an important responsibility to discuss the risks with all female patients before beginning treatment.

TOBACCO SMOKING. Maternal tobacco smoking reduces the chance for a normal pregnancy outcome. Fetal effects include decreased birth weight, birth length, and head circumference, as well as an increased risk for spontaneous abortions, intrauterine fetal death, neonatal death, and prematurity. There is no known increased risk for specific malformations or mental retardation. However, some concern has been raised over the combined use of tobacco and alcohol or other drugs. It is possible that the interactive effects result in a more potent teratogenic effect. Pregnant women should be counseled to reduce smoking as much as possible.

Infectious Agents

The exact frequency of significant infection during pregnancy is not known, but it is probably between 15 and 25 percent. Viruses, bacteria, and parasites may have serious effects on the fetus, including fetal death, growth delay, congenital malformations, and mental deficiency. A full discussion of infectious diseases occurring during pregnancy is given in Chapter 15.

Radiation

Much attention has been directed to the potential adverse effects of radiation during pregnancy. Prenatal ultrasound and ionizing radiation exposure occur frequently as a result of therapeutic or diagnostic medical and dental procedures. When delivered under very specific conditions, ultrasound may affect subcellular materials. However, present evidence does not support any causal relationship between diagnostic ultrasound and birth defects in humans.

The medical effects of ionizing radiation are dose-dependent and include teratogenesis, mutagenesis, and carcinogenesis. The most critical time period appears to be from about two to six weeks after conception. Exposures prior to two weeks either produce a lethal effect or produce no effect at all. Teratogenicity is still a possibility after five weeks, but the risk for deleterious consequences is relatively small.

Theoretically, any dose of ionizing radiation at a critical time could cause fetal damage. However, the incidence of serious effects is significant only at doses greater than 50 rad to the fetus. If a pregnant woman receives more than 10 rad, available data indicate that abortion should be recommended; if exposure is between 5 to 10 rad, termination of pregnancy should be considered, particularly if exposure occurs during the period of organogenesis. Teratogenic effects may include pregnancy loss, growth retardation, eye malformations, and central nervous system defects. Radiation doses of 5 to 15 rad to the pelvis increase the risk of an anomaly by an additional 1 to 3 percent over a background rate of 3 to 4 percent. Radiation doses less than 5 rad are not associated with fetal abnormalities, and patients should be reassured

that their risk is not increased above that of the general population.

The mutagenic effect of radiation is also well known. It is thought that even doses around 5 rad may produce mutations in an exposed fetus. However, it is estimated that a dose of 50 rad would be required to double the spontaneous mutation rate. Thus, the chance that prenatal radiation will produce a genetic disease in the exposed fetus is extremely small.

Ionizing radiation has been shown to be related to the development of leukemia in exposed individuals. It is generally accepted that doses lower than 10 rad increase the chance of leukemia from 1 in 3000 to 1 in 2000.

Fortunately, under ordinary circumstances, only therapeutic levels of radiation present a significant risk to the fetus. Most diagnostic studies deliver substantially less than 5 rad. For example, an upper and lower gastrointestinal series, an IVP, an extra abdominal film, and a lower pelvic study would together deliver a total of less than 3 rad to the fetus. Therefore, in most cases, women exposed to diagnostic radiation can be counseled that the risk is extremely small.

SUGGESTED READING

Allen RW Jr, Ogden B, Bently FL, et al: Fetal hydantoin syndrome, neuroblastoma, and hemorrhagic disease in a neonate. JAMA 244:1464, 1980.

Brent RL: Radiation teratogenesis. Teratology 21:281, 1980.

Brunnell PA: Fetal and neonatal varicella-zoster infections. Semin Perinatol 7:47, 1983.

Hall JG, Pauli RM, Wilson KM: Maternal and fetal sequelae of anticoagulation during pregnancy. Am J Med 68:122, 1980.

Hanson JL: Teratogenetic agents. In Emery AE, Rimoin DL (eds): Principles and Practice of Medical Genetics. Edinburgh, Churchill Livingstone, 1983, pg. 127

Heinonen OP, Stone D, Shapiro S: Birth Defects and Drugs in Pregnancy. Littleton, CO, Publishing Sciences Group, 1977.

Jones KL, Smith DW, Ulleland N, et al: Pattern of malformation in offspring of chronic alcoholic mothers. Lancet 1:1267, 1973.

Kline J, Shrout P, Stein Z, et al: Drinking during pregnancy and spontaneous abortion. Lancet 1:176, 1980.

Nora JJ, Nora AH, Sommerville RJ, et al: Maternal exposure to potential teratogens. JAMA 12:91, 1976.

Saxen I: Associations between oral clefts and drugs taken during pregnancy. Int J Epidemiol 4:37, 1975.

occipitoanterior position. It extends from the undersurface of the occipital bone at the junction with the neck to the center of the anterior fontanelle.

2. Occipitofrontal (11 cm)—the presenting A-P diameter when the head is deflexed, as in an occipitoposterior presentation; it extends from the external occipital protuberance to the glabella.

3. Supraoccipitomental (13.5 cm)—the presenting A-P diameter in a brow presentation and the longest A-P diameter of the head; it extends from the vertex to the chin.

4. Submentobregmatic (9.5 cm)—the presenting A-P diameter in face presentations; it extends from the junction of the neck and lower jaw to the center of the anterior fontanelle.

The transverse diameters of the fetal skull are:

1. Biparietal (9.5 cm)—the largest transverse diameter; it extends between the parietal bones.

2. Bitemporal (8 cm)—the shortest transverse diameter; it extends between the temporal bones.

The average circumference of the term fetal head, measured in the occipitofrontal plane, is 34.5 cm.

PELVIC ANATOMY

Bony Pelvis

The bony pelvis is made up of four bones: the sacrum, coccyx, and two innominates (composed of the ilium, ischium, and pubis). These are held together by the sacroiliac joints, the symphysis pubis, and the sacrococcygeal joint. The union of the pelvis and the vertebral column stabilizes the pelvis and allows weight to be transmitted to the lower extremities.

The sacrum consists of five fused vertebrae. The anterior superior edge of the first sacral vertebra is called the promontory, which protrudes slightly into the cavity of the pelvis. The anterior surface of the sacrum is usually concave. It articulates with the ilium at its upper segment, with the coccyx at its lower segment, and with the sacrospinous and sacrotuberous ligaments laterally.

The coccyx is composed of three to five rudimentary vertebrae. It articulates with the

sacrum forming a joint, and, occasionally, there is fusion between the bones.

The pelvis is divided into the false pelvis above and the true pelvis below the linea terminalis. The false pelvis is bordered by the lumbar vertebrae posteriorly, an iliac fossa bilaterally, and the abdominal wall anteriorly. Its only obstetric function is to support the pregnant uterus.

The true pelvis is a bony canal and is formed by the sacrum and coccyx posteriorly and by the ischium and pubis laterally and anteriorly. Its internal borders are solid and relatively immobile. The posterior wall is twice the length of the anterior wall. The true pelvis is the area of concern to the obstetrician because at times its dimensions are not adequate to permit passage of the fetus.

Pelvic Planes

The pelvis is divided into the following four planes for descriptive purposes:

1. The pelvic inlet
2. The plane of greatest diameter
3. The plane of least diameter
4. The pelvic outlet

These planes are imaginary, flat surfaces extending across the pelvis at different levels. Except for the plane of greatest diameter, each plane is clinically significant.

The *plane of the inlet* is bordered by the pubic crest anteriorly, the iliopectineal line of the innominate bones laterally, and the promontory of the sacrum posteriorly.

The *plane of greatest diameter* is the largest part of the pelvic cavity. It is bordered by the midpoint of the pubis anteriorly, the upper part of the obturator foramina laterally, and the junction of the second and third sacral vertebrae posteriorly.

The *plane of least diameter* is the most important from a clinical standpoint, since most instances of arrest of descent occur at this level. It is bordered by the lower edge of the pubis anteriorly, the ischial spines and sacrospinous ligaments laterally, and the lower sacrum posteriorly.

The *plane of the pelvic outlet* is formed by two triangular planes with a common base at the level of the ischial tuberosities. The anterior triangle is bordered by the subpubic angle at the apex, the pubic rami on the sides, and the bituberous diameter at the base. The posterior triangle is bordered by the sacrococcygeal joint at its apex, the sacrotuberous ligaments on the sides, and the bituberous diameter at the base.

Pelvic Diameters

The diameters of the pelvic planes represent the amount of space available at each level. The key measurements for assessing the capacity of the maternal pelvis include:

1. The obstetric conjugate of the inlet
2. The bispinous diameter
3. The bituberous diameter
4. The posterior sagittal diameter at all levels
5. The curve and length of the sacrum
6. The subpubic angle

The average lengths of the diameters of each pelvic plane are listed in Table 9–1.

Pelvic Inlet. The pelvic inlet has five important diameters (Fig. 9–3). The anteroposterior diameter is described by one of two measurements. The *true conjugate* (anatomic conjugate) is the anatomic diameter, and extends from the middle of the sacral promontory to the superior surface of the pubic symphysis. The *obstetric conjugate* represents the actual space available to the fetus, and extends from the middle of the sacral promontory to the closest point on the convex posterior surface of the symphysis pubis.

The *transverse diameter* is the widest distance between the iliopectineal lines. Each *oblique diameter* extends from the sacroiliac joint to the opposite iliopectineal eminence.

The *posterior sagittal diameter* extends from the A-P and transverse intersection to the middle of the sacral promontory.

Plane of Greatest Diameter. The plane of greatest diameter has two noteworthy diameters. The *A-P diameter* extends from the midpoint of the posterior surface of the pubis to the junction of the second and third sacral vertebrae. The *transverse diameter* is the widest distance between the lateral borders of the plane.

Plane of Least Diameter (Mid-Plane). The plane of least diameter has three important diameters. The *A-P diameter* extends from the lower border of the pubis to the junction of the fourth and fifth sacral vertebrae. The *transverse (bispinous) diameter* extends between the ischial spines. The *posterior sagittal diameter* extends from the bispinous diameter to the junction of the fourth and fifth sacral vertebrae.

Pelvic Outlet. The pelvic outlet has four important diameters (Fig. 9–4). The *anatomic A-P diameter* extends from the inferior margin of the pubis to the tip of the coccyx, while the *obstetric A-P diameter* extends from the inferior margin of the pubis to the sacrococcygeal joint. The *transverse (bituberous) diameter* extends between the inner surfaces of the ischial tuberosities, and the *posterior sagittal diameter* extends from the middle of the transverse diameter to the sacrococcygeal joint.

PELVIC SHAPES

Based upon the general bony architecture, the pelvis may be classified into four basic types (Fig. 9–5).

Gynecoid

This is the classical female type of pelvis and is found in approximately 50 percent of women. It has the following characteristics:

1. Round at the inlet, with the widest transverse diameter only slightly greater than the A-P diameter
2. Side walls straight
3. Ischial spines of average prominence
4. Well-rounded sacrosciatic notch
5. Well-curved sacrum
6. Spacious subpubic arch, with an angle of approximately 90 degrees

TABLE 9–1   AVERAGE LENGTH OF PELVIC PLANE DIAMETERS

PELVIC PLANE	DIAMETER	AVERAGE LENGTH (cm)
Inlet	True conjugate	11.5
	Obstetric conjugate	11
	Transverse	13.5
	Oblique	12.5
	Posterior sagittal	4.5
Greatest diameter	A-P	12.75
	Transverse	12.5
Mid-plane	A-P	12
	Bispinous	10.5
	Posterior sagittal	4.5 – 5
Outlet	Anatomic A-P	9.5
	Obstetric A-P	11.5
	Bituberous	11
	Posterior sagittal	7.5

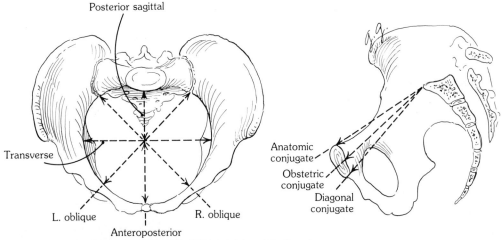

Figure 9–3 Pelvic inlet and its diameters.

These features create a cylindrical shape that is spacious throughout. The fetal head generally rotates into the occipitoanterior (OA) position in this type of pelvis.

Android

Although this is the typical male type of pelvis, it is found in approximately 30 percent of women and has the following characteristics:

1. Triangular inlet with a flat posterior segment and the widest transverse diameter closer to the sacrum than in the gynecoid type
2. Convergent side walls with prominent spines

3. Shallow sacral curve
4. Long and narrow sacrosciatic notch
5. Narrow subpubic arch

This type of pelvis has limited space at the inlet and progressively less space as one moves down the pelvis due to the funneling effect of the side walls, sacrum, and pubic rami. Thus, the amount of space is restricted at all levels. The fetal head is forced to be in the occipitoposterior (OP) position in order to conform to the narrow anterior pelvis. Arrest of descent is common at the midpelvis.

Anthropoid

This type of pelvis resembles that of the anthropoid ape. It is found in approximately

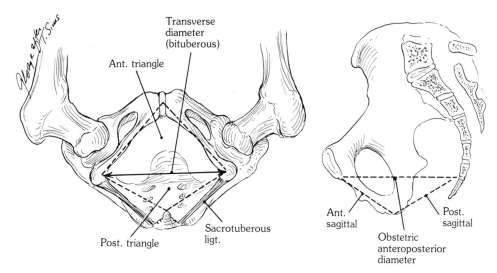

Figure 9–4 Pelvic outlet and its diameters.

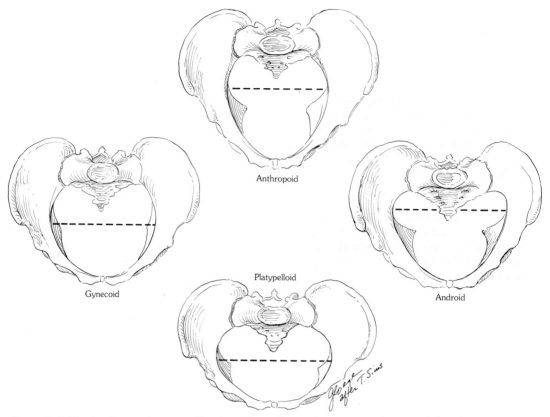

Figure 9–5 The four basic pelvic types. The dotted line indicates the transverse diameter of the inlet. Note that the widest diameter of the inlet is posteriorly situated in an android or anthropoid pelvis.

20 percent of women and has the following characteristics:

1. A much larger A-P than transverse diameter, creating a long narrow oval at the inlet
2. Side walls that do not converge
3. Ischial spines that are not prominent, but are close, due to the overall shape
4. Variable, but usually posterior inclination of the sacrum
5. Large sacrosciatic notch
6. Narrow, outwardly shaped subpubic arch

The fetal head can only engage in the A-P diameter and usually does so in the OP position, since there is more space in the posterior pelvis.

Platypelloid

This pelvis is best described as being a flattened gynecoid pelvis. It is found in only 3 percent of women and it has the following characteristics:

1. A short A-P and wide transverse diameter creating an oval shaped inlet
2. Straight or divergent side walls
3. Posterior inclination of the sacrum
4. A wide bispinous diameter
5. A wide subpubic arch

The overall shape is that of a gentle curve throughout. The fetal head has to engage in the transverse diameter.

ENGAGEMENT

Engagement occurs when the widest diameter of the fetal presenting part has passed through the pelvic inlet. In cephalic presentations, the widest diameter is the biparietal; in breech presentations it is the intertrochanteric.

The *station* of the presenting part in the pelvic canal is defined as its level above or below the plane of the ischial spines. The level of the ischial spines is assigned as "zero" station and each centimeter above or below this level is given a minus or positive designation, respectively.

In the majority of women, the bony presenting part is at the level of the ischial spines when the head has become engaged. This is not true in women with a deep pelvis, in whom the presenting part may be up to 1 cm above the spines, even though engagement has taken place. When the presenting part is out of the pelvis (−3 station or higher) and is freely movable, it is considered to be *floating*. When it has passed through the plane of the inlet but is not yet engaged, it is considered to be *dipping*.

The fetal head usually engages with its sagittal suture in the transverse diameter of the pelvis. The head position is considered to be *synclitic* when the biparietal diameter is parallel to the pelvic plane and the sagittal suture is midway between the anterior and posterior plane of the pelvis. When this relationship is not present, the head is considered to be *asynclitic* (Fig. 9–6).

When the posterior parietal bone is lower in the pelvis than the anterior parietal bone, the sagittal suture is closer to the pubis than the sacrum. This is called *posterior asynclitism*. Synclitism comes about as contractions force the head downward and into lateral flexion and the posterior parietal bone pivots against the sacral promontory. The reverse is found in *anterior asynclitism,* in which contractions force the head to pivot against the pubis.

There is a distinct advantage to having the head engage in asynclitism in certain situations. In a synclitic presentation, the biparietal diameter entering the pelvis measures 9.5 cm; but when the parietal bones enter the pelvis in an asynclitic manner, the presenting diameter measures 8.75 cm. Therefore, asynclitism permits a larger head to enter the pelvis than would be possible in a synclitic presentation.

PELVIMETRY

Clinical

It is not possible to assess all of the pelvic dimensions by clinical mensuration. The diameters that can be clinically evaluated should be assessed at the time of the first prenatal visit, in order to screen for obvious pelvic contractions.

Some obstetricians believe that it is better to wait until later in pregnancy when the soft

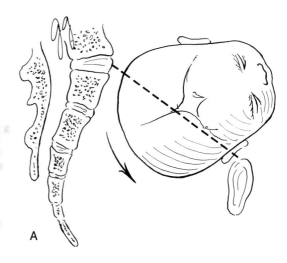

A

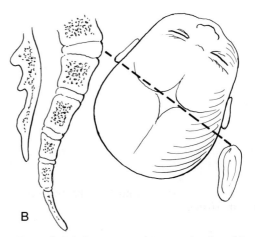

B

Figure 9–6 A, Anterior asynclitism entering the pelvis, and (B) synclitism in the pelvis.

tissues are more distensible and the examination is less uncomfortable and possibly more accurate. It should be remembered that the clinical examination is only an estimate, and there may be a considerable discrepancy from the measurements obtained via x-ray pelvimetry.

The clinical evaluation is started by assessing the *pelvic inlet*. The pelvic inlet can be evaluated clinically for its A-P diameter, while the transverse diameter can be assessed only by x-ray. The obstetric conjugate, previously described under pelvic anatomy, can be estimated from the diagonal conjugate, which is obtained on clinical examination.

The *diagonal conjugate* is approximated by measuring from the lower border of the pubis to the sacral promontory using the tip of the

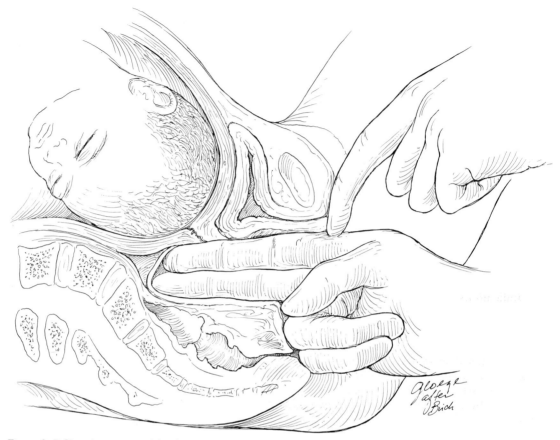

Figure 9–7 Clinical estimation of the diagonal conjugate diameter of the pelvis.

second finger and the point where the index finger meets the pubis (Fig. 9–7). The *obstetric conjugate* is then estimated by subtracting 1.5 to 2 cm, depending on the height and inclination of the pubis. Often the middle finger of the examining hand cannot reach the sacral promontory; thus the obstetric conjugate is considered adequate. If the diagonal conjugate is greater than or equal to 11.5 cm, the A-P diameter of the inlet is considered to be adequate. The transverse diameter of the inlet cannot be evaluated clinically because of the inability to reach this area of the pelvis.

The anterior surface of the sacrum is then palpated in order to assess its curvature. The usual shape is concave. A flat or convex shape may indicate A-P constriction throughout the pelvis.

The *midpelvis* cannot accurately be measured clinically in either the A-P or transverse diameter. However, a reasonable estimate of the size of the midpelvis can be obtained as follows. The pelvic side walls can be assessed

to determine if they are convergent rather than having the usual, almost parallel, configuration. The ischial spines are palpated carefully to assess their prominence, and several passes are made between the spines to approximate the bispinous diameter. The length of the sacrospinous ligament is assessed by placing one finger on the ischial spine and one finger on the sacrum in the midline. The average length is three finger breadths. If the sacrosciatic notch located lateral to the ligament can accommodate two and a half fingers, the posterior midpelvis is most likely of adequate dimensions. A short ligament suggests a forward inclination of the sacrum and a narrowed sacrosciatic notch.

Finally, the *pelvic outlet* is assessed. This is done by first placing a fist between the ischial tuberosities. An 8-cm distance is considered to indicate an adequate transverse diameter. The infrapubic angle is assessed by placing a thumb next to each inferior pubic ramus and then estimating the angle where they meet. An angle of less than 90 degrees is associated with a contracted transverse diameter in the mid-plane and outlet.

X-Ray Pelvimetry

The purpose of x-ray pelvimetry is to aid in determining the need for a cesarean section. However, it can only be used to assess the bony landmarks and, as such, should be considered one piece of information among many variables. Other factors determining the need for a cesarean section include the fetal head size, the force of contractions, the presentation and position of the fetus, and the degree of molding of the fetal head.

The advantage of x-ray over clinical pelvimetry is that it provides more accurate measurements and information about clinically unobtainable measurements.

Indications. There are numerous indications in the obstetric literature for performing x-ray pelvimetry. The most important of these include:

1. Clinical evidence or obstetric history suggestive of pelvic abnormalities
2. A history of pelvic trauma
3. A breech or other abnormal presentation

It should always be questioned whether or not the results obtained with x-ray pelvimetry will have sufficient influence on the patient's management to make the investigation worthwhile.

Dangers. There have been a number of epidemiologic studies purporting a greater risk of leukemia or other cancers in children exposed to x-rays *in utero*. Other studies have refuted these findings, and, at the present time, there are arguments both for and against with no proven data for either side. In light of the present knowledge, it has been decided that if the circumstances dictate the procedure, the risk to the fetus is justifiable.

Method. There are a number of x-ray pelvimetry techniques. If the same reference points of measurement are used, the results from the various techniques should be the same.

The procedure requires two separate films. One is a lateral view, which is used for the A-P measurements; the other is an inlet view, which is used for the transverse diameter. It is important that the landmarks of the pelvis be well visualized. Rotation results in distortion and should be avoided. Since there is distortion of the diameters due to the distance from the x-ray plate, a correction must be made. This can be done by placing a centimeter grid at the same plane as the pelvis. Doses of radiation to the fetus from the pelvimetry range from 0.5 to 1 rad.

SUGGESTED READING

Caldwell WE, Moloy HC: Anatomic variations in the female pelvis and their effect in labor with a suggested classification. Am J Obstet Gynecol 26:479, 1933.

Caldwell WE, Moloy HC: More recent conceptions of the pelvic architecture. Am J Obstet Gynecol 40:558, 1940.

Hannah WG: X-ray pelvimetry—A critical appraisal. Am J Obstet Gynecol 1:333, 1940.

Oppenheim BC, Greim ML: The effects of diagnostic x-ray exposure on the human fetus: An examination of the evidence. Radiology 114:529, 1975.

Oxorn H, Foote R: Human Labor and Delivery. 4th ed. East Norwalk, CT, Appleton-Century-Crofts, 1981.

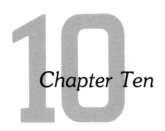

Chapter Ten

NORMAL LABOR, DELIVERY, AND THE PUERPERIUM

MICHAEL G. ROSS, CALVIN J. HOBEL, and SUHA H. N. MURAD

Labor is a physiologic process that permits a series of extensive changes in the mother to allow for the delivery of her fetus through the birth canal. It is defined as progressive cervical effacement and/or dilatation resulting from regular uterine contractions occurring at least every five minutes and lasting 30 to 60 seconds.

The role of the birth attendant is to anticipate and manage complications that may occur to either the mother or the fetus. When a decision is made to intervene, it must be considered carefully; each intervention carries not only potential benefits, but also potential risks. In the vast majority of cases, the best management may be "cautious observation."

PREPARATION FOR LABOR

Before actual labor begins, a number of physiologic preparatory events commonly occur.

Lightening

Two or more weeks before labor, the fetal head in most primigravid women settles into the brim of the pelvis. In multigravid women, this often does not occur until early in labor. Lightening may be noted by the mother as a flattening of the upper abdomen and an increased prominence of the lower abdomen. Compression of the bladder often results in increased frequency of urination.

False Labor

During the last four to eight weeks of pregnancy, the uterus undergoes irregular contractions that normally are painless. Such contractions appear unpredictably and sporadically and can be rhythmic and of mild intensity. In the last month of pregnancy, these contractions may occur more frequently, sometimes every 10 to 20 minutes, and with greater intensity. These "Braxton Hicks" contractions are considered false labor in that they are not associated with progressive cervical dilatation or effacement. However, they may serve a physiologic role in preparing the uterus and cervix for true labor. When Braxton Hicks contractions occur early in the third trimester of pregnancy, it is important to distinguish them from true preterm labor.

Cervical Effacement

Prior to the onset of parturition, the cervix is frequently noted to soften as a result of increased water content and collagen lysis. Simultaneous effacement, or thinning of the cervix, occurs as it is taken up into the lower uterine segment (Fig. 10–1). Consequently, patients often present in labor with a cervix that is already partially effaced. As a result of cervical effacement, the mucous plug within the cervical canal may be released. The onset of labor may thus be heralded by

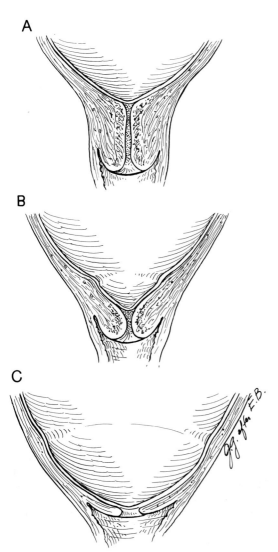

A

B

C

Figure 10–1 *A,* The absence of cervical effacement prior to labor. *B,* Cervix being progressively taken up into the lower segment of the uterus (approximately 50 percent effaced). *C,* Cervix fully taken up; that is, cervix is completely effaced.

the passage of a small amount of blood-tinged mucus from the vagina ("bloody show").

STAGES OF LABOR

There are four stages of labor, each of which is considered separately. These stages in actuality are definitions of progress during labor, delivery, and the puerperium.

The *first stage* is from the onset of true labor to complete dilatation of the cervix. The *second stage* is from complete dilatation of the cervix to the birth of the baby. The *third stage* is from the birth of the baby to delivery of the placenta. The *fourth stage* is from delivery of the placenta to stabilization of the patient's condition, usually at about six hours postpartum.

First Stage of Labor

Phases. The first stage of labor consists of two phases: a *latent phase* during which cervical effacement and early dilatation occur, and an *active phase* during which more rapid cervical dilatation occurs (Fig. 10–2). Although cervical softening and early effacement may occur prior to labor, during the first stage of labor the entire cervical length is retracted into the lower uterine segment as a result of myometrial contractile forces and pressure exerted by either the presenting part or fetal membranes.

Length. The length of the first stage may vary in relation to parity; primiparous patients generally experience a longer first stage than multiparous patients (Table 10–1). Because the latent phase may overlap considerably with the preparatory phase of labor, its duration is highly variable. It may also be influenced by other factors, such as sedation and stress. The duration of the latent phase has little bearing on the subsequent course of labor. The active phase begins when the cervix is 3 to 4 cm dilated in the presence of regularly occurring uterine contractions. The minimal dilatation during the active phase of the first stage is nearly the same for primiparous and multiparous women: 1 and 1.2 cm per hour, respectively. Progress slower than this must be evaluated for uterine dysfunction, fetal malposition, or cephalopelvic disproportion.

Measurement of Progress. During the first stage, the progress of labor may be measured in terms of cervical effacement, cervical dilatation, and the descent of the fetal head. The clinical pattern of the uterine contractions alone is not an adequate indication of progress. After completion of cervical dilatation, the second stage commences. Thereafter, only the descent of the presenting part is available to assess the progress of labor.

Clinical Management of the First Stage

Certain steps should be taken in the clinical management of the patient during the first stage of labor.

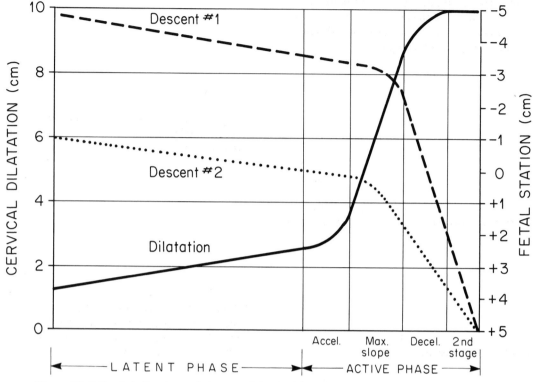

Figure 10–2 Cervical dilatation and descent of the fetal head during labor. The first descent curve represents a fetus with a floating presenting part at the onset of labor, while the second represents a fetus with the presenting part fixed in the pelvis prior to labor. (Modified with permission from Friedman EA: Labor: Evaluation and Management, 2nd ed. East Norwalk, CT, Appleton-Century-Crofts, 1978, p 41.)

Maternal Position. The mother may ambulate during the first stage provided that intermittent monitoring assures fetal well-being and the presenting part is engaged in patients with ruptured membranes. The mother may choose to sit or recline. If she is lying in bed, the lateral recumbent position should be encouraged to assure perfusion of the uteroplacental unit. The supine position should be discouraged.

Administration of Fluids. Due to decreased gastric emptying during labor, oral fluids are best avoided. Placement of a 16- to 18-gauge venous catheter is advisable during the active phase of labor. This intravenous route is used to hydrate the patient with crystalloids during labor, to administer oxytocin after the delivery of the placenta, and for the treatment of any unanticipated emergencies.

Preparing the Patient. Although once considered routine procedures for delivery, the use of enemas, pubic and vulvar shaves, and skin preparations may be individualized by physicians and patients. An enema should be considered in patients who are constipated and in those who have large amounts of stool palpable in the rectum during the pelvic examination.

Investigations. Every woman admitted in labor should have a hematocrit or hemoglobin measured and a blood clot held in the event that a cross-match is needed. Blood

TABLE 10–1 CHARACTERISTICS OF NORMAL LABOR

CHARACTERISTIC	PRIMIPARA	MULTIPARA
Duration of first stage:	6–18 hr	2–10 hr
Rate of cervical dilatation during active phase:	1 cm/hr	1.2 cm/hr
Duration of second stage:	30 min to 3 hr	5–30 min
Duration of third stage:	0–30 min	0–30 min

group, rhesus type, and an antibody screen should be done if these are not known. Additionally, a voided urine specimen should be checked for protein and glucose.

Maternal Monitoring. Maternal pulse rate, blood pressure, respiratory rate, and temperature should be recorded every one to two hours in normal labor and more frequently if indicated. Fluid balance, particularly urine output and intravenous intake, should be monitored carefully.

Analgesia. Adequate analgesia, discussed in Chapter 12, is important during the first stage of labor.

Fetal Monitoring. Auscultation of the fetal heart rate should occur every 15 minutes, immediately following a contraction. The fetal heart rate can also be monitored continuously using either Doppler equipment (external monitoring) or a fetal scalp electrode (internal monitoring). Continuous fetal heart rate monitoring is not necessary in uncomplicated pregnancies.

Uterine Activity. Uterine contractions should be monitored every 30 minutes by palpation for their frequency, duration, and intensity. For high-risk pregnancies, uterine contractions should be monitored continuously along with the fetal heart rate. This can be achieved electronically using either an external tocograph or an internal pressure catheter in the amniotic cavity. The latter is recommended when a patient's labor is being augmented with oxytocin (Pitocin).

Vaginal Examination. During the latent phase, particularly when the membranes are ruptured, vaginal examinations should be done sparingly to decrease the risk of an intrauterine infection. In the active phase, the cervix should be assessed approximately every two hours to determine the progress of labor. Cervical effacement and dilatation, the station and position of the presenting part, and the presence of molding or caput in vertex presentations should be recorded. Additional examinations may be performed if the patient reports the urge to push (to determine if full dilatation has occurred) or if a significant fetal heart rate deceleration occurs (to examine for a prolapsed umbilical cord).

Amniotomy. The artificial rupture of fetal membranes may provide information on the volume of amniotic fluid and the presence or absence of meconium. In addition, rupture of the membranes may cause an increase in uterine contractility. However, amniotomy incurs risks of chorioamnionitis if labor is prolonged, and umbilical cord compression or cord prolapse if the presenting part is not engaged. It should not be routinely performed unless internal monitoring is indicated.

Second Stage of Labor

At the beginning of the second stage, the mother usually has a desire to bear down with each contraction. This abdominal pressure together with the uterine contractile force combines to expel the fetus. During the second stage of labor, fetal descent must be monitored carefully to evaluate the progress of labor. Descent is measured in terms of progress of the presenting part through the birth canal.

In cephalic presentations, the shape of the fetal head may be altered during labor, making the assessment of descent more difficult. *Molding* is the alteration of the relationship of the fetal cranial bones to each other as a result of the compressive forces exerted by the bony maternal pelvis. Some molding is necessary for delivery under normal circumstances. If cephalopelvic disproportion is present, the amount of molding will be more pronounced. *Caput* is a localized, edematous swelling of the scalp caused by pressure of the cervix on the presenting portion of the fetal head. The development of both molding and caput can create a false impression of fetal descent.

The second stage generally takes from 30 minutes to 3 hours in primigravidae, and from 5 to 30 minutes in multigravidae. The median duration is 50 minutes in a primipara and slightly under 20 minutes in a multipara. These times may vary, depending on the type of analgesia.

Mechanism of Labor. Six movements of the baby enable it to adapt to the maternal pelvis: descent, flexion, internal rotation, extension, external rotation, and expulsion (Fig. 10–3). These movements are discussed below for both an occipitoanterior and occipitoposterior position at engagement. The mechanism of labor for other presentations is discussed in Chapter 18.

DESCENT. Descent is brought about by the force of the uterine contractions, maternal bearing-down efforts, and gravity if the patient is upright. A variable degree of fetal descent occurs before the onset of labor in primigravidae and during the first stage in

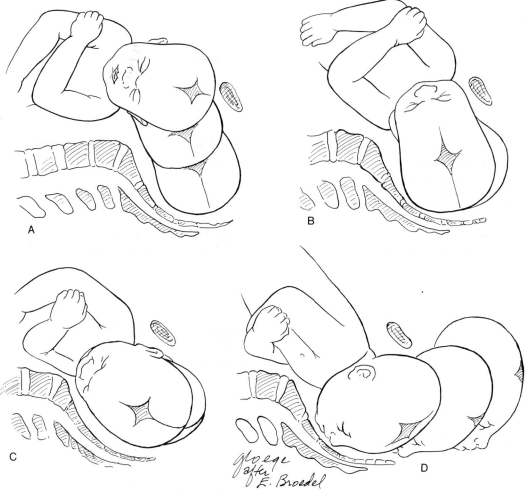

Figure 10–3 Mechanism of labor for a vertex presentation in the left occipitotransverse position. *A,* Flexion and descent; *B* and *C,* continued descent and commencement of internal rotation; *D,* completion of internal rotation to the occipitoanterior position, followed by delivery of the head by extension.

both primigravidae and multigravidae. Descent continues progressively until the fetus is delivered; the other movements are superimposed on it.

FLEXION. Partial flexion exists prior to labor as a result of the natural muscle tone of the fetus. During descent, resistance from the cervix, walls of the pelvis, and pelvic floor cause further flexion of the cervical spine with the baby's chin approaching its chest. In the occipitoanterior position, the effect of flexion is to change the presenting diameter from the occipitofrontal to the smaller suboccipitobregmatic (see Fig. 9–2). In the occipitoposterior position, complete flexion may not occur, resulting in a larger presenting diameter, which may contribute to a longer labor.

INTERNAL ROTATION. In the occipitoan-

terior positions, the fetal head, which enters the pelvis in a transverse or oblique diameter, rotates so that the occiput turns anteriorly toward the symphysis pubis. Internal rotation probably occurs as the fetal head meets the muscular sling of the pelvic floor. It is often not accomplished until the presenting part has reached the level of the ischial spines (zero station), and therefore is engaged. In the occipitoposterior positions, the fetal head may rotate posteriorly so the occiput turns toward the hollow of the sacrum. Alternatively, the fetal head may rotate greater than 90 degrees, positioning the occiput under the pelvic symphysis, and thus converting to an occipitoanterior position. Approximately 75 percent of the fetuses commencing labor in the occipitoposterior position rotate to the occipitoanterior position during flexion and descent. In either case, the sagittal suture normally orients in the anteroposterior axis of the pelvis.

EXTENSION. The flexed head in an occipitoanterior position continues to descend within the pelvis. Since the vaginal outlet is directed upwards and forward, extension must occur before the head can pass through it. As the head continues its descent, there is bulging of the perineum followed by crowning. *Crowning* occurs when the largest diameter of the fetal head is encircled by the vulvar ring. At this time, the vertex has reached station +5. An incision in the perineum (episiotomy) may aid in reducing perineal resistance as well as in preventing tearing and stretching of perineal tissues. The head is born by rapid extension as the occiput, sinciput, nose, mouth, and chin pass over the perineum.

In the occipitoposterior position, the head is born by a combination of flexion and extension. At the time of crowning, the posterior bony pelvis and the muscular sling encourage further flexion. The forehead, sinciput, and occiput are born as the fetal chin approaches the chest. Subsequently, the occiput falls back as the head extends, and the nose, mouth, and chin are born.

EXTERNAL ROTATION. In both the occipitoanterior and occipitoposterior positions, the delivered head now returns to its original position at the time of engagement to align itself with the fetal back and shoulders. Further head rotation may occur as the shoulders undergo an internal rotation to align themselves anteroposteriorly within the pelvis.

EXPULSION. Following external rotation of the head, the anterior shoulder delivers under the symphysis pubis, followed by the posterior shoulder over the perineal body, then the body of the child.

Clinical Management of the Second Stage

As in the first stage, certain steps should be taken in the clinical management of the second stage of labor.

Maternal Position. With the exception of avoiding the supine position, the mother may assume any comfortable position for effective bearing down. If the birth is to occur in another room, primiparous patients should be moved at the beginning of crowning. Multiparous patients should be brought to the delivery room at the time of complete cervical dilatation.

Bearing Down. With each contraction, the mother should be encouraged to bear down with expulsive efforts. This is particularly important for patients with regional anesthesia, as their reflex sensations may be impaired.

Fetal Monitoring. During the second stage, the fetal heart rate should be monitored either continuously or after each contraction. Early fetal heart rate decelerations with prompt recovery following the uterine contraction may occur during this stage.

Vaginal Examination. Progress should be recorded approximately every 30 minutes during the second stage. Particular attention should be paid to the descent and flexion of the presenting part, the extent of internal rotation, and the development of molding or caput.

Delivery of the Fetus. When delivery is imminent, the patient is usually placed in the lithotomy position, and the skin over the lower abdomen, vulva, anus, and upper thighs is cleansed with an antiseptic solution. Appropriate sterile leggings and drapes are applied. Uncomplicated deliveries, particularly in multiparous women, may be carried out in the supine position. The left lateral position may be used to deliver patients with hip or knee joint deformities that prevent adequate flexion, or for patients with a superficial or deep venous thrombosis in one of the lower extremities.

As the perineum becomes flattened by the crowning head, an *episiotomy* is usually performed, especially in the nulliparous patient, to prevent perineal lacerations and probable permanent relaxation of the pelvic outlet.

To facilitate delivery of the fetal head, a Ritgen's maneuver is performed (Fig. 10–4). The right hand, draped with a towel, exerts upward pressure through the distended perineal body, first to the supraorbital ridges and then to the chin. This upward pressure, which increases extension of the head and prevents it from slipping back between contractions, is counteracted by downward pressure on the occiput with the left hand. The downward pressure prevents rapid extension of the head and allows a controlled delivery.

Once the head is delivered, the airway is cleared of blood and amniotic fluid using a bulb suction. The oral cavity is cleared ini-

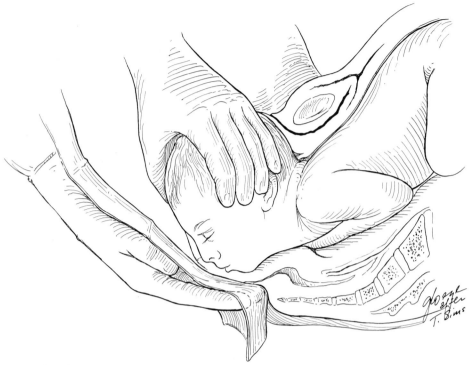

Figure 10–4 Ritgen's maneuver. The right hand is used to extend the head, while counterpressure is applied to the occiput by the left hand to allow a controlled delivery of the fetal head.

tially, and then the nares. Suction of the nares is not performed if fetal distress or meconium stained liquor is present, because it may result in gasping and aspiration of pharyngeal contents. A second towel is used to wipe secretions from the face and head.

After the airway has been cleared, an index finger is used to check whether or not the umbilical cord encircles the neck. If so, the cord can usually be slipped over the infant's head. If the cord is too tight, it can be cut between two clamps.

Following delivery of the head, the shoulders descend and rotate into the anteroposterior diameter of the pelvis and are delivered (Fig. 10–5). Delivery of the anterior shoulder is aided by gentle downward traction on the head. The brachial plexus may be injured if too much force is used. The posterior shoulder is delivered by elevating the head. Finally, the body is slowly extracted by traction on the shoulders.

After delivery, blood will be infused from the placenta into the newborn, provided the baby is held below the introitus. It is therefore usual to wait 15 to 20 seconds before clamping and cutting the umbilical cord. The newborn is then placed under an infant warmer.

Third Stage of Labor

Immediately after the baby's delivery, the cervix and vagina should be thoroughly inspected for lacerations and surgical repair performed if necessary. The cervix, vagina, and perineum may be more readily examined prior to the separation of the placenta, as there should be no uterine bleeding to obscure visualization at this time.

Delivery of the Placenta. Separation of the placenta generally occurs within 5 to 10 minutes of the end of the second stage. Squeezing of the fundus to hasten placental separation is not recommended, as it may increase the likelihood of fetal-maternal transfusion.

Signs of placental separation are as follows: (1) a fresh show of blood from the vagina; (2) the umbilical cord lengthens outside the vagina; (3) the fundus of the uterus rises up; and (4) the uterus becomes firm and globular. Only when these signs have appeared should the assistant attempt traction on the cord. With gentle traction, maternal bearing down, and counterpressure between the symphysis and fundus, the placenta is delivered.

Following delivery of the placenta, attention should be paid to any uterine bleeding that may originate from the placental implan-

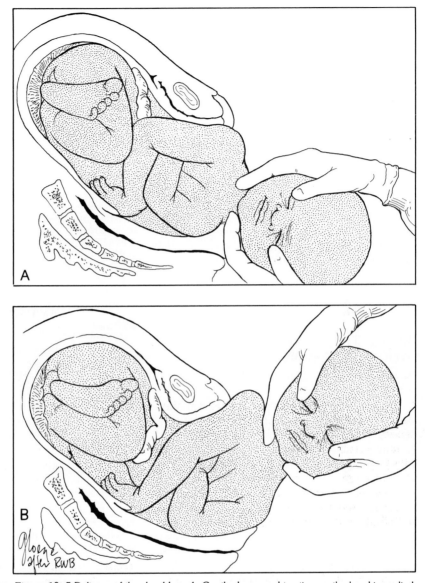

Figure 10–5 Delivery of the shoulders. *A,* Gentle downward traction on the head is applied to deliver the anterior shoulder, and *B,* gentle upward traction is used to deliver the posterior shoulder.

tation site. Uterine contractions, which reduce this bleeding, may be hastened by uterine massage and the use of oxytocin. It is routine to add 20 units of oxytocin to the intravenous infusion after the baby has been delivered. The placenta should be examined to assure its complete removal. If the patient is at risk for postpartum hemorrhage (e.g., because of anemia, prolonged oxytocic augmentation of labor, multiple gestation, or hydramnios), manual removal of the placenta and/or manual exploration of the uterus may be necessary.

Perineal Lacerations. Perineal lacerations, with or without episiotomy, may be classified as follows:

First degree: A laceration involving the vaginal mucosa or perineal skin.

Second degree: A laceration extending into the submucosal tissues of the vagina or perineum with or without involvement of the muscles of the perineal body.

Third degree: A laceration involving the anal sphincter.

Fourth degree: A laceration involving the rectal mucosa.

The birth attendant should perform a digital rectal examination after delivery to be certain there is no undiagnosed rectal tear and that sutures from the episiotomy repair have not penetrated the rectal mucosa.

Fourth Stage of Labor

The hour immediately following delivery requires close observation of the patient. Blood pressure, pulse rate, and uterine blood loss must be monitored closely. It is during this time that postpartum hemorrhage commonly occurs, usually because of uterine relaxation, retained placental fragments, or undiagnosed lacerations. Occult bleeding (e.g., vaginal hematoma formation) may present with complaints of pelvic pain. There may be an increase in pulse rate, often out of proportion to any decrease in blood pressure.

INDUCTION AND AUGMENTATION OF LABOR

Induction of labor is the process whereby labor is initiated by artificial means; *augmentation* is the artificial stimulation of labor that has begun spontaneously.

The natural onset of labor at term involves complex interactions between the fetus and mother which are discussed in Chapter 45. Oxytocin is identical to the natural pituitary peptide, and it is the only drug used for induction and augmentation of labor. Pitocin and Syntocinon are the synthetic preparations. Currently, prostaglandin E_2 (PGE_2) is being investigated as a possible cervical ripening agent, but it has not yet been approved by the Food and Drug Administration.

Indications and Contraindications

The physician must be fully aware of both the indications and contraindications for the use of oxytocin (Table 10–2). In general, induction of labor before term is indicated only when the continuation of pregnancy represents significant risk to the fetus or mother. In some situations, induction may be indicated at term, as in the case of premature rupture of the membranes. Induction at term for convenience is not appropriate unless the

TABLE 10–2 INDICATIONS AND CONTRAINDICATIONS FOR INDUCTION AND AUGMENTATION OF LABOR

INDICATIONS	
Induction	**Augmentation**
Maternal	Abnormal labor (in the
Pre-eclampsia	presence of inadequate
Diabetes mellitus	uterine activity)
Heart disease	—prolonged latent
	phase
	—prolonged active
	phase
Fetoplacental	
Prolonged pregnancy	Abruptio placentae
Intrauterine growth	
retardation	
Fetal distress	
Rh incompatability	
Fetal abnormality	
Premature rupture of	
membranes	
Chorioamnionitis	

CONTRAINDICATIONS	
Maternal	
Absolute	Same contraindications,
Contracted pelvis	except that augmenta-
Prior uterine surgery	tion is occasionally
—classic or lower seg-	done in a patient with
ment cesarean sec-	spontaneous onset of
tion	labor and previous
—complete transec-	lower transverse cesar-
tion of uterus (my-	ean section
omectomy, recon-	
struction)	
Relative	
Overdistended uterus	
Grand multiparity	
Advanced maternal	
age	
Fetoplacental	
Preterm fetus without	
lung maturity	
Acute fetal distress	
Abnormal presentation	

patient has a history of previous precipitous delivery (less than three hours) or lives an unusually long distance from the hospital.

In general, any condition that makes normal labor dangerous for the mother or fetus is a contraindication to induction or augmentation of labor. The most common contraindication is prior uterine surgery in which there has been complete transection of the uterine wall. Even though a lower transverse uterine incision is no longer considered a contraindication to a trial of spontaneous labor, induction of labor would be contraindicated. In selected cases, however, augmentation is permissible.

Induction of labor prior to term for maternal or fetal indications must not be undertaken without the assessment of fetal pulmonary maturity, provided that a delay will not jeopardize the mother or fetus. Fetal lung maturity can most often be accelerated within 24 to 48 hours by the use of glucocorticoids.

Technique for Induction and Augmentation

A hospital obstetrical service must have guidelines for the proper use of oxytocin for induction and augmentaiton. In general, an assessment and plan of management must be outlined in the progress notes of the patient's medical record. Indications for induction of labor should be clearly stated. It is helpful to assess the likelihood of success by a careful pelvic examination to determine the *Bishop Score,* which evaluates the status of the cervix and the station of the fetal head (Table 10–3). A high score (9 to 13) is associated with a high likelihood of a vaginal delivery, whereas a low score (less than 5) is associated with a decreased likelihood of success (65 to 80 percent). Prior to beginning induction, the patient must have her blood typed and screened for antibodies. A blood specimen should be held in the laboratory in case crossmatching becomes necessary (see Complications). Continuous electronic monitoring of the fetal heart rate and uterine activity is required during induction. An internal uterine catheter for monitoring uterine pressure is suggested if intensity cannot be adequately assessed.

Oxytocin Infusion. There are several principles that should be followed when oxytocin is used to induce or augment labor.

1. Oxytocin must be given intravenously in order to allow the health care team to quickly discontinue its use if a complication such as uterine hypertonus or fetal distress develops. Since oxytocin has a half-life of 3 to 5 minutes, its physiologic effect will diminish within 15 to 30 minutes after discontinuation.

2. A dilute infusion must be used and piggybacked into the main intravenous line so that it can be stopped quickly if necessary, without interrupting the main intravenous route.

3. The drug is best infused with a calibrated infusion pump that can be easily adjusted to accurately effect the required infusion rate.

4. The induction of labor for a specific indication should not exceed 72 hours. In patients with a low *Bishop Score,* it is not unusual for an induction to progress slowly. If the cervix effaces and dilates, it is recommended that the membranes be ruptured on the third day. If adequate progress is not made within 12 hours of rupturing the membranes, a cesarean section should be performed.

5. If adequate labor is established, the infusion rate and the concentration can almost always be reduced by one half, especially during the second stage of labor. This principle avoids the risk of hyperstimulation and fetal distress from excessive stimulation, which frequently occur once labor has been established.

6. Oxytocic augmentation should not exceed 12 hours in any 24-hour period.

The protocol for oxytocic induction or augmentation of labor is shown in Table 10–4.

Amniotomy. Amniotomy alone is rarely used to induce labor. In general, induction with oxytocin facilitates the application of the presenting part to the lower uterine segment, thus reducing the likelihood for cord prolapse when the membranes are later ruptured. Amniotomy reduces the uterine volume, which is thought to increase uterine sensitivity and facilitate the induction of labor. However, loss of amniotic fluid significantly increases the likelihood of cord compression and possibly increases the likelihood of fetal distress.

Complications

There are three major complications from the use of oxytocin for the induction and

---

TABLE 10–3 BISHOP SCORE TO ASSESS LIKELIHOOD OF SUCCESSFUL INDUCTION OF LABOR

PHYSICAL FINDINGS	RATING			
	0	1	2	3
Cervix				
Position	Posterior	Mid	Anterior	—
Consistency	Firm	Medium	Soft	—
Effacement (%)	0–30	46–50	60–70	≥80
Dilatation (cm)	0	1–2	3–4	≥5
Fetal head				
Station	−3	−2	−1, 0	+1, +2

0 - 4   80% vaginal delivery
5 - 9   95%
≥ 9   100%

TABLE 10–4 METHOD OF OXYTOCIN
INFUSION FOR
INDUCTION/AUGMENTATION

Solution
  10 units of oxytocin in 1000 ml of 5% dextrose or
  balanced salt solution (10 mU/ml)
Administration
  a. Piggyback into main I.V. line
  b. Administer solution by infusion pump
  c. Initial rate is 0.5–1.0 mU/min
  d. Increase every 15 min (every 20–30 min may be
     more appropriate for augmentation)
  e. Maximum dose is 20 mU/min
  f. Dosage progression as follows:
       0.5 mU/min
       1 mU/min
       2 mU/min
       5 mU/min
       7.5 mU/min
       10 mU/min
       15 mU/min
       20 mU/min

augmentation of labor. First, an excessive infusion rate can cause *hyperstimulation* and thereby cause fetal distress. In rare situations, a tetanic contraction can occur and lead to *rupture of the uterus*. Second, since oxytocin has a similar structure to antidiuretic hormone, it has an intrinsic *antidiuretic effect* and will increase water reabsorption from the glomerular filtrate. Severe *water intoxication* with convulsions and coma can rarely occur when oxytocin is infused continuously for more than 24 hours—hence, the reason for limiting its use to a 12-hour period. Third, prolonged oxytocin infusions can result in *uterine muscle fatigue* (nonresponsiveness) and *post-delivery uterine atony* (hypotonus), which can increase the risk of postpartum hemorrhage.

PUERPERIUM

The puerperium consists of the period following delivery of the baby and placenta to approximately six weeks postpartum. During the puerperium, the reproductive organs and maternal physiology return toward the prepregnancy state.

Anatomic and Physiologic Changes

Involution of the Uterus. Through a process of tissue catabolism, the uterus rapidly decreases in weight from about 1000 gm at delivery to 50 gm at approximately three weeks postpartum. The cervix similarly loses its elasticity and retains its prepregnancy firmness. For the first few days after delivery, the uterine discharge (lochia) appears red (*lochia rubra*) due to the presence of erythrocytes. After three to four days, the lochia becomes paler (*lochia serosa*), and, by the tenth day, it assumes a white or yellow/white color (*lochia alba*). Foul smelling lochia suggests, but is not diagnostic of, endometritis.

Vagina. Although the vagina never returns to its prepregnancy state, the supportive tissues of the pelvic floor gradually regain their former tone.

Cardiovascular System. Immediately following delivery, there is a marked increase in peripheral vascular resistance due to the removal of the low-pressure uteroplacental circulation. The cardiac work and plasma volume gradually return to normal during the first two weeks of the puerperium. Due to the loss of plasma volume and the diuresis of extracellular fluid, there is a marked weight loss in the first week. A significant granulocytic leukocytosis may be seen in the immediate postpartum period.

Psychosocial. It is fairly common for women to exhibit a mild degree of depression a few days following delivery. The "postpartum blues" are probably due to both emotional and hormonal factors. With understanding and reassurance from both family and physician, this usually resolves without consequence.

Return of Menstruation and Ovulation. In women who do not nurse, menstrual flow will usually return by six to eight weeks following delivery, although this is highly variable. Although ovulation may not occur for several months, particularly in nursing mothers, contraceptive counseling and use should be emphasized during the puerperium to avoid unwanted pregnancy (see Chapter 40).

BREAST FEEDING

There are many advantages to breast feeding. First, breast milk is the ideal food for the newborn, is inexpensive, and is usually in good supply. Second, nursing accelerates the involution of the uterus, because suckling stimulates the release of oxytocin, thereby causing increased uterine contractions. Third, and probably most important, there are immunological advantages for the baby from breast feeding. Various types of maternal antibodies are present in breast milk. The predominant immunoglobulin is secretory IgA, which provides protection in the infant's gut by preventing attachment of bacteria (e.g., *Escherichia coli*) to cells on the mucosal surface. This prevents the bacteria from penetrating the bowel wall. It is also thought that maternal lymphocytes pass through the infant's gut wall and initiate immunologic processes not yet well understood. Breast feeding thereby provides the newborn with passive immunity against certain infectious diseases until its own immune mechanisms become fully functional by three to four months.

Lactation

Various hormones, such as estrogen, progesterone, human chorionic gonadotropin, cortisol, insulin, prolactin, and placental lactogen play an important role in preparing the breasts for lactation. At delivery, two events are instrumental in initiating lactation. First, the drop in placental hormones allows lactation to occur. (Prior to delivery, these hormones interfere with the lactogenic action of prolactin.) Second, suckling stimulates the release of prolactin and oxytocin. The latter causes contraction of the myoepithelial cells in the alveoli and milk ducts. The suckling stimulus is thought important for milk production, as well as the ejection of colostrum and milk.

On approximately the second day after delivery, colostrum is secreted. Its content is comprised mostly of protein, fat, and minerals. It is the colostrum that contains secretory IgA. After about three to six days, the colostrum is replaced by mature milk. The content of milk varies considerably depending upon the nutritional status of the mother and the gestational age at the time of delivery. In general, the major components of breast milk are proteins, lactose, water, and fat. The major proteins synthesized in the human breast, which are unique and not found in cows' milk, are casein, lactoalbumin, and beta-lactoglobulin. Essential amino acids are delivered from the mother's blood, and some of the nonessential amino acids can be synthesized in the breast. Lactose and fatty acids are synthesized in the breast.

Lactation Suppression

When the mother chooses not to breast feed, lactation suppression is indicated. The simplest, and probably safest, method to accomplish this is to use a tightfitting bra to prevent breast distention. If breast distention does occur, pumping only makes the situation worse. Ice packs should be applied and the discomfort managed with analgesics. Drugs, such as estrogens in combination with testosterone, are frequently used to suppress lactation but must be given immediately after delivery to be effective, and there is concern that they may increase the risk of thromboembolism. Bromocriptine (Parlodel), a dopamine agonist, stimulates the production of prolactin inhibitory factor, which results in a fall in prolactin levels and inhibition of lactation. Therapy with bromocriptine should be started only after the patient's vital signs have stabilized and not sooner than four hours after delivery. The dosage is 2.5 mg twice daily for 14 days.

Complications of Breast Feeding

Cracked Nipples. If the nipples of the breast become fissured, nursing may become difficult. Since fissures are also a portal of entry for bacteria, they should be managed aggressively with a nipple shield and an appropriate cream, such as lanolin or Masse Breast Cream. Further breast feeding should be temporarily stopped. Milk can be expressed manually until the nipples heal, at which time breast feeding can be resumed.

Mastitis. This is an uncommon complication of breast feeding and usually develops two to four weeks after beginning breast feeding. The first symptoms are usually slight fever and chills. These are followed by redness of a segment of the breast, which becomes indurated and painful. The etiologic agent is usually *Staphylococcus aureus*, which originates from the infant's oral pharynx. Milk should be obtained from the breast for culture and sensitivity, and the mother should be started on antibiotics immediately. Since the majority of staphylococcal organisms are penicillinase-producing, a penicillinase-resistant antibiotic, such as cloxacillin, should be used. Breast feeding should be discontinued and an appropriate antibiotic should be continued for seven to ten days. A breast pump can be used to maintain lactation until the infection has cleared, but the milk should be discarded. The infant, as well as other family members, should be evaluated for staphylo-

TABLE 10–5 EFFECTS OF MATERNAL DRUG INGESTION ON BREAST FEEDING INFANTS

DRUG	REPORTED INFANT EFFECTS
Sedative-hypnotics	
Diazepam	Sedation
Meprobamate	Effects not known
Antipsychotics	
Chlorpromazine	No adverse effects reported
Haloperidol	No adverse effects reported
Non-narcotic analgesics	
Acetaminophen	No adverse effects reported
Salicylates	No known adverse effects; theoretical risk of platelet dysfunction
Naproxen	Effects not known
Anticonvulsants	
Phenobarbital	Sedation
Phenytoin	Sedation, decreased sucking
Narcotics	
Heroin	May cause addiction
Methadone	One infant death reported
Meperidine	No adverse effects reported
Antibiotics	
Penicillin	May modify bowel flora, cause allergy, or interfere with sepsis work-up
Ampicillin	Same as for penicillin
Erythromycin	Same as for penicillin
Nitrofurantoin	Theoretical risk of hemolytic anemia in infants with G6PD deficiency
Tetracycline	Same as for penicillin; theoretical risk of discoloration of teeth and inhibition of bone growth
Digoxin	No adverse effects reported
Thyroid drugs	
Thyroxine	May interfere with screening for hypothyroidism
Propylthiouracil	Nodular goiter
Antihypertensives	
Methyldopa	No adverse effects reported
Propranolol	No adverse effects reported
Theophylline	One case of infant irritability following maternal administration of a rapidly absorbed oral preparation

coccal infections that may be a source of reinfection if breast feeding is resumed.

Drug Passage to the Newborn. Since an infant may ingest up to 500 ml of breast milk per day, maternally administered drugs that pass into breast milk may have a significant effect on the infant. The amount of drug found in breast milk depends on the maternal dose, the rate of maternal clearance, the physicochemical properties of the drug, and the breast milk composition with respect to fat and protein. The gestational age of the infant may also be a determinant of the ultimate drug effect. Table 10–5 lists selected drugs with their reported newborn effects.

SUGGESTED READING

Bishop EN: Pelvic scoring for elective induction. Obstet Gynecol 24:266, 1964.

Briggs GG, Bodendorfer TW, Freeman RK, et al: Drugs in Pregnancy and Lactation, Baltimore, Williams & Wilkins, 1983.

Friedman EA: Labor: Evaluation and Management. 2nd ed. East Norwalk, CT, Appleton-Century-Crofts, 1978.

Goldman AS, Smith CW: Host resistance factors in breast milk. J Pediatr 82:1082, 1973.

Harrison RG: Suppression of lactation. Semin Perinatol 3:287, 1979.

Herxheimer A (ed): Drugs which can be given to nursing mothers. Drug and Therapeutic Bulletin, London, Consumer's Association, 1983, p 5.

Hughey MJ, McElin TW, Bird CC: An evaluation of preinduction scoring systems. Obstet Gyneol 48:635, 1976.

McNeilly AS, Robinson ICA, Houston MJ, et al: Release of oxytocin and prolactin in response to suckling. Br Med J 286:257, 1983.

Oxorn H, Foote WR (eds): Human Labor and Birth. 3rd ed. East Norwalk, CT, Appleton-Century-Crofts, 1975.

Pritchard JA, MacDonald PC (eds): Obstetrics. 6th ed. East Norwalk, CT, Appleton-Century-Crofts, 1980.

Rovinsky JJ: Management of normal labor and delivery. In Sciarra JJ, Gerbie AB (eds): Gynecology and Obstetrics. Vol 2. Philadelphia, Harper & Row Publishers, 1984.

Sandberg EC: Synopsis of Obstetrics. 10th ed. St. Louis, CV Mosby Co, 1978.

Tyson JE, Friesen HG, Anderson MS: Human lactational and ovarian response to endogenous prolactin release. Science 177:897, 1972.

RESUSCITATION OF THE NEWBORN

CALVIN J. HOBEL

Improved surveillance using antenatal and intrapartum fetal heart rate monitoring, real time ultrasound, and fetal scalp blood sampling, have allowed the clinician to recognize the fetus at risk who may need special care at birth. A problem-oriented assessment during prenatal visits allows identification of those patients who will need special assessment during labor.

PREPARATION FOR EXTRAUTERINE LIFE

Reaching maturity is the most important step for the fetus *in utero*. Prematurity is the leading cause of poor neonatal outcome because the fetus has not yet progressed through complete stages of anatomic development and biochemical maturation. Even the fetus delivered at term undergoes changes prior to and with the onset of labor.

During pregnancy, fetal thyroxine (T_4) is converted to reverse triiodothyronine (rT_3), which is metabolically inactive. Several days prior to the onset of term labor, cortisol levels increase in the fetus and induce a change in thyroid hormone dynamics. Cortisol induces the enzyme system allowing the conversion of T_4 to triiodothyronine (T_3), which is metabolically more active and necessary for neonatal thermogenesis. At birth, there is a surge of thyroid stimulating hormone (TSH), and at no time during life does this hormone reach such high levels as it does 30 minutes after birth. This is followed by a hyperthyroid

neonatal state for several days, which is necessary for the newborn to maintain its body temperature.

A second change that occurs with the onset of labor is a change in fetal breathing activity. Fetal breathing, as observed by real time ultrasound, is rarely observed once labor is established. This is thought to be associated with a decrease in pulmonary fluid dynamics that may be important for the onset of respiration after delivery and the retention of surfactant in the lungs.

Finally, labor is a stress to the fetus that stimulates the release of catecholamines. The latter may be responsible for the mobilization of glucose, lung fluid absorption, alterations in the perfusion of organ systems, and, possibly, the onset of respiration. Only at times of severe stress later in life do levels of catecholamines reach levels as high as those at birth.

ETIOLOGY OF NEONATAL CARDIORESPIRATORY DEPRESSION

At term, 0.5 percent of infants will require vigorous resuscitation (positive pressure ventilation for more than one minute). At earlier stages of gestation, almost all infants require some type of supportive care.

Table 11–1 lists the antepartum and intrapartum factors that must be recognized during pregnancy in order to identify the fetus at risk.

TABLE 11–1 PRENATAL AND INTRAPAR-
TUM CONDITIONS LIKELY TO
PREDISPOSE TO ASPHYXIA
NEONATORUM

ANTEPARTUM PROBLEMS	INTRAPARTUM PROBLEMS
Past Medical Problems	Preterm labor
Chronic hypertension	Premature rupture of
Diabetes mellitus	membranes
Renal disease	Fetal distress
Hyperthyroidism	Abnormal labor
Epilepsy	Prolonged labor
Pulmonary disease	Precipitous labor
	Abruptio placentae
Developing Problems	Amnionitis
Inaccurate gestational	Anesthetic problems
dates	Hypotension
Multiple pregnancy	Hypertension
Intrauterine growth	Operative delivery
retardation	
Fetal macrosomia	
Prolonged pregnancy	
Congenital anomalies	
Pregnancy-Induced Problems	
Hypertension	
Gestational diabetes	

FACILITATING NEONATAL ADAPTATION

The physician performing the delivery must delegate the responsibility for neonatal resuscitation. All nurses working in the delivery room must be trained in techniques of neonatal assessment and resuscitation. If risk factors increase the likelihood of delivering a depressed infant, a pediatrician trained in neonatal resuscitation should be summoned.

Following delivery of a normal newborn, attention should be directed toward the following important steps to assure optimal neonatal adaptation.

Clear the Airway

Descent through the birth canal causes compression of the chest wall, resulting in the discharge of fluid from the mouth and nose. When the head emerges from the vagina, the physician should use a towel or gauze pad to remove secretions from the face. In addition, a bulb suction may be used to aspirate secretions from the oral pharynx. The bulb suction should not be used to suction the nose because nasal stimulation may initiate a gasp and cause bradycardia. Also, nasal stimulation may cause aspiration of meconium, if present.

Dry the Newborn

An important part of neonatal adaptation is the initiation of thermogenesis. Excessive cooling from exposure of the wet skin is detrimental to all preterm infants and to depressed full-term infants. The physician should dry off the infant with a towel prior to cutting the cord. This serves to stimulate the onset of respiration.

Clamp the Cord

The umbilical arteries usually close spontaneously within 45 to 60 seconds of birth, while the umbilical vein remains patent for three to five minutes or longer. Delayed cord clamping significantly increases the neonatal blood volume, which increases the likelihood of neonatal jaundice and tachypnea. The ideal time for clamping the cord is 20 to 30 seconds after birth.

Assure Onset of Respiration

The onset of respiration is usually within a few seconds of birth but may be delayed for up to 60 seconds. In the absence of clinical data to suggest a biochemical abnormality (hypoxia-acidosis), it is usually best to adopt an expectant policy of standing back and giving the infant a chance to breathe spontaneously.

THE APGAR SCORE

This is an excellent tool for assessing the overall status of the newborn soon after birth (one minute) and after a brief period of observation (five minutes) (Table 11–2). A normal Apgar score is 7 or greater at one minute, and 9 or 10 at five minutes.

RESUSCITATION OF THE ASPHYXIATED INFANT

The delivery of an asphyxiated infant should be predictable, based on a careful clinical assessment of those factors associated with biochemical abnormalities. During the past five years, increasing emphasis has been

TABLE 11-2   THE APGAR SCORE FOR DETERMINING THE CONDITION OF A NEWBORN INFANT

SIGN	0	1	2
Heart rate	Absent	Below 100	Over 100
Respiratory effort	Absent	Slow, weak cry	Good, strong cry
Muscle tone	Limp	Some flexion of extremities	Active motion
Reflex irritability (response to stimulation of sole of foot)	None	Grimace	Strong cry
Color	Pale, blue	Body: pink Extremities: blue	Completely pink

placed on transferring the mother with a high risk pregnancy to a tertiary care regional center before labor, rather than transferring the sick neonate after delivery. The mother is considered to be a better and safer transport incubator.

Ideally, at the time of delivery, a segment of cord should be doubly clamped to allow blood gas determinations on cord arterial and venous blood. These serve as a baseline to assess the severity of the neonatal hypoxia and acidosis.

A stepwise sequence of procedures is necessary to enable a smooth transition to a normal metabolic state. This sequence is referred to as the ABCs of resuscitation and is summarized in Figure 11-1.

Establish an Airway

In any infant with a high likelihood of asphyxia, suctioning of the airway must be initiated after the delivery of the head. The asphyxiated neonate usually has meconium present in the upper airway, which must be cleared with an oral suction catheter prior to delivery of the shoulders. Immediately following the delivery of the infant, an endotracheal tube should be inserted to remove thick mucus or meconium from the trachea and upper airway.

Initiate Breathing

With an established airway, either bag-mask ventilation or ventilation via an endo-

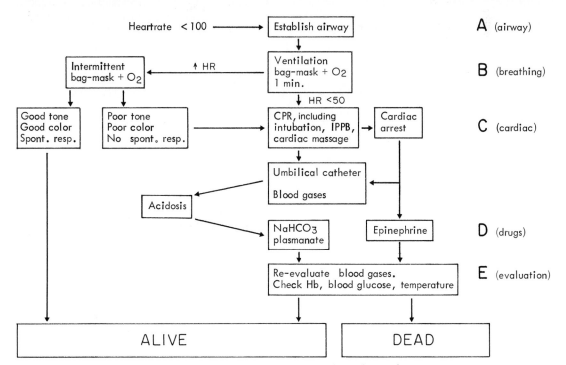

Figure 11-1 The ABC's of resuscitation for the asphyxiated neonate.

tracheal tube must be initiated in order to deliver oxygen to the lungs. Usually, the heart rate increases rapidly after the apnea is corrected, and intermittent bag-mask ventilation with supplemental oxygen can be given until spontaneous respiration commences.

Assure Cardiac Performance

If cardiac performance is poor (heart rate less than 50 beats per minute after 1 minute), external cardiac massage must be initiated. The best technique for cardiac massage in the newborn is to compress the middle third of the sternum with two fingers at a rate of 100 times per minute. The middle finger and either the index or ring finger should be used (Fig. 11–2). The sternum should be depressed approximately 2 cm. Placement of the other hand beneath the infant's back can facilitate compression of the heart between the sternum and spine. Cardiac arrest is rare. If cardiac massage and artificial ventilation are not successful in reestablishing cardiac function, an intracardiac injection of a dilute solution of epinephrine may be given through the chest wall.

Correct Biochemical Abnormalities

Acidosis. In the case of a very sick newborn, an umbilical arterial catheter is placed and blood gases obtained to monitor the severity of the acidosis and the effectiveness of the resuscitation. Severe acidosis can be corrected by the infusion of sodium bicarbonate.

Anemia. On rare occasions, the newborn may have abnormal perfusion secondary to blood loss (for example, from vasa previa or abruptio placentae), which can be corrected only by immediate transfusion with blood from the mother, a blood bank, or a walk-in donor. A solution of plasmanate can be used to temporarily maintain an adequate vascular volume.

Narcotic Depression. Respiratory depression secondary to medication is unusual in today's practice of natural childbirth. If respiratory depression from excessive use of narcotics is suspected, naloxone (Narcan) is effective. It is just as effective and more easily administered intramuscularly than intravenously. There is a very high toxic ratio of neonatal naloxone, so dosage is less critical than for most drugs. Table 11–3 lists the drugs commonly used in resuscitation and their dosages.

Hypoglycemia. Hypoglycemia can also contribute to unsuccessful resuscitation, especially in infants with intrauterine growth retardation or those with diabetic mothers. Glucose administration should be considered after the other issues have been addressed. The use of high concentrations of glucose (for example, 25 to 50 percent) is contrain-

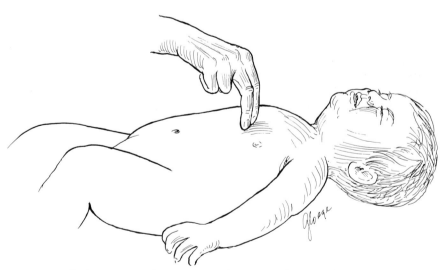

Figure 11–2 Technique for cardiac massage in the neonate. Note that the middle third of the sternum is depressed with two fingers of the physician's right hand. The infant's back may be supported with the left hand if necessary.

TABLE 11–3 DRUGS USED TO RESUSCITATE THE NEONATE

DRUG	DOSE	ROUTE	VOLUME
Sodium Bicarbonate	1–3 mEq/kg	UA UV	Dilute 1:1 with sterile water to 0.5 mEq/cc Dosage 2–6 cc/kg
Epinephrine	0.1 mg/kg	IV	0.1 cc/kg of a 1:10,000 solution
Naloxone	0.01 mg/kg	IM or IV	Neonatal dosage: 0.5 cc/kg of a 0.02 mg/cc solution Maternal dosage: .025 cc/kg of a 0.4 mg/cc solution
Plasmanate		IV	4–5 cc/kg

UA = umbilical artery; UV = umbilical vein
IV = intravenous; IM = intramuscular

dicated in asphyxiated newborns because in the absence of oxygen, the glucose is converted to lactic acid, which may increase the likelihood of brain damage.

Evaluate Other Factors

Following a systematic resuscitation effort, it is necessary to search for other contributing factors if cardiorespiratory depression persists. *Hypothermia* is one of the most critical aggravating factors, and temperature control must be continuously supported. A *pneumothorax* is not uncommon following a difficult resuscitation (especially with intubation). It must be recognized promptly and decompressed with a chest tube.

LONG-TERM OUTCOME

Recent data have indicated that low birth weight (less than 2500 gm), whether due to prematurity or intrauterine growth retardation, is an independent risk factor for cerebral palsy. By contrast, for infants weighing more than 2500 gm, Apgar scores less than or equal to 3 at five minutes are not associated with an increased risk of cerebral palsy, provided there is no associated obstetric complication. If both a low Apgar score and an obstetric complication are present, there is an increased risk of cerebral palsy.

SUGGESTED READING

Apgar V, James LS: Further observations on the newborn scoring system. J Dis Child 104:419, 1962.

Cordero J, Hon EG: Neonatal bradycardia following nasopharyngeal stimulation. J Pediatr 78:441, 1971.

Gregory GA, Gooding CA, Phibbs RA, et al: Meconium aspiration in infants—a prospective study. J Pediatr 85:848, 1974.

Hobel CJ: Management of the high risk fetus and neonate. In Bolognese RJ, Schwarz RH, Schneider J (eds): Perinatal Medicine. 2nd ed. Baltimore, Williams & Wilkins, 1982, p 3.

Hobel CJ, Hyvarinen MA, Okada DM, et al: Prenatal and intrapartum high-risk screening. Am J Obstet Gynecol 117:1, 1973.

Hobel CJ, Oh W, Hyvarinen MA, et al: Early versus late treatment of neonatal acidosis in low birth weight infants: Relation to respiratory distress syndrome. Pediatrics 81:1178, 1972.

MacDonald HM, Mulligan JC, Allen AC, et al: Neonatal asphyxia. I. Relationship of obstetric and neonatal complications to neonatal mortality in 38,405 consecutive deliveries. J Pediatr 96:898, 1980.

Milner AD, Vyas H: Lung expansion at birth. J Pediatr 101:879, 1982.

Modanlou H, Yeh SY, Hon EH, et al: Fetal and neonatal biochemistry and Apgar scores. Am J Obstet Gynecol 117:942, 1973.

Myers RE: Experimental models of perinatal brain damage: Relevance to human pathology. In Gluck L (ed): Intrauterine Asphyxia and the Developing Fetal Brain. Chicago, Yearbook Medical Publishers Inc, 1977, p 37.

Nelson KB, Ellenberg JH: Obstetrical complications as risk factors for cerebral palsy or seizure disorders. JAMA 251:1843, 1984.

Rudolph AM: The changes in the circulation after birth. Circulation 41:343, 1970.

Todres ID, Rogers MC: Methods of external cardiac massage in the newborn infant. J Pediatr 86:781, 1975.

Chapter Twelve

OBSTETRIC ANALGESIA AND ANESTHESIA

KENNETH A. CONKLIN

During labor and vaginal delivery, analgesia can be achieved with nonpharmacologic approaches, systemic medication, inhalational agents, or regional analgesic techniques. For cesarean section, regional or general anesthesia may be used (Table 12–1). Important considerations discussed in this chapter include placental drug transfer, the

effects of obstetric analgesia on uterine blood flow and uterine activity, and the analgesic agents and techniques used for labor and vaginal delivery, cesarean section, and complicated obstetric situations.

PLACENTAL TRANSFER OF DRUGS

The effects of a maternally administered drug upon the embryo, fetus, or neonate depend upon the amount of the drug that reaches the fetal circulation. The fetal to maternal ratio (FMR) of the drug concentration is utilized to assess placental drug transfer. This ratio is determined by measuring the drug levels in samples of fetal and maternal blood obtained simultaneously (e.g., at the time of delivery). A high FMR suggests a high degree of placental transfer.

Although all drugs cross the placenta to some extent, the degree of transfer is determined by maternal and fetal blood flow to the placenta, as well as by factors that determine drug passage across the placental barrier itself.

Maternal Circulation of the Placenta

Maternal blood flow to the placenta is governed by the total uterine blood flow and the fraction that perfuses the intervillous space. Anything that reduces uterine blood flow, such as uterine contractions or maternal

TABLE 12–1 ANALGESIC AND ANESTHETIC TECHNIQUES FOR OBSTETRICS

I. Labor and Delivery
  A. Nonpharmacologic approaches
    1. Lamaze
    2. Le Boyer
    3. Acupuncture
    4. Hypnosis
  B. Regional anesthetic techniques
    1. Local infiltration for episiotomy
    2. Epidural
    3. Spinal
    4. Caudal
    5. Paracervical
    6. Pudendal
  C. Systemic Medications
    1. Narcotics
    2. Sedative-tranquilizers
  D. Inhalation analgesics
    1. Nitrous oxide
    2. Penthrane
    3. Ethrane

II. Cesarean Section
  A. Regional anesthesia
    1. Epidural
    2. Spinal
  B. General anesthesia

hypotension, reduces drug delivery to the placenta.

Drug Transfer Across the Placenta

Nearly all drugs cross the placenta by passive diffusion. The amount of transfer is proportional to the concentration gradient of the drug across the placenta. However, the tendency of a drug to cross the placenta depends on its diffusion constant. This is determined by the physicochemical properties of the drug, which include molecular weight, spatial configuration, lipid solubility, degree of ionization, and amount of drug binding to maternal plasma proteins. In general, if the molecular weight is under 1000, the size and spatial configuration do not affect placental transfer. As the amount of protein binding increases, transfer decreases, since only unbound drug can cross the placenta. A highly ionized drug will also exhibit limited placental transfer. Finally, drugs with high lipid solubility tend to cross the placenta readily.

Fetal Circulation of the Placenta

Fetal-placental blood flow via the umbilical arteries has been estimated to be approximately 50 percent of the combined ventricular output. Fetal circulation of the placenta increases with fetal asphyxia, and this may increase placental drug transfer. Fetal asphyxia is also accompanied by a reduced pH of fetal blood, which results in the phenomenon of "ion trapping." In this situation, a lower pH causes a drug that is a weak base (e.g., a narcotic or local anesthetic) to become more highly ionized, thus trapping it in the fetal circulation. This may further increase drug delivery to the fetus during fetal asphyxia.

Evaluating Drug Effects in Newborns

A reduced Apgar score may occur in association with obstetric analgesia or anesthesia, particularly if there is marked hypotension with a spinal or epidural block, or if a high dose of narcotic is administered during labor. However, subtle effects of maternal medication or birth asphyxia may be missed entirely by the Apgar score. Therefore, more sophisticated techniques have been developed for evaluating neurologic and behavioral parameters of the neonate that are controlled by higher central nervous system functions. These evaluations include the Brazelton Neonatal Behavioral Assessment Scale, the Early Neonatal Neurobehavioral Scale, and the Neurologic and Adaptive Capacity Score.

EFFECTS OF OBSTETRIC ANESTHESIA ON UTERINE ACTIVITY AND BLOOD FLOW

Analgesia and anesthesia must be administered to the parturient in a manner that neither reduces uterine activity, which may alter the progress of labor, nor reduces uterine blood flow, which may result in fetal distress.

Effects on Uterine Activity and Labor

The uterus has alpha and beta-2 adrenergic receptors. Alpha adrenergic stimulants increase uterine tone. Conversely, agents with beta-2 adrenergic stimulating properties reduce uterine activity. Epinephrine, a potent beta-2 agonist, can be released from the adrenal glands during the pain and stress of labor, and this may reduce uterine contractility and slow the progress of labor.

Systemic Medication. Narcotics administered during the latent phase of the first stage of labor generally reduce uterine contractions. If given during the active phase, these agents increase or have no effect on uterine activity. Improvement of uterine contractility, when it occurs, is most likely attributable to decreased maternal epinephrine secretion. Tranquilizing agents have little effect on uterine activity when administered during the active phase of labor.

Inhalation Anesthetics. In circumstances such as therapy for a tetanic uterine contraction or for intrauterine manipulations, uterine relaxation is required. The most reliable technique for rapidly producing this effect is with general anesthesia using a high concentration of a halogenated anesthetic (halothane or enflurane). These agents produce a dose-dependent decrease in uterine resting tone, uterine contractility, and uterine responsiveness to oxytocin. These actions, however, can also markedly increase uterine blood loss. Therefore, when these agents are needed for uterine relaxation, they are used for as short a period of time as possible.

Regional Anesthesia. The effect of well-conducted epidural analgesia on uterine activity depends upon whether it is administered during the latent or the active phase of the first stage of labor. When given during the latent phase, epidural analgesia generally reduces uterine activity. Although it is uncertain as to the mechanism involved, interruption of oxytocin release in response to cervical dilatation (Ferguson's reflex) may cause uterine inhibition. During the active phase of the first stage of labor, epidural analgesia has either no significant effect or causes enhanced uterine activity. These beneficial effects are most likely due to reduced maternal epinephrine secretion from blockade of the sympathetic preganglionic innervation of the adrenal glands.

Improperly administered epidural or spinal anesthesia during labor or vaginal delivery may have adverse effects. Hypotension, for example, will reduce uterine activity and slow the process of labor. Excessive anesthesia during the first stage of labor relaxes the pelvic musculature and may interfere with flexion and internal rotation of the fetal head. This can prolong the second stage. The second stage may also be prolonged if the patient's abdominal muscles are relaxed by anesthesia. When this occurs, the parturient is unable to bear down efficiently. In some patients, this problem is compounded by the reduced desire to push when perineal analgesia is produced. In the parturient who is motivated to bear down and is properly instructed, the appropriate use of regional anesthesia without excessive motor blockade will not prolong the second stage of labor.

Effects on Uterine Blood Flow

Normal fetal respiratory gases depend on the maintenance of uterine blood flow (UBF). A drop in UBF due to a decrease in uterine perfusion pressure (UPP) or an increase in uterine vascular resistance may result in hypoxia, hypercarbia, and acidosis in the fetus.

UPP is the difference between uterine arterial pressure (UAP) and uterine venous pressure (UVP). UAP, which is proportional to maternal blood pressure, is reduced by maternal hypotension. This may occur from blockade of the sympathetic nervous system during regional anesthesia if the parturient is not adequately hydrated or if deep general anesthesia with halothane (Fluothane) or enflurane (Ethrane) is administered. These effects may be enhanced by aortocaval compression, which produces the following effects: (1) compression of the inferior vena cava, which elevates UVP and reduces venous return to the heart, thereby causing a fall in cardiac output, maternal blood pressure, and UAP; (2) compression of the aorta above the origin of the uterine arteries, which further reduces UAP.

Intrinsic uterine vascular resistance may be increased when the concentration of local anesthetics in the uterine circulation is very high. This may occur with a paracervical block or if an unintentional intravascular injection is given when attempting epidural anesthesia. Vasopressor drugs that directly stimulate alpha-adrenergic receptors (for example, norepinephrine, epinephrine, and phenylephrine) also increase intrinsic vascular resistance. This effect is not seen with ephedrine (the vasopressor indicated for obstetric use), which possesses direct beta-adrenergic stimulating effects on the heart (beta-1), but only indirect alpha-stimulating effects (release of norepinephrine from sympathetic nerve terminals). Intrinsic vascular resistance may also be increased by release of endogenous cathecholamines when sympathetic nervous system activity is high. Extrinsic uterine vascular resistance is determined by uterine tone.

PAIN PATHWAYS OF PARTURITION

Pain is the sensation of discomfort resulting from stimulation of specialized nerve endings. During labor and vaginal delivery, pain is caused by uterine contractions, dilatation of the cervix, and distension of the perineum. The visceral afferent nerve fibers that carry the sensory impulses from the uterus enter the spinal cord at the tenth, eleventh, and twelfth thoracic and first lumbar spinal segments (T10 to L1). Pain from the perineum travels via somatic afferent nerve fibers, primarily in the pudendal nerve, and reaches the spinal cord through the second, third, and fourth sacral segments (S2 to S4) (Fig. 12–1). These sensory fibers from the uterus and perineum make synaptic connections in

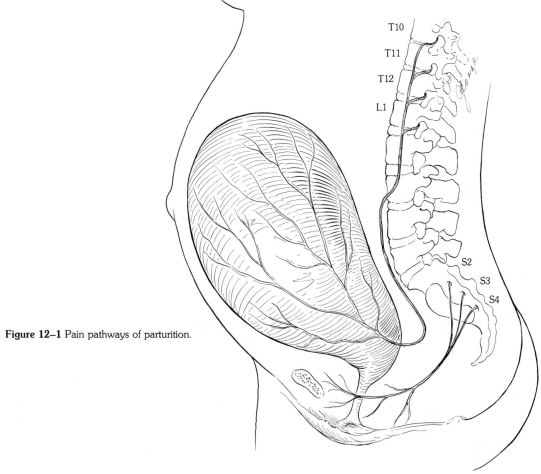

Figure 12–1 Pain pathways of parturition.

the dorsal horn with cells that provide axons that make up the spinothalamic tracts. During the early part of the first stage of labor, pain arises primarily from the uterus. During the latter part of the first stage and throughout the second stage of labor, pain impulses arise not only from the uterus but also from the perineum as the fetal presenting part passes through the pelvis.

SELECTION OF LOCAL ANESTHETICS FOR OBSTETRIC USE

The agents used clinically for regional anesthesia possess the general structure shown in Figure 12–2. The linkage between the aromatic portion and the intermediate chain separates these agents into two groups with important distinctions. Although a rare occurrence, an ester-linked drug (e.g., chloroprocaine, procaine, or tetracaine) is more likely to be associated with allergic reactions

than is an amide-linked agent (e.g., lidocaine or bupivacaine). The ester-linked local anesthetics are rapidly metabolized by plasma cholinesterase, which markedly reduces the potential for maternal systemic toxicity, as well as limits fetal drug exposure and neonatal effects. The amide-linked local anesthetics are slowly degraded by the liver, thus allowing a greater degree of placental transfer.

Placental transfer of the amide-linked local anesthetics, as reflected by fetal/maternal ratios (Table 12–2), is most affected by their degree of ionization and percentage of protein binding in maternal plasma. The low molecular weight (all under 350) and relatively high lipid solubility of these drugs do not significantly impair their passage across the placenta. The FMR of bupivacaine is 0.25, which is considerably lower than that of lidocaine (0.55). This is because the drug is more highly ionized and has a greater degree of protein binding. However, despite

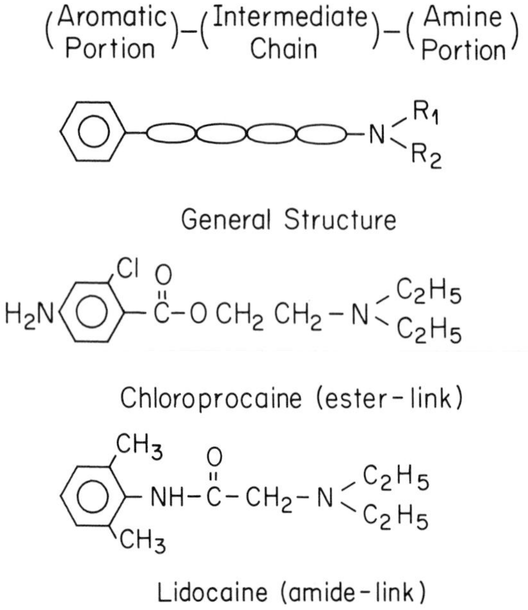

$$\left(\genfrac{}{}{0pt}{}{\text{Aromatic}}{\text{Portion}}\right) - \left(\genfrac{}{}{0pt}{}{\text{Intermediate}}{\text{Chain}}\right) - \left(\genfrac{}{}{0pt}{}{\text{Amine}}{\text{Portion}}\right)$$

General Structure

Chloroprocaine (ester–link)

Lidocaine (amide–link)

Figure 12–2 Structure of local anesthetics. The aromatic portion is primarily responsible for the lipophilic property (lipid solubility) of the local anesthetic, although this property is also affected by the -R groups. The intermediate chain serves to link the aromatic and amine portions of the molecule. The amine portion (generally a tertiary amine) confers upon the local anesthetic the property of being a weak base and is responsible for the hydrophilic property (water solubility) of the drug.

the difference in placental transfer, use of either lidocaine or bupivacaine for well-conducted epidural blocks during labor or cesarean section does not affect Apgar scores or neurobehavioral performance. Therefore, since neonatal outcome is also unaffected by chloroprocaine because of rapid metabolism, the choice of local anesthetic for epidural analgesia or anesthesia is based upon the onset and duration of action of the drugs, as shown in Table 12–2.

ANALGESIA AND ANESTHESIA FOR LABOR AND VAGINAL DELIVERY

Selection of the appropriate analgesic technique for labor and vaginal delivery depends upon the desires of the parturient, the skills of available personnel, the stage of labor, and whether or not contraindications to a particular technique exist.

Systemic Medication

Systemic medication is more easily administered than spinal or epidural blocks but introduces potential adverse effects that are not seen with regional analgesia. Maternal awareness may be depressed, making the parturient less able to participate in the birth process. Systemic medications rapidly cross the placenta and may result in neonatal depression. Additionally, these agents do not provide the degree of analgesia that can be easily achieved with a regional technique. Despite these limitations, systemic medication is still an appropriate means of providing analgesia, especially in situations when an anesthesiologist is unavailable, regional analgesia is contraindicated (in the presence of coagulopathy, skin infection, and certain neurologic and musculoskeletal disorders), or the patient is fearful of regional anesthesia.

Narcotics. Meperidine (Demerol) is the most popular narcotic for the parturient during labor. It is generally administered in doses of 25 to 50 mg intravenously (IV) or 50 to 100 mg intramuscularly (IM). After IV injection, the peak effect is seen in 7 to 8 minutes with a duration of action of 1.5 to 3 hours.

TABLE 12–2 PROPERTIES OF LOCAL ANESTHETICS

PROPERTY	CHLOROPROCAINE	TETRACAINE	LIDOCAINE	BUPIVACAINE
Trade name(s)	Nesacaine	Pontocaine	Xylocaine	Marcaine, Sensorcaine
pKa	8.7	8.2	7.9	8.1
% Ionized (pH 7.4)	95	86	76	83
% Protein bound	—	76	64	95
FMR	—	—	0.55	0.25
Potency	0.7	4	1	4
Use	Epidural	Spinal	Epidural	Epidural
Onset	Rapid	Rapid	Intermediate	Slow
Duration	Short	Long	Intermediate	Long

pKa: Dissociation constant for the drug
FMR: Fetal/maternal ratio

The peak effect and duration of action after an IM dose are 45 minutes and 3 to 4 hours, respectively. Alphaprodine (Nisentil), which is structurally similar to meperidine but much more lipid soluble, is also frequently used. When given IV (two 10-mg doses 5 minutes apart), the peak effect is seen within 1 to 2 minutes (of each injection) with a duration of action of 30 minutes. Alphaprodine can also be given subcutaneously in a dose of 30 mg (peak effect in 20 minutes). A recently introduced narcotic agonist-antagonist, butorphanol (Stadol), is also effective for providing analgesia during labor (1 mg IV or IM). Morphine is rarely used because it is associated with a greater degree of neonatal respiratory depression.

Although narcotics provide both analgesia and sedation, they may be associated with maternal, fetal, or neonatal side effects (Table 12–3). Most side effects can be reversed, however, with naloxone (Narcan), a narcotic antagonist.

Sedative-Tranquilizers. These agents are generally given in combination with a narcotic. The phenothiazine promethazine (Phenergan), 25 mg IM or 12.5 mg IV, relieves anxiety, controls nausea and vomiting, and reduces narcotic requirements during labor. Hydroxyzine (Vistaril), 50 mg IM, has similar properties. These drugs are without significant maternal, fetal, or neonatal side effects when used in recommended doses. Diazepam (Valium) is rarely used in current obstetric practice because it is associated with significant neonatal side effects, including reduced Apgar scores, impaired neurobehavioral status, impaired thermogenesis (hypothermia

TABLE 12–3   POTENTIAL SIDE EFFECTS OF NARCOTICS

I. Maternal
  A. Orthostatic hypotension
  B. Nausea and vomiting
  C. Delayed gastric emptying (increases aspiration risk)
  D. Slowing of labor (if given too early)
  E. Respiratory depression

II. Fetal
  A. Reduced beat-to-beat variability of fetal heart rate

III. Neonatal
  A. Respiratory depression
  B. Decreased Apgar score
  C. Altered neurobehavioral status

when the infant is cold-stressed), and reduced feeding. Fetal tachycardia and reduced beat-to-beat variability are also seen when doses as small as 2.5 mg are given during labor.

Inhalation Analgesia

This technique, which is infrequently used in the United States, involves the administration of subanesthetic concentrations of inhalation agents to provide analgesia during the first and second stages of labor. These drugs are administered with a mask or mouthpiece in a manner such that the parturient remains awake, cooperative, and in control of her airway so as to prevent pulmonary aspiration of gastric contents. Although not comparable with the degree of analgesia or safety of epidural anesthesia, the use of inhalation analgesia is associated with less risk of neonatal depression when compared with narcotics.

Nitrous oxide (N_2O) is the most commonly used inhalation agent. When administered for labor or vaginal delivery, the parturient intermittently breathes a 50 percent concentration of N_2O in oxygen. Intermittent inhalation of methoxyflurane (Penthrane), 0.1 to 0.3 percent in oxygen, or enflurane (0.5 percent in oxygen) are alternative, but less popular, techniques.

Regional Analgesia and Anesthesia

Regional analgesic and anesthetic techniques for labor and delivery include peripheral (paracervical and pudendal) and central (lumbar epidural, caudal, and spinal) nerve blocks. *Epidural anesthesia* is the ideal anesthetic for the obstetric patient. It provides excellent analgesia during labor and anesthesia for vaginal delivery. Should it become necessary, an epidural block initiated during labor can be supplemented to provide anesthesia for cesarean section. A *paracervical block,* which is rarely used, provides analgesia during labor, but only for pain of uterine contractions and only during the early first stage of labor. A *pudendal block* provides perineal analgesia and is appropriate to administer for vaginal delivery as an alternative to an epidural block. A *caudal anesthetic* produces anesthesia that is comparable to spinal anesthesia for delivery but is infrequently used because a spinal block can be more quickly and easily administered.

Paracervical Block. This technique anesthetizes the sensory nerves of the uterus (T10 to L1) by the transvaginal injection of local anesthetic just lateral to the cervix on each side. Although the block is relatively easy to perform and does not produce maternal hypotension, it is associated with a high incidence of fetal distress due to vasoconstriction of the uterine artery caused by the close proximity of the local anesthetic. Additionally, maternal toxicity from intravascular injection (e.g., a local anesthetic-induced seizure), or hematoma formation from uterine artery damage, may occur.

Pudendal Block. A pudendal block for perineal analgesia may be administered shortly before delivery (Fig. 12–3). The pudendal nerve (S2 to S4) is blocked as it travels just posterior to the junction of the ischial spine and sacrospinous ligament. About 10 ml of 1 percent lidocaine or 2 percent chloroprocaine are injected on each side after aspirating to avoid intravascular injection. The analgesia produced in the lower birth canal and perineum allows for low forceps delivery and episiotomy.

A pudendal block is easy to administer, is not associated with maternal hypotension, and is rarely associated with fetal distress. Disadvantages include incomplete analgesia at the time of delivery, since the pain of uterine contractions is unaffected, and incomplete perineal analgesia, especially if vaginal delivery is difficult or if there is extension of the episiotomy. This is because the perineum has sensory innervation from nerves other than the pudendal nerve. Analgesia may be improved by local anesthetic infiltration of the perineum in combination with the pudendal block. Complications include systemic toxic reactions, puncture of the rectum, hematoma formation, and sciatic nerve block if the needle is inserted too deeply.

Epidural Anesthesia. A continuous lumbar epidural analgesic should not be initiated until labor is well established. This is generally when dilatation of the cervix is 4 to 5 cm in a multipara or 5 to 6 cm in a nullipara, uterine contractions are strong and regular, and the fetal head is engaged. A 19- or 20-

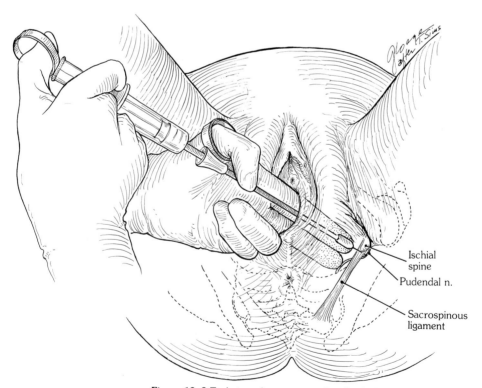

Ischial spine

Pudendal n.

Sacrospinous ligament

Figure 12–3 Technique for transvaginal pudendal block.

gauge indwelling catheter is inserted into the epidural space at the L3–4 interspace through a special needle (e.g., Touhy).

During the early active phase of labor, relatively small doses of local anesthetic (e.g., 6 to 8 ml of 0.25 percent bupivacaine) provide adequate segmental analgesia (T10 to L1) for pain arising from the uterus. During the latter part of the first stage, the level of analgesia should be extended (T10 to S5) so that perineal discomfort is also relieved. This is accomplished by increasing the anesthetic dose (e.g., 8 to 12 ml of 0.25 percent bupivacaine) and elevating the patient's head 20 to 30 degrees. This technique can also be utilized to provide analgesia during the second stage of labor. Shortly before vaginal delivery, anesthesia from T10 to S5 is generally accomplished by injection of 10 to 12 ml of 3 percent chloroprocaine. To achieve perineal analgesia and muscle relaxation, the anesthetic is injected with the parturient in the sitting position. Chloroprocaine is used in this situation because of its rapid onset and short duration of action.

Certain precautions must be taken when administering an epidural anesthetic. After negative aspiration for blood and cerebrospinal fluid (CSF), an initial test dose of 3 ml is given, and any evidence of a spinal block (e.g., the rapid onset of sensory loss) is checked for. Assuming that the initial test dose does not produce a spinal block, a second test dose of 5 ml is given to exclude the possibility of intravascular injection. If signs of intravascular injection, such as dizziness or tinnitus, do not occur, the remaining dose of local anesthetic is administered at the rate of 5 ml per minute. If the local anesthetic solution contains epinephrine (5 μg/ml), tachycardia occurring after a test dose also indicates an intravascular injection. A balanced salt solution must be administered IV concomitantly with an epidural anesthetic to prevent maternal hypotension.

Spinal (Subarachnoid) Anesthesia. A subarachnoid block is generally administered shortly before delivery by injecting a small amount of local anesthetic (e.g., 4 mg of tetracaine or 30 mg of lidocaine) through a spinal needle placed in the L3–4 interspace. To prevent the anesthetic level from ascending too high, the local anesthetic solution is made hyperbaric (with respect to CSF) by the addition of 10 percent dextrose, and the injection is made with the parturient in the sitting position. The anesthetic level should extend to T10. As with an epidural block, an IV crystalloid solution (600 to 800 ml) must be given to prevent hypotension. Although some have advocated the use of a "saddle block" (a spinal anesthetic of S1 to S5) for vaginal delivery, this procedure does not provide complete pain relief, since the sensory nerves from the uterus are not anesthetized.

The main disadvantage of spinal anesthesia is the occurrence of a postspinal headache, a complication that is more likely in the pregnant than the nonpregnant patient. The etiology of the headache is loss of CSF through the hole in the dura, creating traction on the meninges. The incidence of this complication can be minimized by using either a small gauge spinal needle (25 or 26 gauge) or a special spinal needle (Whitacre type) that separates, but does not cut, the longitudinal fibers of the dura.

Caudal Anesthesia. This type of anesthesia is performed by injecting local anesthetic into the sacral epidural space. Entrance to this space is gained by placing an epidural needle through the sacrococcygeal membrane that covers the sacral hiatus. One advantage of a caudal block is that good perineal anesthesia can be achieved without placing the parturient in the sitting position. Disadvantages are the larger dose of local anesthetic needed to produce anesthesia (compared with a spinal or lumbar epidural block) and the technical difficulty that is commonly encountered when performing the procedure.

General Anesthesia

General anesthesia is not administered electively for vaginal delivery because the parturient is at substantial risk of pulmonary aspiration of gastric contents when unconscious. However, if an emergency arises in which rapid anesthesia is necessary, such as for shoulder dystocia, undiagnosed twins, or breech presentation, general anesthesia is indicated. A high concentration of halothane (2 percent) or enflurane (4 percent) is used when uterine relaxation is necessary.

ANESTHESIA FOR CESAREAN SECTION

The choice of anesthetic technique for cesarean section depends upon the desire of the patient, the skills of the anesthesiologist, and the reason for the operation. Regional anesthesia is generally considered to be superior to general anesthesia. It allows the parturient to be awake and the father to be present, reduces blood loss, is associated with less risk of maternal aspiration of gastric contents, and reduces neonatal drug effects.

Although either a spinal or epidural block is appropriate, the latter technique has several advantages. With epidural anesthesia, hypotension is less likely to occur because the sympathetic nervous system is blocked more slowly. Anesthesia is more controllable if an epidural catheter is placed, since additional anesthetic doses can be given if necessary. Furthermore, a headache does not occur postoperatively, since the dura is not punctured. A spinal anesthetic is technically easier to administer, and the anesthetic takes effect much more quickly. It would be indicated when it is desirable to use regional anesthesia for a cesarean section, but time does not permit placement of an epidural block.

Compared with regional anesthesia, general anesthesia has the advantage of greater cardiovascular stability (i.e., less hypotension) and more rapid institution of anesthesia. It would thus be indicated when urgent cesarean section is required, such as for maternal hemorrhage or profound fetal distress.

Regardless of the anesthetic technique selected, certain precautions should be taken to reduce maternal risk and to optimize fetal well-being and neonatal outcome. A clear, nonparticulate antacid (e.g., 30 ml of 0.3 molar sodium citrate) should be administered 30 to 60 minutes prior to anesthesia to reduce the maternal risk of pulmonary aspiration of acidic gastric contents. The maternal blood pressure and electrocardiogram (EKG) should be monitored throughout the procedure. Left uterine displacement should be used to prevent aortocaval compression.

If regional anesthesia is selected, 1500 to 2000 ml of a balanced salt solution containing 0.5 to 1 percent dextrose must be administered IV to prevent hypotension. Ephedrine should be available for treatment of hypotension, and supplemental oxygen should be given to the mother to increase placental oxygen transfer and reduce the chance of fetal distress if hypotension does occur.

If the anesthetic is appropriately administered, whether it be general or regional, Apgar scores will be unaffected, regardless of the time from induction of anesthesia to delivery. Apgar scores after cesarean section are depressed, however, with prolonged uterine incision to delivery times (that is, greater that 90 seconds). Neurobehavioral status, which is unaffected by regional anesthesia, is temporarily impaired when general anesthesia is used. This is due to the thiopental or ketamine administered for induction of general anesthesia. The other drugs used for general anesthesia do not affect infant outcome, either because of the low concentration used (N_2O and halothane) or because of very limited placental transfer (as with muscle relaxants, which are fully ionized quaternary ammonium compounds).

Epidural Anesthesia

The local anesthetics used for cesarean section include lidocaine (1.5 or 2 percent), chloroprocaine (3 percent), and bupivacaine (0.5 percent). A very large dose (20 ml) of local anesthetic is used, and the precautions previously described must be taken. The desired level of anesthesia is T4 to S5.

Spinal Anesthesia

The block is generally performed with the patient in the lateral position. After identifying the subarachnoid space, 7 to 9 mg of tetracaine or 60 to 70 mg of lidocaine is slowly injected. The local anesthetic solution is made hyperbaric by the addition of dextrose (final concentration 5 percent), and a small dose of epinephrine (e.g., 50 μg) may be added to prolong the duration of anesthesia. The patient is then immediately turned supine and a right hip wedge placed so that anesthesia will be achieved bilaterally. Some anesthesiologists administer 25 mg of ephedrine 15 minutes before performing the block for prophylaxis against hypotension.

General Anesthesia

There are two primary concerns during induction of general anesthesia. The first is for maternal aspiration of acidic gastric contents, a risk that results from loss of the protective laryngeal reflexes during induction. This risk is reduced by antacid administration and by application of pressure on the cricoid cartilage to occlude the esophagus until the airway is secured with a cuffed endotracheal tube. The second concern is for maternal and fetal oxygenation. When apneic, as during induction of anesthesia, the pregnant patient becomes hypoxic much more rapidly than a nonpregnant individual because of the increased oxygen consumption and reduced functional residual capacity. Therefore, the patient must breathe 100 percent oxygen for at least five minutes before induction of anesthesia.

Induction of general anesthesia is accomplished with intravenous injection of thiopental (Pentothal), 3 to 4 mg/kg. In certain circumstances, such as maternal hemorrhage, ketamine (0.75 mg/kg) is used for induction of anesthesia because it causes less depression of the maternal cardiovascular system. Endotracheal intubation is facilitated by injection of the depolarizing muscle relaxant, succinylcholine (Anectine, 1.5 mg/kg), immediately following the thiopental or ketamine. Anesthesia is maintained until delivery of the fetus with 50 percent N_2O in oxygen. A low concentration of halothane (0.5 percent) or enflurane (1 percent) is also administered to increase the depth of anesthesia, thus reducing maternal blood levels of catecholamines and maintaining better uteroplacental perfusion. Following delivery of the fetus, it is common practice to discontinue the halothane (or enflurane) and deepen the anesthetic by administration of a narcotic. Muscle relaxation is maintained during the procedure with succinylcholine or a nondepolarizing muscle relaxant, such as curare, metocurine, or pancuronium.

ANESTHESIA FOR COMPLICATED OBSTETRICS

Pregnancy-Induced Hypertension

Continuous lumbar epidural anesthesia is the technique of choice during labor and vaginal delivery. Once active labor begins, or earlier if labor is being augmented with oxytocin, the epidural catheter is placed, provided that there is no contraindication. Epidural analgesia, which should be continuous throughout labor and vaginal delivery, provides optimal patient comfort, improves uterine blood flow, helps control blood pressure,

and reduces the chance of seizures (low blood levels of local anesthetics depress the CNS).

When cesarean section is necessary, epidural anesthesia provides the greatest maternal and fetal safety. Spinal anesthesia is less desirable, since hypotension is more likely, although the risk of hypotension is less during regional anesthesia in a pre-eclamptic patient than in a normal parturient.

General anesthesia introduces several factors that increase maternal and fetal risk. Maternal blood pressure can increase significantly, causing a decrease in cardiac index and uterine blood flow; it may also result in left ventricular failure with pulmonary edema or intracranial hemorrhage. Therefore, use of a potent vasodilator, such as IV nitroglycerin or sodium nitroprusside, is necessary to prevent exacerbation of maternal hypertension. Care must also be taken with the administration of muscle relaxants, since magnesium, which is commonly used to treat preeclampsia, enhances their action. Because of the increased maternal risk during general anesthesia, invasive hemodynamic monitoring of blood pressure (intra-arterial catheter) and possibly cardiac filling pressures (central venous or pulmonary artery catheter) are indicated. Additionally, fluid administration should be somewhat restricted with either regional or general anesthesia to reduce the risk of pulmonary edema.

Heart Disease

The choice of analgesic or anesthetic technique for the parturient with heart disease depends, in general, upon whether or not the hemodynamic changes brought about by a lumbar epidural block will be tolerated. Patients with aortic stenosis or coarctation of the aorta have a fixed obstruction to ejection of left ventricular output that prevents increases in stroke volume. Thus, they may not be able to compensate for the reduction of venous return and systemic vascular resistance that occur with epidural anesthesia, and hypotension may result. Patients with right-to-left shunts (tetralogy of Fallot, Eisenmenger's syndrome) also may not tolerate epidural anesthesia, since a fall in systemic vascular resistance will increase the shunt. Finally, patients with primary pulmonary hypertension do not tolerate decreases in preload. Therefore, in patients with these cardiac lesions, labor is likely to be most safely managed with systemic medication and a pudendal block for delivery. General anesthesia is perferred for cesarean section.

The clinical course of parturients with other cardiac lesions may actually be improved when epidural anesthesia is used. For example, patients with mitral stenosis, mitral regurgitation, aortic regurgitation, patent ductus arteriosus, and atrial or ventricular septal defects (with left-to-right shunts) may not tolerate the cardiovascular changes associated with pain and increased sympathetic activity during labor and delivery. Thus, lumbar epidural analgesia is the technique of choice. Generally, with these cardiac lesions, cesarean section is also best managed with epidural anesthesia, and if indicated, hemodynamic monitoring.

Breech Presentation

Systemic medication during labor and pudendal block at the time of delivery (to preserve maximum ability to push) may be used for breech presentations. Epidural anesthesia is an alternative that provides superior analgesia without the side effects of systemic agents. With proper coaching and the use of appropriate local anesthetic doses during the second stage, the parturient can push effectively. At the time of delivery, the epidural block can provide perineal relaxation for delivery of the fetal head. Regardless of the technique employed, the anesthesiologist must be prepared to utilize general anesthesia to facilitate a difficult breech delivery.

Multiple Gestation

Use of continuous epidural anesthesia reduces infant mortality, shortens the interval between delivery of the first and second twin, facilitates forceps deliveries when indicated, and may allow for version and extraction when necessary. General anesthesia with halothane may be necessary to provide uterine relaxation should rapid delivery of the second twin become necessary.

SUGGESTED READING

Amiel-Tison C, Barrier G, Shnider SM, et al: A new neurologic and adaptive capacity scoring system for evaluating obstetric medications in full term newborns. Anesthesiology 56:340, 1982.

Apgar V: A proposal for a new method of evaluation of the newborn infant. Anesth Analg 32:260, 1953.

Caton D: Obstetric anesthesia and concepts of placental transport: A historical review of the nineteenth century. Anesthesiology 46:132, 1977.

Conklin KA, Murad SHN: Pharmacology of drugs in obstetric anesthesia. Semin Anesth 1:83, 1982.

Datta S, Alper MH: Anesthesia for cesarean section. Anesthesiology 53:142, 1980.

Ralston DH, Shnider SM: The fetal and neonatal effects of regional anesthesia in obstetrics. Anesthesiology 43:34, 1978.

Scanlon JW, Brown WU, Weiss JB, et al: Neurobehavioral responses of newborn infants after maternal epidural anesthesia. Anesthesiology 40:121, 1974.

Wright JP: Anesthetic considerations in pre-eclampsia-eclampsia. Anesth Analg 62:590, 1983.

ANTEPARTUM HEMORRHAGE

JUAN J. ARCE and JOHN MORRIS

Vaginal bleeding in the second half of pregnancy occurs in less than 5 percent of pregnancies. The incidence of prematurity and the perinatal mortality rate are at least quadrupled in pregnancies complicated by bleeding during the second and third trimesters. The causes of antepartum hemorrhage are listed in Table 13–1.

In the presurgical era, maternal mortality was as high as 50 percent and fetal mortality as high as 90 percent. At that time, most patients with severe antepartum bleeding were treated expectantly. Subsequently, some cases were treated with rather ingenious but questionable maneuvers, including external or internal version and traction on the fetal skull with the Willet scalp clamp to tamponade the source of bleeding. These maneuvers decreased maternal mortality when practiced by skilled obstetricians.

Early in the present century, cesarean section became the cornerstone of management for placenta previa and significantly decreased both maternal and fetal mortality. The utilization of blood transfusions in the 1940s allowed the obstetrician to prolong the pregnancy in order to overcome the problems of prematurity.

INITIAL EVALUATION

Unless the bleeding is profuse and the patient hemodynamically unstable, the initial evaluation of a patient with an antepartum hemorrhage should consist of a history, physical examination, and special investigations designed to establish the cause of bleeding.

History

The nature and duration of the bleeding should be determined, and any associated symptoms, such as pain or uterine contractions, should be elicited. The medical record should be reviewed to determine whether or not a Pap smear was performed during the present pregnancy. If a recent Pap smear was negative, cervical cancer as a cause for the bleeding is unlikely. It is also important to review the time of the last menstrual period, onset of fetal movements, time of first fetal heart tones, previous ultrasonic examinations, and fundal height measurements in order to determine the gestational age accurately.

TABLE 13–1 CAUSES OF ANTEPARTUM HEMORRHAGE

Unknown etiology
Placental
 Placenta previa
 Abruptio placentae
 Vasa previa
Cervical
 Carcinoma
 Erosion
 Polyp
Vaginal
 Varicose veins
 Lacerations
Uterine
 Fibromyomata
Bowel or bladder bleeding

Physical Examination

The amount of bleeding should be noted, and the patient's color, pulse rate, and blood pressure recorded. Uterine tenderness or contractions should be noted, as should the presence or absence of fetal heart sounds. Sterile speculum examination should be performed to rule out a vaginal or cervical cause for the bleeding, but digital pelvic examinations should be avoided until placenta previa has been excluded by ultrasonography.

Investigations

A complete blood count should be obtained and compared with previous evaluations to help assess the amount of blood loss. The most important step in the initial evaluation is to carry out an immediate ultrasonic examination to determine the location of the placenta (Fig. 13–1). In addition to determining its location, the characteristics of the placenta are also carefully assessed, although retroplacental clots are rarely visualized in the presence of a placental abruption. Occasionally, uterine fibroids are seen, but these rarely cause vaginal bleeding. The ultrasonic assessment should include measurement of the biparietal diameter (BPD) and femur length to confirm the gestational age.

Principles of Management

The patient should be admitted to the hospital and blood should be sent for cross-matching. If there is any hypotension, immediate resuscitation with intravenous crystalloids, colloids, and packed red blood cells is indicated. Uterine activity and fetal heart rate should be monitored to establish fetal well-being and to rule out labor. If the pregnancy is preterm (less than 37 weeks), efforts are directed towards expectant management if the bleeding is not excessive. Beyond 37 weeks, delivery of the fetus is usually appropriate. The management of cervical cancer in pregnancy is discussed in Chapter 53.

PLACENTA PREVIA

Placenta previa implies implantation of part or all of the placenta in the lower uterine segment. The condition is associated with an increased perinatal mortality, principally because of prematurity and intrauterine hypoxia. Maternal mortality is also increased, principally because of hemorrhage and infection.

Classification

The classification of placenta previa is based upon the location of the placenta in relation to the internal cervical os (Fig. 13–2). The classification is made on the basis of findings at the initial examination, since as labor progresses and the lower segment retracts, the findings may change.

Central or Complete Placenta Previa. The placenta is implanted centrally so as to com-

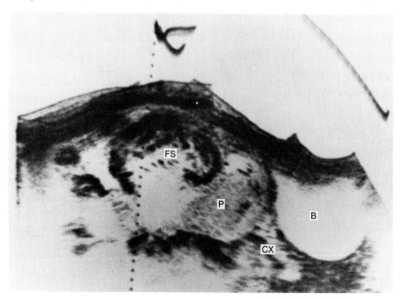

Figure 13–1 Ultrasonic examination of a patient with an antepartum hemorrhage caused by placenta previa. Fetal shoulder (FS), placenta (P), cervix (CX), and bladder (B) are indicated.

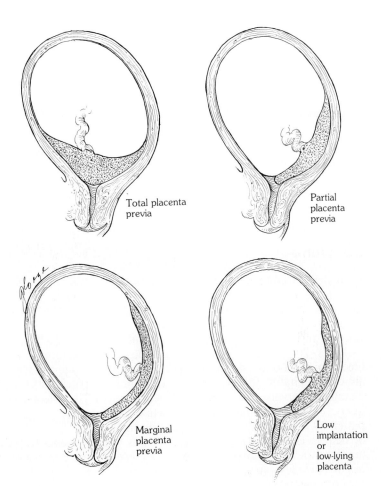

Figure 13–2 Types of placenta previa.

pletely cover the internal cervical os. Approximately 25 percent of the cases will have a central implantation, and this is by far the most dangerous location.

Partial Placenta Previa. This occurs when the cervical os is partially covered by placental tissues.

Marginal Placenta Previa. The edge of the placenta extends to the margins of the internal os.

Low Lying Placenta. A portion of the placenta is implanted into the lower uterine segment, but the lower edge is away from the internal os.

Ventral and Dorsal Implantation. Placental localization may be further defined as either anterior (ventral) or posterior (dorsal). Posterior implantation is particularly troublesome in that the placental mass may obstruct the engagement of the presenting part during labor.

Incidence

Placenta previa occurs in approximately 1 in 250 live births, and accounts for about 20 percent of cases of antepartum hemorrhage. The true incidence is difficult to assess because some patients with a low-lying placenta will remain asymptomatic throughout the pregnancy. In addition, placental migration, the so-called peripatetic placenta, alters the incidence figures. Recurrent placenta previa occurs in up to 6 percent of patients.

Etiology

Low implantation occurs 10 to 20 times more frequently in association with spontaneous abortion than with term or preterm pregnancies. Placenta previa tends to be associated with fetal abnormalities, twin gestation, and placenta accreta. In addition, patients with placenta previa may give a history of multiple uterine curettages.

Advanced maternal age, previous cesarean section, and grand multiparity have also been associated with this entity. Perhaps this is the result of the change in size and contour of the uterine cavity, predisposing to lower implantation of the fertilized ovum.

The bleeding is caused by separation of the placenta as the lower uterine segment lengthens during late pregnancy. The blood is maternal in origin.

Symptoms

Painless, bright red vaginal bleeding in the third trimester is the most important symptom and should be regarded as due to placenta previa until proven otherwise. In occasional instances, the bleeding is evident as early as 20 weeks. Once one episode of bleeding has occurred, subsequent episodes almost inevitably follow, usually at unpredictable intervals, but with increasing frequency. The bleeding may occur while the patient is at rest, and may be relatively light or heavy. The initial bleeding rarely leads to maternal or fetal mortality; however, subsequent episodes can be extremely dangerous for both the mother and her fetus. In contrast to placental abruption, bleeding from a placenta previa is never occult, and thus, clinical signs of hypovolemia bear a relationship to the severity of the bleeding.

Physical Examination

On abdominal examination, the uterus is typically nontender and nonirritable. The fetus is easily outlined, and an abnormal lie, such as transverse or oblique, may be present. If a longitudinal lie is present, the presenting part is high above the inlet.

Although the definitive diagnosis is made by palpating the placenta through the cervical os, digital examination should be avoided until a decision must be made regarding the method of delivery, as such examination may precipitate profuse bleeding.

Placental Localization

In the past, diagnostic methods included soft tissue radiography, angiography, and am-

niography. Later, radioisotope techniques using radiolabelled human serum albumin were popular. In the last decade or so, ultrasonic techniques have been used exclusively for placental localization and have a 95 percent accuracy. The use of ultrasound during the first or second trimester has become very popular, and placental localization is part of the standard ultrasonic evaluation. Even if the placenta is found to be centrally located during the second trimester, less than 15 percent of such cases will have a persistent placenta previa at term. The apparent migratory change in placental position (the so-called peripatetic placenta) is believed to be secondary to elongation of both the upper and lower uterine segments. Accordingly, reassessment as to location is indicated every four to six weeks.

If the placenta is implanted on the posterior wall of the uterus, its lower margin may be obscured, especially when the vertex of the fetus is located in this area. Under these circumstances, the diagnosis of the type of placenta previa can only be confirmed with a "double set-up" examination (see below).

Management

General Measures. On admission, immediate measures to correct apparent or potential hypovolemic shock must be initiated. A wide-bore catheter is inserted into an appropriate vein. Blood is drawn for estimation of hemoglobin and hematocrit and for crossmatching of at least two units of blood. A central venous pressure line or preferably a Swan-Ganz catheter will help to evaluate the hemodynamic status of the patient.

Little change in vital signs may occur, despite a brisk vaginal hemorrhage. The usual signs of hypovolemia are blunted because of the 35 percent increase in blood volume that characterizes normal pregnancy. A fall in hematocrit is usually the first alteration observed, as extravascular fluid is absorbed through the microcirculation to maintain blood volume. Hypotension and tachycardia are more serious signs. The amount of blood loss is often underestimated.

Specific Measures. Prior to fetal maturity, prolongation of the pregnancy is desirable, provided the bleeding settles and the fetus is healthy. The concept of expectant management developed in the 1940s when blood transfusions became available and the first episode of bleeding due to placenta previa was reported to be rarely fatal to either the mother or fetus. The patient should be carefully monitored for fetal distress and uterine activity in a tertiary care center.

When the fetus reaches maturity, a *double set-up examination* remains the standard of care, especially when the lowermost margin of the placenta cannot be adequately assessed with ultrasonic examination. The following requirements must be observed for this examination:

1. Fetal maturity must be confirmed either by amniocentesis or by ultrasonography.

2. The procedure must be conducted in an operating room; all personnel needed for a possible cesarean section must be in attendance, including the anesthesiologist and pediatrician.

3. The patient must be prepped and draped for abdominal surgery.

4. At least 2 liters of crossmatched blood must be available.

When these conditions are met, a speculum is carefully inserted to inspect the cervix. If no local source of bleeding is seen, the speculum is removed and the fornices manually palpated to determine whether or not there is placental tissue between the cervix and the presenting part. A cushionlike sensation will indicate the presence of placenta. At this point, a finger is inserted carefully into the cervical canal and gently advanced towards the internal os. If placental tissue is palpated, the procedure is terminated and a cesarean section done. If no tissue is palpated at the internal os, the finger is advanced to assess the presenting part, whereupon the membranes may be stripped away from the lower segment in order to feel for the margins of the placenta.

Fewer double set-up examinations are performed today than in the past because of accurate localization of the placenta by ultrasound; however, the procedure still has its place in modern obstetrics.

Cesarean section is the preferred method of delivery in all cases of complete and partial placenta previa and in many cases of marginal or low-lying placenta. In the latter situation, the obstetrician may elect amniotomy and a trial of induction of labor, provided the cervix is favorable. While there is no ideal method of anesthesia for this particular complication of pregnancy, most authorities recommend general anesthesia for cesarean section. A low vertical incision in the uterus is preferred over a transverse incision, except in those patients in whom the placenta is implanted posteriorly or in whom the lower uterine segment has thinned out.

Special precautions must be taken to avoid excessive blood loss when entering the uterine cavity. Incising an anterior placenta is acceptable but should be avoided if possible. It is preferable to manually dissect the upper pole of the placenta off the uterus, rupture the membranes, and deliver the fetus. Immediate cord clamping avoids fetal blood loss.

Complications

At delivery, *placenta accreta* may be encountered. It is most common in cases of multiparity and especially in cases with a history of previous uterine surgery. This condition may require emergency hysterectomy.

Postpartum hemorrhage due to the diminished contractile capacity of the lower uterine segment may create profuse blood loss. Under these circumstances, measures to correct this problem will include massage of the uterus, and administration of intravenous oxytocin, ergonovine (Ergotrate), and/or 15-methylprostaglandin F_2-alpha. When these agents fail, bilateral uterine artery ligation or total hysterectomy may be necessary. Complications associated with massive blood loss include *transfusion reactions*, *serum hepatitis*, and *pituitary insufficiency*. Puerperal infection is more common in patients with placenta previa because of the close proximity of the placental site to the vaginal flora.

ABRUPTIO PLACENTAE

Definition and Classification

Abruptio placentae is the clinical term used to describe the partial or complete detachment of the placenta from its normal site of implantation. The condition is sometimes referred to as an *accidental hemorrhage*. Lesser degrees of separation, particularly those sometimes identified as marginal separations or marginal sinus bleeds, are not true abruptions. Abruptio placentae complicates about 1 in 200 deliveries and accounts for about 30 percent of cases of antepartum hemorrhage. As with placenta previa, it is associated with a significantly increased perinatal and maternal mortality.

Classification of the degree of placental separation is usually based upon the percentage of the maternal surface of the placenta covered with adherent clot.

Etiology

The etiology of premature separation of the placenta is uncertain and speculative. Rarely, a traumatic origin seems probable, such as blunt or sharp abdominal trauma or acute velocity changes associated with automobile accidents. However, most separations are spontaneous and nontraumatic. Factors associated with the entity include gestational hypertension, acute decompression of an overdistended uterus (twins, hydramnios), short umbilical cord, uterine anomaly or tumor, folic acid deficiency, multiparity, and advanced maternal age. Most of these associated factors are not good predictors and, therefore, do not afford the clinician a method of predicting which patients will develop placental abruption.

Pathophysiology

While the causes of the focal placental separation are not known, much less the mechanisms by which it is usually self-limiting, the maternal bleeding into the decidua basalis leads to a decidual (retroplacental) hematoma. Whether this is due to some inherent weakness in the anchoring villi or in the fibrous septae or to an anomaly in the spiral arterioles is uncertain.

As the abruption evolves, blood coagulates and slowly dissects between the decidua and the fetal membranes. If the blood dissects upwards toward the fundus, the hemorrhage will remain concealed. If the blood dissects downward and eventually escapes through the cervix, the bleeding becomes revealed. In severe cases, hemoglobin penetrates the chorionic and amniotic membranes to discolor the amniotic fluid. Blood also infiltrates the myometrium. This can be quite extensive, and the clinical appearance of the uterus at the time of cesarean section is referred to as a *"Couvelaire"* uterus. Rarely does this uterus fail to contract, either postpartum or postoperatively.

If profound hypotension occurs, the patient may become anuric because of *acute tubular necrosis* (which is usually reversible) or *bilateral renal cortical necrosis* (which is usually irreversible).

Tissue thromboplastin from the disrupted placenta and the subplacental decidua enters the blood stream and initiates a consumption coagulopathy or *disseminated intravascular coagulation*. Fibrinogen, platelets, and other clotting factors, particularly factors V, VIII, and XIII, are consumed. Simultaneously, fibrinolysis produces fibrin degradation (split) products.

Symptoms

The clinical presentation of vaginal bleeding and uterine pain should immediately suggest the diagnosis of placental abruption. The clinical manifestations are usually proportional to the degree of separation, but the actual volume of blood loss may not be apparent because the bleeding may be concealed as a retroplacental clot. A combination of both revealed and concealed bleeding is not unusual, and the diagnosis may be totally unsuspected and made only on postpartum inspection of the placenta. In contrast to the bright red bleeding associated with placenta previa, the revealed blood of abruptio placentae is usually dark because it has been retained in the uterus for some time.

Physical Examination

The patient may exhibit tachycardia and hemorrhagic shock out of proportion to the amount of revealed hemorrhage. In contrast to placenta previa, the uterus is usually hypertonic and tender to palpation. An increasing fundal height, determined by periodic measurements, may give an indication of continued concealed bleeding. The fetus may be difficult to outline. The fetal lie is usually longitudinal, and the presenting part may be deep in the pelvis. Fetal heart tones may be normal in mild cases or completely absent in severe cases.

Management

The clinical management is highly variable and depends upon factors such as gestational age, fetal distress, cervical dilatation, hemodynamic status, and the presence or absence of a coagulopathy. Nevertheless, therapeutic priorities are the replacement of lost blood and the safe and timely termination of the pregnancy for both mother and fetus. The immediate priorities are:

1. To secure one or more intravenous lines and resuscitate the patient. A central venous pressure catheter or a Swan-Ganz catheter may be required in complicated, hemodynamically unstable cases.

2. To determine fetal well-being using electronic fetal monitoring.

3. To assess uterine activity using external tocography. A uterine pressure tracing that reflects *both* uterine hypertonicity and tachysystole is almost diagnostic of premature separation of the placenta (Fig. 13–3). Abnormal fetal heart rate patterns usually accompany the abnormal uterine contractions.

4. To establish fetal age, fetal maturity, and placental localization using real-time ultrasound.

Concurrently, blood should be drawn for crossmatching, and a clot observation test carried out. If the blood does not clot, or if an unstable clot forms and disintegrates, a clotting defect can be diagnosed. A peripheral Wright stained blood smear should be examined for platelets, and a microhematocrit performed. Laboratory tests for disseminated intravascular coagulation should be ordered, including prothrombin time, activated partial thromboplastin time, fibrinogen level, and fibrin degradation products.

A Foley catheter may be necessary in the "moderate" and "severe" cases of placental separation to assess urine output accurately while initiating appropriate fluid replacement. The latter should initially be a Ringer's lactate solution or normal saline, followed by crossmatched whole blood or packed red blood cells when available. If crossmatched blood is not readily available, a colloid solution such as plasmanate should be used. If hypofibrinogenemia is evident (no clot retraction in 30 minutes), cryoprecipitate is useful. Terminating the pregnancy is the only way to reverse the coagulopathy.

If the bleeding is heavy or the pregnancy is beyond about 36 weeks, rupture of the membranes is required to induce labor as soon as possible. This is usually done at the time of a double set-up to exclude placenta previa. Oxytocin may be utilized to augment labor if necessary. Vaginal delivery is the route of choice in the absence of fetal distress or in the presence of a dead fetus. Even though the cervix is uneffaced, the uterus is usually sufficiently irritable that vaginal delivery can be expeditiously accomplished, particularly in multiparae. Cesarean section is indicated if labor does not ensue promptly in spite of amniotomy and oxytocic stimulation.

VASA PREVIA

Vasa previa occurs with velamentous insertion of the cord and implies the presence of

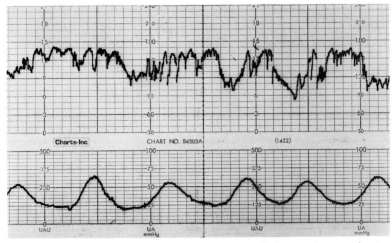

Figure 13–3 Recording of strip monitor from a patient with abruptio placentae showing an internal reading of intra-amniotic pressure and fetal heart rate. Note the increased uterine tone and failure of the uterus to relax between contractions. Note also the tachysystole and the increased vagal response of the fetal heart rate.

fetal blood vessels in the membranes overlying the internal os and in front of the fetal presenting part. The vessels may be palpated or demonstrated at amnioscopy. Since bleeding from vasa previa is from the fetus, only a relatively small amount of blood loss can occur before the fetus exsanguinates. A Kleihauer-Betke test on the blood demonstrates the presence of fetal red cells (see Chapter 25). Unless immediate vaginal delivery can be expedited, urgent cesarean section is indicated. In either case, fetal prognosis is poor.

BLEEDING OF UNKNOWN ETIOLOGY

This represents the largest single etiologic group. The diagnosis is made only after exclusion of other known causes. Patients in this category generally have spotting or minimal bleeding only. Some of these patients may have minor degrees of separation, either of the placenta or of an undiagnosed accessory lobe. Others may be bleeding from a marginal sinus, although the existence of this entity is controversial.

SUGGESTED READING

Benedetti TJ, Cotton DB, Reed JC, et al: Hemodynamic observations in severe pre-eclampsia with a flow-directed pulmonary artery catheter. Am J Obstet Gynecol 136:465, 1980.

Brenner BF, Edelman DA, Hendricks CH: Characteristics of patients with placenta previa and results of "expectant management." Am J Obstet Gynecol 132:180, 1978.

Cotton DB, Reed JA, Paul RH, et al: The conservative aggressive management of placenta previa. Am J Obstet Gynecol 137:687, 1980.

DeValera E: Abruptio placentae. Am J Obstet Gynecol 100:599, 1968.

Hibbard LT: Fetal mortality in placenta previa. Obstet Gynecol 8:163, 1956.

Hynes DM: Premature separation of placenta: Ten years' experience. Am J Obstet Gynecol 96:660, 1966.

King DL: Placental migration demonstrated by ultrasonography. Radiology 109:167, 1973.

Knab DR: Abruptio placentae: An assessment of the time and method of delivery. Obstet Gynecol 52:625, 1978.

Page EW, King EB, Merrill JA: Abruptio placentae: Dangers of delays in delivery. Obstet Gynecol 3:385, 1964.

Pedowitz P: Placenta previa: An evaluation for expectant management and the factors responsible for fetal wastage. Am J Obstet Gynecol 93:16, 1965.

Pritchard JA, Brekken AL: Clinical and laboratory studies on severe abruptio placentae. Am J Obstet Gynecol 97:681, 1967.

Silver R, Depp R, Sabbagha RE, et al: Placenta previa: Aggressive expectant management. Am J Obstet Gynecol 150:15, 1984.

Chapter Fourteen

HYPERTENSIVE DISORDERS OF PREGNANCY

CHARLES R. BRINKMAN III

The hypertensive disorders of pregnancy are major contributors to maternal and perinatal morbidity and mortality. Complications from hypertensive disorders of pregnancy currently represent the single most common cause of maternal death in virtually all developed countries. The reported incidence depends upon the criteria for diagnosis, and there is a distinct lack of uniformity. In Great Britain, with primarily a Caucasian population, some form of hypertension occurs in 25 percent of pregnancies. In the United States, the incidence reported by the Task Force on Toxemia of the Collaborative Perinatal Project was 28 percent for whites and 36 percent for blacks.

CLASSIFICATION AND DEFINITIONS

The classification of hypertensive disorders recommended by the American College of Obstetricians and Gynecologists is outlined in Table 14–1. The general term toxemia should not be used, since it represents the entire spectrum of hypertensive disorders of pregnancy and, on occasion, may also include patients with only proteinuria.

The clinical criteria for the diagnosis of hypertension in pregnancy merit some discussion. There is uniform agreement that an absolute blood pressure of 140/90 mm Hg is abnormal because the normal resting arterial pressure is lower in pregnant than in nonpregnant subjects. An increase of 30 mm Hg in the systolic pressure or 15 mm Hg in the diastolic pressure also represents a pathologic change. The problem with this latter criterion is the lack of a standardized baseline from which the increase should be calculated if the patient is first seen after the fifth or sixth month of pregnancy. Because of the many potential errors associated with the clinical determination of blood pressure, the diagnosis of hypertension should be reserved for those having an abnormal reading, taken with the patient at rest on two occasions at least six hours apart.

Pre-eclampsia–Eclampsia

This acute syndrome is peculiar to pregnancy and is referred to as *pregnancy-induced hypertension* (PIH) or *acute hypertensive disease of pregnancy*. Pre-eclampsia is primarily, although not exclusively, confined to the young woman in her first pregnancy. It most commonly occurs during the last trimester of pregnancy. When it arises in the early second

TABLE 14–1 CLASSIFICATION OF HYPERTENSIVE DISORDERS OF PREGNANCY*

1. Pre-eclampsia–eclampsia (hypertension peculiar to pregnancy)
2. Chronic hypertension (of whatever cause)
3. Chronic hypertension with superimposed pre-eclampsia
4. Late or transient hypertension

*Recommended by the American College of Obstetricians and Gynecologists.

trimester (14 to 20 weeks), a hydatidiform mole or choriocarcinoma may be present.

The diagnosis of pre-eclampsia is made by the presence of pathologic edema (hands and face), hypertension, and proteinuria. Edema per se is not essential for the diagnosis of pre-eclampsia; hydrostatic edema of the lower extremities occurs frequently in normal pregnancy. Hypertension is absolutely essential for the diagnosis of pre-eclampsia. There is agreement that the combination of hypertension and proteinuria is diagnostic. When either hypertension or proteinuria is present alone, it is difficult to be certain whether or not the patient has pre-eclampsia in its early stage of development or a hypertensive disorder unrelated to pregnancy.

Pre-eclampsia is divided into mild and severe forms, depending on the height of the blood pressure and the degree of proteinuria (Table 14–2). The position of the patient when the blood pressure is taken and the criteria used for the diastolic pressure are of some importance. The arterial blood pressure should preferably be recorded while the patient is lying down on her side, and with the cuffed arm at heart level. Even when recorded in the sitting position, care should be taken to place the arm with the blood pressure cuff at heart level. In taking the diastolic pressure, Korotkoff's fourth phase (muffling) should be recorded.

In addition to the blood pressure and proteinuria criteria for severe pre-eclampsia listed in Table 14–2, any of the following conditions arising in a mild pre-eclamptic patient would place her in the severe category:

1. Oliguria (less than 400 ml/24 hrs)
2. Altered consciousness, headache, scotomata, or blurred vision
3. Pulmonary edema or cyanosis

4. Epigastric or right upper quadrant pain
5. Significantly altered liver function
6. Significant thrombocytopenia

Eclampsia

Eclampsia is defined as the addition of grand mal seizures to either the mild or severe pre-eclamptic syndrome. Patients with severe pre-eclampsia are at greater risk to develop seizures, but 25 percent of eclamptic patients have only mild pre-eclampsia. In general, 25 percent of eclamptic patients develop the syndrome prior to labor, 50 percent during labor, and 25 percent after delivery.

Chronic Hypertension

The diagnosis of chronic hypertension is made in those patients in whom hypertension is known to antedate pregnancy or in whom hypertension is first noted prior to the twentieth gestational week. These patients may have any of the diseases that cause hypertension, including essential hypertension, acute and chronic glomerulonephritis, chronic pyelonephritis, and collagen vascular diseases, particularly systemic lupus erythematosus. It is not uncommon for the physiologic stress of pregnancy to bring to clinical attention for the first time a previously inapparent or subclinical vascular or renal disease. In these situations, it may be very difficult to determine whether one is dealing with a pregnancy-induced (pre-eclampsia) or aggravated (chronic hypertension) condition.

Chronic Hypertension with Superimposed Pre-eclampsia

Pre-eclampsia may become superimposed on chronic hypertensive disease. In most instances, there is an underlying hypertensive

TABLE 14–2 CRITERIA FOR DETERMINING THE SEVERITY OF PREGNANCY-INDUCED HYPERTENSION

CONDITION	BLOOD PRESSURE	PROTEINURIA	EDEMA
Pre-eclampsia Mild	140/90 to 160/110 or Systolic: ≥30 mm Hg increase Diastolic: ≥15 mm Hg increase	<5 gm/24 hr 1 to 2 plus	Hands and/or face
Severe	>160/110	>5 gm/24 hr 3 to 4 plus	Hands and/or face
Eclampsia	Any of the above with seizures		

disorder of renal or other origin, and the process is aggravated by pregnancy. If the diagnosis of superimposed pre-eclampsia is to be used, it should be reserved for those chronic hypertensive patients who either have a marked increase in preexisting proteinuria during the pregnancy, or demonstrate significant proteinuria for the first time in the latter half of pregnancy. The perinatal risk is greatly increased in these patients.

Late or Transient Hypertension

Also called gestational hypertension, this confusing hypertensive syndrome occurs in the second half of pregnancy, during labor, or within 48 hours of delivery, without significant proteinuria (less than 300 mg/L). It is extremely difficult to differentiate this condition from pre-eclampsia. The diagnosis should be made only in retrospect, when the pregnancy has been completed without the development of proteinuria. Even then, renal disease should be ruled out first.

PRE-ECLAMPSIA–ECLAMPSIA

Etiology

Pre-eclampsia-eclampsia is justly called a disease of theories. Despite extensive interest and investigation, no definite cause has been identified. As the term "toxemia" indicates, the search for a toxin has been long, arduous, and fruitless. An infectious etiology has also been sought unsuccessfully.

Because of the prompt resolution of the disease following delivery, most attention has been focused upon the placenta and its membranes and the fetus. A *hormonal etiology* has been postulated, but no hormone or combination of hormones has been experimentally proven to produce pre-eclampsia.

Currently three hypotheses are in the forefront of investigation. The first hypothesis relates pre-eclampsia to an *immunologic factor* or deficiency. Suggestions have been made for both excessive compatibility and excessive incompatibility between mother and fetus. The second hypothesis relates the syndrome to *prostaglandins* and proposes an imbalance between the vasodilators PGE_2 and prostacyclin and the vasoconstrictor PGF series.

The third hypothesis, which relates the disease to *uteroplacental ischemia*, suggests the following:

1. Pre-eclampsia begins with uteroplacental ischemia, which is thought to be related to various factors. One is an increased intramural resistance in the myometrial vessels, which could be related to a heightened myometrial tension produced by a large fetus in a primipara, twins, or hydramnios. Alternatively, ischemia could be due to underlying vascular changes such as occur in chronic hypertensive disease.

2. The uteroplacental ischemia leads to the production of a vasoconstrictor substance, which, upon entering the circulation, produces renal vasoconstriction; this latter condition leads to the increased production of renin-angiotensin and aldosterone.

3. The renin-angiotensin produces a generalized vasoconstriction and aggravates further the uteroplacental ischemia.

4. Aldosterone leads to water and electrolyte retention and generalized edema, including edema of the intima of the arterioles. These changes produce arteriolar stiffness, which increases sensitivity to angiotensin. Further vasoconstriction leads to capillary hypoxia and increased permeability of the glomerular membrane, leading to proteinuria and further edema. Vasoconstriction and hypoxia in certain areas of the brain would produce convulsions and coma.

In favor of the hypothesis relating the disease to uteroplacental ischemia is the more frequent occurrence of pre-eclampsia in primiparae with large babies and in patients with multiple pregnancy, polyhydramnios, or hydatidiform mole. In all of these conditions, there is increased distension of the uterine walls, which probably increases vascular resistance. However, opposing the hypothesis are the following findings:

1. No vasoconstrictor substance has been isolated from the blood of patients with pre-eclampsia, even when the blood is collected from the uterine veins.

2. Blood levels of renin-angiotensin and aldosterone are not significantly different in patients with pre-eclampsia from those with a normal pregnancy.

The search for the cause or causes of pre-eclampsia is hampered by the lack of an animal model. All efforts to reproduce the human disease in animals have been unsuccessful.

Pathophysiology

Although the etiology of the pregnancy-induced hypertensive syndrome is unknown, it is well accepted that the underlying pathophysiologic abnormality is a *generalized arteriolar constriction*. A rise in blood pressure can be elicited by an increase in either cardiac output or systemic vascular resistance. Cardiac output in pregnant patients with pre-eclampsia and eclampsia is not significantly different from that of normal pregnant subjects in the last trimester of pregnancy. On the other hand, the systemic vascular resistance has been shown to be significantly elevated.

Renal blood flow and glomerular filtration rate (GFR) in patients with pre-eclampsia and eclampsia are significantly lower than those in patients with a normal pregnancy of a comparable gestational period. The decrease in renal blood flow has been shown to be related to constriction of the afferent arteriolar system. This afferent vasoconstriction may eventually lead to damage to the glomerular membranes, thereby increasing their permeability to proteins. The renal vasoconstriction and the decrease in GFR could also account for the oliguria.

The few studies that have been done on cerebral hemodynamics have shown that the cerebral vascular resistance is always high in patients with pre-eclampsia and eclampsia. In hypertensive patients without convulsions, cerebral blood flow may remain within normal limits due to autoregulatory phenomena. However, in convulsive cases, cerebral blood flow and oxygen consumption are below those of normal pregnant subjects. Likewise, the few studies that have been done in human subjects on uteroplacental circulation have shown a decreased blood flow and increased vascular resistance in pre-eclamptic patients.

Pathology and Pathogenesis

There are three major pathologic lesions primarily associated with pre-eclampsia and eclampsia, namely (1) *hemorrhage and necrosis* in many organs, presumably secondary to arteriolar constriction, (2) *glomerular capillary endotheliosis,* and (3) *lack of decidualization of the myometrial segments of the spiral arteries*. Arteriolar vasospasm of relatively short duration (one hour) may cause hypoxia and necrosis of sensitive parenchymal cells.

Vasospasm of longer duration (three hours) may cause infarction in vital organs, such as the liver, placenta, and brain. In the liver, periportal necrosis and hemorrhage may occur, with a subcapsular hematoma a rare complication. In the brain, focal areas of hemorrhage and necrosis may occur. In the retina, the clinical window to the arterial vasculature, vasospasm may be visualized on ophthalmoscopic examination. Retinal hemorrhage is considered to be an extremely ominous sign, since it may signal similar phenomena in other vital organs.

The typical renal lesion of pre-eclampsia-eclampsia is "*glomerular capillary endotheliosis,*" which is best seen by electron microscopy. This disorder is manifested by marked swelling of the glomerular capillary endothelium, with deposits of fibrinoid material in and beneath the endothelial cells. On light microscopy, the glomerular diameter is increased, with protrusion of the glomerular tufts into the neck of the proximal tubules and variable degrees of endothelial/mesangial cell swelling.

The uteroplacental pathology in pre-eclampsia-eclampsia is characterized by a *lack of "decidualization" of the myometrial segments of the spiral arteries*. Under normal circumstances, the invasion of trophoblast results in the replacement of the muscular and elastic layers of the spiral arteries by fibrinoid and fibrous tissue, resulting in large tortuous channels that extend through the myometrium. In pre-eclampsia, this change is limited to the decidual segments of the vessels and may result in a 60 percent reduction in the diameter of the myometrial segment of a spiral artery. The extent of placental infarction is increased in almost all hypertensive pregnancies.

Clinical and Laboratory Manifestations

Many of the clinical manifestations of pre-eclampsia and eclampsia can be explained on the basis of vasospasm.

Angiotensin Sensitivity

One of the earliest signs of developing pre-eclampsia is an increased vascular sensitivity to angiotensin administration. Patients destined to develop pre-eclampsia respond to an intravenous infusion of angiotensin with a greater rise in diastolic blood pressure than normal pregnant patients. The rise is usually 20 mm Hg or more in at-risk patients.

Weight Gain and Edema

Abnormal weight gain and edema occur early and reflect an expansion of the extravascular fluid compartment. This latter is related to the increased capillary permeability produced by the arteriolar vasoconstriction. The increased capillary permeability allows fluid to diffuse from the intravascular space with resultant expansion of the extracellular space.

Excessive weight gain and edema, especially if confined to the lower extremities, do not establish a diagnosis of pre-eclampsia. Edema that includes the face and hands is of more concern, but is still not diagnostic.

Elevation of Blood Pressure

The next sign usually detected is an elevation of blood pressure, particularly the diastolic pressure (greater than 90 mm Hg), which more closely mirrors changes in peripheral vascular resistance. In the antepartum period, the blood pressure changes may occur days to weeks after the onset of fluid retention.

Proteinuria

Proteinuria completes the classic clinical triad of pre-eclampsia. In the antepartum period, this sign may occur days or weeks after the onset of hypertension. If the disease first manifests during labor or in the immediate postpartum period, this progression of events is compressed into hours and sometimes minutes. The proteinuria of pre-eclampsia-eclampsia can be explained on the basis of afferent arteriolar constriction with increased glomerular permeability to protein.

Renal Function

It is usually only during the stage of renal involvement, clinically denoted by proteinuria, that detectable changes in renal function appear. The earliest change may be an increase in serum uric acid concentration. Creatinine clearance may decrease, and serum creatinine and blood urea nitrogen may increase; the hematocrit may also increase, reflecting the relative hypovolemia. Renal involvement may progress to significant oliguria and frank renal failure.

Liver and Placental Function

In the liver, vasospasm may produce focal hemorrhages and infarctions. Therefore, elevated serum enzyme levels are usually present. Thrombocytopenia and disseminated intravascular coagulation may occur, reflecting an increased platelet destruction. Spasm in the uteroplacental vascular bed results in placental infarcts, which may become extensive and lead to a retroplacental hemorrhage. The indirect evidence for a reduced uteroplacental blood flow is the increased incidence of placental infarctions and intrauterine fetal growth retardation.

Central Nervous System (CNS) Effects

Visual disturbances, such as blurred vision, spots, and scotomata, represent degrees of retinal vasospasm. Increased reflex irritability or hyperreflexia are extremely worrisome signs of CNS involvement and may denote imminent seizures related to cerebral vasospasm and hypoxia.

Diagnosis and Evaluation

In the prenatal history and physical examination, particular attention should be directed to any previous history of hypertension and/or proteinuria in either the pregnant or nonpregnant state. Review of medical records from previous hypertension or proteinuria evaluations or from previous hypertensive pregnancies is frequently helpful in establishing a working diagnosis and in guiding further evaluation and management. During the initial physical examination, particular attention should be given to the funduscopic examination in order to record baseline findings. Blood pressure taken in both arms may point toward the rare aortic coarctation.

For the purposes of clinical diagnosis and further evaluation, patients may be divided into two working groups: chronic hypertension and pre-eclampsia. The chronic hypertension group includes most multiparae, those with a previous history of hypertension, and those developing hypertension prior to 20 weeks. Pre-eclampsia is predominantly limited to those women in their first pregnancy who develop the syndrome after 20 weeks.

Table 14–3 outlines the baseline studies recommended for those patients falling into the chronic hypertension group. Table 14–4 outlines the baseline tests to be performed once the diagnosis of pre-eclampsia is suspected. While some of these tests will result in a low yield, the establishment of normality

TABLE 14–3 INITIAL EVALUATION OF A PATIENT WITH CHRONIC HYPERTENSION

BLOOD	URINE	OTHER
Electrolytes	Sediment	EKG
Blood urea nitrogen (BUN)	Culture	Obstetric ultrasound
Creatinine	24-hour protein	
Antinuclear antibody (ANA)	24-hour creatinine	

or abnormality as early in the course as practical may be very helpful as the pregnancy progresses.

Management of Pre-eclampsia

The management of pre-eclampsia should begin at the first sign of abnormality, well before the diagnosis is confirmed. When excessive weight gain or fluid retention is documented in the absence of other pathognomonic changes, a brief dietary history should be obtained, looking for indiscretions and excesses. Appropriate counseling should follow. The patient should be advised of the concerns and be requested to practice bed rest, preferably in the left lateral position. For the following 48 hours, activity out of bed should be limited to eating meals (not preparing them) and using the bathroom. A no-added salt diet may be prescribed. More severe sodium restriction is contraindicated for all but those in frank renal failure. Follow-up is requested 48 hours later in order to confirm continued normal blood pressure and to determine the efficacy of treatment for the weight gain and fluid retention. Successful treatment dictates no further intervention other than perhaps the continuation of the no-added salt diet. If there has been no weight loss, continued reduction of activity with periods of bed rest and more frequent prenatal visits are indicated.

The treatment of hypertension depends to a great extent on the duration of the pregnancy and the height of the blood pressure. At the lowest end of the hypertensive spectrum, namely 140/90, and in the absence of proteinuria, outpatient management is possible. Mild salt reduction (no added salt) and bed rest in the left lateral position are again advised. The patient and her family should be counseled regarding warning symptoms of deterioration. Follow-up should occur no later than 48 hours. Many patients in this category respond to bed rest with a normalization of their blood pressure. These women merely require more frequent follow-up than usual.

For the nonresponders, the next step should be a trial of bed rest and a no-added salt diet in the more controlled environment of the hospital. If blood pressure normalizes, observation should be continued for an additional 24 to 48 hours and the patient discharged on a continued regimen of bed rest and diet with frequent follow-up. Nonresponders who are greater than 36 gestational weeks should be considered for induction of labor. Those less than 37 weeks should continue bed rest and diet in the hospital for several days, while undergoing the work-up detailed in Table 14–4. Patients with continued mild hypertension (not greater than 150/100) without proteinuria and with normal laboratory values may be considered for discharge and close follow-up.

The advent of proteinuria in the hypertensive primigravida confirms the diagnosis of pre-eclampsia and requires prompt hospitalization and evaluation (Table 14–4). For those meeting the criteria for mild pre-eclampsia (Table 14–2) who are less than 37 gestational weeks, a period of bed rest, no-added salt diet, and observation, during which appropriate laboratory tests are carried out, is indicated. For those greater than 36 weeks, induction of labor is the treatment of choice, since delivery is the ultimate treatment for this disease.

Patients meeting the criteria for severe pre-eclampsia should have a period of evaluation and stabilization prior to a final management decision. Those with persistent blood pressure greater than or equal to 160/110 are

TABLE 14–4 INITIAL EVALUATION OF A PATIENT WITH PRE-ECLAMPSIA

BLOOD	URINE
Electrolytes	Sediment
Blood urea nitrogen (BUN)	24-hour protein
Creatinine	24-hour creatinine
Uric acid	
Platelet count	
Liver function studies	

TABLE 14–5   ANTIHYPERTENSIVE THERAPY DURING PREGNANCY

AGENT	ROUTE	ACTION	PEAK RESPONSE	SIDE EFFECTS	COMMENT
Hydralazine (Apresoline)	IV or PO	Direct vasodilator	20–30 min 1–2 hr	Headache, palpitations, lupus-like syndrome	Increases cardiac output and probably uterine and renal blood flow Drug of choice for short-term control
Methyldopa (Aldomet)	PO	False neurotransmitter	3–5 days	Postural hypotension, drowsiness, fluid retention	Frequently used for long-term control of mild hypertension
Diazoxide (Hyperstat)	IV	Direct vasodilator	2–4 min	Hypotension, hyperglycemia	Hard to control; may cause rapid decrease in blood pressure
Prazosin (Minipress)	PO	Alpha$_1$ blocker (postsynaptic)	1–3 hr	Hypotension (especially first dose), drowsiness	Limited obstetric experience reported
Atenolol (Tenormin)	PO	Selective beta$_1$ blocker	1–2 wk	Lassitude, breathlessness	Limited experience
Labetalol (Trondate)	PO	Nonselective beta$_1$ and alpha$_1$ blocker	2 hr	Tremulousness, headache	Increasing experience and efficacy reported May be drug of choice in future
Nitroprusside (Nipride)	IV	Direct vasodilator	1–2 min	Hypotension, cyanide toxicity in fetus	Useful for only short-term control in hypertensive crisis

candidates for antihypertensive therapy (Table 14–5). Prompt response to therapy may allow temporization in those pregnancies of less than 37 weeks. Patients greater than 36 weeks should be delivered, along with those who fail to stabilize and improve, regardless of gestational age. Intrapartum fetal monitoring is mandatory for all patients (see Chapter 20).

Antihypertensive Therapy. Antihypertensive therapy has two main objectives in both pregnancy-induced and pregnancy-aggravated hypertension: (1) to reduce the maternal morbidity and mortality associated with cerebral vascular accidents, and (2) to reduce the perinatal morbidity and mortality associated with intrauterine growth retardation, placental infarcts, and placental abruption. In the absence of underlying abnormalities in the maternal cerebral vasculature, arterial pressures below 160/100 probably do not need therapy for maternal indications. Acute elevations in maternal blood pressure above that level should be promptly brought under control with an intravenous agent, such as hydralazine, or, in a very critical or refractory situation, nitroprusside.

Caution must always be exercised not to lower the arterial pressure too far or too rapidly, for either may result in a decreased uteroplacental blood flow and fetal distress. While the fetus may certainly derive some benefit from the antihypertensive therapy instituted for maternal indications, it is within the diastolic range of 90 to 100 mm Hg that

therapy has been instituted primarily for fetal indications. Controversy continues to exist as to whether or not effective antihypertensive therapy improves perinatal outcome, although the weight of evidence is increasing in favor of such treatment.

In the near-term and laboring patient, short-term control can best be achieved with intravenous hydralazine. In the patient in whom long-term control is the objective, one of the oral agents is the treatment of choice. Current preference is for methyldopa (Aldomet), although evidence is accumulating that beta blockers such as atenolol (Tenormin) and labetalol (Trondate) may be more efficacious. There is some concern that beta blockers that cross the placenta may cause intrauterine growth retardation.

Anticonvulsant Therapy. Because of the risk of seizures and their attendant morbidity and even mortality, a great deal of attention must be given to the level of central nervous system irritability. Peripheral reflexes, particularly of the patella and ankle, are most frequently used as determinants of increased instability.

Seizure prophylaxis should be instituted in all pre-eclamptics during labor and delivery and continued for 12 to 24 hours following delivery. All severe pre-eclamptics should have seizure prophylaxis instituted upon admission and continued during the period of evaluation and observation. Magnesium sulfate is the agent of choice because of its efficacy and associated low neonatal morbid-

TABLE 14–6 MAGNESIUM SULFATE THERAPY

TYPE OF TREATMENT	IM	IV
Prophylactic		
Loading	5 gm each buttock	4 gm over 10 min
Maintenance	5 gm/4 hr	1–2 gm/hr
Therapeutic (for seizure treatment)	—	1 gm/min until seizure controlled; 4–6 gm maximum

ity. Both intramuscular and intravenous routes are effective.

Table 14–6 outlines the protocols for magnesium administration, while Table 14–7 reviews the relationship of serum concentrations to clinical response. The magnesium ion is excreted exclusively through the kidneys, so caution must be exercised in those patients with compromised renal function.

Management of Fluid Balance. The management of fluid balance is of major importance in all hypertensive patients receiving intravenous therapy. Accurately recorded intake and output data must be kept in order to calculate requirements. These patients are vasoconstricted and may have some relative degree of reduced intravascular volume, both of which may reduce urinary output. In addition, they may be receiving several different therapeutic infusions, such as magnesium sulfate and oxytocin, which have a direct or indirect effect on urinary output.

The most common errors that occur in the management of these patients are volume overload and water intoxication. The conservative approach is to replace documented output plus insensible loss with an appropriate electrolyte-containing fluid. Because of the multifaceted pathophysiology of this disease, central hemodynamic monitoring may aid in the management of the more severe

TABLE 14–7 CLINICAL CORRELATES OF SERUM MAGNESIUM SULFATE LEVELS

SERUM CONCENTRATION (mg/dl)	(mEq/L*)	OBSERVED RESPONSE
1.2–1.8	1.5–2.1	Normal
3–8	2.5–6.7	Therapeutic range
6–8	5–6.6	CNS depression
8–10	6.6–8.3	Absent reflexes
12–17	10–14.2	Respiratory depression
13–17	10.8–14.2	Coma
19–20	15.8–16.6	Cardiac arrest

*1 mEq/L = 1.2 mg/dl

cases. Pulmonary artery and pulmonary capillary wedge pressures are more helpful in guiding fluid therapy than is central venous pressure, which on occasion may be misleading.

Management of Eclampsia

If the patient develops convulsive seizures at home, she is usually brought to the hospital in a comatose condition. The management of these patients should be carried out by a team of physicians and well-trained nurses in an isolated labor room, with minimum noise and not too much light. As with any epileptic condition, the initial requirement is to clear the airway and give oxygen by face mask to relieve airway obstruction and hypoxia. Blood pressure should be recorded every 10 minutes with the patient in the lateral position. An intravenous line should be placed for drawing blood and administering drugs and fluids. Intravenous fluids should be limited to sufficient 5 percent dextrose in water to replace urine output, plus about 700 ml per day to replace insensible losses. An indwelling catheter should be placed in the bladder, urine sent to the laboratory for urinalysis, and all urine output recorded.

Pharmacologic management necessitates an antihypertensive drug (hydralazine) to lower blood pressure and relieve vasoconstriction. The aim is to decrease the diastolic pressure by 25 to 30 percent from the hypertensive values. Magnesium sulfate is given intravenously to decrease hyperreflexia and prevent further convulsions (Table 14–6). Agents such as diazepam (Valium) may also be used.

If the patient is prenatal, no attempt should be made to deliver her either vaginally or by cesarean section until the acute phase of convulsive eclampsia and coma has passed. Interference during the acute phase may aggravate the oliguria and other manifestations of the disease. When the urine output increases and the coma and convulsions are controlled, delivery should be expedited, preferably by the vaginal route. If this is not feasible, cesarean section is indicated.

Management of Chronic Hypertension

The management of pregnancy-aggravated or chronic hypertension is in many ways more clear-cut. Despite the fact that the blood pressure of these patients may be "normal" in the first and second trimesters, existing antihypertensive medication should be stopped only for unusually low pressures or other strong indications. Those women who are not taking antihypertensive agents should be started once the diastolic pressure is consistently greater than 90 mm Hg. The foundations of conservative management include reduced physical activity and bed rest.

Because these women have a high incidence of intrauterine fetal growth retardation, both early and serial ultrasonic examinations are indicated. The early ultrasound (16 to 20 weeks) is primarily for confirmation of pregnancy dates, while serial ultrasonic examinations (every three weeks from 24 to 28 weeks) are of great assistance in detecting growth retardation. Significant growth retardation may be an indication for early delivery.

Because of the concern for chronic uteroplacental insufficiency in this group of patients, the various tests for fetal well-being are indicated (see Chapter 6). Depending on the clinical circumstances, fetal monitoring may start as early as 28 weeks and, in all hypertensive patients, should be commenced by 36 weeks.

A significant increase in hypertension or the addition of proteinuria to a previously nonproteinuric chronic hypertensive patient is of great concern. Many would regard these as signs of superimposed pre-eclampsia. The incidence of superimposed pre-eclampsia varies from 15 to 25 percent. These patients should undergo further laboratory evaluation, as outlined in Table 14–4. Management should follow that outlined for severe pre-eclampsia.

In general, the timing of delivery in the chronic hypertensive group is more difficult. For those without fetal growth retardation in whom the blood pressure is well controlled and proteinuria is not present, a full-term gestation may be allowed, provided there is normal fetal well-being. Any progression beyond the fortieth week should be very carefully considered. The presence of growth retardation or blood pressure deterioration or the advent of proteinuria may dictate earlier delivery. If delivery is desirable but not imperative prior to 37 weeks, confirmation of fetal lung maturity should be initially obtained. There is no contraindication to vaginal delivery in the hypertensive patient, and therefore, the route of delivery should be decided on obstetric criteria.

Sequelae and Outcome

There are essentially no long-term maternal sequelae to an episode of uncomplicated pre-eclampsia or eclampsia in the primigravid patient. Such patients are at no greater risk of subsequently developing hypertensive cardiovascular disease than any other individual. Interestingly, their female offspring do have an increased risk of pre-eclampsia in their own pregnancies. Similarly, pregnancy does not seem to affect the subsequent course of a patient with chronic hypertension. Some of the more serious complications of both pregnancy-induced and pregnancy-aggravated hypertension, such as cerebro-vascular accidents and renal failure, may have long-term maternal sequelae.

Fetal and neonatal sequelae are more difficult to determine, since some of the prenatal morbidity and mortality of these hypertensive syndromes are related to intrauterine growth retardation and acute and chronic fetal distress. All of these may have long-term central nervous system effects.

SUGGESTED READING

Assali NS (ed): Pathophysiology of gestation. In Maternal Disorders. Vol 1. New York, Academic Press, 1972.

Brosens IA, Robertson WB, Dixon HG: The role of the spiral arteries in the pathogenesis of pre-eclampsia. Obstet Gynecol Annu 1:117, 1972.

Chamberlain G, Philipp E, Howlett B, et al: British Births, 1970. In Obstetric Case. Vol 2. London, Heinemann, 1978.

Chesley LC: Hypertensive Disorders in Pregnancy. New York, Appleton-Century-Crofts, 1978, p 57.

Gant NF, Chand S, Worley RJ, et al: A clinical test useful for predicting the development of acute hypertension in pregnancy. Am J Obstet Gynecol 120:1, 1974.

Gant NF, Daley GL, Chand S, et al: A study of angiotensin II pressor response throughout primigravid pregnancy. J Clin Invest 52:2682, 1973.

Michelson EL, Fuschman WH: Labetalol: An alpha- and beta-adrenoceptor blocking drug. Ann Intern Med 99:553, 1983.

Report on Confidential Enquiries into Maternal Deaths in England and Wales, 1973–1975. Report on Health and Social Subjects. Department of Health and Social Security, 1975.

Rubin PC, Butters L, Clark DM, et al: Placebo-controlled trial of atenolol in treatment of pregnancy-associated hypertension. Lancet 1(8322):431, 1983.

Sheehan HL, Lynch JB: Pathology of Toxemia of Pregnancy. Baltimore, Williams & Wilkins, 1973.

Symonds EM: Etiology of pre-eclampsia: A review. J Royal Soc Med 73:871, 1980.

Vollman RF: Study design, population and data characteristics. In Friedman MA (ed): Progress in Clinical and Biological Research. Blood Pressure, Edema and Proteinuria in Pregnancy. Vol 7. New York, Alan R Liss Inc, 1976.

15

Chapter Fifteen

INFECTIONS IN PREGNANCY

GARY OAKES

Infections in pregnancy have become a common and important cause of maternal and neonatal morbidity. This chapter summarizes etiologic factors, clinical manifestations, treatment, and prognosis for the more common infectious disease entities complicating pregnancy.

BACTERIAL INFECTIONS

Urinary Tract Infections

Urinary tract infection occurs more frequently during pregnancy and the postpartum period, and the increased incidence is apparently due to a combination of hormonal and mechanical factors. There is a functional decrease in ureteral tone and motility combined with mechanical compression of the ureters at the pelvic brim, resulting in dilatation of the upper ureter, renal pelvis, and calyceal system. The bladder is also compressed by the enlarging uterus, and there may be distortion or distension of the ureteral orifices. As a result of these factors, urinary stasis occurs throughout the urinary tract, providing a medium for bacterial proliferation. There may also be vesicoureteral reflux allowing contamination of the upper urinary tract with infected urine from the bladder.

Clinical Manifestations. Urinary tract infections during pregnancy usually manifest as asymptomatic bacteriuria, acute cystitis, or acute pyelonephritis.

Asymptomatic bacteriuria occurs in 2 to 10 percent of all pregnant women, particularly those in the lower socioeconomic group. It is usually present at the first prenatal visit and

uncommonly occurs subsequent to an initial negative urine culture. The diagnosis of asymptomatic bacteriuria requires the recovery of 100,000 or more organisms of the same species per milliliter of urine from an asymptomatic patient. This can usually be accomplished by obtaining a clean-catch midstream urine specimen for culture. Routine bladder catheterization increases the risk of infection and should be avoided.

Approximately 25 percent of women with asymptomatic bacteriuria during pregnancy subsequently develop acute symptomatic urinary infection later in that pregnancy. This can be prevented by the elimination of asymptomatic bacteriuria with antibiotic therapy. There is an increased incidence of premature delivery in those patients with bacteriuria who subsequently develop symptomatic pyelonephritis, which further supports the need to identify and treat asymptomatic bacteriuria.

Acute cystitis is characterized by dysuria, frequency, and urgency. Systemic signs and symptoms are absent. The urine usually contains bacteria and an abnormal number of leukocytes. The incidence of cystitis during pregnancy has been reported to be 1 to 2 percent.

Acute pyelonephritis is the most frequent medical complication of pregnancy necessitating hospitalization. The incidence increases with advancing gestation, and it is reported to occur in about 2 percent of pregnancies. Acute pyelonephritis is usually characterized by a history of fever, shaking chills, and flank pain associated with nausea, vomiting, urinary frequency, urgency, and dysuria. On physical examination, there is fever and costovertebral angle tenderness. The urinalysis generally reveals pyuria and bacteriuria. A positive blood culture may be found occasionally.

Treatment. Asymptomatic bacteriuria should be treated with antimicrobial agents to prevent the development of more serious urinary tract infection. Ideally, the agent utilized should be based on the antimicrobial sensitivity of the microorganism, but in practice, ampicillin, cephalexin, nitrofurantoin, and sulfisoxazole have been used safely and successfully. Short-term treatment, combined with surveillance for recurrent bacteriuria, is nearly as effective as continuous antimicrobial administration.

While asymptomatic bacteriuria and cystitis can usually be treated in an outpatient situation, acute pyelonephritis during pregnancy is generally best treated in the hospital because of the potential for maternal sepsis and shock. Intravenous antibiotics are begun initially using ampicillin or cefazolin and are subsequently altered or adjusted, depending upon the antimicrobial sensitivities or clinical condition. Therapy is switched to oral administration when the patient is afebrile and the flank pain has disappeared. Therapy should continue for a total of 10 to 14 days. Subsequent surveillance for bacteriuria is important because of the high risk of recurrent pyelonephritis. Patients who develop recurrent pyelonephritis during pregnancy should have an intravenous pyelogram (IVP) performed postpartum to evaluate the urinary tract for abnormalities.

Group B Streptococcus

Group B streptococcus can be cultured from the vaginal canal of 5 to 25 percent of pregnant women, and the rate does not appear to be affected by race, age, socioeconomic status, or parity. Approximately 50 percent of infants born to mothers with positive cultures at the time of labor become colonized with group B streptococcus, but the incidence of neonatal infection is only 2 per 1000 live births. However, these early-onset infections are frequently severe and result in neonatal death in up to 50 percent of cases.

Maternal colonization is frequently transient or intermittent, and the pattern a particular patient will follow is unpredictable. Thus, a patient with a prior positive culture may have a negative culture at the onset of labor, while another patient who was previously cultured as negative may demonstrate colonization when labor begins. The bacterial reservoir for this colonization has not been established, but the gastrointestinal tract appears likely. Because of these factors, the eradication of maternal colonization with group B streptococcus during the third trimester with intermittent antibiotic therapy has been largely unsuccessful. Moreover, it appears that the rate of neonatal colonization is not altered if intramuscular penicillin is used at birth for routine eye prophylaxis.

Clinical Manifestations. Group B streptococcus can cause significant maternal morbidity. *Postpartum endometritis* associated with a spiking fever in the first 24 hours after delivery is the usual presentation. Whether or not group B streptococcal infection causes preterm labor is unclear, but *premature rupture of the membranes* does appear to be increased in colonized patients. Preterm delivery is a frequent accompaniment of premature membrane rupture, suggesting at least an indirect association with maternal group B streptococcal colonization.

Neonatal disease is manifest as two differing clinical syndromes. Early onset sepsis is characterized by the onset of symptoms within the first day of life. The symptoms include respiratory distress, apnea, hypotension, and seizures. Early diagnosis is critical but often difficult because the symptoms are nonspecific. The streptococci associated with early-onset disease are acquired from the maternal genital tract. Late onset infections commonly present as meningitis at four to seven days of age and appear to be unassociated with prior obstetric events.

Treatment. Maternal colonization prior to labor does not appear to warrant antibiotic therapy because of lack of success in eradicating the organism. However, these patients should probably receive a course of antibiotics at the onset of labor, and penicillin is the drug of choice. The possibility of group B streptococcal infection should be sought in all patients with preterm labor or premature rupture of membranes by obtaining a cervical/vaginal culture.

Neonatal sepsis should be treated aggressively at the first suspicion. Current opinion suggests a combination of penicillin and an aminoglycoside as optimal antibiotic treatment.

Listeria

Listeria monocytogenes is a pathogen that is found infrequently in humans, but is an important contributor to perinatal infection. The gram-positive bacillus, which is frequently traced to unpasteurized milk, has also been implicated as a potential etiologic agent in habitual abortion.

Clinical Manifestations. When maternal infection occurs, the symptoms are frequently nonspecific and include fever, malaise, and upper respiratory or gastrointestinal complaints. The illness is usually brief, self-limiting, and seldom-diagnosed. However, maternal listeriosis can be associated with preterm labor and/or congenital infection. Fetal infection can occur either transplacentally or from ascending spread, frequently in the presence of intact membranes. Severe fetal infection can cause intrauterine fetal death or may produce severe sepsis at birth, with respiratory distress and shock. Neonatal infection can present as pneumonitis, conjunctivitis, skin rash, or meningitis in the newborn period.

Treatment. *L. monocytogenes* demonstrates *in vitro* sensitivity to a wide range of antibiotics, including penicillin, erythromycin, chloramphenicol, sulfonamides, and tetracycline. A combination of ampicillin and an aminoglycoside is generally recommended for treatment of listeriosis in either the mother or the newborn infant.

Chlamydia

Chlamydiae are obligatory, intracellular bacteria. Of the two species, only *Chlamydia trachomatis* has been implicated in human perinatal infections. Chlamydial cervical infection has been reported to occur in up to 30 percent of pregnant women, and prevalence rates appear to be highest in the lower socioeconomic group. Infants delivered vaginally to women with chlamydial infection of the cervix have a 60 to 70 percent risk of acquiring the infection during passage through the birth canal. Cesarean section appears to decrease the risk of acquiring chlamydial infection except when there has been premature rupture of the membranes.

Clinical Manifestations. The most frequent maternal manifestation of chlamydial infection is *cervicitis*. There is a hypertrophic cervical erosion associated with a mucopu-

rulent endocervical discharge. In addition, there appears to be an increased risk for developing late onset *endometritis* following vaginal delivery.

Chlamydial infection has been implicated as an etiologic factor in spontaneous abortion, preterm delivery, and intrauterine fetal demise, but these associations are unproven.

Neonatal infection is generally manifest as either *conjunctivitis* or *pneumonia*. Between 25 and 50 percent of exposed neonates develop early conjunctivitis, and 10 to 20 percent of infants develop late pneumonia. Chlamydial conjunctivitis develops 5 to 14 days after birth, beginning with conjunctival hyperemia and progressing rapidly to produce a mucopurulent discharge. In contrast, chlamydial pneumonia usually presents between 4 and 18 weeks of age. Upper respiratory symptoms such as nasal congestion and stuffiness predominate, with minimal fever. Tachypnea and staccato cough may be present. A chest x-ray usually reveals hyperexpansion, with bilateral symmetric interstitial infiltrates.

Treatment. Chlamydiae are sensitive to antibiotics, particularly erythromycin and tetracycline. Maternal cervicitis and neonatal conjunctivitis and pneumonia respond to systemic erythromycin administration. Because silver nitrate eye prophylaxis does not prevent the development of chlamydial conjunctivitis, there is growing support for erythromycin ointment as the routine agent for ocular prophylaxis at birth.

Mycoplasma

Two commonly isolated genital mycoplasmas are *Mycoplasma hominis* and *Ureaplasma urealyticum*. Genital mycoplasmas can be frequently isolated from pregnant women and from their neonates after vaginal delivery.

Clinical Manifestations. Maternal genital tract infections with mycoplasma have been seen in association with *spontaneous abortion, low birth weight infants,* and *postpartum fever.* Specifically, mycoplasma have been the most common organisms isolated from spontaneous second trimester abortuses. No firm association has been made with first trimester abortions.

Mycoplasma appears to be the responsible agent for approximately 10 percent of maternal postpartum fevers and may occasionally be recovered in blood cultures. Genital mycoplasma is found more frequently among mothers who deliver infants weighing less than 2500 gm. Moreover, when mycoplasma is isolated from the mother, the birth weight of the infant is lower than when the microorganism is not present, independent of other risk factors for low birth weight. The mechanism for this effect is not known and requires further investigation. Isolated case reports of serious neonatal infection with mycoplasma exist, but these are very uncommon.

Treatment. Recognized mycoplasma infection can be treated with either erythromycin or tetracycline, although the clinical course is usually self-limiting. Further study is necessary to evaluate the role of antenatal treatment of mycoplasma, as well as the long-term effects of neonatal colonization without treatment.

Tuberculosis

Active tuberculosis is currently an uncommon disease in pregnancy, albeit a potentially serious one. Approximately 3 percent of young adults are tuberculin-positive, but the incidence of active disease is significantly lower, ranging from 0.06 to 0.4 percent of the population. The highest incidence is seen in malnourished, low socioeconomic, or minority group individuals.

Clinical Manifestations and Diagnosis. All pregnant patients seen for prenatal care should be screened for tuberculosis with an intradermal tuberculin skin test, unless there is known previous positive reactivity. The skin test reactivity is not specifically altered by pregnancy. A standard chest x-ray with abdominal shielding should be performed on those patients with a positive skin test to evaluate for the presence of active disease. Routine screening by chest x-ray need not be done. Active untreated pulmonary tuberculosis can result in increased pregnancy wastage and/or congenital tuberculosis. However, in patients receiving adequate antituberculosis chemotherapy, this increased risk is eliminated. Pregnancy does not appear to increase the likelihood of progression or reactivation of tuberculosis.

Treatment. Patients with recent skin test conversion and negative chest x-rays should probably be treated with isoniazid for one year beginning in the third trimester. Follow-up in a public health tuberculosis control program can provide the serial assessments necessary to maintain the duration of therapy.

Patients with a positive or suspicious chest x-ray should have serial sputum cultures taken for bacteriologic confirmation of the disease and drug sensitivities. Because of the long interval frequently required for growth of *Mycobacterium tuberculosis* in culture, chemotherapy is usually begun before the results are obtained. Isoniazid and ethambutol in combination are the usual drugs of choice in pregnancy. No teratogenesis has been established, but their use during the first trimester should be avoided.

Other drug therapy may be required when the sensitivities of the organism are known. Rifampin has been associated with congenital malformations in rodents, but teratogenesis in humans has not been reported. Streptomycin given in early pregnancy may cause vestibular and auditory damage, while ethionamide is a potent teratogen.

After the onset of labor, the pregnant patient with active tuberculosis should be isolated so that labor, delivery, and recovery all occur in the same room, if possible. Congenital tuberculosis does occur, so an infant delivered of a patient with active tuberculosis should be thoroughly evaluated. Since placental involvement is more common than fetal disease, histologic examination of the placenta can provide important information regarding the probability of neonatal infection.

After birth, a healthy newborn infant should be separated from a mother with active tuberculosis until the mother is bacteriologically negative. Similarly, breast feeding should be allowed only when the mother's sputum is negative. Because of the very high risk of developing active tuberculosis, infants born to mothers with active disease should receive either isoniazid chemoprophylaxis for one year or bacillus Calmette-Guérin (BCG) vaccination.

SPIROCHETE INFECTIONS

Syphilis

At their initial prenatal visit, all pregnant patients should have a serologic screening test for syphilis, such as the Venereal Disease Research Laboratory (VDRL) slide test or the rapid plasma reagin (RPR) test. If positive, a treponema-specific test, such as the fluorescent treponemal antibody absorption test (FTA-ABS), should be done to confirm the diagnosis. This confirmatory test is essential because of the possibility of biologic false-positive reactions to the reagin tests, which can occur in many medical conditions, including pregnancy itself.

Clinical Manifestations. The clinical manifestations of syphilis during pregnancy are similar to those in the nonpregnant state (see Chapter 33), with the asymptomatic primary chancre and secondary dermatologic forms of the disease predominantly seen.

Congenital syphilis is a systemic infection usually resulting from transplacental passage of the spirochete. It is now known that this can occur as early as six weeks' gestation, but clinical manifestations of the disease in the fetus are not usually apparent unless maternal infection is present after 16 weeks' gestation. Congenital syphilis can occur with all stages of maternal disease, although the fetus is more likely to be involved when the mother has been recently infected. Fetal infection can result in abortion, intrauterine fetal demise, intrauterine growth retardation, preterm delivery, neonatal death, or infectious sequelae.

At birth, there may be no evidence of disease or there may be severe manifestations, including hepatosplenomegaly, generalized lymphadenopathy, hemolytic anemia, periostitis and osteochondritis of the long bones, and a cutaneous bullous eruption from which spirochetes can be seen on darkfield microscopy. "Snuffles," a rhinitis resulting from nasal mucosal involvement, is frequently seen.

Diagnosis. The serologic diagnosis of neonatal syphilis can be difficult because of passive placental transfer of material antibodies. Frequently, the infant's titer is significantly elevated over the mother's level, suggesting neonatal involvement. If there is no neonatal involvement, the reagin titer should become negative within three to four months of delivery. If there are clinical manifestations of disease at birth, the diagnosis is more readily made.

Treatment. Long-acting penicillin is the antibiotic treatment of choice. The current recommendation during pregnancy is 2.4 million units of benzathine penicillin administered intramuscularly weekly for three weeks.

For patients who are allergic to penicillin, erthyromycin is used. However, there is concern that the fetus may not be adequately treated with erythromycin because of the poor placental transfer.

Women treated for syphilis during pregnancy should undergo careful follow-up consisting of a monthly determination of the reagin titer to assess the effectiveness of therapy. In addition, sexual contacts and the delivered neonate need immediate evaluation and probable treatment.

VIRAL INFECTIONS

Herpes Simplex

It is estimated that approximately 1 to 2 percent of pregnancies are complicated by herpes infection, the vast majority of which are recurrent infections.

Clinical Manifestations. The clinical manifestations of herpes genitalis are discussed in Chapter 33. Genital infection during pregnancy secondary to herpes simplex virus types I and II may lead to disastrous consequences for the neonate. If the fetus passes through the birth canal in the presence of herpes virus, the risk of acquiring the virus and developing disseminated neonatal herpetic infection from 7 to 21 days after delivery is high. The treated mortality rate in neonates with disseminated herpes infection is approximately 50 percent, with as many as two thirds of surviving infants suffering severe neurologic sequelae. If, in the presence of active genital herpes, delivery occurs by cesarean section prior to rupture of the membranes, there is very little risk of neonatal infection. Very rare cases of transamniotic infection have been reported.

Diagnosis and Treatment. The primary goal for treatment of herpetic infections during pregnancy is the prevention of neonatally acquired infection. Thus, pregnant patients who have a history of genital herpes or a partner with such a history must be monitored closely in the third trimester to rule out active infection, asymptomatic disease, or viral shedding. This is best done by obtaining serial cultures of the cervix and external genital area. As many as 50 percent of neonatal herpetic infections occur when there is minimal or no maternal genital symptoms at birth. In the presence of active genital lesions or positive cultures, cesarean section should be performed. If active infection has occurred close to the time of delivery, a negative culture must have been obtained subsequent to the infection if vaginal delivery is to be considered. The risks of *acyclovir* in pregnancy have not been evaluated, so its use should be postponed until more information is available.

Cytomegalovirus

Cytomegalovirus (CMV), a DNA virus in the herpes virus family, causes more congenital infections than any other agent.

Clinical Manifestations and Diagnosis. The overwhelming majority of maternal CMV infections are asymptomatic. When present, the symptoms most often resemble a mononucleosis-like illness with fever, malaise, myalgia, pharyngitis, atypical lymphocytosis, lymphadenopathy, and a negative heterophil reaction. Maternal CMV infections may be primary or recurrent, with the latter the more common. Viral excretion persists for a long period after an infectious episode, despite high CMV antibody titers, making identification of infants at-risk difficult.

In asymptomatic patients, the cervix appears to be the most frequently involved site, with viral recovery demonstrated in about 10 percent of pregnant patients. Other sites include the urinary tract in about 5 percent, the pharynx in 2 percent, and breast milk in postpartum women in about 15 percent of cases. The virus is readily isolated in fibroblast tissue culture from sites of excretion. Pregnancy, per se, does not appear to increase the risk of CMV acquisition, but there is an increasing rate of viral excretion as pregnancy progresses; the virus can be isolated from the cervix in about 3 percent of patients in the first trimester, 5 percent in the second trimester, and 8 percent in the third trimester.

Up to 2.5 percent of all live births are congenitally infected with CMV, the highest frequency occurring when the mother is young and/or poor. In contrast to many other viral infections, congenital CMV infection frequently results from recurrent maternal CMV infection. About 90 to 95 percent of infants with congenital CMV infection are asymptomatic at birth, but the virus can be cultured from the child's urine. Even asymptomatic infections can produce neurologic or perceptual sequelae during the preschool years in 10 to 15 percent of affected individuals.

While only 5 to 10 percent of congenital CMV infection is manifest symptomatically at birth, when present it is potentially catastrophic as 90 percent of these infants develop major sequelae, including mental retardation, optic atrophy, blindness, epilepsy, spastic diplegia, and sensorineural hearing loss. For reasons not understood, nonneural organs are relatively unaffected, and intrauterine death is rare.

In addition to the congenital infections, another 3 to 5 percent of neonates acquire CMV infection at or shortly after birth, usually from exposure to infected cervical secretions or ingestion of infected breast milk. Infants infected by these routes may shed virus for several years, but long-term risks have not been well-elucidated.

Treatment. There is no effective treatment for CMV infections. Antiviral chemotherapy has been disappointing. Even prevention is difficult because of the problems of diagnosis and lack of specific antibody immunity. Any patient who develops a heterophil-negative mononucleosis-like syndrome should be evaluated for CMV infection. Consideration should be given to pregnancy termination if the gestational age permits it.

Rubella

Approximately 85 percent of pregnant patients demonstrate immunity to rubella virus. Thus, 15 percent are susceptible to this RNA virus, which causes relatively mild disease in adults but potentially catastrophic teratogenesis in the fetus. The epidemiology of rubella has been significantly altered since vaccines were introduced in 1969. The incidence has declined, and the most common age for acquisition of disease has risen from childhood to young adulthood.

Clinical Manifestations. When rubella is acquired, about half of the cases are subclinical or asymptomatic. When symptoms manifest, there is an incubation period of 14 to 21 days, which is followed by the appearance of lymphadenopathy in the suboccipital, postauricular, and/or posterior cervical regions; mild fever; and malaise. Four to six days later, a macular rash develops on the face, neck, trunk, and extremities. These symptoms usually resolve in two to three days. Complications are rare, although adult females may have a transient arthritis/arthralgia syndrome.

In contrast, the congenital rubella syndrome includes multiorgan manifestations. Up to 50 percent of newborns will manifest some abnormality attributable to rubella if maternal infection is acquired in the first eight weeks of gestation. Commonly, cataracts, patent ductus arteriosus, and hearing impairment are seen in a small-for-gestational age neonate, but thrombocytopenic purpura, hepatosplenomegaly, microcephaly, jaundice, mental retardation, pneumonitis, radiolucencies of the long bones, peripheral pulmonic stenosis, and ventricular septal defects can occur. The majority of newborns with congenital rubella syndrome have active viral shedding for months to years after birth. The virus can be isolated from a nasopharynx or throat washing.

Diagnosis. The diagnosis of rubella is most commonly made serologically. Hemagglutination inhibiting (HAI) antibodies (IgG) and specific rubella antibodies (IgM) rise sharply after the onset of the rash. The HAI antibodies persist, while the IgM antibodies disappear after six to eight weeks. Complement-fixing antibodies do not appear until seven to ten days or more after the onset of disease. Thus, the diagnosis can be made by noting a fourfold HAI rise in paired sera one to two weeks apart, or by evaluating the relationship of the other antibody fractions to each other. Rubella can also be diagnosed from culture and isolation of the virus during the acute phase. Similarly, congenital rubella can be confirmed by viral culture or the demonstration of rubella-specific IgM antibodies in cord or neonatal blood.

Treatment. There is no specific treatment for rubella, and the use of gamma globulin after rubella exposure does not prevent congenital rubella syndrome. The best approach is prevention. A specific vaccine exists, which yields a high response rate. Those patients found to be seronegative at the first prenatal visit are candidates for postpartum immunization. Up to 20 percent of patients who are immunized postpartum may not develop an adequate antibody response, so follow-up antibody titers should be obtained. Breastfeeding is not a contraindication to rubella immunization.

Hepatitis B

In general, the incidence and clinical course of hepatitis B (HB) is no different during pregnancy than in the nonpregnant state. Teratologic damage to the fetus has not been demonstrated. However, infants born of mothers who acquire hepatitis B late in pregnancy or who are chronic carriers of hepatitis B surface antigen (HBsAg) are at risk to become congenitally infected.

Certain population groups, such as Asians, American Indians, Eskimos, South Pacific immigrants, parenteral drug users, and patients with a past history of hepatitis B, have a high carrier rate of HBsAg. Patients in these categories should be screened for HBsAg during pregnancy. The Centers for Disease Control recommend that newborns of HBsAg-positive mothers receive passive immunization with a single dose (0.5 ml, intramuscularly) of specific hepatitis B immune globulin (HBIG) within 12 hours of birth, together with HB vaccination (0.5 ml, intramuscularly) within seven days and repeated at one and six months. HBIG alone is only about 75 percent effective, whereas the HBIG-HB combination increases effectiveness to about 90 percent.

Varicella

The acquisition of varicella or chicken pox during pregnancy can be serious for both mother and baby. Adult chicken pox is a potentially fatal disease, overwhelming pneumonia being the usual cause of death. Disseminated neonatal chicken pox may follow maternal infection, the greatest risk occurring when birth takes place within five days of the onset of varicella in the mother. Infants delivered within five days of the onset of maternal varicella should receive passive immunization with varicella-zoster immune globulin.

PARASITIC INFESTATIONS

Toxoplasmosis

Toxoplasmosis is a systemic disease caused by the protozoan *Toxoplasma gondii*. The infection is usually acquired by ingestion of undercooked meat or contamination from infected cat feces.

Clinical Manifestations. Primary maternal infection is usually asymptomatic, but can occasionally manifest as a mononucleosis-like syndrome with cervical lymphadenopathy. Of patients acquiring toxoplasmosis during pregnancy, about one-half of the neonates are congenitally affected. The frequency of congenital toxoplasmosis increases and the severity decreases as pregnancy progresses.

Congenital toxoplasmosis is usually asymptomatic in the newborn period. When overt, congenital toxoplasmosis produces micropthalmia, hydrocephaly, chorioretinitis, convulsions, jaundice, hepatosplenomegaly, lymphadenopathy, pneumonitis, rash, and mental retardation. The majority of affected infants who are asymptomatic at birth develop some sequelae by school age, usually chorioretinitis or other neurologic manifestations. The classic triad of hydrocephalus, intracranial calcifications, and chorioretinitis is not frequently seen at birth.

Diagnosis. Screening blood tests include the Sabin-Feldman dye test and indirect fluorescent antibody tests for both IgG and IgM. Toxoplasmosis can be diagnosed when there is documented seroconversion; a fourfold rise in titer in paired, serial blood samples; or an initial high IgM titer.

Treatment. Although pharmacologic treatment with pyrimethamine (Daraprim), sulfadiazine, and folinic acid for one month is standard therapy, preventive measures are most desirable. Pregnant women should avoid eating undercooked meat, particularly beef, pork, and lamb, and drinking raw goat's milk. Handling cat litter boxes or raw meat should be avoided unless gloves are used and thorough handwashing follows.

TORCH TITERS

Torch titers (Table 15–1) should be obtained on any woman who has an unexplained stillbirth or a fetus with severe intrauterine growth retardation. The routine screening of all pregnant patients is not cost-effective.

TABLE 15–1   TORCH TESTS

T	Toxoplasmosis
O	Other (syphilis)
R	Rubella
C	Cytomegalovirus
H	Herpes simplex

SUGGESTED READING

Alfond CA: Rubella. In Remington J, Klein J (eds): Infectious Diseases of the Fetus and Newborn. Philadelphia, WB Saunders Co, 1976, p 71.

Anthony BF, Okada DM, Hobel CJ: Epidemiology of group B streptococcus: Longitudinal observations during pregnancy. J Infect Dis 137:524, 1978.

Braun P, Lee YH, Klein JO, et al: Birth weight and genital mycoplasmas in pregnancy. N Engl J Med 284:167, 1971.

Charles D: Syphilis. Clin Obstet Gynecol 26:125, 1983.

Desmonts F, Couvreur J: Congenital toxoplasmosis: A prospective study of 378 pregnancies. N Engl J Med 290:1110, 1974.

Grossman JH: Herpes simplex virus (HSV) infections. Clin Obstet Gynecol 25:555, 1982.

Harris RE, Thomas UL, Shelokov A: Asymptomatic bacteriuria in pregnancy: Antibody-coated bacteria, renal function, and intrauterine growth retardation. Am J Obstet Gynecol 126:20, 1976.

Nahmias AJ, Roizman B: Infection with herpes simplex virus 1 and 2. N Engl J Med 289:667, 1973.

Regan JA, Chao S, James LS: Premature rupture of membranes, preterm delivery, and group B streptococcal colonization of mothers. Am J Obstet Gynecol 141:184, 1981.

Schachter J, Holt J, Goodner E, et al: Prospective study of chlamydial infection in neonates. Lancet 2(8139):377, 1979.

Schaefer G, Zervoudakis IA, Fuchs FF, et al: Pregnancy and pulmonary tuberculosis. Obstet Gynecol 46:706, 1975.

Stagno S, Pass RF, Dworsky ME, et al: Maternal cytomegalovirus infection and perinatal transmission. Clin Obstet Gynecol 25:563, 1982.

Whalley PJ, Cunningham FC: Short-term versus continuous antimicrobial therapy for asymptomatic bacteriuria in pregnancy. Obstet Gynecol 49:262, 1977.

Chapter Sixteen

MEDICAL COMPLICATIONS OF PREGNANCY

BAHIJ NUWAYHID

Physiologic adaptation to pregnancy involves the cardiovascular, pulmonary, endocrine, hematologic, neurologic, renal, and gastrointestinal systems. In a normal, healthy pregnant woman, the adaptive responses are appropriate and well-tolerated. When there is underlying pathology, the responses of the different organ systems are less well-tolerated, and organ failure may occur. Physiologic changes in pregnancy are discussed in Chapter 4 and only briefly summarized in this chapter.

CARDIOVASCULAR SYSTEM

Physiologic Changes During Pregnancy

During human pregnancy, cardiac output increases by almost 40 percent. Most of this increase is due to an increase in stroke volume, since heart rate increases by only about 10 beats per minute during the third trimester. Cardiac output peaks at around 28 to 32 weeks and then stabilizes. Because of the increase in cardiac output, grade 2 systolic flow murmurs may be frequently heard at the left sternal border, with no radiation. Additionally, a third heart sound might be heard, with wide splitting of S1. Diastolic murmurs should be considered pathologic and investigated. Because of the increased venous return, cardiac fullness, and hypertrophy, the heart is displaced superiorly, laterally, and

anteriorly, and the point of maximum impulse is shifted superiorly and laterally. Electrocardiographic changes include a left axis deviation and a flattened T wave.

Heart Disease

Heart disease in pregnancy can be divided into two categories: *rheumatic* and *congenital*. Rheumatic heart disease has traditionally accounted for about 90 percent of cases, but in recent years this percentage has been dropping because of better treatment of rheumatic fever and decreased pathogenicity of the organism. On the other hand, the number of females with congenital heart disease reaching childbearing age with unimpaired fertility has increased. In a modern tertiary referral center, approximately 35 percent of patients may have congenital heart disease.

Rheumatic Heart Disease. The most common lesion with rheumatic heart disease is mitral stenosis. Irrespective of the specific valvular lesion, these patients are at higher risk of developing heart failure, pulmonary edema, subacute bacterial endocarditis, and thromboembolic disease. They also have a high rate of fetal wastage.

Pure mitral stenosis is found in about 90 percent of rheumatic heart disease patients. During pregnancy, the cardiac output increases, and the mechanical obstruction worsens. Asymptomatic patients may develop symptoms of cardiac decompensation or pulmonary edema.

Atrial fibrillation is more common in patients with severe mitral stenosis, and its onset during pregnancy is ominous. Nearly all women who develop atrial fibrillation during pregnancy experience congestive heart failure. On the other hand, if atrial fibrillation predates pregnancy, only half of the women will develop pulmonary congestion and heart failure.

Patients with mitral insufficiency or aortic stenosis are in less danger of having cardiac decompensation in the third trimester of pregnancy. The myocardium of these young women is able to increase its workload without decompensation.

Congenital Heart Disease. This entity includes patients with atrial or ventricular septal defects, primary pulmonary hypertension (Eisenmenger's syndrome), and cyanotic heart disease. If the anatomic defect has been corrected during childhood with no residual damage, the patient will go through pregnancy with no apparent complications. Patients with persistent atrial or ventricular septal defects and those with tetralogy of Fallot with complete surgical correction tolerate pregnancy well. On the other hand, patients with primary pulmonary hypertension or cyanotic heart disease with residual pulmonary hypertension are in danger of decompensating during pregnancy. Pulmonary hypertension from any cause is associated with a 25 to 50 percent maternal mortality during pregnancy or in the immediate postpartum period. In all these patients, care should be taken to avoid overloading the circulation and precipitating pulmonary congestion, heart failure, or hypotension with reversal of the left-right shunt, conditions that will lead to hypoxia and sudden death.

Cardiac Arrhythmias. Paroxysmal atrial tachycardia is the most common cardiac arrhythmia. Usually it is benign and not associated with underlying heart disease. It is generally provoked by strenuous exercise. Atrial fibrillation and atrial flutter are more serious and usually associated with underlying cardiac disease.

Peripartum and Postpartum Cardiomyopathy. This entity is very rare, but is exclusively associated with pregnancy. These patients have no underlying cardiac disease, and symptoms of cardiac decompensation appear during the last weeks of pregnancy or 2 to 20 weeks postpartum. Pregnant individuals at risk to develop cardiomyopathy are those with a history of pre-eclampsia or hypertension and those with poor nutrition. No etiologic factor has been found, although Coxsackie B virus and fetal antimyocardial antibodies have been incriminated.

Management of Cardiac Disease During Pregnancy

The New York Heart Association's functional classification of heart disease is of value in assessing the risk of pregnancy for a patient with cardiac disease and in determining the optimal management during pregnancy, labor, and delivery (Table 16–1). In general, the maternal and fetal risks for patients with Class I and II disease are small, while they are greatly increased with Class III and IV disease. This does not imply that less attention should be given to the former group. Pulmonary edema leading to maternal death has been reported in patients with Class I and II cardiac disease.

Prenatal Management. As a general principle, all pregnant cardiac patients should be managed with the help of a cardiologist. Frequent prenatal visits are indicated, and frequent hospital admissions may be needed, especially for patients with Class III and IV cardiac disease. It is important to keep in mind a number of guidelines during the prenatal period.

AVOIDANCE OF EXCESSIVE WEIGHT GAIN AND EDEMA. Cardiac patients should be placed on a low-sodium diet (2 gm per day) to prevent excessive expansion of blood volume. They should be encouraged to rest in the lateral decubitus position for at least one hour every morning, afternoon, and evening to promote diuresis, especially during the latter part of gestation. Adequate sleep should be encouraged.

TABLE 16–1 NEW YORK HEART ASSOCIATION'S FUNCTIONAL CLASSIFICATION OF HEART DISEASE

Class I	No signs or symptoms of cardiac decompensation
Class II	No symptoms at rest, but minor limitation of physical activity
Class III	No symptoms at rest, but marked limitation of physical activity
Class IV	Symptoms present at rest, discomfort increased with any kind of physical activity

AVOIDANCE OF STRENUOUS ACTIVITY. All cardiac patients should avoid strenuous activity. Individuals with heart disease are unable to increase their cardiac output to the same extent as healthy individuals to meet the increased metabolic demands associated with exercise. Consequently, they tend to extract more oxygen from the arterial blood, resulting in a larger arteriovenous oxygen difference. With strenuous exercise and/or tissue hypoxia, blood is shifted from the uteroplacental circulation to other organs.

AVOIDANCE OF ANEMIA. With anemia, the oxygen-carrying-capacity of the blood decreases. This is compensated for by an increase in cardiac output, brought about mainly by an increase in heart rate. An increase in heart rate, especially with mitral stenosis, leads to a decrease in left ventricular filling time, so pulmonary congestion and edema may result. Another factor that might lead to cardiac decompensation is the inability of the right ventricle to pump all of the venous return.

EARLY DETECTION OF A PROBLEM. During every prenatal visit, the patient should be carefully examined to exclude infection, cardiac decompensation, pulmonary congestion, and cardiac arrhythmias.

Aside from the increased metabolic demands and cardiac output associated with a febrile illness, *bacteremia* may lead to the development of bacterial endocarditis.

With *heart failure,* the pulse increases to a rate greater than 100 beats per minute; the neck veins become congested; and the liver and spleen become enlarged and tender. Excessive weight gain is usual, and generalized edema might be present. Digitalization and diuretics will be required if heart failure develops.

With *pulmonary congestion,* a history of dyspnea and orthopnea might be elicited, and pulmonary rales and crepitations are usually present. Vital capacity, which can be measured in clinic, is decreased.

The apical heart rate should be auscultated because the peripheral pulse may not be sensitive to changes in cardiac rhythm. The onset of *dysrhythmias,* a change in the character of a murmur, or a change in heart sounds necessitates further cardiac work-up and specific treatment.

Although *cardiac decompensation* may occur at any phase of pregnancy, it is most likely to occur during the period of peak increase in cardiac output (28 to 32 weeks), during labor, during delivery, or during the immediate postpartum period. A pregnant patient with sufficient cardiac reserve to tolerate the peak increase in cardiac output without cardiac decompensation has a good chance of continuing the pregnancy without complications.

Management of Labor. During labor, cardiac output increases by about 40 to 50 percent when compared with pre-labor levels and by about 80 to 100 percent when compared with pre-pregnancy levels. Although part of the increase in cardiac output during labor is due to catecholamine release brought about by pain and apprehension, most of the increase is due to abdominal and uterine muscle contraction. In order to minimize the increase in cardiac output, assurance, sedation, and epidural anesthesia are encouraged early in labor. Prophylactic antibiotics (penicillin and gentamicin) against subacute bacterial endocarditis are started once labor is established and continued for 48 hours postpartum. In order to reduce the risk of supine hypotension and increase the oxygen-carrying-capacity of the blood, patients should be nursed on the side and given oxygen by mask.

In patients with severe cardiac disease (Class III and IV, pulmonary hypertension), monitoring of the cardiovascular status is essential during labor and delivery. Arterial and Swan-Ganz catheters should be inserted to monitor arterial pressure and cardiac output, together with right atrial, main pulmonary artery, and pulmonary wedge pressures. The cardiac rhythm should be monitored continuously. Fluid intake and urine output, arterial blood gases, hemoglobin concentration, and electrolytes are also monitored. Labor monitoring may be accomplished by external or internal means, depending on the obstetric needs, although the former is preferred. It is desirable to limit the number of pelvic examinations and to avoid the use of the intrauterine catheter in order to reduce the incidence of intrauterine infection.

Management of Delivery and the Immediate Postpartum Period. Cardiac patients should be delivered vaginally unless there are obstetric indications for cesarean section. It is important to shorten the second stage of labor by performing an outlet forceps delivery. The patient should be instructed to avoid pushing during uterine contractions because the associated increase in intra-abdominal pressure increases venous return and cardiac output and might lead to cardiac decompensation.

The immediate postpartum period presents special risks to the cardiac patient. After delivery of the placenta, the uterus contracts and about 500 ml of blood is added to the effective blood volume. In order to minimize the risk of overloading the circulation, the lower extremities are kept at the level of the body by lowering the stirrups, the uterus is not massaged to expedite placental separation, and pitocin is not given after delivery of the placenta. A small postpartum hemorrhage is frequently desirable, and if cardiac decompensation occurs, phlebotomy and/or rotating tourniquets should be considered.

Thromboembolic Disorders

These disorders include superficial thrombophlebitis, deep venous thrombosis, and pulmonary embolism. The overall incidence of these disorders during pregnancy is about 1.4 percent. About 80 percent occur during the postpartum period.

Superficial Thrombophlebitis. The incidence of superficial thrombophlebitis during pregnancy is 1 in 600 during the antepartum period and 1 in 95 in the immediate postpartum period. It is more common in patients with varicose veins, obesity, and limited physical activity. In most patients, superficial thrombophlebitis is limited to the calf area, and symptoms include swelling and tenderness of the involved extremity. On physical examination, there is erythema, tenderness, warmth, and a palpable cord over the course of the involved superficial veins.

Superficial thrombophlebitis is not life-threatening and does not lead to pulmonary embolization. However, if not treated promptly and adequately, the inflammatory process might extend to the deep veins. Pain medications, local application of heat (thermal blanket), and elevation of the lower extremities to promote improved venous flow are often sufficient treatment. There is no need for anticoagulants or anti-inflammatory agents. After five to seven days of bedrest and when symptoms disappear, the patient may be ambulated gradually. Postrecovery residual effects frequently persist in the form of valvular incompetence. Patients should be instructed to avoid standing for prolonged periods of time and to wear support hose to help avoid a repeat infection, which is prone to occur during pregnancy and the immediate postpartum period.

Deep Venous Thrombosis. The incidence of deep venous thrombosis is 1 in 2000 antepartum and 1 in 700 postpartum. The risk of pulmonary embolization is high, and immediate treatment is indicated. Vascular injury, infection, or tissue trauma, coupled with the hypercoagulability and venous stasis of pregnancy are the triggering factors for deep venous thrombosis.

CLINICAL FEATURES. The clinical diagnosis of deep venous thrombosis is difficult. Pain in the calf areas in association with dorsiflexion of the foot (positive Homan's sign) is a clinical sign of deep venous thrombosis in the calf veins. Acute swelling and pain in the thigh area, plus tenderness in the femoral triangle, are suggestive of ileofemoral thrombosis.

INVESTIGATIONS. Noninvasive techniques such as Doppler ultrasound and plethysmography are helpful, but a negative result does not exclude the diagnosis. Iodine-125 labeled fibrinogen and technetium-99 scans are sensitive to calf and iliac thrombosis, respectively. However, they are infrequently used because of unavailability or radiation hazard. The best single test for the diagnosis of deep venous thrombosis is a well-performed venogram. Although some iliac lesions are missed and there is a 2 percent incidence of phlebitis induced by the dye, the greatest concern is about radiation exposure, which is about 1 rad. This test should be done if the diagnosis is uncertain.

TREATMENT. When a clinical diagnosis of deep venous thrombosis is made, anticoagulant therapy should be started and further diagnostic work-up delayed several hours until adequate heparin levels have been reached. If the work-up fails to identify any ileofemoral or calf thrombosis, heparin may be discontinued.

Many obstetricians and patients are not willing to accept the risks and limitations of a venogram and maintain anticoagulant therapy on the basis of clinical findings. Such an empiric approach is not without risks. In addition, these patients will forever carry such a diagnosis, necessitating special precautions during any subsequent pregnancy or surgical procedure.

Treatment of active deep venous thrombosis during pregnancy is initiated with intravenous heparin therapy. An initial dose of 10,000 units followed by a continuous infusion of intravenous heparin at a rate of about 1000 units per hour is maintained for five to seven days, or until symptoms disappear. For the first one to two days, the heparin dose should be increased or decreased to keep the prothrombin time (PT) at 2 to 2.5 times the normal control values. Since anticoagulant therapy must be continued for the duration of pregnancy and up to six weeks postpartum, either subcutaneous full dose heparin or warfarin (Coumadin) by mouth might be given. If warfarin is chosen, a partial thromboplastin time (PTT) should be obtained weekly. PTT values should be maintained in the range of 2 to 2.5 times control.

Heparin is a high molecular weight substance that does not cross the placental barrier, so there are no untoward effects for the fetus and neonate. Heparin therapy may be continued until the onset of labor, stopped during active labor and delivery, and resumed 6 to 12 hours postpartum. If prothrombin time remains prolonged during labor, 5 gm of protamine sulfate are enough to reverse the action of heparin. There is no evidence to suggest increased postpartum uterine bleeding or bleeding from the episiotomy site when patients are restarted on anticoagulant therapy. Additionally, heparin is not secreted in breast milk. Complications of long-term therapy include (1) hemorrhage, (2) heparin-associated thrombocytopenia, and (3) heparin-induced osteoporosis.

Warfarin has a low molecular weight and crosses the placental barrier. If it is given during the period of fetal organogenesis, it is teratogenic. Late in gestation and with the onset of uterine contractions, fetal ecchymoses and intracranial bleeding may occur. Warfarin may, therefore, be given during the second trimester and up until 36 weeks of gestation. Thereafter, heparin is reinstituted and continued until the onset of labor. During the postpartum period, warfarin may be resumed.

Pulmonary Embolism. The incidence of pulmonary embolism during pregnancy is about 1:2500. The maternal mortality is less than 1 percent if treated early and greater than 80 percent if left untreated. In about 70 percent of cases, deep venous thrombosis is the instigating factor.

CLINICAL FEATURES. Clinical and laboratory findings parallel the degree of insult but may be deceptively nonspecific. Suggestive symptoms include pleuritic chest pain, shortness of breath, air hunger, palpitations, hemoptysis, and syncopal episodes. Suggestive signs include tachypnea, tachycardia, low-grade fever, a pleural friction rub, chest splinting, pulmonary rales, an accentuated pulmonic valve second heart sound, and even signs of right heart failure. In most obstetric patients, the signs and symptoms of a pulmonary embolus are subtle.

INVESTIGATIONS. An electrocardiogram might show sinus tachycardia with or without premature heart beats or right ventricular axis deviation. Cardiac enzymes are not helpful. On chest x-ray, atelectasis, pleural effusion, obliteration of arterial shadows, and elevation of the diaphragm might be present. Arterial blood gases taken on room air show an oxygen tension below 80 mm Hg. If there is any doubt about the diagnosis, a technetium-99 ventilation-perfusion scan has a sensitivity of 95 percent in detecting pulmonary embolism, provided there is no heart failure, obstructive or constrictive lung disease, or pulmonary infiltrate. It can be performed with minimal risk to the fetus. Pulmonary angiography is rarely required, but its main value is to diagnose a large embolus in patients on whom embolectomy is planned.

Treatment of acute episodes and follow-up during pregnancy, labor, delivery, and the postpartum period are the same as for deep venous thrombosis.

PROPHYLACTIC ANTICOAGULANT THERAPY. In pregnant patients with a history of a pulmonary embolus or deep venous thrombosis during a previous pregnancy, prophylactic anticoagulants are given during pregnancy and the immediate postpartum period. Most patients are given full-dose anticoagulation but some studies have suggested that minidose heparin (10,000 to 15,000 units per day) might be given. For patients with a history of deep venous thrombosis or pulmonary embolism not related to pregnancy, prophylactic minidose heparin might also be given, although there are no firm data to support such an approach.

PULMONARY DISORDERS

Obstructive Lung Disease

Bronchial Asthma. The incidence of bronchial asthma in pregnancy is approximately 1 percent, and about 15 percent of these individuals develop one or more severe attacks during gestation. Although the effect of pregnancy on bronchial asthma is variable, severe asthma is associated with a high abortion rate and an increased incidence of intrauterine fetal death and fetal growth retardation because of intrauterine hypoxia. Pulmonary function studies done during an acute episode show (1) increased airway resistance; (2) increased residual volume, functional residual capacity, and total lung capacity; (3) decreased inspiratory and expiratory reserve volume; (4) decreased vital capacity; and (5) decreased one-second forced expiratory volume (FEV_1), peak expiratory flow rate, and maximum midexpiratory flow rate.

OBSTETRIC MANAGEMENT. Pregnant asthmatics should be followed closely during pregnancy to assure adequate maternal and fetal assessment. In most asthmatics, no drug treatment is needed. Adequate bedrest, the avoidance of dehydration, early and aggressive treatment of respiratory infections, and the avoidance of hyperventilation, excessive physical activity, and allergins are sufficient to prevent an exacerbation of symptoms. Additionally, minimal studies are needed to assess respiratory status. Cough medications containing iodine should be used with care because of the risk of causing a congenital goiter in the fetus.

In moderately affected asthmatics, baseline pulmonary function studies and a chest x-ray (with abdominal shielding) are essential to assess cardiopulmonary status. Follow-up studies are repeated as clinically indicated, although vital capacity may be assessed in the clinic at every visit. Most of these patients will respond well to beta-adrenergic receptor stimulant inhalers, such as epinephrine and isoproterenol (Isuprel), used two to three times per day. If symptoms persist or the inhalers are needed more than three to four times per day, one of the xanthine derivatives should be given, such as theophylline (Theo-Dur), 100 to 500 mg orally, twice daily. Selective beta$_2$ receptor stimulants, such as terbutaline (2.5 mg every four to six hours), may be added to the above regimen if symptoms persist.

Patients with more complicated cases should be managed in consultation with pulmonary internists and respiratory therapists. If glucocorticoids are needed, every effort should be made to taper the dose gradually and then stop it. If continuous steroids are deemed necessary, 5 to 10 mg of prednisone every other day is usually sufficient.

For severe attacks, hospitalization is usually necessary. If patients are not already on xanthine preparations, a loading dose of aminophylline (5 to 6 mg/kg) is given intravenously over a period of 30 minutes, followed by a maintenance dose of 0.5 to 0.9 mg/kg/hr. Blood levels of aminophylline should be maintained at 12 to 20 μg/ml. Epinephrine (1:1000) in a dose of 0.3 to 0.5 ml or terbutaline, 0.25 to 0.5 mg, may be administered subcutaneously if there is inadequate response to aminophylline. Corticosteroids may be administered intravenously in a dose equivalent to prednisone 60 mg/day. Once the acute episode is over, oral aminophylline and beta-sympathomimetic preparations are substituted and steroids tapered gradually.

Since most of the medications the mother receives during pregnancy cross the uteroplacental barrier, the potential of added risk to the fetus must be emphasized to parents. Although xanthines seem to be safe for the fetus, epinephrine usage during pregnancy is associated with a slight increase in the rate of congenital anomalies. Glucocorticoids are associated with fetal intrauterine growth retardation.

Antepartum monitoring of the fetus to assess growth and development is essential. Early and serial pelvic ultrasounds, together with nonstress or oxytocin challenge tests, as indicated, are usually employed.

The timing of delivery is dependent on the status of both the mother and the fetus. If pregnancy is progressing well, there is no need for early intervention, and it is advisable to await the spontaneous onset of labor. If the maternal condition is deteriorating or there is fetal growth retardation, planning for an early delivery is recommended.

MANAGEMENT OF LABOR AND DELIVERY. If the patient has been taking oral steroids during pregnancy, the intravenous administration of glucocorticoids is recommended during labor, delivery, and the postpartum period. A selective epidural block during labor benefits the patient in that it reduces pain, anxiety, hyperventilation, and respiratory work, all of which are known to aggravate the disease or precipitate an attack. Vaginal delivery should be anticipated, but if cesarean section is indicated for obstetric reasons, general anesthesia is desirable. Endotracheal intubation represents the most common stimulus precipitating asthma during general anesthesia. Spinal or epidural anesthesia for cesarean section poses potential hazards to the asthmatic patient. The supine position will limit respiration, while the high thoracic level of the block might impair coughing and the sensation of breathing and lead to increased patient anxiety. Additionally, the high sympathetic nerve blockade may lead to parasympathetic dominance and bronchoconstriction. Nausea, vomiting, and coughing may develop with peritoneal traction during surgical manipulation.

Other Forms of Obstructive Lung Disease. The most severe form of obstructive lung disease observed during pregnancy is in patients with *cystic fibrosis.* The abnormal mucus results in airway plugging, inflammation, bronchiectasis, and recurrent pulmonary infections. Approximately half of these patients develop serious and progressive pulmonary decompensation during and after pregnancy. Although fetal outcome depends on the severity of the maternal disease, available data suggest excellent fetal survival rates. *Chronic bronchitis* and *emphysema* are not common in women of childbearing age.

Restrictive Lung Disease

Tuberculosis. The incidence of tuberculosis in the indigent population varies from 0.6 to 4.8 percent. About 10 to 12 percent of these cases are active. Tuberculosis during pregnancy is discussed in Chapter 15.

ENDOCRINE DISORDERS

Only the most common endocrine disorders are discussed in this section. Emphasis is on diabetes mellitus and thyroid disease.

Diabetes Mellitus

Incidence and Classification. The incidence of diabetes mellitus in pregnancy is less than 0.5 percent. In addition to the uniform classification of diabetes during the nonpregnant state (Table 16–2), White's classification of diabetes during pregnancy is used and is of more prognostic value (Table 16–3).

Complications. Fetal and maternal complications associated with diabetes mellitus during pregnancy are listed in Table 16–4.

Diagnosis. Screening for diabetes mellitus

TABLE 16–2 CLASSIFICATION OF DIABETES MELLITUS (NONPREGNANT)

A. Diabetes mellitus
   1. Type I —Insulin-dependent
           Ketosis-prone
   2. Type II—Noninsulin-dependent
           Ketosis-resistant
   3. Diabetes associated with certain conditions or syndromes
B. Impaired glucose tolerance
C. Gestational diabetes

is discussed in Chapter 6. If the fasting and one-hour or two-hour screening plasma glucose levels are abnormal, a glucose tolerance test may not be required. For borderline screening tests, a three-hour glucose tolerance test should be performed, preceded by a special diet containing about 300 gm of carbohydrate for the previous three days (Table 16–5). If any two values are abnormal, excluding the fasting blood glucose, the patient is classified as having gestational diabetes Class A. If the fasting blood sugar is also abnormal, she is classified as having Class B or Class A/B.

TABLE 16–3 WHITE'S CLASSIFICATION OF DIABETES IN PREGNANCY

CLASS	DESCRIPTION
A	Gestational diabetes. Glucose intolerance developing during pregnancy; fasting blood glucose is normal
A/B	Gestational diabetes with fasting plasma glucose greater than 105 mg/dl; or 2-hour postprandial plasma glucose greater than 120 mg/dl
B	Overt diabetes developing after age 20 and duration less than 10 years
C	Overt diabetes developing before age 20 or duration greater than 10 years
D	Overt diabetes developing before age 10 or duration greater than 20 years and/or background retinopathy
E	Overt diabetes at any age or duration with calcified pelvic vessels
F	Overt diabetes at any age or duration with nephropathy
R	Overt diabetes at any age or duration with proliferative retinopathy
RF	Overt diabetes at any age or duration with both retinopathy and nephropathy
H	Overt diabetes at any age or duration with arteriosclerotic heart disease
T	Overt diabetes at any age or duration with a renal transplant

TABLE 16–4 MATERNAL AND FETAL COMPLICATIONS OF DIABETES MELLITUS

ENTITY	MONITORING
A. MATERNAL COMPLICATIONS	
1. Obstetric complications	
a. Polyhydramnios	Close prenatal surveillance; ultrasound
b. Pre-eclampsia	
2. Diabetic emergencies	Blood glucose monitoring; insulin and dietary adjustment; check for infection, including urine culture every six weeks
a. Hypoglycemia	
b. Ketoacidosis	
c. Diabetic coma	
3. Vascular and end organ involvement or deterioration	
a. Cardiac	EKG, first visit and as needed
b. Renal	Renal function studies, first visit and as needed
c. Ophthalmic	Funduscopic evaluation, first visit and as needed
d. Peripheral vascular	Check for ulcers, foot sores; noninvasive Doppler studies as needed
4. Neurologic	
a. Peripheral neuropathy	Neurologic and gastrointestinal consultations as needed
b. Gastrointestinal disturbance	
B. FETAL COMPLICATIONS	
1. Macrosomia with traumatic delivery	Repeat pelvic ultrasound prior to delivery
2. Delayed organ maturity (pulmonary, hepatic, neurologic, pituitary-thyroid axis)	Amniocentesis for lung profile
3. Congenital anomalies	
a. Cardiovascular	Prior to 22 weeks' gestation, maternal serum alphafetoprotein; Hgb A1C monthly; pelvic ultrasound and fetal echocardiogram; amniocentesis and genetic counseling, if necessary
b. Neural tube defects	
c. Caudal regression syndrome	
4. Intrauterine growth retardation	
a. Intrauterine fetal death	Repeat ultrasound every 4 weeks; NST and OCT; biophysical profile weekly or biweekly
b. Abnormal FHR patterns	
c. Small-for-dates babies	

TABLE 16–5 THREE-HOUR GLUCOSE TOLERANCE TEST*

TEST	NORMAL PLASMA GLUCOSE (mg/dl)
fasting	105
1 hour	190
2 hours	165
3 hours	145

*100 gm of oral glucose given after an overnight fast.

The best time to screen for diabetes is between 26 and 28 weeks' gestation, because peripheral insulin resistance and insulin response to a glucose load start to increase at that time.

Management—Diabetic Team. Management of the gestational diabetic requires patient teaching and counseling, medical-nursing assessments and interventions, strategies to achieve maternal euglycemia, and avoidance of fetal-neonatal compromise. A diabetic team works together to achieve these objectives. This team includes the patient, obstetrician, clinical nurse specialist, dietitian, psychosocial worker, and neonatologist.

PATIENT. The most significant change in diabetic management during pregnancy has been the inclusion of the patient as an active participant in formulating management strategies. In addition to teaching the patient survival skills, such as the identification and management of hypo- and hyperglycemic episodes, she is taught the techniques for home glucose monitoring, insulin administration, and dietary adjustments.

OBSTETRICIAN. The obstetrician, as the head of the diabetic team, coordinates its activities and presents a unified concept of medical care strategies to the patient. This physician plays a very important role in the prevention and early identification of prognostically poor indices, such as hypertension, infection, poor control of blood glucose, polyhydramnios, and/or fetal macrosomia.

CLINICAL NURSE SPECIALIST. The clinical nurse specialist is involved in teaching the patient basic concepts about the pathophysiology of diabetes during pregnancy, assessing patient compliance and well-being, and teaching the patient methods of insulin administration, home glucose monitoring, and survival skills.

PSYCHOSOCIAL WORKER. The psychosocial worker helps the patient to deal emotionally with her diabetes and explores the avenues to help her avoid stress.

DIETITIAN. The dietitian evaluates the patient's knowledge about the American Diabetic Association's (ADA) diet and food exchange lists and provides dietary information as necessary.

Achieving Euglycemia. In recent years, the importance of stricter metabolic control in decreasing perinatal morbidity and mortality has been appreciated. In order to achieve euglycemia, diet, insulin, and exercise must be regulated.

DIET. An ADA diet with at least 1800 calories should be prescribed. Caloric requirements are calculated on the basis of 16 calories per pound of ideal body weight, plus 300 calories for anticipated weight gain during pregnancy. For an obese patient, additional calories are needed to prevent starvation ketonemia, while for an underweight patient, additional calories are needed for an appropriate weight gain during pregnancy. In general, 50 to 60 percent of the caloric requirements are given as carbohydrates, 18 to 22 percent as protein, and the remainder (about 25 percent) as fat. Inclusion of a high-fiber content in the diet is recommended.

A comprehensive meal plan must be devised for the patient. It is particularly important in the pregnant diabetic to have a bedtime snack.

INSULIN. Oral hypoglycemic agents are not recommended during pregnancy, since they cross the placental barrier and may induce fetal and neonatal hypoglycemia. Short, intermediate or long-acting insulin may be used in a combination of dosage schedules to effect maternal euglycemia. The peak action of short-acting (regular) insulin is about 4 hours, intermediate-acting insulin (neutral protamine Hagedorn (NPH)) about 12 hours, and long-acting insulin 14 to 20 hours. For tight diabetic control during pregnancy, long-acting insulins are rarely used, but a combination of short and intermediate insulins are given as a split morning and evening dose. A method for calculating insulin dosage is shown in Table 16–6. Beef and pork combinations or pork insulin alone may be used. These are now available as purified insulin products (less than 50 particles/million of impurities). Pork insulins are more expensive but less antigenic. They are recommended for patients using insulin for short periods of time, during pregnancy, or for those with

TABLE 16–6 METHOD FOR CALCULATION OF STARTING DOSE OF INSULIN

Insulin units = body weight (kg) × 0.6 (First trimester)
  0.7 (Second trimester)
  0.8 (Third trimester)

Dosage schedule: Give ⅔ in AM and ⅓ in PM.
  AM ⅔ NPH, ⅓ regular
  PM ½ NPH, ½ regular

high-circulating beef antibody titers. Recently, synthetic human insulin has been introduced; its promise lies in reducing the antibody production, which increases insulin resistance.

Blood glucose levels drawn at specified hours to coincide with the peak action of insulin are utilized to assess the adequacy of insulin therapy. For a split (morning and evening), mixed (NPH and regular) dose of insulin, blood sugar levels are drawn at 7:00 A.M., 11:00 A.M., 4:00 P.M., and 10:00 P.M.—prior to breakfast, lunch, dinner, and evening snack, respectively. The 7:00 A.M. and 4:00 P.M. blood glucose levels reflect the adequacy of evening and morning NPH dosage, respectively. Similarly, the 11:00 A.M. and 10:00 P.M. levels reflect the adequacy of morning and evening regular insulin dosages. In some individuals, 2:00 A.M. blood glucose levels might be indicated to adequately adjust the insulin dosage and avoid nocturnal hypoglycemia. A mean daily serum glucose level of less than 100 mg/dl is encouraged, with fasting and premeal blood sugars between 70 to 80 mg/dl and postprandial levels between 100 and 120 mg/dl.

Adjusting the insulin dosage to achieve euglycemia is facilitated by careful home glucose monitoring. It is important to keep the following principles in mind:

1. Initial adjustment should be directed toward achieving a fasting plasma glucose level of 70 to 80 mg/dl.

2. Only one change in insulin dosage should be attempted at any given time; additionally, at least 24 hours should be allowed after a dosage change to evaluate blood sugar response adequately.

3. Prior to changing the insulin schedule, careful attention should be given to compliance with diet, change in physical activity, or other temporary mitigating factors, such as stress or infection, that alter insulin requirements.

EXERCISE. Diabetic patients should be encouraged to exercise about half an hour after meals. Use of a stationary bike or mild to moderate aerobic exercises are adequate. A hospitalized, sedentary patient who achieves euglycemia during her hospital stay may encounter frequent episodes of hypoglycemia once she is discharged and returns to her usual daily activities.

Antepartum Obstetric Management. Aside from achieving euglycemia, adequate surveillance should be maintained during pregnancy to avoid maternal complications and to assure fetal growth and development. A maternal serum alpha-fetoprotein level should be obtained at 16 to 20 weeks to alert the obstetrician to the possibility of an open neural tube defect in the fetus. Maternal renal, cardiac, and ophthalmic function are closely monitored. The glycosylated hemoglobin levels (Hgb A1C) are monitored monthly. The percentage of Hgb A1C has been shown to correlate with long-term (up to four weeks) blood glucose levels. Elevated levels of Hgb A1C suggest that diabetic control is not adequate. Regular electronic, biochemical, and ultrasonographic fetal monitoring should be performed, as shown in Figure 6–1 (Chapter 6). For diabetic Classes A, B, and C, fetal macrosomia should be sought, while for Classes D, E, and F, fetal growth retardation is more commonly found.

Timing of Delivery. Recent advances in the management of the diabetic patient, such as tight metabolic control, availability of the fetal lung profile, and fetal biophysical profile determinations have obviated the need for early delivery. If the maternal state is stable, blood glucose is in the euglycemic range, and fetal studies indicate continued growth of a healthy baby, delivery may be delayed until fetal lung maturity is achieved. Early intervention is indicated if these conditions are not met. For macrosomic babies, increased birth trauma to both mother and fetus should be kept in mind, and judicious use of cesarean section is preferable to early induction of labor when the cervix is still unfavorable. Prolonged serial induction of labor should not be pursued in a diabetic patient unless maternal and fetal monitoring are carefully carried out.

Intrapartum Management. Adequate intrapartum management of a diabetic patient requires maternal euglycemia during labor, which may be achieved by giving a continuous infusion of regular insulin in 5 per cent dextrose at a rate of 0.5 to 2 units of insulin per hour. Plasma glucose levels are measured every 2 hours and insulin dosage adjusted accordingly to maintain a plasma glucose level of between 80 and 100 mg/dl. In calculating the 24-hour insulin requirements, the ratio of insulin requirements to total caloric intake per day may be used as a rough estimate. This ratio multiplied by caloric intake during labor (600 calories) yields an estimate of anticipated total insulin requirements for the day. Provided plasma glucose is monitored frequently and insulin administered when plasma glucose exceeds 100 mg/dl, not all insulin-dependent patients will require exogenous insulin during labor.

Fetal monitoring is recommended for all diabetic patients, especially for those who are insulin-dependent. Internal monitoring is advised if there is any doubt about the fetal status or the progression of labor.

Standard obstetric criteria should guide the individual as to the mode of delivery. Irrespective of mode of delivery, a neonatologist should be available in the labor area for immediate neonatal evaluation.

Postpartum Period. After delivery of the fetus and placenta, insulin requirements drop sharply because the placenta, which is the source of many insulin antagonists, has been removed. Most insulin-dependent diabetic patients do not require exogenous insulin for the first 48 to 72 hours after delivery. Plasma glucose levels should be obtained every 6 hours and regular insulin given when plasma glucose levels exceed 150 mg/dl. Prior to hospital discharge, patients may be restarted on two thirds of their prepregnancy insulin dosage, and gradual adjustments made as necessary.

Patients should be counseled about changes in diet. Except for gestational Class A diabetics, the ADA diet with the same distribution of carbohydrates, proteins, and fat should be maintained. If the mother is breast feeding, 700 calories per day should be added to the maintenance diet.

Contraceptive counseling is an important aspect of total patient care, especially in the diabetic patient (see Chapter 40). Tubal ligation is recommended for patients who are desirous of permanent sterilization or for those with advanced vascular involvement.

Thyroid Diseases

Normal Thyroid Physiology During Pregnancy. With the increase in glomerular filtration rate that occurs during pregnancy, the renal excretion of iodine increases, and plasma inorganic iodine levels are nearly halved. Whether or not goiter ensues depends on the ability of the thyroid gland to compensate, which in turn depends on the concentration of plasma inorganic iodine and dietary iodine intake. Goiters due to iodine deficiency are not likely if plasma inorganic iodine levels are greater than 0.08 μg/dl. Only in patients who have plasma inorganic iodine levels that are borderline prior to pregnancy is there an increased incidence of goiter during pregnancy. Inorganic iodine supplementation up to a total of 250 μg per day is sufficient to prevent goiter formation during pregnancy.

THYROID FUNCTION TESTS. The *free thyroxine concentration* is the only direct method of estimating thyroid function that compensates for changes in thyroxine-binding globulin (TBG) capacity. Although serum levels of bound triiodothyronine (T_3) and thyroxine (T_4) are increased during pregnancy (as discussed in Chapter 4), free thyroxine levels remain within the normal range. The uptake of triiodothyronine by resin (T_3 resin uptake), which is an indirect measure of thyroxine-binding capacity, tends to be in the hypothyroid range during pregnancy, an indication that more binding sites are available. Since serum thyroxine increases and the T_3 resin uptake decreases, the free thyroxine index remains the same during pregnancy. Since determination of free thyroxine levels is time-consuming, difficult, and expensive, the *free thyroxine index* may be used as an indirect approximation of the free thyroxine concentration during pregnancy. Values of thyroid function tests during pregnancy are shown in Table 16–7.

FETAL THYROID FUNCTION. Prior to 10 weeks' gestation, no organic iodine is present in the fetal thyroid. By 11 to 12 weeks, the fetal thyroid is able to produce iodothyronines and thyroxine, and by 12 to 14 weeks it is able to concentrate iodine. Fetal thyroid-stimulating hormone (TSH), thyroxine, and free thyroxine levels suggest that a mature, autonomous, thyroid-pituitary axis exists as early as 12 weeks of gestation.

In the amniotic fluid, T_4 and reverse T_3 concentrations reach a peak at 25 to 30 weeks and then decrease, while T_3 concentrations continue to increase throughout pregnancy. Whether or not amniotic fluid levels of thyroid hormone activity reflect the fetal compartment is unknown, although levels of T_3 in the amniotic fluid have been used for the prenatal diagnosis of fetal thyroid abnormalities.

PLACENTAL TRANSFER OF THYROID HORMONE. There is minimal transfer of thyroxine and triiodothyronine across the placenta. Thyroid hormone analogues, with smaller molecular weights, decreased protein binding, and increased fat solubility cross the placental barrier much more easily and could potentially be used to affect the fetal status without producing maternal thyrotoxicosis.

Maternal Hyperthyroidism. The incidence of maternal thyrotoxicosis is about 1 per 500 pregnancies. Although the incidence of fetal wastage is not increased, there is an increased

TABLE 16–7 THYROID FUNCTION TESTS IN NONPREGNANT WOMEN AND IN MATERNAL AND CORD BLOOD AT TERM

TEST	NONPREGNANT	PREGNANT	CORD
Serum thyroxine (μg/dl)	5–12	10–16	6–13
Free thyroxine (ng/dl)	1.0–2.3	2.5–3.5	1.5–3.0
Serum triiodothyronine (ng/dl)	110–230	150–250	40–60
Reverse triiodothyronine (ng/dl)	—	35–65	80–360
Resin T_3 uptake (percent)	20–30	10	10–15
TBG (μg/dl)	12–28	40–50	10–16
Serum TSH (μU/ml)	1.9–5.4	0–6	0–20

Note: Absolute values for these tests may vary according to the method used, but the ratio between maternal and cord values should remain constant. Modified with permission from Burrow GN, Ferris T (eds): Medical Complications During Pregnancy. Philadelphia, W B Saunders Co, 1972, p. 194.

incidence of prematurity and intrauterine growth retardation and a higher neonatal morbidity and mortality.

Graves' disease or toxic diffuse goiter is the most common cause of hyperthyroidism associated with pregnancy. Other causes of hyperthyroidism in pregnancy include hydatidiform mole and toxic nodular goiter. Patients with Graves' disease tend to have a remission during pregnancy and an exacerbation during the postpartum period. There is evidence to suggest that the increased immunologic tolerance during pregnancy may lead to a decrease in thyroid antibodies and amelioration of symptoms.

CLINICAL FEATURES. The clinical diagnosis of hyperthyroidism in pregnancy is difficult because many signs and symptoms of the hyperdynamic circulation associated with hyperthyroidism are present in a normal euthyroid pregnant individual. A resting pulse rate greater than 100 beats per minute that fails to slow with a Valsalva maneuver, eye changes, loss of weight, and heat intolerance are all helpful in making the clinical diagnosis.

INVESTIGATIONS. A total serum thyroxine level of greater than 15 µg/dl or a greatly elevated free thyroxine index are diagnostic. Since the free thyroxine index is not an actual measure of free thyroxine concentration, free thyroxine levels are helpful in confirming the diagnosis.

THERAPY. Since *radioactive iodine* treatment is *contraindicated* during pregnancy, either medical treatment or partial surgical ablation of the thyroid gland is utilized.

The mainstay of antithyroid therapy is thioamides, which block the synthesis but not the release of thyroid hormone. It usually takes about one week for amelioration of symptoms and four to six weeks for full control. *Propylthiouracil* (PTU) and *methimazole* (Tapazole) have been used interchangeably, although PTU has the added advantage of blocking conversion of T_4 to T_3.

Once a diagnosis of hyperthyroidism has been made, the patient should be started on 100 to 150 mg of PTU every eight hours. After the symptoms have subsided and serum levels of thyroxine have returned toward normal, the dose of PTU should be lowered gradually to about 100 mg/day and maintained for the duration of pregnancy. Postpartum, the dose might be increased to about 300 mg/day to avoid an exacerbation of symptoms.

Since PTU crosses the placenta without difficulty, a major concern during maternal treatment is the development of fetal goiter and hypothyroidism. Clinical follow-up of these patients suggests that only 1 to 5 percent of children exposed to PTU develop goiter. The neonatal goiter associated with PTU therapy is not large and obstructive, and there is no conclusive evidence that PTU treatment can lead to cretinism. Children exposed to thioamides *in utero* attain full physical and intellectual development and have normal thyroid function studies. PTU excretion in breast milk does not exceed 0.025 percent of the administered daily maternal dose, and no changes occur in the thyroid function tests of breast-fed neonates.

Recently, there has been interest in the use of beta-receptor blockers in conjunction with PTU. *Propranolol* in a dose of 40 mg every six hours may be used. However, there are scattered reports implicating propranolol as an etiologic agent in intrauterine growth retardation, fetal demise, impaired fetal responses to hypoxic stress, and postnatal hypoglycemia and bradycardia. Therefore, the drug should be used only in acute situations to control symptoms until PTU achieves its effect.

Surgical management of the hyperthyroid pregnant patient is recommended only if medical treatment fails. Nowadays, few patients undergo subtotal thyroidectomy during pregnancy. It is advisable to delay surgery until the second trimester, since the rate of spontaneous abortion is highest during the first trimester. For rapid control of thyrotoxicosis prior to surgery, the addition of propranolol, 40 mg every six hours, and potassium iodide, 100 mg per day for five to seven days, usually results in a marked improvement within a week.

Thyroid Storm. The major risk for a pregnant patient with thyrotoxicosis is the development of a thyroid storm. Precipitating factors include infection, labor, cesarean section, or noncompliance with medication. The maternal mortality exceeds 25 percent in spite of good medical management. The signs and symptoms associated with a thyroid storm include: hyperthermia, marked tachycardia, perspiration, and severe dehydration. Specific treatment is directed at (1) blocking beta-adrenergic activity with propranolol, 40 mg every six hours; (2) blocking secretion of thyroid hormone with sodium iodide, 1 gm IV; and lithium, 300 mg three times daily;

(3) blocking synthesis of thyroid hormone and conversion of T_4 to T_3 with 1200 mg PTU given in divided doses; (4) further blocking the deamination of T_4 to T_3 with 8 mg dexamethazone per day; (5) replacing fluid losses with at least 5 liters of fluid; and (6) rapidly lowering the temperature with hypothermic techniques.

Neonatal Thyrotoxicosis. About 1 percent of pregnant women with a history of Graves' disease give birth to children with thyrotoxicosis. Although it is transient and lasts less than two to three months, it is not a benign condition, since it is associated with a neonatal mortality rate of about 16 percent.

Neonatal thyrotoxicosis is most likely related to placental transfer of thyroid-stimulating immunoglobulins of the 7S (IgG) variety such as long-acting thyroid stimulator (LATS). The presence of LATS in maternal and cord blood and the decline in neonatal serum concentrations of LATS as neonatal thyrotoxicosis improves gives credence to the above hypothesis. Recently it has been found that LATS protector is more commonly found in the serum of mothers whose infants develop thyrotoxicosis, and levels of LATS-P exceeding 20 units/ml are almost always associated with neonatal thyrotoxicosis.

Hypothyroidism. Hypothyroidism is relatively uncommon during pregnancy.

MATERNAL HYPOTHYROIDISM. Hypothyroid pregnant patients have a higher incidence of spontaneous abortions, stillbirths, and offspring with retarded neonatal sexual differentiation. However, most infants of hypothyroid mothers are healthy.

The most important laboratory finding to confirm the diagnosis of hypothyroidism is an elevated TSH level. Other findings include low levels of serum triiodothyronine and thyroxine and a decreased T_3 resin uptake.

Once a diagnosis of hypothyroidism has been made in a pregnant woman, thyroid replacement should be started immediately. L-thyroxine in a dose of 0.15 mg every eight hours is usually sufficient to ameliorate the symptoms. Later adjustments in the dosage schedule depend on the increase in serum T_3 and T_4 levels and the decrease in TSH.

Not infrequently, pregnant women are encountered who are receiving maintenance doses of thyroxine for obscure reasons. While some physicians have recommended discontinuation of thyroid treatment for five to six weeks to allow for a reevaluation of thyroid function, most have opted for continuation of treatment during pregnancy and reevaluation during the postpartum period.

NEONATAL HYPOTHYROIDISM. Thyroid hormone deficiency during the fetal and early neonatal periods leads to generalized developmental retardation. The severity of symptoms depends on the time of onset and the severity of the deprivation. If the disease is diagnosed and treated during the early neonatal period, the damage may be greatly minimized.

The incidence of congenital hypothyroidism (*cretinism*) is about 1 in 4000 births. The etiologic factors include thyroid dysgenesis, inborn errors of thyroid function, and drug-induced endemic hypothyroidism. The most common cause of neonatal goiter is maternal ingestion of iodides present in cough syrup. The goiters associated with maternal iodine ingestion are large and obstructive, unlike those associated with maternal PTU treatment.

The clinical diagnosis of neonatal hypothyroidism is very difficult. Hypothyroidism should be suspected in a large neonate with respiratory and feeding difficulties, an umbilical hernia, and rough dry skin. Today, screening of all neonates prior to discharge with serum thyroxine and serum TSH levels should identify almost all affected infants.

HEMATOLOGIC DISORDERS

Anemia

Physiologic Anemia in Pregnancy. During pregnancy, the blood volume increases by 40 to 50 percent. The red cell mass increases by 25 percent, so there is a relative increase in plasma volume, compared to red cell mass. The hematocrit and hemoglobin concentrations decrease. The term "physiologic anemia of pregnancy" is applied to this drop in hematocrit. The serum iron levels decrease slightly but remain within the normal range, while the total iron binding capacity increases by about 15 percent. Hemoglobin levels less than 10 gm/dl indicate the presence of anemia. Only hemoglobin levels less than 6 gm/dl are associated with an increased incidence of stillborn and premature infants.

Iron Deficiency Anemia. Primary iron deficiency is responsible for about 80 percent of nonphysiologic anemias during pregnancy. Approximately 1000 mg of additional iron is required during pregnancy for the expanded maternal red cell mass, for fetal hemoglobin, and for iron lost through bleeding at the time of delivery. Therefore, at least 4 mg of elemental iron are needed per day. This amount exceeds the 1.3 to 2.6 mg per day that is absorbed from a normal diet, even in an iron-deficient person. As a result, iron supplementation during pregnancy is necessary. A 325-mg ferrous sulfate tablet taken daily (60 mg of elemental iron) is usually sufficient for prophylactic purposes, although more is needed with iron deficiency anemia.

Laboratory findings depend on the severity and chronicity of anemia. Initially, the iron stores are depleted, followed by a decrease in the serum iron and an increase in the total iron-binding capacity. Finally, morphologic changes in the red cells occur. Serum ferritin levels less than 10 ng/ml, serum iron levels less than 60 μg/dl, and transferrin saturation rates (total iron binding capacity/serum iron) less than 16 percent are suggestive of iron deficiency anemia. A peripheral smear may show microcytosis, hypochromia, and a reticulocyte count that is low for the degree of anemia. If the diagnosis of iron deficiency anemia is equivocal or the patient is not responding to iron supplementation, bone marrow aspiration is recommended. The absence of stainable iron on a bone marrow aspirate is diagnostic for iron deficiency.

The *thalassemia trait* must be differentiated from iron deficiency anemia, since both entities exhibit microcytic, hypochromic red blood cells. With the thalassemia trait, the serum iron, total iron-binding capacity, and stainable iron on bone marrow aspirate are within normal limits. The hemoglobin A_2 level is elevated.

Up to 1 gm of oral ferrous sulfate per day (180 mg of elemental iron) is usually sufficient to reverse the anemia. Occasionally, when more rapid iron supplementation is required in a severely anemic patient at or close to term, intramuscular or intravenous administration of iron has been suggested. This latter approach is not recommended, since side effects are numerous.

Folic Acid Deficiency Anemia. The incidence of folic acid deficiency anemia varies from 0.5 to 25 percent, depending on the region of the country, the population, and the diet. Where leafy green vegetables are available all year around, the incidence of folate deficiency is low, while the reverse is true in cold, mountainous, and isolated areas. Nonnutritional factors also contribute to folate deficiency, including (1) chronic hemolytic anemias with increased red blood cell turnover; (2) medications, such as phenytoin (Dilantin) and methotrexate; (3) malabsorption entities, such as sprue; and (4) increased demand, as in a twin gestation. Rarely, folic acid deficiency presents as a single entity, but more commonly it is found in association with iron deficiency anemia.

In about 50 per cent of patients, anemia develops in the latter part of pregnancy or during the postpartum period, since it takes about 18 weeks of a folate-deficient diet to produce anemia. Initially, the serum folate level decreases, followed by hypersegmentation of neutrophils. Much later, the red blood cell folate levels fall, urinary formiminoglutamic acid (FIGLU) excretion increases after a histidine load, and megaloblastic anemia develops. A bone marrow aspirate showing megaloblasts is diagnostic, although it is rarely used.

For prophylactic and treatment purposes, 0.7 to 1 mg of folic acid may be given daily, either alone or with ferrous sulfate. Patients with chronic hemolytic anemia or those on antifolate medications might require 2 mg of folic acid per day.

Combined Iron and Folate Deficiency. In this group of patients, the diagnosis of either entity is difficult, since laboratory findings are equivocal, and changes in red blood cell morphology are inconsistent. A complete hematologic response does not occur until both iron and folic acid are given. If the anemia is severe, and there is a partial response to treatment, a bone marrow aspirate is indicated.

Hemoglobinopathies

Careful medical, family, and obstetric histories are usually helpful in uncovering hemoglobinopathies. However, the presence of severe anemia or failure to respond to iron and folic acid supplementation should alert the physician to look for these disorders. Hemoglobin electrophoresis differentiates normal adult hemoglobin A from sickle hemoglobin S, fetal hemoglobin F, and hemoglobin C.

Sickle-Cell Disease. This entity includes sickle-cell anemia, which has a homozygous S-S pattern, sickle-cell trait (S-A), sickle-cell beta-thalassemia (S-B-Thal), and sickle-cell hemoglobin C disease (S-C). The maternal mortality-morbidity and the fetal complication rate reflect the percentage of S hemoglobin and the degree of anemia in the pregnant patient. Patients with S-A and S-B-Thal tolerate pregnancy well with lower rates of maternal-fetal complications, since the hemoglobin A level is higher than the hemoglobin S level. The incidence of sickle-cell anemia (S-S) in blacks is about 1:2000, while the incidence of sickle-cell trait is about 1:11.

Maternal mortality in patients with sickle-cell disease is about 2 percent. Morbidity rates still average about 80 percent and involve sickle-cell crises, pyelonephritis, severe anemia, neurologic manifestations, and sickle-cell lung syndrome. Fetal wastage is highest during a sickle-cell crisis, and even if the fetus survives, the incidence of intrauterine growth retardation is increased. Pregnancy has an adverse effect on sickle-cell disease.

ANTEPARTUM MANAGEMENT. Pregnant patients with sickle-cell disease should seek early prenatal care, be seen frequently, and be informed of the maternal-fetal risks associated with their pregnancy. Recommended initial studies include (1) early ultrasound to assess fetal viability and exclude gross congenital anomalies; (2) hemoglobin electrophoresis to assess the percentage of hemoglobin S; (3) a complete blood and reticulocyte count with red blood cell indices to assess the degree of anemia; (4) serum iron, total iron-binding capacity, and serum folate to assess iron and folic acid stores; (5) renal function studies, including microscopic urine analysis and culture; and (6) pulmonary function studies in patients with frequent episodes of respiratory infection.

Supplemental iron should not be given to patients with a history of repeated blood transfusions or those with a diagnosis of hemochromatosis. Supplements of folic acid (1 to 2 mg/day) are recommended.

Several studies have suggested that prophylactic simple or exchange transfusions might be of value in preventing sickle-cell crises, fetal growth retardation, perinatal mortality, premature labor, and maternal infection. The theoretic benefits are (1) an increase in the oxygen-carrying capacity of the blood; (2) a reduction in the percentage of sickled hemoglobin; and (3) suppression of production of cells with S-S hemoglobin. However, the *National Institutes of Health Consensus Report* does not support the use of prophylactic transfusions. At UCLA, sickle-cell patients are transfused (1) when hemoglobin levels fall below 9 gm/dl in spite of iron and folic acid supplementation *and* the patient becomes symptomatic; (2) when the patient is having a sickle-cell crisis and not responding to supportive measures; (3) late in the third trimester or prior to labor and delivery to raise the hemoglobin above 10 gm/dl; and (4) postpartum in the presence of severe infection.

Maternal surveillance studies are repeated at least every four to six weeks. Episodes of sickle-cell crisis and urinary or pulmonary infections are treated aggressively. During the third trimester, fetal surveillance studies (pelvic ultrasound, stress, and nonstress testing) are indicated to assess fetal growth and development.

INTRAPARTUM CARE. Labor and delivery pose additional maternal and fetal risks for an individual with sickle-cell disease. The risk of development of a sickle-cell crisis is increased if oxygen and fluid demands are not met. Similarly, the growth-retarded fetus might not tolerate the stress of labor due to uteroplacental insufficiency. To safeguard against these complications, the following measures are indicated:

1. Oxygen supplementation to the mother
2. Administration of intravenous fluids
3. Reassurance and early sedation to prevent excessive anxiety
4. Adequate fetal monitoring
5. Avoidance of a prolonged and/or traumatic labor and delivery
6. Administration of prophylactic antibiotics if an operative delivery is necessary

Disorders of Blood Coagulation and Platelets

The presence of ecchymoses and hematomas is usually associated with a deficient coagulation mechanism, while petechial lesions are associated with platelet disorders. A drug history is important, since certain drugs might affect coagulation factors, platelets, and blood vessels. Simple tests, such as a prothrombin time (PT) and partial thromboplastin time (PTT), are appropriate for the initial diagnosis of coagulation disorders, while a platelet count is sufficient for differentiation of thrombocytopenic and non-thrombocytopenic purpura.

Inherited Disorders of Plasma Coagulation Factors. The most common inherited plasma coagulation disorders are: hemophilia A (factor VIII deficiency), hemophilia B (factor IX deficiency), and von Willebrand's disease. Hemophilias A and B are x-linked recessive disorders and the typical female carrier is not clinically affected.

Von Willebrand's disease accounts for about 10 percent of the inherited coagulation disorders and can lead to a hemorrhagic diathesis in the pregnant patient. The laboratory diagnosis of von Willebrand's disease is based on (1) factor VIII, procoagulant (VIII:C) and related antigen (VIII R:Ag) deficiency; (2) prolonged bleeding time; (3) positive tourniquet test; (4) delayed response to infused plasma with production of new factor VIII *in vivo*. Treatment for von Willebrand's disease is with fresh frozen plasma or cryoprecipitate.

Thrombocytopenia. With thrombocytopenia, the bleeding time becomes prolonged, clot retraction becomes decreased, and the tourniquet test becomes positive. Although a peripheral smear is sufficient for determining the platelet count, a bone marrow aspirate is needed to quantitate the megakaryocytes. Idiopathic thrombocytopenic purpura and thrombotic thrombocytopenic purpura are discussed in Chapter 4.

Disseminated Intravascular Coagulopathy (DIC). The factors usually responsible for DIC in pregnancy are varied and may be grouped into several categories: (1) abruptio placentae; (2) severe pre-eclampsia or eclampsia; (3) intrauterine fetal demise; (4) sepsis; (5) transfusion reaction; and (6) amniotic fluid embolism.

Impaired clot retraction, decreased serum fibrinogen, decreased platelet count, and an increase in fibrin split products, prothrombin time, and partial thromboplastin time are diagnostic of DIC.

Treatment is directed at resolving the underlying etiologic factor. In most obstetric situations, emptying the uterus is sufficient to reverse the process. Occasionally, fresh frozen plasma, cryoprecipitate, and whole blood and platelet transfusions are needed to establish hemostasis, especially if delivery is not imminent or a cesarean section is planned. Continuous heparin infusion may be useful in reversing DIC occurring in association with an intrauterine fetal death, but heparin is contraindicated in an actively bleeding patient.

Circulating Anticoagulants. Circulating anticoagulants are acquired inhibitors of blood coagulation. Most of these inhibitors are against factor VIII, although inhibitors against other blood factors may occur. Inhibitors of factor VIII have been reported in antepartum and postpartum patients and in various individuals with immunologic disorders, such as rheumatoid arthritis, ulcerative colitis, and systemic lupus erythematosus (SLE). Another circulating anticoagulant that is detected more frequently in patients with SLE is an inhibitor of the activation of prothrombin. Most patients with this anticoagulant do not bleed abnormally.

NEUROLOGIC DISORDERS

Seizures

Since there are no specific neurologic disorders related to pregnancy, only seizure disorders are discussed in this section.

Seizure frequency during pregnancy may increase, decrease, or remain the same. It is difficult to relate the worsening of seizure control during pregnancy to the lower plasma levels of anticonvulsant drugs, since seizure control improves in more than 50 percent of patients. Rarely, grand mal seizure may occur for the first time during pregnancy or in the puerperium and must be distinguished from eclampsia.

Treatment

The two most commonly used drugs for seizure treatment are diphenylhydantoin (Dilantin) and phenobarbital. Initial treatment with a single drug is preferred, and phenobarbital is the better choice in pregnancy, since its teratogenic effects are less severe. A dose of 100 to 250 mg per day of phenobarbital may be given in divided doses. The serum levels are monitored, and the dose is increased gradually until a therapeutic level (10 to 40 µg/ml) is reached. If such a drug regimen proves inadequate, Dilantin may be tried, either alone or in addition to the phenobarbital. Other anticonvulsant drugs, such as clonazepam (Clonopin) and carbamazepine (Tegretol), should be used with care. Valproic acid (Depakene) poses special risks to the mother and fetus and should be avoided.

Megaloblastic anemia due to folic acid deficiency occurs as a rare complication of anticonvulsant therapy. Most of the reported cases have followed the administration of Dilantin. The use of folic acid supplementation during pregnancy in the epileptic patient is controversial. Folic acid supplements are known to reduce the plasma levels of Dilantin, so if folic acid supplements are used, careful attention should be paid to plasma levels of Dilantin. Similarly, antacids and antihistamines should be avoided, since they also lower plasma levels of Dilantin and may precipitate a seizure attack.

For the treatment of *status epilepticus*, immediate hospitalization is required. Patency of the airway should be ascertained. After blood is drawn for plasma levels of anticonvulsants, 10 mg of intravenous diazepam (Valium) should be given slowly, followed by 200 to 500 mg of diphenylhydantoin. If seizure patterns continue, 500 mg of amobarbital sodium may be added. If the above measures fail, general anesthesia may be employed. Therapeutic levels of diphenylhydantoin, 10 to 20 mEq/ml, must be maintained during the rest of the pregnancy and postpartum period.

The management of labor and delivery follows obstetric indications. During labor and in the immediate postpartum period, anticonvulsant drugs may be given intravenously. Cord blood should be sent for the measurement of prothrombin time because of the possibility of a coagulopathy in the neonate. Postpartum, the dose of the anticonvulsant drug may be lowered, provided a therapeutic level is maintained. Although anticonvulsants are excreted in breast milk in small amounts, breast feeding is not contraindicated.

Complications

Pregnant patients with epilepsy have a twofold increase in such maternal complications as pre-eclampsia, vaginal bleeding, hyperemesis, prolonged labor, and premature labor.

In the fetus, there is a high incidence of intrauterine fetal demise, coagulopathy, and congenital anomalies. In the neonate, higher rates of coagulopathy, drug withdrawal symptoms, and neonatal morbidity and mortality are reported. (Teratogenic effects of anticonvulsants are discussed in Chapter 8). Anticonvulsants alone may not be responsible for the two- to threefold increase in the rate of congenital anomalies. Other risk factors include the occurrence of frequent convulsions during pregnancy, the increased incidence of maternal complications during pregnancy, and the socioeconomic status of the pregnant epileptic.

RENAL DISORDERS

Acute Renal Failure

Acute renal failure during pregnancy or in the postpartum period may be due to deterioration of renal function secondary to a pre-existing renal disease or to a pregnancy-related disorder. The underlying causative factors may be prerenal, renal, or postrenal. With *prerenal causes*, a history of blood or fluid loss is usually elicited from the patient or implied from reviewing the medical history. *Renal causes* are usually suspected in a patient with a history of pre-existing renal disease or with a hypercoagulable state, such as thrombotic thrombocytopenic purpura or hemolytic uremic syndrome. With prolonged hypotension, acute cortical necrosis or acute tubular necrosis may occur. *Postrenal* causes are less common, but should be suspected in situations where urologic obstructive lesions are present or where there is a history of kidney stones.

Laboratory Studies. Laboratory tests are directed at assessing renal function, cardiovascular status, and patency of the urologic tract.

RENAL STUDIES. These include urine output, BUN-creatinine ratio, fractional excretion of sodium, and urine osmolality.

Oliguria is defined as *urine output* of less than 25 ml/hr, while anuria is the cessation of urine output. With acute renal failure, the urine output may not decrease, although oliguria or anuria are usually present. Not infrequently, a decrease in urine output alerts the physician to an impending crisis.

During pregnancy, the serum values of BUN and creatinine decrease, but the *BUN-creatinine ratio* remains about 20:1. A ratio greater than 20:1 suggests tubular hypoperfusion (prerenal failure).

The *fractional excretion of sodium* (FE$_{Na}$) is calculated as follows:

$$FE_{Na} = \frac{\text{Urine sodium/plasma sodium}}{\text{Urine creatinine/plasma creatinine}} \times 100$$

An FE$_{Na}$ less than 1 percent is suggestive of hypovolemia and tubular hypoperfusion. Alternatively, a value greater than 3 percent is highly indicative of tubular damage.

Urine osmolality greater than 500 mOsm per liter or a urine/plasma osmolality ratio greater than 1.7:1 is highly suggestive of renal hypoperfusion. Urine specific gravity is of limited value, especially when there is protein or hemolyzed blood in the urine.

CARDIOVASCULAR STUDIES. Acute blood and fluid loss are usually associated with orthostatic hypotension, tachycardia, decreased skin turgor, and reduced sweating. In a pregnant hypertensive or pre-eclamptic patient who is in labor, many of these signs are overlooked. A Swan-Ganz catheter introduced through the external jugular vein into the pulmonary artery allows monitoring of right and left ventricular filling pressure, cardiac output, and pulmonary capillary wedge pressure. Systemic vascular resistance may be calculated. This can help to distinguish between congestive heart failure, cardiac tamponade, and volume depletion, any of which can lead to acute renal failure.

UROLOGIC TRACT STUDIES. A Foley catheter and renal sonogram are usually sufficient to diagnose obstructive lesions. Rarely, a one-shot intravenous pyelogram is needed.

Treatment. PRERENAL CAUSES. Restoration of intravascular volume, cardiac output, and arterial pressure to normal values is sufficient to reverse oliguria. Careful attention should be given to electrolyte imbalance when large amounts of crystalloids are infused.

RENAL CAUSES. Acute tubular necrosis, acute cortical necrosis, or both may be present. Because acute cortical necrosis is generally irreversible, treatment is directed toward preventing further damage. A trial of diuretic therapy to increase urinary output appears to decrease the duration and severity of acute tubular necrosis and increase survival rates. Intravenous administration of 25 gm of mannitol and 40 mg of furosemide (Lasix) is given initially and then repeated every four to six hours for 48 hours in the presence of adequate urinary response. If the diuretic therapy fails to increase the urine output, an oliguric fluid regimen is initiated. Fluid intake should be limited to replacement of urine output and insensible water loss, and renal function studies should be monitored on a daily basis. For the first few days after the renal ischemic episode, renal function may worsen; however, within 7 to 10 days, most patients with acute tubular necrosis show marked improvement. If renal function deteriorates rapidly or fails to recover, hemodialysis is recommended.

In some patients in whom acute renal failure is accompanied by oliguria, a diuretic phase coincides with the recovery period. The urine output might exceed 10 liters per day, and if fluid and electrolyte losses are not replaced promptly, death ensues.

About 50 percent of obstetric patients who develop acute renal failure during pregnancy or the postpartum period will recover enough renal function during the first year to survive without dialysis.

POSTRENAL CAUSES. In many instances, simple measures, such as turning the patient to the side to displace the gravid uterus from the ureters or inserting a Foley catheter into the bladder to overcome urethral obstruction, will resolve the problem. In situations in which a ureteral or renal pelvic obstruction is present (e.g., stones) surgical intervention is indicated to relieve the obstruction.

Chronic Renal Failure

The outcome of pregnancies complicated by chronic renal disease is less favorable. Good pregnancy outcome may be expected in nonhypertensive pregnant patients who have serum creatinine levels below 1.5 mg/dl prior to conception. When the serum creatinine levels exceed 3 mg/dl, continuation of pregnancy until fetal viability is rare. Hypertensive individuals with chronic renal disease do not fair as well as normotensive patients with the same degree of renal impairment.

Pregnancy has no effect on the natural course of the renal disease in patients who have mild impairment of renal function and are normotensive. The deterioration in renal function, superimposition of hypertension, and substantial increase in proteinuria seen during pregnancy subside after delivery. Patients with nephrotic syndrome do well during pregnancy in spite of the massive urinary protein losses. In most of these individuals, proteinuria partially abates postpartum.

Pregnancy Following Renal Transplants

Pregnancy after renal transplantation should not be considered before a thorough assessment of maternal, fetal, and neonatal risk factors. Fetal complications include steroid-induced adrenal and hepatic insufficiency, prematurity, and intrauterine growth retardation. Decrease in thymus size, lymphopenia, and lethargy have been reported. In addition, the infant may inherit the primary disease of the mother or other family members.

The criteria shown in Table 16–8 may be used to identify renal transplant patients who are good candidates for pregnancy.

GASTROINTESTINAL DISORDERS

Nausea and Vomiting During Pregnancy

About 60 to 80 percent of pregnant women complain of nausea and vomiting during the first 8 to 12 weeks of gestation. The symptoms are usually mild and disappear during the early part of the second trimester. In a small number of patients, the severity of the symptoms necessitates hospital admission.

TABLE 16–8   CRITERIA FOR SELECTING
             SUITABLE RENAL
             TRANSPLANT PATIENTS
             FOR PREGNANCY

1. Two years post-transplant with good health
2. Anatomic status compatible with good obstetric outcome
3. No proteinuria
4. No significant hypertension
5. No evidence of active allograft rejection
6. No evidence of pelvicalyceal distension on recent IVP
7. Serum creatinine less than 2 mg/dl
8. Prednisone dosage 15 mg/day or less and azathioprine dosage 2 mg/kg/day or less

Adapted with permission from Davison JM, Lindheimer MD: Pregnancy in renal transplant recipients. J Reprod Med 27:613, 1982.

The underlying causes of nausea and vomiting during pregnancy are not well delineated. Several hypotheses are proposed:

1.   Psychic events. Patients under emotional stress are more likely to experience nausea and vomiting.

2.   Neuroendocrine alterations. The appearance of nausea and vomiting parallels the increase in serum chorionic gonadotropin. Additionally, vomiting is more common and frequently more severe in pregnancies where serum levels of chorionic gonadotropin are greatly elevated, as in a twin gestation or molar pregnancy. Neuroendocrine alterations of the emetic threshold may be implicated.

3.   Adrenal and pituitary dysfunction. Patients with Addison's disease or adrenocortical insufficiency following adrenalectomy complain of nausea and vomiting. Administration of ACTH to patients with hyperemesis gravidarum often produces a therapeutic response. However, both glands function normally in the hyperemetic patient.

4.   Hyperthyroxinemia. Hyperthyroxinemia is present in about 70 percent of patients with hyperemesis.

5.   Sex steroid imbalance. Progesterone deficiency and estrogen excess have been implicated, although no data substantiate either claim.

6.   Drugs. Drugs and chemicals may evoke nausea and vomiting through their alteration of the chemoreceptors in the base of the fourth ventricle. Prostaglandins, chemotherapeutic and noxious agents, and cardiac glycosides are thought to work through such a mechanism.

Hyperemesis Gravidarum. This term is reserved for the intractable nausea and vomiting that occurs in a few gravidas; the overall incidence is about 1 percent. Cultural, racial, and personality factors are known to influence the prevalence of this disorder. It is more commonly found in the Caucasian population, and less frequently seen in blacks, Eskimos, and some African tribes. It is also seen in oppressive cultural environments and in individuals stereotyped as having an immature personality. The disorder appears more frequently with first pregnancies, but tends to recur with subsequent pregnancies. Pregnancy outcome is usually good, with no added risk to mother or neonate.

Clinical diagnosis is based on history and physical findings. A history of intractable vomiting and inability to retain food and fluid intake is usually elicited. Physical findings of weight loss, dry and coated tongue, and decreased skin turgor are very suggestive. The initial laboratory work-up includes urine tests for ketonuria and blood tests for electrolytes and acetone. Electrolyte disturbances may include hypokalemia, hyponatremia, and hypochloremic alkalosis.

Additional laboratory work-up should include hematologic, renal, and hepatic studies. Although the condition is self-limiting, occasionally severe complications result from metabolic deterioration with hepatic or renal involvement.

Treatment. Nonhospital management includes dietary alterations and avoidance of spicy foods and other foods that induce emesis. Patients are encouraged to take small, frequent meals and to eat solid foods. Antiemetic drugs such as prochlorperazine (Compazine) are discouraged; their use should be limited to patients who are well-informed about the potential fetal risks and in whom conservative approaches fail.

If electrolyte disturbances are present, patients are admitted to the hospital for further work-up and treatment. Intravenous hydration, correction of electrolyte and acid-base imbalance, and psychologic counseling are instituted. Frequently, stressful life events are identified, and intervention may facilitate improvement. Gastroscopy may sometimes be indicated to rule out gastric pathology. In refractory cases where there is persistent weight loss and starvation ketosis, parenteral hyperalimentation may be necessary.

Reflux Esophagitis

During pregnancy, physiologic alterations occur that increase the potential for esophageal reflux. Early in pregnancy, the lower esophageal sphincter tone remains unchanged, but the responses to pharmacologic and humoral manipulations are reduced. During late pregnancy, with the increase in serum progesterone levels, the sphincter tone decreases. Additionally, during pregnancy, the intragastric pressure increases and the intraesophageal pressure decreases. Gastric pH and gastric acid output remain unchanged.

Reflux esophagitis or heartburn is a common complaint during pregnancy. It occurs in about 70 percent of gravidas and gets worse during the latter part of gestation.

Symptoms and Diagnosis. The main symptoms include substernal discomfort aggravated by meals and the recumbent position and occasional hematemesis. An unusual symptom peculiar to reflux esophagitis is water brash, which is best described as the sudden filling of the mouth with clean, watery material that has a salty taste and produces a nauseous sensation.

The diagnosis of reflux esophagitis is usually based on symptoms and response to treatment. In severe cases, in those with atypical clinical manifestations, and in those that are unresponsive to treatment, endoscopy is indicated.

Treatment. Treatment is usually symptomatic. Patients are instructed to refrain from eating large and late meals; to avoid the recumbent position, especially after meals; and to use an extra pillow to elevate the head when sleeping. Patients with more severe symptoms also require liquid antacids, which should be taken one to three hours after meals.

Other medications should be reserved for the more severe and refractory cases. Cimetidine, an H_2 histamine receptor antagonist, inhibits gastric acid secretion but has no effect on gastric volume, gastric emptying, or lower esophageal sphincter tone. The drug has been associated with cardiac arrhythmias, cardiac arrest, and an increased risk of gastric carcinoma. It crosses the placenta and reaches the fetus in substantial quantities. Another drug that has been used successfully in Europe for treatment of reflux esophagitis during pregnancy is metoclopramide (Reglan), which is a potent dopamine antagonist. In addition to its antiemetic effects, it promotes gastric emptying and increases lower sphincter tone. Side effects include psychosis, extrapyramidal symptoms, and galactorrhea.

Peptic Ulcer

Pregnancy conveys relative protection against the development of peptic ulceration and may ameliorate an already present ulcer. Gastric acid secretion is probably not altered during pregnancy, although some studies suggest modest suppression.

Diagnosis. The diagnosis of ulcer disease is mainly based on symptomatic improvement in response to conservative treatment. Endoscopy is reserved for those cases that do not respond to antacid treatment, have more severe gastrointestinal symptoms, or manifest significant gastrointestinal hemorrhage. Radiographic studies, such as a barium swallow or upper gastrointestinal series, have no advantage over endoscopy and are unnecessary, especially during pregnancy.

Treatment. Treatment involves avoiding caffeine, alcohol, tobacco, and spicy foods, all of which stimulate acid secretion. Liquid antacids with a low sodium content are recommended and should be continued for at least six weeks. These include Maalox TC Suspension, Mylanta II liquid, and Gelusil II liquid. Cimetidine should be reserved for complicated, recurrent, and refractory cases.

Acid Aspiration Syndrome (Mendelson's Syndrome)

The pregnant patient in labor is at an increased risk of having acid aspiration because of (1) delayed gastric emptying, which is made worse when associated with increased anxiety or the use of sedatives, narcotics, and anticholinergic agents; (2) increased gastric acidity; and (3) increased intra-abdominal and intragastric pressure, making regurgitation more likely. Damage to the pulmonary tissue is greatest when the pH of the aspirated fluid is less than 2.5 or the volume of the aspirate is greater than 25 ml.

Preventive efforts are directed at decreasing the acidity of the gastric contents or decreasing the acid secretion by the stomach. Liquid magnesium and aluminum antacids given every three to four hours during labor decrease the gastric acidity but increase the volume of the gastric acid-antacid emulsion. In addition, particulate matter within the antacid acts as a focus for infection within the lung parenchyma.

The signs and symptoms of acid aspiration syndrome vary depending on the volume, acidity, and consistency of the aspirate. Solid aspirates may obstruct the tracheobronchial tree and lead to cyanosis, atelectasis, and mediastinal shift. Liquid aspirates tend to produce segmental rather than lobar signs, affect the right lung more than the left, and produce a burn-like injury to the lung parenchyma. Increased airways resistance, decreased lung compliance, and pulmonary edema may be present.

Gastrointestinal Bypass and Pregnancy

A pregnant patient with a jejunoileal bypass poses special problems. The overall capacity for nutrient and mineral absorption is drastically reduced because of anatomic diversion and decreased transit time. The overall absorption of fat is reduced 30 to 80 percent, with profound effects on water and electrolyte absorption. Serum triglycerides, cholesterol, calcium, magnesium, and fat-soluble vitamins (A, D, E, and K) are usually low. Hepatic dysfunction may occur due to deposition of fat in the liver parenchyma. Dietary counseling is aimed at emphasizing the need for the pregnant patient to ingest enough calories and nutrients to avoid weight loss and mineral and vitamin deficiency. If this conservative approach fails, total parenteral nutrition is recommended.

The outcome of pregnancy in patients with a jejunoileal bypass is usually good, provided specific metabolic and nutritional deficiencies are corrected.

Chronic Inflammatory Bowel Disease

The two entities described under this disorder are Crohn's disease (regional enteritis) and ulcerative colitis. In about 25 percent of patients with inflammatory bowel disease, differentiation between these two disorders is difficult.

Patients with inflammatory bowel disease do well during pregnancy, provided there are no acute exacerbations. It seems unlikely that the natural history of the disease changes during pregnancy. Patients with regional enteritis are thought to have higher rates of abortion and fetal loss than normal individuals or patients with ulcerative colitis. This difference might be related to the fact that patients with regional enteritis are usually thin and debilitated.

Treatment. Treatment of an acute exacerbation of inflammatory bowel disease is the same for pregnant and nonpregnant patients, although some of the more experimental drugs should not be used during pregnancy. If diarrhea is the main complaint, dietary restriction of lactose, fruits, and vegetables is necessary. If a lactose-free diet is used, calcium supplementation is needed. Constipating agents, such as Pepto-Bismol and psyllium hydrophilic mucilloid (Metamucil), may be used daily and are quite effective. The use of diphenoxylate/atropine (Lomotil) or loperamide (Imodium) should be restricted to cases where conservative management fails. For those patients with mild to moderate symptoms, sulfasalazine may be beneficial. Although its action is not well understood, current views suggest that it inhibits prostaglandin synthesis. The usual daily dose is 2 to 12 gm, although lower dosage is recommended during pregnancy. If sulfasalazine is to be used during pregnancy, it is probably wise not to use it during the third trimester, since it may induce neonatal kernicterus by binding to serum albumen and displacing bilirubin.

Steroid treatment is indicated when there is excessive weight loss, anorexia, partial intestinal obliteration, or persistent rectal bleeding. Prednisone, 20 to 40 mg daily, may be given and the dose tapered gradually when symptoms resolve. Prednisone crosses the placenta, and possible steroid teratogenicity should be explained to the patient. Other more experimental drugs, such as azathioprine and 6-mercaptopurine, should be avoided during pregnancy.

HEPATIC DISORDERS

In this section, liver disorders that are peculiar to pregnancy are discussed.

Intrahepatic Cholestasis of Pregnancy

Although the pathogenesis of this syndrome is not known, some distinctive features are present: (1) cholestasis and pruritus without other major liver dysfunction; (2) a tendency to recur with each pregnancy; (3) an association with oral contraceptives; and (4) a benign course in that there are no maternal hepatic sequelae. The disease may be inherited as an autosomal dominant disorder.

The main symptom in a patient with cholestasis of pregnancy is itching, which may occur early in pregnancy. Jaundice may be observed late in pregnancy, although it is rare. Laboratory tests are variable and of little help except that all patients have an elevated serum bile acid level at some point during pregnancy.

Treatment. Treatment is partially effective in relieving the itching. Cholestyramine, which binds the bile acids in the gut, has been used with mixed results. The recommended dose is 12 gm per day taken in divided doses with meals. Since this resin binds fat soluble vitamins (A, D, E, and K), oral daily supplements of vitamin K should be given. Phenobarbital to induce liver enzymes has been used in the treatment of this syndrome with a minor degree of success. Termination of pregnancy is the only effective cure. Itching disappears within hours or days of delivery.

Complications. Although this entity is benign in nature and leaves no maternal sequelae, the outcome of pregnancy is not as favorable. The incidence of prematurity and stillbirth is increased, possibly due to decreased maternal fat absorption. At term, and especially during labor, prothrombin time should be checked. If prolonged, vitamin K should be given parenterally to decrease the risk of postpartum hemorrhage.

Hepatic Toxemia

As the name implies, this entity refers to hepatic end organ involvement as part of the pre-eclamptic syndrome. Frequently, hepatic disease is not suspected, and only an abnormality in the liver function tests suggests this diagnosis. Typically, the transaminase levels (SGOT and SGPT) are elevated, and, on rare occasions, bilirubin levels are also increased.

Although the course of the disease may be benign and the liver function tests may return to normal after delivery, more serious complications can occur. Thrombocytopenia in association with microangiopathic hemolytic anemia and disseminated intravascular coagulation is more common in pre-eclamptic patients with hepatic involvement.

The treatment of hepatic toxemia is the same as that of pre-eclampsia. In mild cases, expectant management is desirable, while in severe cases immediate delivery is recommended. For patients with right upper quadrant or epigastric pain, abnormal liver enzymes, and thrombocytopenia, immediate delivery is recommended, irrespective of the degree of hypertension or proteinuria. Such patients should also be observed and evaluated to exclude the presence of an hepatic hematoma or rupture of the liver capsule.

Acute Fatty Liver Atrophy

This is a very serious complication that is peculiar to pregnancy. It most commonly occurs in the third trimester of pregnancy or the early postpartum period. Although the etiology is unknown, many physicians tend to regard it as a form of severe hepatic toxemia. Presentation is variable, with abdominal pain, nausea and vomiting, jaundice, and increased irritability. Invariably these patients go into hepatic coma. Laboratory findings include an increase in prothrombin and partial thromboplastin time, hyperbilirubinemia, hyperammonemia, and a moderate elevation of the transaminases.

Prognosis is very poor, and about 80 percent of patients die while in coma. Treatment is mainly directed at supportive measures for the postpartum patient and immediate delivery of the pregnant individual. Dietary restriction of protein and administration of lactulose by mouth to yield two to three stools per day is the main form of treatment. For the coagulopathy of hepatic failure, vitamin K supplementation is not effective, and fresh frozen plasma should be given. Survivors of liver failure have no hepatic sequelae. Even subsequent pregnancies in these patients have progressed well with no increased maternal or fetal risks.

SUGGESTED READING

Burrow GN: The thyroid gland in pregnancy. In Friedman E (ed): Major Problems in Obstetrics and Gynecology. Vol 3. Philadelphia, W B Saunders Co, 1972.

Burrow GN, Ferris T (eds): Medical Complications in Pregnancy. Philadelphia, W B Saunders Co, 1982.

Creasy B, Resnik R: Maternal and Fetal Medicine. Philadelphia, W B Saunders Co, 1984.

Davison JM, Lindheimer M: Pregnancy in renal transplant recipients. J Reprod Med 27:613, 1982.

Gabbe SG, Mestmoun JG, Freeman RK, et al: Management and outcome of Class A diabetes mellitus. Am J Obstet Gynecol 127:465, 1977.

Gabbe SG, Mestmoun JG, Freeman RK, et al: Management and outcome of pregnancy in diabetes mellitus, Classes B to R. Am J Obstet Gynecol 129:723, 1977.

Malkosian GD Jr, Moller KL, Aoro LA, et al: Miscellaneous medical complications. In Iffy L, Kaminelzky H (eds): Principles and Practice of Obstetrics and Perinatology. New York, Wiley Medical Publishers, 1981.

Metcalfe J, Ueland K: Maternal cardiovascular adjustments to pregnancy. Prog Cardiovasc Dis 16:363, 1974.

Merkatz IR, Adam PAJ: Pregnancy in diabetes. Semin Perinatol 2:287, 1978.

Skyler JS, Mintz DH, O'Sullivan MJ: Management of diabetes and pregnancy. In Rifkin H, Raskin P (eds): Diabetes Mellitus. Vol, 5. Bowie, MD, Robert J Brady Co, 1981, p 161.

Szekely P, Snaith L (eds): Heart Disease and Pregnancy. Edinburgh, Churchill-Livingstone, 1974.

Chapter Seventeen

CONDITIONS REQUIRING SURGERY DURING PREGNANCY

WILLIAM J. DIGNAM

Surgical procedures other than those performed directly on the uterus have no deleterious effect on pregnancy. Some authors have noted an increased incidence of abortion or premature labor in patients who undergo such procedures, but this finding has not been corroborated by others. It is likely that undesirable outcomes are related to the underlying disease rather than the surgical procedure itself. Spontaneous abortions commonly occur during the first trimester of pregnancy, so it is best to postpone all operations, except urgent ones, until after this time to avoid any suggestion that an abortion may have been related to the surgical procedure. During abdominal operations, the uterus should be manipulated as little as possible.

Anesthesia is an important consideration. Although there is no evidence that any of the commonly employed anesthetic agents produce harmful effects on the fetus, it is preferable to avoid all drugs during the period of organogenesis. Patients should be well oxygenated at all times, and hypotension should be avoided. Antibiotics to be avoided are tetracyclines throughout pregnancy and sulfonamides and chloramphenicol in late pregnancy.

ANATOMIC AND PHYSIOLOGIC ALTERATIONS

An awareness of anatomic and physiologic alterations during pregnancy is important to enable the physician to properly interpret the history and physical findings. Changes in anatomy are most often due to the markedly enlarged uterus and the accompanying enlargement and upward displacement of attached structures, such as the broad ligaments, tubes, ovaries, and vascular pedicles. Changes in physiology of particular importance include dilatation and diminished peristalsis of the urinary and gastrointestinal systems and dilatation of the venous system with stasis of the blood. These physiologic changes are apparently caused by progesterone and, therefore, take place well before the enlarging uterus would logically produce them. Altered laboratory results due to normal pregnancy are shown in Table 4–1.

EMERGENCY OPERATIONS

Some conditions, all of which are uncommon, may require urgent surgical treatment

165

during pregnancy, regardless of the gestational age.

Acute Abdominal Emergencies

Appendicitis. The diagnosis of acute appendicitis during pregnancy is notoriously difficult, so great care should be taken in the evaluation of pregnant patients with abdominal pain. A delay in diagnosis is common and explains the continuing maternal mortality associated with this disease. The fetal death rate is also increased because of the increased rate of prematurity associated with perforation of the appendix. The common symptoms of appendicitis, such as anorexia, nausea, vomiting, and intermittent lower abdominal pain, also occur during normal pregnancy, thus creating diagnostic confusion. The enlarging uterus pushes the appendix higher in the abdomen so that the pain may occur in a different location than in nonpregnant women. In addition, the broad ligament may cover the appendix, making the findings during abdominal examination less obvious. For these reasons, palpation of the lateral portion of the abdomen may be more successful in eliciting tenderness and muscle spasm. The changing positions of the right colon and appendix are depicted in Figure 17–1.

If the possibility of appendicitis cannot be excluded, laparotomy should be carried out. If the diagnosis seems certain, a transverse incision is best; if there is uncertainty, a vertical incision should be employed to permit appropriate management if other conditions are found. If appendicitis is encountered near the end of pregnancy, the inflamed appendix should be treated appropriately, but cesarean section should not be performed. Labor is not harmful to a laparotomy incision, even if it is a very recent one.

Gallbladder Disease. Cholecystitis is more common in pregnancy. There is an increase in serum cholesterol and an increase in the secretion of cholesterol into the bile. These occurrences, in conjunction with the biliary stasis due to the increased emptying time of the gallbladder, lead to the formation of stones, obstruction of the ducts, and cholecystitis.

Possible confusing factors include the leukocytosis of normal pregnancy and the normal increase in alkaline phosphatase. The

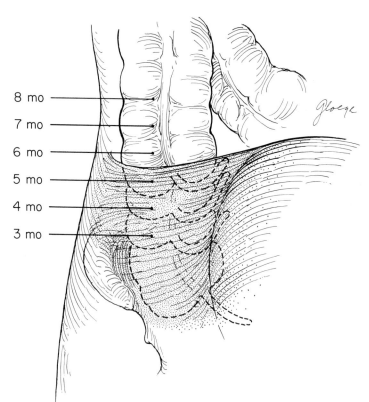

8 mo

7 mo

6 mo

5 mo

4 mo

3 mo

Figure 17–1 The changing position of the right colon and appendix due to the enlarging uterus.

nausea and vomiting of normal pregnancy may also be a source of confusion. The location of pain in the right upper quadrant and the tenderness and muscle spasm in that area are not significantly different from those symptoms noted in nonpregnant patients. However, examination of the area may be more difficult, particularly during late pregnancy, because of the distension of the abdomen by the enlarging uterus. In addition to the usual conditions that may simulate cholecystitis, it is important to be aware of the possible confusion introduced by the distended tender liver of patients with severe hypertensive disorders of pregnancy.

Cholecystitis is primarily treated medically during pregnancy, but occasionally this modality is unsuccessful. If signs of progressive peritonitis develop, cholecystectomy becomes necessary.

Pancreatitis. The incidence of acute pancreatitis in pregnant patients is lower than that in nonpregnant patients, but the mortality rate is significantly higher. The marked increase in fetal mortality is attributed to prematurity. Most nonpregnant patients with pancreatitis have gallstones or use alcohol to excess. For pregnant patients, it is very important to seek a history of excessive intake of alcohol because of the potential effects on the fetus. However, published reports indicate that many of these patients have idiopathic pancreatitis.

The symptoms of pancreatitis include nausea and vomiting, which are present in many normal pregnant women, particularly in early pregnancy. Patients with pancreatitis experience epigastric pain and develop tenderness and muscle spasm in the epigastric area. It may be difficult to evaluate that area, particularly in late pregnancy, because of muscle tension produced by the enlarged uterus.

Serum amylase and lipase may be elevated in patients with pancreatitis. However, these findings may be difficult to evaluate because an elevation of either one may be present in patients with other diseases of the gastrointestinal system. Serum amylase may be elevated in normal pregnancy.

Conservative management is the treatment of choice for patients with pancreatitis. This includes bed rest and nasogastric suction. Intravenous fluid replacement is of major importance, and careful attention to electrolyte balance is necessary. Analgesia with meperidine hydrochloride (Demerol) may well

be required. Usually pancreatitis subsides spontaneously in a few days, but if the digestion of pancreatic tissue is extensive, the patient may become critically ill with the production of large amounts of peritoneal fluid. In these instances, peritoneal lavage or laparotomy with subsequent drainage may be indicated.

Peptic Ulcer. Peptic ulcer is most common in men and older women. When present in younger women, there is a tendency for the symptoms to subside during pregnancy. This may be related to the increase in histaminase of placental origin during pregnancy.

Epigastric pain is a common symptom. Although many pregnant women complain of epigastric discomfort, they usually describe it as a feeling of pressure, rather than the burning or boring sensation of a peptic ulcer. Bleeding is a common occurrence and may result in anemia, which is also common in pregnant women.

X-rays should be avoided for diagnosis because of possible damage to the fetus. Endoscopic procedures are preferred.

Treatment consists of antacid therapy and anticholinergic drugs. The latter are safe to use after the first trimester. Histamine analogues such as cimetidine have not been studied adequately during pregnancy and should be used only in extreme circumstances.

The complications of peptic ulcer include hemorrhage and perforation. The hemorrhage may be profuse, and the resultant hypotension is a threat to the fetus. Endoscopic procedures may be successful in controlling the bleeding. However, if there is any question about their efficacy, laparotomy should be performed immediately. Perforation should also be managed by laparotomy and appropriate surgical procedures.

Bowel Obstruction. Bowel obstruction in pregnant patients is usually due to the presence of adhesions, as is true in nonpregnant individuals in the same age group. Volvulus may occasionally be responsible. It is most common in late pregnancy, possibly due to traction on pre-existing adhesions by the enlarging uterus.

The symptoms and signs of bowel obstruction during pregnancy are similar to those noted in nonpregnant individuals. The nausea and vomiting encountered in early normal pregnancy may be a source of confusion, as may the abdominal pain noted at varying times in normal pregnancy. The pain due to bowel obstruction is more colicky in nature, however, and is usually accompanied by high-pitched bowel sounds that come in rushes. After the obstruction has been present for a number of hours, the abdomen may become quite silent.

Usually an upright film of the abdomen will show the dilated loops of bowel with characteristic air-fluid levels. The radiation exposure should be kept to a minimum.

Treatment consists of nasogastric suction, correction of fluid and electrolyte abnormalities, and laparotomy through a vertical incision if the obstruction persists. Appropriate intestinal surgery should be carried out and the pregnancy left undisturbed.

Torsion of Adnexal Structures. The supporting structures for the tubes and ovaries are elongated during pregnancy. Torsion of these organs can more easily occur, therefore, particularly if the organ is not adherent to surrounding structures. Ovarian cysts, such as cystic teratomata, may easily undergo torsion, as may a hydrosalpinx.

Typically, these events are characterized by sudden and usually quite severe pain in either lower quadrant, which may radiate along the flank in a cephalad direction. Such discomfort has been described as reverse renal colic. At times, the pain is less obvious, and, as with appendicitis, the abdominal tenderness may be less easy to detect if the broad ligament has been drawn up over the mass. After complete torsion has been present for more than 24 hours, the pain may paradoxically diminish, apparently due to devitalization of the sensory nerves. There is some associated leukocytosis, but it is not more than that associated with normal pregnancy.

Ordinarily, a tender mass is palpable on pelvic examination, particularly during the rectovaginal examination. Sonographic examination may be helpful. The corpus luteum functions for about five weeks after ovulation, but corpus luteum cysts have been noted in more advanced pregnancies. However, a cystic mass of the ovary which persists more than eight weeks after ovulation is much less likely to be a corpus luteum cyst.

Appropriate management consists of prompt surgical removal. A vertical incision permits better exposure, and gentle handling of the uterus is important. If the ovary containing the corpus luteum is removed later than five weeks after ovulation, progesterone replacement therapy is not necessary.

Tubo-Ovarian Abscess. Infections of the tubes and ovaries are very uncommon during pregnancy, probably because the developing pregnancy prevents the ascent of the infectious organisms from the cervix and vagina. These infections do occasionally occur, however, and must be considered in the differential diagnosis of acute appendicitis.

The pain is usually located in either lower quadrant and may develop gradually. It may at first be confused with the lower abdominal pain noted by many normal pregnant women. Patients with infection have more steady pain, however, which gradually becomes severe. The patient becomes obviously ill, with a high fever and a leukocytosis much greater than that seen in normal pregnancy. The erythrocyte sedimentation rate is not of much assistance because it can be quite high in normal pregnancy.

Physical examination may not be as helpful as desired because some of these masses are carried cephalad by the enlarging broad ligament. The pocket provided by the large uterus and broad ligament may mask signs of rupture. Sonographic examination may be of assistance.

Treatment is not different from that advised for nonpregnant women. The patients must be kept under close observation in hospital. Since multiple organisms are involved, parenteral treatment with broad-spectrum antibiotics, such as gentamicin and clindamycin, is recommended. If signs of advancing peritonitis develop, laparotomy through a vertical incision should be carried out.

Abdominal Trauma. Major abdominal trauma is uncommon during pregnancy. It does occur, however, and motor vehicle accidents are the major cause. The use of seat belts for pregnant women is somewhat controversial. A shoulder restraint is advisable at all times to prevent a head injury to the mother. A lap belt is desirable early in pregnancy, but after the first trimester there is some possibility of damage to the fetus. The recommendation of the American College of Obstetricians and Gynecologists is that pregnant women should wear seat belts properly designed for them throughout pregnancy.

The principles of management of abdominal trauma are the same as those pertaining to nonpregnant individuals. Generally, surgery is required to control bleeding or to repair damage to the gastrointestinal tract. Lacerations or wounds of the uterus should be repaired.

TABLE 18–1 CRITERIA FOR VAGINAL DELIVERY OF A BREECH PRESENTATION

1. The fetus must be in a frank breech presentation.
2. The gestational age must be at least 36 weeks.
3. The estimated fetal weight should be between 2500 and 3800 gm.
4. The fetal head must be flexed.
5. The maternal pelvis must be adequately large, as assessed by x-ray pelvimetry.
6. There must be no other maternal or fetal indication for cesarean section.

Management During Labor

Vaginal Delivery. The intrapartum management of a breech presentation depends upon the type of breech and the gestational age. The standard of care in most communities is to routinely deliver all breech presentations by cesarean section in order to avoid the increased perinatal morbidity and mortality that occur with vaginal delivery secondary to umbilical cord prolapse, birth asphyxia, and birth trauma. However, the incidence of umbilical cord prolapse with frank breech presentations approaches that for vertex presentations, so the management of the term frank breech is controversial.

Strict criteria for allowing a trial of labor and vaginal delivery of a term breech are summarized in Table 18–1. These are directed toward minimizing the possibility of umbilical cord prolapse, birth trauma, and asphyxia. In addition, sonography must be performed to exclude the presence of fetal anomalies. If a fetal anomaly is found that is incompatible with life, such as anencephaly, the patient should not be delivered by cesar-

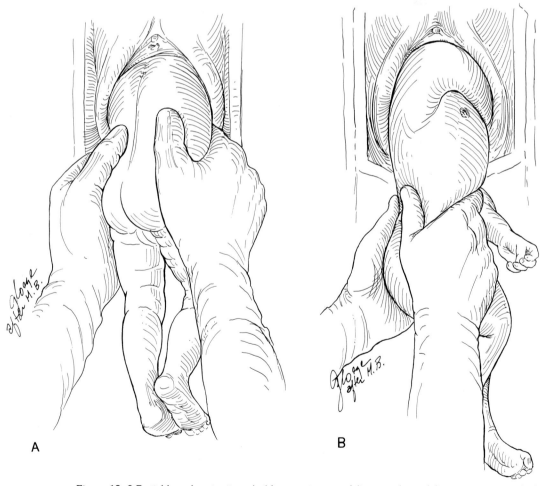

A

B

Figure 18–2 Partial breech extraction. *A,* After spontaneous delivery to the umbilicus, traction is applied to the infant's pelvis. When the scapulae are visible, rotation of the trunk allows delivery of the anterior shoulder. *B,* Delivery of the anterior shoulder by downward traction.

Illustration continued on following page

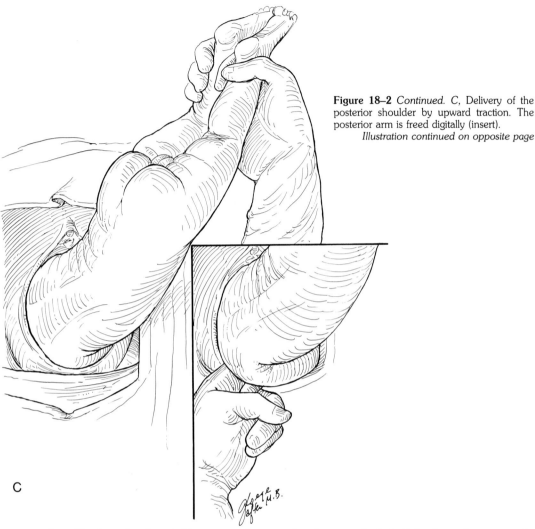

Figure 18–2 *Continued. C,* Delivery of the posterior shoulder by upward traction. The posterior arm is freed digitally (insert).
Illustration continued on opposite page

C

ean section. On the other hand, if an anomaly is found that would predispose the fetus to jeopardy if delivered vaginally, such as hydrocephalus, delivery should be accomplished by cesarean section. Utilizing these criteria, term frank breeches may be delivered vaginally without affecting the perinatal mortality rate. However, there is a greater incidence of birth trauma, particularly brachial plexus injuries, in those fetuses delivered vaginally as opposed to those delivered by cesarean section.

There are three types of vaginal breech delivery. *Spontaneous breech delivery* occurs when the fetus delivers spontaneously without any manipulation by the obstetrician other than that of supporting the fetus. With a *partial (or assisted) breech extraction*, the fetus is allowed to deliver spontaneously until the fetal umbilicus is at the introitus at which

point the remainder of the fetus is extracted. A *total breech extraction* occurs when the obstetrician extracts the entire body of the fetus. The preferred method of vaginal delivery is the partial breech extraction, although total breech extraction is often used for delivery of the second twin.

Partial Breech Extraction (Fig. 18–2). Once the fetus has delivered spontaneously to the umbilicus, the thumbs of the obstetrician are placed over the fetal sacrum and the fingers over the fetal hips. Gentle downward traction is exerted until the scapulas appear at the introitus. After delivery of the scapulas, the anterior axilla becomes visible, and, at this time, the shoulders are ready to deliver. By rotating the trunk, such that the bisacromial diameter is in the anteroposterior plane, the anterior shoulder and arm will usually deliver first. Subsequent rotation of

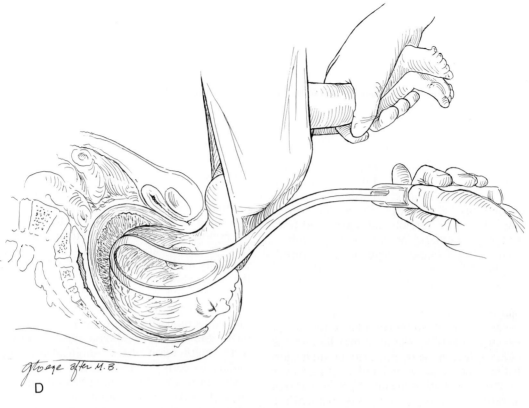

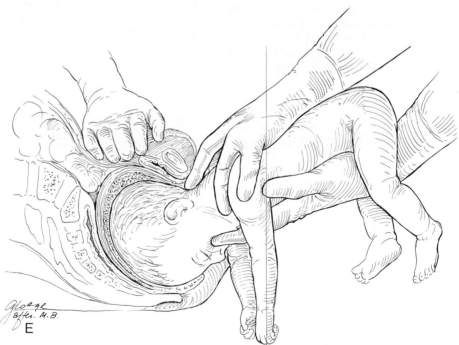

Figure 18–2 *Continued. D*, Delivery of the aftercoming head using Piper forceps. *E*, Delivery of the aftercoming head using the Mauriceau-Smellie-Veit maneuver. Every effort is made to maintain flexion of the head.

the trunk in the opposite direction will facilitate delivery of the other shoulder. If the shoulders do not deliver by trunk rotation, the posterior arm and shoulder are delivered by splinting the fetal elbow with the fingers and sweeping the arm across the fetal chest. Subsequent gentle downward traction on the fetal trunk will then facilitate delivery of the other shoulder and arm. Occasionally, one or both arms are located around the back of the neck (nuchal arm). Delivery in this instance may be facilitated by rotation of the trunk through 180 degrees. Should rotation of the fetus fail to deliver the nuchal arm, it may have to be forcibly extracted, and fracture of the humerus or clavicle may result.

Once the shoulders have been delivered, the head is delivered utilizing either the Mauriceau-Smellie-Veit maneuver or Piper forceps. With the Mauriceau-Smellie-Veit maneuver, the child is straddled over one forearm. The obstetrician places the index and ring fingers on the fetal maxilla and the middle finger in the mouth to maintain flexion of the head. The other hand is placed over the shoulders so that the middle finger presses upward on the occiput to aid flexion while the index and ring fingers apply traction to the shoulders. Utilizing this maneuver, the fetal neck is kept in a flexed position and delivery of the head is accomplished by gentle downward traction. Suprapubic pressure by an assistant will help to maintain flexion of the fetal head. Some obstetricians use Piper forceps routinely, since this method has been shown to effect delivery of the head with the least amount of trauma to the fetus.

Cesarean Section. Premature breeches should be delivered by cesarean section because of the large disparity between the size of the fetal head and that of the fetal trunk, the head being much larger. Therefore, if labor and vaginal delivery occur, successively larger parts of the fetus deliver, with the largest part, the fetal head, delivering last. The fetal lower extremities, abdomen, and trunk may deliver through an incompletely dilated cervix, with the larger head becoming trapped against the cervix. When this occurs, the umbilical cord may be compressed in the birth canal. This may lead to fetal asphyxia, and birth trauma may occur in an attempt to rapidly deliver the head, which has no time to mold to the shape of the maternal pelvis.

With complete and incomplete term breeches, delivery should be accomplished by cesarean section for two reasons. First, the incidence of umbilical cord prolapse is about 10 percent for these types of breeches, as opposed to about 2 percent for a frank breech. Second, with an incomplete breech, the fetal lower extremities, abdomen, and trunk may deliver through an incompletely dilated cervix, resulting in entrapment of the aftercoming head against the cervix.

Complications and Outcome

Perinatal morbidity and mortality are increased with breech presentation. The perinatal mortality of all breech fetuses is approximately 25 percent, versus 2 to 3 percent for nonbreeches. When prematurity and multiple gestation are excluded, the perinatal mortality for breeches is still about four times that of nonbreeches.

Factors that contribute to the increased perinatal morbidity and mortality include lethal congenital anomalies, birth trauma, and birth anoxia. Birth anoxia usually results from compression of the umbilical cord secondary to cord prolapse during labor or entrapment of the aftercoming head during vaginal delivery. Birth trauma usually occurs with vaginal delivery as opposed to cesarean section and generally results from forceful traction being placed on the fetus. Fetal organs most likely to be injured are the brain, spinal cord, liver, adrenal glands, and spleen. Other sites of injury include the brachial plexus, pharynx, bladder, and sternocleidomastoid muscle. Maternal mortality and morbidity are increased with breech presentation secondary to the widespread use of cesarean section as the mode of delivery.

FACE PRESENTATION

Face presentation occurs when the fetal head is hyperextended such that the fetal face, between the chin and orbits, is the presenting part. The incidence is about 1 in 500 deliveries.

Etiology

Controversy exists as to the etiologic factors. Normally, the attitude of the fetal head is one of flexion due to the greater tone of the flexor muscles in the neck. It is generally agreed that high maternal parity may predispose to hyperextension of the fetal neck in that the pendulous maternal abdomen and unengaged fetal head allow the back of the fetus to sag forward in the same direction as the occiput. Other factors that may predispose to hyperextension of the fetal neck that are not universally agreed upon include a contracted maternal pelvis and fetal macrosomia. Most authorities are of the opinion that the hyperextension is intrinsic to the fetus.

Diagnosis

The diagnosis of a face presentation may be made by Leopold examination, the fetal cephalic prominence lying on the same side as the spine with a deep groove between them. In reality, the diagnosis is usually made at the time of vaginal examination during labor with palpation of the fetal mouth, nose, malar bones, and orbital ridges. Such a presentation may be confirmed by sonography or x-ray if sonography is not available. Since anencephalic fetuses in the cephalic presentation, by definition, present face first, this diagnosis must be ruled out when a face presentation is suspected.

Mechanism of Labor

The position of the presenting face is classified according to the location of the fetal chin (mentum). Approximately 60 percent of face presentations are mentoanterior at the time of diagnosis, while 15 percent are mentotransverse, and 25 percent mentoposterior. The mechanism of labor with a face presentation is such that the submentobregmatic diameter presents into the maternal pelvis. This is the same length as the suboccipitobregmatic diameter that presents with vertex presentations (see Chapter 9). Labor occurs by internal rotation, which places the fetal chin under the symphysis with delivery occurring by subsequent flexion of the head (Fig. 18–3). The chin and mouth appear at the vulva initially, followed by the nose, eyes, and brow.

Management and Outcome

The intrapartum management of a face presentation is expectant, since about 75 percent deliver by normal spontaneous delivery or low forceps. Vaginal delivery can only occur once the head rotates to a mentoanterior position. With a persistent mentoposterior position, vaginal delivery cannot occur because the mentum would have to deliver under the symphysis by extension, and the fetal neck is already hyperextended. Approximately half of the mentoposterior presentations will spontaneously rotate to a mentoanterior position. The majority of mentotransverse presentations will also rotate spontaneously to a mentoanterior position. Face presentation is not a contraindication to augmentation of labor with pitocin.

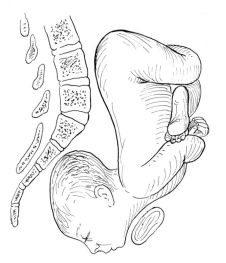
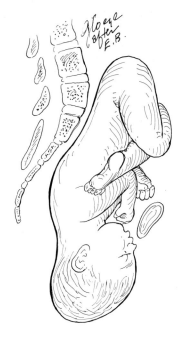

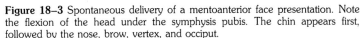

Figure 18–3 Spontaneous delivery of a mentoanterior face presentation. Note the flexion of the head under the symphysis pubis. The chin appears first, followed by the nose, brow, vertex, and occiput.

Cesarean section is indicated when dilatation and descent do not progress despite adequate uterine activity, as occurs with persistent mentotransverse or mentoposterior positions. Midpelvic delivery by vacuum or forceps and maneuvers to attempt to convert the face presentation to a vertex presentation are contraindicated, since they result in increased perinatal morbidity and mortality. When delivered by spontaneous vaginal delivery or low forceps (Fig. 18–4), perinatal morbidity and mortality for face presentations are similar to those for vertex presentations.

BROW PRESENTATION

Brow presentation occurs when the presenting part of the fetus is between the facial orbits and anterior fontanelle (Fig. 18–5). This type of presentation arises as the result of extension of the fetal head such that it is midway between flexion (vertex presentation) and hyperextension (face presentation). The incidence is about 1 in 1400 deliveries. With a brow presentation, the presenting diameter is the supraoccipitomental, which is much longer than the presenting diameter for a face or a vertex presentation (see Chapter 9).

Etiology

The etiology is the same as that for face presentation. The brow presentation is usually unstable or transitional and probably occurs when the head is in the process of

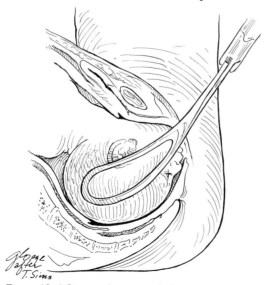

Figure 18–4 Simpson forceps applied to a mentoanterior face presentation.

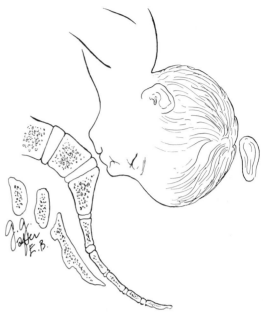

Figure 18–5 Brow presentation. Note the large presenting diameter (supraoccipitomental).

converting from a vertex to a face presentation or vice versa.

Diagnosis

The diagnosis of a brow presentation can be made by Leopold examination, with the examiner being able to palpate both the fetal chin and occiput. As with face presentation, the diagnosis is usually made by vaginal examination during labor by palpating the anterior fontanelle, orbital ridges, and eyes. The position of the presenting part is classified according to the location of the brow (frontum).

Management and Outcome

The intrapartum management is expectant. As mentioned previously, the brow presentation is an unstable one. Fifty to 75 percent will convert to either a face presentation, through extension, or a vertex presentation, through flexion, and will subsequently deliver vaginally. With a persistent brow presentation, the large presenting diameter makes vaginal delivery impossible, unless the fetus is very small or the maternal pelvis very large, and delivery must be accomplished by cesarean section. There is an increased incidence of both prolonged labor (30 to 50 percent) and dysfunctional labor (30 percent). As with face presentations, midpelvic delivery and methods to convert the brow presentation to a vertex presentation are contraindicated.

Perinatal morbidity and mortality are similar to those for vertex presentations.

SHOULDER PRESENTATION

Shoulder (or acromion) presentation occurs when the long axis of the fetus is perpendicular or at an acute angle to the long axis of the mother, as occurs with a transverse or oblique lie (Fig. 18–6). The oblique lie is unstable and usually converts to a longitudinal or transverse lie. Shoulder presentation is rare and occurs with an incidence of 0.3 percent.

Etiology

Etiologic factors include unusual relaxation of the maternal abdominal wall (which results from high parity), prematurity, placenta previa, multiple gestation, hydramnios, and contracted maternal pelvis.

Diagnosis

The diagnosis is readily made by Leopold examination, with no fetal pole detected at the fundus or above the pubic symphysis. The fetal head lies in either the right or left maternal iliac fossa. X-ray or sonographic examination will readily confirm the diagnosis. The diagnosis can, at times, be made by vaginal examination if enough dilatation of the cervix has occurred. In this situation, one may palpate the fetal ribs, scapula, and clavicle. With advanced labor, the shoulder becomes wedged into the maternal pelvis, and

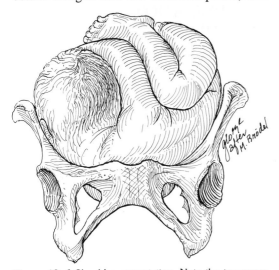

Figure 18–6 Shoulder presentation. Note the transverse lie of the fetus with the back down.

the fetal hand and arm frequently prolapse into the vagina.

Management

With such a presentation, vaginal delivery is impossible unless the fetus is extremely small (that is, extremely immature), since the fetal head and trunk would have to enter the maternal pelvis at the same time. If the diagnosis is made prior to labor, external cephalic version may be successful. Otherwise, cesarean section must be performed. If the fetal feet occupy the fundal region, which occurs with a back down transverse lie, a vertical uterine incision is recommended in order to provide enough room for the operator to reach up inside the uterus to the fundus, grasp the feet, and deliver the fetus by total breech extraction.

COMPOUND PRESENTATION

Compound presentation occurs when a fetal extremity prolapses alongside the presenting part and both parts enter the maternal pelvis at the same time. This type of presentation occurs more frequently with premature gestations. The incidence of a hand or arm prolapsing alongside the presenting fetal head is 1 in 700 deliveries. It is much less common for both hands to present alongside the fetal head or for a hand to present alongside a breech.

The etiology is obscure, and the management of such a presentation is expectant. Usually, the prolapsed part of the fetus does not interfere with labor. If the arm prolapses, it is best to wait to see if it moves out of the way as the head descends. If it does not, the arm may be gently pushed upward while the head is simultaneously pushed downward by fundal pressure. If the complete extremity prolapses and the fetus then converts to a shoulder presentation, delivery must be accomplished by cesarean section.

SUGGESTED READING

Collea JV: Current management of breech presentation. Clin Obstet Gynecol 23(2):525, 1980.

Collea JV, Rabin SC, Weghorst GR, et al: The randomized management of term frank breech presentations: Vaginal delivery vs cesarean section. Am J Obstet Gynecol 131:186, 1978.

Cruikshank DP, Cruikshank JE: Face and brow presentation: A review. Clin Obstet Gynecol 24(2):333, 1981.

Cruikshank DP, White CA: Obstetric malpresentations: Twenty years' experience. Am J Obstet Gynecol 116:1097, 1973.

19

Chapter Nineteen

MULTIPLE GESTATION

JAMES R. SHIELDS and ARNOLD L. MEDEARIS

Multiple gestation may be defined as any pregnancy in which two or more embryos or fetuses exist simultaneously. It is of utmost importance to recognize multiple gestation as a complication of pregnancy. The perinatal mortality and morbidity in multiple gestation exceed that of singleton gestations in a disproportionate manner, and maternal morbidity is increased. Although this chapter is devoted primarily to twin gestations, since they are the most common, the information presented also generally applies to pregnancies involving three or more fetuses.

ETIOLOGY AND CLASSIFICATION OF TWINNING

Multiple gestation may occur as the result of the division of a fertilized egg, fertilization of more than one egg by more than one sperm, or a combination of the two processes. The former process results in *monozygotic (identical) twins,* while the latter results in *dizygotic (fraternal) twins.* Since dizygotic twins arise from two fertilized eggs, they will always have two amnions and two chorions; the placentas may be either separate or fused, and the sexes may be different. With dizygotic twinning, the eggs may not be fertilized at the same time. *Superfecundation* may occur in which two ova are fertilized within a short period of time but not at the same coitus.

Monozygotic twins may arise from cleavage of a fertilized egg at various stages during embryogenesis, and the relationship of the fetal membranes depends upon the time at which the embryo divides (Table 19–1). If division occurs within the first 72 hours of fertilization, before differentiation of the amnion and chorion, the result will be *diamnionic, dichorionic,* monozygous twins with either separate or fused placentas. If division occurs four to eight days after ovulation, the chorion has already become differentiated and the result will be *diamnionic, monochorionic,* monozygous twins. If division occurs after eight days, both amnion and chorion have differentiated, and the result will be *monoamnionic, monochorionic,* monozygous twins. Of all monozygotic twins, 70 percent are monochorionic, and of these, the vast majority are diamnionic. The remaining 30 percent are diamnionic, dichorionic (Fig. 19–1).

DETERMINATION OF ZYGOSITY

After delivery of twins, an attempt should be made to determine the zygosity. In 80

TABLE 19–1 THE RELATIONSHIP BETWEEN THE TIMING OF CLEAVAGE AND THE NATURE OF THE MEMBRANES IN TWIN GESTATIONS

TIME OF CLEAVAGE*	NATURE OF THE MEMBRANES
0–72 hours	Diamnionic, dichorionic
4–8 days	Diamnionic, monochorionic
9–12 days	Monoamnionic, monochorionic

*Time interval between ovulation and cleavage of the egg.

Monochorionic Twin Placentation

Dichorionic Twin Placentation

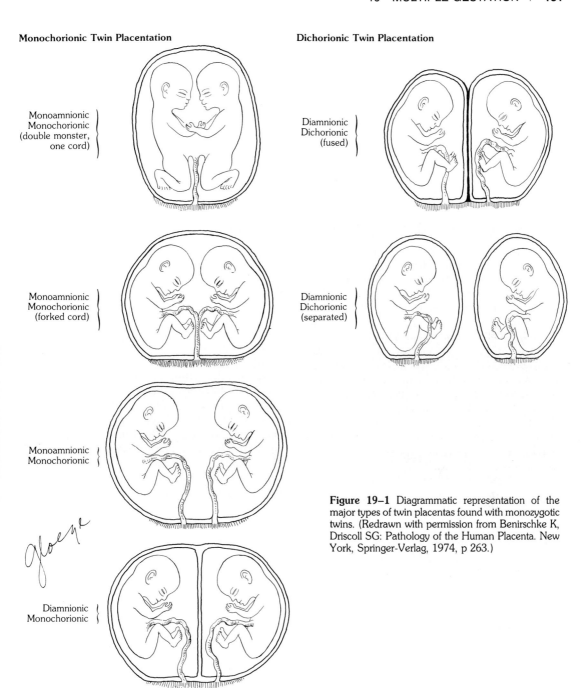

Monoamnionic
Monochorionic
(double monster,
one cord)

Diamnionic
Dichorionic
(fused)

Monoamnionic
Monochorionic
(forked cord)

Diamnionic
Dichorionic
(separated)

Monoamnionic
Monochorionic

Diamnionic
Monochorionic

Figure 19–1 Diagrammatic representation of the major types of twin placentas found with monozygotic twins. (Redrawn with permission from Benirschke K, Driscoll SG: Pathology of the Human Placenta. New York, Springer-Verlag, 1974, p 263.)

percent of twins, this may be done relatively easily by determining the relationship of the fetal membranes, fetal sex, and major and minor blood groupings. Thirty percent of twins will be of different sex and are, therefore, dizygotic. Twenty three percent will have monochorionic placentas and are, therefore, monozygotic. Twenty seven percent will have the same sex, dichorionic placentas, but different blood groupings and must be, therefore, dizygotic. Twenty percent will have the same sex, dichorionic placentas, and identical blood groupings. For this latter group, further studies, such as HLA typing or the acceptance or rejection of reciprocal skin grafts, allow determination of zygosity.

INCIDENCE AND EPIDEMIOLOGY

The frequency of multiple gestation is not constant throughout the world, but varies according to race, hereditary factors, maternal age, maternal parity, and the use of fertility agents. Dizygotic twinning increases with a maternal history of twinning, increasing maternal age, and increasing maternal parity. In North America, twinning occurs with a frequency of 1 in 90 gestations. In approximately one third of these twin gestations, the fetuses are monozygotic, or identical; the remaining two thirds are dizygotic, or fraternal. In contrast, twinning in western Nigeria occurs with a frequency of 1 in 22 gestations, the difference being due to a higher rate of dizygotic twinning. The incidence of multiple gestation with the use of clomiphene is about 10 percent versus about 30 percent following gonadotropin therapy.

Rates of multiple gestation are usually expressed as occurrences per births, as opposed to occurrences per conception. The actual rate per conception is difficult to analyze, since the abortion rate in twins is higher than that in singletons.

ABNORMALITIES OF THE TWINNING PROCESS

Abnormalities in the twinning process are common and may result in conjoined twins, placental vascular anastomoses, twin-twin transfusion syndrome, and fetal malformations. These abnormalities occur only in monochorionic (monozygotic) twins.

Conjoined Twins

If division of the embryo occurs after the embryonic disc has formed, that is, about 13 days after fertilization, cleavage of the embryo is incomplete and results in conjoined ("Siamese") twins. This is a very rare event, occurring once in 70,000 deliveries. Conjoined twins are classified according to the anatomic location of the joining: thoracopagus (anterior), pyopagus (posterior), craniopagus (cephalic), or ischiopagus (caudal). The majority of such twins are thoracopagus.

Placental Vascular Anastomoses

Placental vascular anastomoses occur very frequently in monochorionic twins. The most common type is arterial-arterial, followed by arterial-venous and then venous-venous. Vascular communications between the two fetuses via the placenta may give rise to a number of problems, including abortion, hydramnios, twin-twin transfusion syndrome, and fetal malformations. The incidence of both minor and major congenital malformations in twins is twice that of singletons, the majority of malformations occurring in monochorionic twins.

Twin-Twin Transfusion Syndrome

The presence of arterial-venous anastomoses in the placenta of monochorionic twins will often lead to the twin-twin transfusion syndrome. Arterial blood from the donor twin enters the placenta and courses through a cotyledon, which is shared by the two twins. The blood then empties into a vein of the recipient twin. As a result of this chronic shunting, the donor twin develops hypovolemia, hypotension, anemia, microcardia, and growth retardation. The recipient twin develops hypervolemia, hyperviscosity, thrombosis, hypertension, cardiomegaly, polycythemia, edema, and congestive heart failure. Hydramnios is also frequent and may result from increased renal blood flow secondary to hypervolemia and/or transudation of fluid across congested chorionic fetal blood vessels. The hyperperfused twin is prone to develop kernicterus during the neonatal period as a result of polycythemia and subsequent hyperbilirubinemia.

Fetal Malformations

Arterial-arterial placental anastomoses may result in a number of fetal malformations. In this situation, the arterial blood from the donor twin enters the arterial circulation in the placenta of the recipient twin and blood flow may become reversed in the recipient twin. Embolization can occur in the recipient twin as trophoblastic tissue enters its circulation. The recipient twin, being perfused in a reverse direction with relatively poorly oxygenated blood, may fail to develop normally.

Umbilical Cord Abnormalities

Abnormalities of the umbilical cord also occur with a higher frequency in twins, primarily the result of abnormalities in monochorionic twins. Absence of one umbilical artery occurs in about 3 to 4 percent of twins, as opposed to 0.5 to 1 percent of singletons. The absence of one umbilical artery is significant because in 30 percent of such cases, it is associated with other congenital anomalies. Marginal and velamentous umbilical cord insertions also occur more frequently, the latter occurring in about 5 percent of twins.

MATERNAL PHYSIOLOGIC RESPONSE

A number of normal maternal physiologic responses to pregnancy are exaggerated with multiple fetuses. On the average, multiple gestation results in a 500-ml increase in blood volume over that of a singleton. The increased blood volume, combined with the increased iron and folate requirements of additional fetuses, may predispose the mother to anemia. Additional physiologic responses may occur secondary to the increased weight of the uterus. Hydramnios occurs in 12 percent of multiple gestations, primarily in monochorionic gestations. This added increase in the size of the uterus may lead to increasing respiratory difficulty as the overdistended uterus causes greater elevation of the diaphragm. The weight of the uterus may cause further compression of the great vessels, resulting in a more pronounced decrease in uterine blood flow secondary to aortic compression and/or supine hypotension. Greater compression of the ureters can also occur, leading to obstructive uropathy and renal failure. These severe complications are more common when acute hydramnios develops.

DIAGNOSIS

Historic factors such as a maternal family history of dizygotic twinning, the recent use of fertility drugs, a maternal sensation of feeling larger than with previous pregnancies, or a sensation of excessive fetal movements increase the suspicion of a multiple gestation. Physical signs include excessive weight gain, abdominal palpation of an excessive number of fetal parts, auscultation of two separate fetal heart rates that differ by more than ten beats per minute, and rapid uterine growth.

Most of the time, twinning will result in a fundal height that is 4 cm larger than expected for a singleton. This is referred to as a size/dates discrepancy.

When a multiple gestation is suspected, confirmation should be established by sonography. Separate gestational sacs may be seen as early as six weeks of gestation. After the tenth week, multiple fetal parts may be visualized. When sonography is not available, a single anteroposterior abdominal x-ray will reveal the fetal skeletal parts that are usually visible at about 16 weeks.

The need for early diagnosis of multiple gestation cannot be overemphasized. In many studies, almost half the twin gestations are not diagnosed until delivery of the first twin. Failure of early diagnosis leads to an increased incidence of intrauterine growth retardation and preterm labor, both of which increase the perinatal morbidity and mortality. In addition, there is an increased likelihood of maternal complications.

ANTEPARTUM MANAGEMENT

Intensive antepartum management serves to prolong gestation, increase birth weight, decrease perinatal morbidity and mortality, and decrease the incidence of maternal complications. The complications of multiple gestation are shown in Table 19–2.

The patient should be seen weekly beginning in the mid-second trimester. The cervix should be assessed frequently, since multiple gestation may lead to early cervical effacement and dilatation. The patient should be examined for the development of nondependent edema, the urine routinely checked for protein, and the blood pressure monitored closely. With multiple gestation, pregnancy-induced hypertension tends to occur more frequently, earlier, and more severely than with singletons. Dietary considerations must not be overlooked, as there is an increased need for calories, iron, vitamins, and folate.

The prevention of prematurity is of utmost importance. Many regimens have been developed, including bed rest, hospitalization, prophylactic beta-sympathomimetic (tocolytic) agents, and/or cervical cerclage. Bed rest during the late second and third trimesters increases birth weight, probably by increasing uterine blood flow. Many studies have shown that bed rest also prolongs gestation and

TABLE 19–2 COMPLICATIONS OF MULTIPLE GESTATIONS

MATERNAL	FETAL
Anemia	Hydramnios
Hypertension	Malpresentation
Premature labor	Placenta previa
Postpartum uterine atony	Abruptio placentae
Postpartum hemorrhage	Premature rupture of the membranes
	Umbilical cord prolapse
	Intrauterine growth retardation
	Congenital anomalies
	Increased perinatal morbidity
	Increased perinatal mortality

decreases perinatal mortality, whereas other studies have failed to demonstrate these additional benefits. Recently, Swedish workers have reported a perinatal mortality rate equal to that of singletons (0.6 percent). Their patients were advised to undergo bed rest at home until the third trimester, when they were hospitalized for additional bed rest. They were subsequently discharged home at 36 weeks, unless complications arose. Pregnancies were not usually permitted to go beyond 38 weeks' gestation.

Fetal surveillance is also crucial in decreasing perinatal morbidity and mortality. Routine sonography should be performed at monthly intervals beginning at 26 to 28 weeks in order to assess fetal growth, since twins have a tendency to suffer from intrauterine growth retardation (IUGR). Assessment of fetal well-being by nonstress testing (NST) should be performed weekly beginning at 38 weeks, unless the pregnancy is complicated by other factors, such as IUGR, hypertension, or hydramnios. If these complications develop, nonstress testing should be instigated immediately and the frequency increased to twice per week. The use of the contraction stress test to rule out uteroplacental insufficiency in the face of a nonreactive NST is relatively contraindicated in multiple gestations, since these pregnancies are already predisposed to develop preterm labor.

INTRAPARTUM MANAGEMENT

Should preterm labor develop (less than 35 weeks), aggressive measures must be taken.

These include treatment with tocolytic agents to arrest labor, assessment of fetal pulmonary maturity, and maternal administration of glucocorticoids when necessary to accelerate fetal lung maturation if the gestational age is less than 34 weeks. Care must be taken to avoid iatrogenic fluid overload. Table 19–3 provides a list of necessary prerequisites for the management of labor in pregnancies complicated by multiple gestation.

Vertex-Vertex Presentations

In order to choose the optimal method of delivery, the presentations of the fetuses must be accurately known. By convention, the presentation is designated as X/Y, in which X is the presenting twin (twin A) and Y is the second twin (twin B). All combinations of presentation are possible. Vertex/vertex occurs most frequently (50 percent of the time), followed by vertex/breech, breech/vertex, and breech/breech.

For *vertex/vertex presentations,* labor is allowed as with a singleton vertex presentation. Both fetal heart rates must be monitored continuously during labor. Oxytocin is not contraindicated for dysfunctional labor, but should be administered in dilute solution with an infusion pump. Uterine contractions should be monitored with an intrauterine pressure catheter. After delivery of the first

TABLE 19–3 PREREQUISITES FOR THE INTRAPARTUM MANAGEMENT OF MULTIPLE GESTATIONS

1. A secondary or tertiary care center
2. A delivery room equipped for immediate cesarean section, if necessary
3. A well functioning large bore intravenous line (e.g., 16 gauge) to administer fluids and blood rapidly, if necessary
4. Two units of typed and cross-matched blood
5. The capability to continuously monitor the fetal heart rates simultaneously
6. An anesthesiologist who is immediately available to administer general anesthesia should intrauterine manipulation or cesarean section be necessary for delivery of the second twin
7. Two obstetricians scrubbed and gowned for the delivery, one of whom is skilled in intrauterine manipulation and delivery of the second twin
8. Imaging techniques, preferably sonography, for determining the precise presentations of the twins
9. Two pediatricians, one of whom is skilled in the immediate resuscitation of the newborn
10. An appropriate number of nurses to assist in the delivery and care of the newborn infants

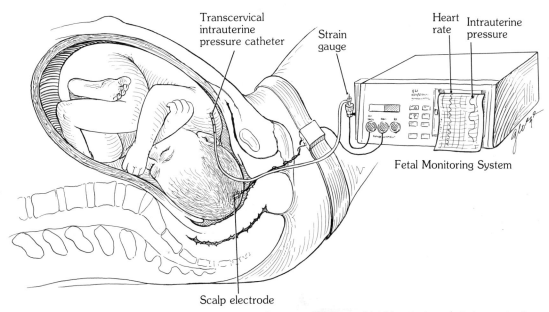

Figure 20–1 Technique for continuous electronic monitoring of fetal heart rate and uterine contractions.

to monitor heart rate and a plastic catheter transcervically into the amniotic cavity to monitor uterine contractions (Fig. 20–1). In order to carry out this technique, the fetal membranes must be ruptured, and the cervix must be dilated to at least 2 cm. Internal monitoring gives better FHR tracings because the rate is computed from the sharply defined R-wave peaks of the fetal electrocardiogram, whereas with the external technique, the rate is computed from the less precisely defined first heart sound obtained with an ultrasonic transducer. The internal uterine catheter allows precise measurement of the intensity of the contractions in millimeters of mercury, whereas the external tocotransducer measures only frequency and duration, not intensity.

In the clinical setting, internal and external techniques are often combined by using a scalp electrode for precise heart rate recording and the external tocotransducer for contractions. This approach minimizes possible side effects from invasive internal monitoring. With increasing evidence of the benefits derived from this technique, the concept of monitoring all patients is gaining support.

ETIOLOGY OF FETAL DISTRESS

The developing fetus presents a paradox. Its arterial blood oxygen tension is only 25 ± 5 torr compared with adult values of about 100 torr. However, the rate of oxygen consumption is twice that of the adult per unit weight, and its oxygen reserve is only enough to meet its metabolic needs for one to two minutes. Blood flow from the maternal circulation, which supplies the fetus with oxygen through placental exchange of respiratory gases, is momentarily interrupted during a contraction. A normal fetus can withstand the stress of labor without suffering from hypoxia because sufficient oxygen exchange occurs during the interval between contractions.

Under normal circumstances, the fetal heart rate is determined by the atrial pacemaker. Modulation of the rate occurs physiologically through innervation of the heart by the vagus (decelerator) and sympathetic (accelerator) nerves. A fetus whose oxygen supply is marginal cannot tolerate the stress of contractions and will become hypoxic. Under hypoxic conditions, baroreceptors and chemoreceptors in the central circulation of the fetus influence the FHR by giving rise to contraction-related or "periodic" FHR changes. The hypoxia will also result in anaerobic metabolism. Pyruvate and lactic acid accumulate causing fetal acidosis. The degree of fetal acidosis can be measured by sampling blood from the presenting part. By definition, fetal distress occurs when the fetus is unable to maintain biochemical homeostasis as assessed by a fetal scalp blood pH of 7.25 or less. Clinical and experimental data indicate

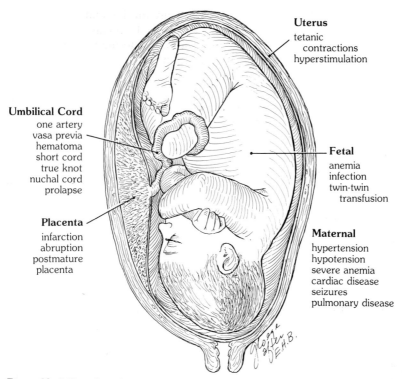

Uterus
tetanic
  contractions
hyperstimulation

Umbilical Cord
  one artery
  vasa previa
  hematoma
  short cord
  true knot
  nuchal cord
  prolapse

Fetal
anemia
infection
twin-twin
  transfusion

Placenta
  infarction
  abruption
  postmature
  placenta

Maternal
hypertension
hypotension
severe anemia
cardiac disease
seizures
pulmonary disease

Figure 20–2 Clinical conditions associated with fetal distress in labor.

that fetal death occurs when 50 percent or more of the transplacental oxygen exchange is interrupted.

Fetal oxygenation can be impaired at different anatomic locations within the uteroplacental-fetal circulatory loop. For example, there may be impairment of oxygen transportation to the intervillous space as a result of maternal hypertension or anemia, oxygen diffusion may be impaired in the placenta because of infarction or abruption, or the oxygen content in the fetal blood may be impaired because of hemolytic anemia in Rh-isoimmunization. Figure 20–2 summarizes the clinical conditions that may be associated with fetal distress during labor.

FETAL HEART RATE PATTERNS

The assessment of the fetal heart rate depends upon an evaluation of (1) the baseline pattern and (2) the periodic changes related to uterine contractions.

Baseline Assessment

This requires determination of the rate in beats per minute (BPM) and the variability. Normal and abnormal rates are listed in Ta-

ble 20–1. Baseline variability can be divided into short-term and long-term intervals. These are described as follows:

1. Short-term or *beat-to-beat variability*. This reflects the interval between either successive fetal electrocardiogram signals or mechanical events of the cardiac cycle. Normal short-term variability fluctuates between 5 and 25 BPM. Variability below 5 BPM is considered to be potentially abnormal. When associated with decelerations, a variability of less than 5 BPM usually indicates severe fetal distress.

2. Long-term variability. These fluctuations may be described in terms of the frequency and amplitude of change in the baseline rate. The normal long-term variability is 3 to 10 cycles per minute. Variability is physiologically decreased during fetal sleep states.

TABLE 20–1 BASELINE FETAL HEART RATES

RATE	BEATS PER MINUTE
Normal	120–160
Abnormal	
Tachycardia	>160
Bradycardia	<120

Periodic FHR Changes

These are changes in baseline fetal heart rate related to uterine contractions. The responses to uterine contractions may be categorized as follows:

1. No change. The FHR maintains the same characteristics as in the preceding baseline FHR.
2. Acceleration. The FHR increases in response to uterine contractions. This is a normal response.
3. Deceleration. The FHR decreases in response to uterine contractions. Decelerations may be early, late, variable, or mixed. All except early decelerations are abnormal.

Types of Patterns

Early Deceleration (Head Compression). This pattern usually has an onset, maximum fall, and recovery that is coincident with the onset, peak, and end of the uterine contraction (Fig. 20–3). The nadir of the FHR coincides with the peak of the contraction. This pattern is seen when engagement of the fetal head has occurred. Early decelerations are not thought to be associated with fetal dis-

tress. The pressure on the fetal head leads to increased intracranial pressure that elicits a vagal response similar to the Valsalva maneuver in the adult. The vagal reflex can be abolished by the administration of atropine, but this approach is not used clinically.

Late Deceleration (Uteroplacental Insufficiency). This pattern has an onset, maximal decrease, and recovery that is shifted to the right in relation to the contraction (Fig. 20–4). The severity of late decelerations is graded by the magnitude of the decrease in FHR at the nadir of the deceleration (Table 20–2). Fetal hypoxia and acidosis are usually more pronounced with severe decelerations. Late decelerations are generally associated with low scalp blood pH values and high base deficits, indicating metabolic acidosis from anaerobic metabolism. The partial pressure of carbon dioxide (PCO_2) in the fetal blood is usually in the normal range, and the fetal blood oxygen partial pressure (PO_2) is only slightly below normal because of the Bohr effect—the shift to the left of the oxygen dissociation curve caused by the acidosis. The PO_2 is, therefore, not a sensitive indicator for monitoring fetal compromise.

Variable Deceleration (Cord Compression). This pattern has a variable time of

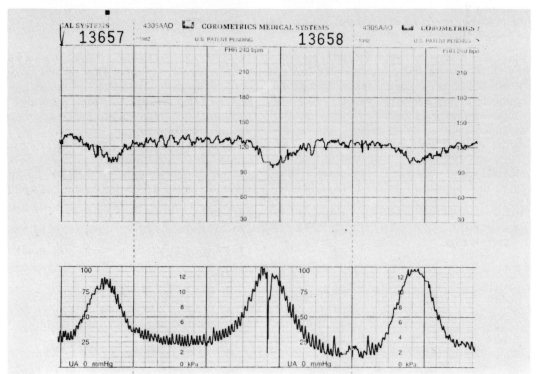

Figure 20–3 Early deceleration. Note that the deceleration starts and ends with the uterine contraction. Good beat-to-beat variability is demonstrated.

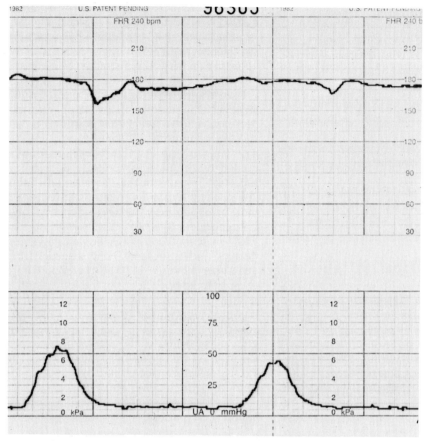

Figure 20-4 Late decelerations in a severely distressed fetus. Note tne tachycardia and lack of beat-to-beat variability in addition to the late decelerations.

onset and a variable form and may be non-repetitive. Variable decelerations are caused by umbilical cord compression. Partial or complete compression of the cord causes a sudden increase in blood pressure in the central circulation of the fetus. The brady-cardia is mediated via baroreceptors. This reflex can be abolished or ameliorated by atropine (e.g., chemical vagotomy). How-ever, this approach is not used clinically.

Fetal blood gases indicate respiratory acidosis with a low pH and high PCO_2 values. When cord compression has been prolonged, hy-poxia is also present, showing a picture of combined respiratory and metabolic acidosis in fetal blood gases.

The severity of variable decelerations is graded by their duration (Table 20-2). When the fetal heart rate falls below 80 BPM during the nadir of the deceleration, there is usually

TABLE 20-2 PRINCIPLES OF GRADING LATE AND VARIABLE DECELERATIONS

CRITERIA OF GRADING	MILD	MODERATE	SEVERE
Late deceleration: amplitude of drop in FHR	<15 BPM	15–45 BPM	>45 BPM
Variable deceleration: duration of deceler-ation	<30 sec duration	30–60 sec	>60 sec

BPM = beats per minute; FHR = fetal heart rate; sec = seconds
Adapted with permission from Kubli FW, Hon EH, Khazin AF, et al: Observations on heart rate and pH in the human fetus during labor. Am J Obstet Gynecol 104:1190, 1969.

a loss of the P-wave in the fetal electrocardiogram, indicating a nodal rhythm or a second-degree heart block.

Combined or Mixed Patterns. These patterns may be difficult to define and may exhibit characteristics of any of the above patterns.

STRATEGIES FOR INTERVENTION

A normal fetal heart rate pattern on the electronic monitor indicates a greater than 95 percent probability of fetal well-being. However, abnormal patterns may occur in the absence of fetal distress. The false-positive rate (i.e., good Apgar scores and normal fetal acid-base status in the presence of abnormal fetal heart rate patterns) is as high as 80 percent. Therefore, electronic fetal monitoring is a screening rather than a diagnostic technique. Failure to appreciate this limitation may lead to inappropriate intervention.

Strategies for intervention always depend upon the clinical circumstances in which fetal distress is seen. When abnormal fetal heart rate patterns are seen, the first step should be a search for the underlying cause. When the cause is identified, such as maternal hypotension, steps should be taken to correct the problem. In general, a term-sized fetus tolerates ominous fetal heart patterns better than a preterm fetus. A fetus with additional risk factors, such as intrauterine infection from chorioamnionitis, may deteriorate sooner than a fetus in a normal parturient. Other considerations in the management of fetal distress include the maternal condition and the stage of labor. Therefore, the management of an abnormal fetal heart rate pattern depends upon the clinical situation in which the fetal heart rate abnormality is seen.

Variable Decelerations

The most frequently encountered FHR pattern is that of variable decelerations. In order to stop fetal pressure on the cord, a change in maternal position to the right or left side generally abolishes the decelerations. One hundred percent oxygen should be given by face mask to the mother. If the pattern is persistent, placing the mother in the Trendelenburg position or elevating the presenting part by vaginal examination may be tried.

If an oxytocic infusion is running, it should be stopped.

Variable decelerations of severe degree are most frequently seen during the second stage of labor, with the patient pushing during uterine contractions. The safest intervention to deliver the fetus with cord compression is often an outlet forceps delivery. When progressive acidosis occurs, as determined by serial scalp blood pH determinations, cesarean section should be performed if vaginal delivery is not imminent. Another circumstance requiring immediate intervention is persistent bradycardia (prolonged bradycardia). This condition is encountered when the fetal heart rate falls to 60 to 90 beats per minute for greater than 2 minutes. Prolonged bradycardia may be a final stage of fetal decompensation.

Late Decelerations

Late decelerations of the fetal heart rate are most commonly seen in pregnancies associated with uteroplacental insufficiency. The following steps are taken in rapid succession in order to alleviate fetal distress and to determine the underlying cause (Fig. 20–5):

1.   Change the maternal position from supine to left or right lateral; the supine hypotension syndrome is caused by compression of the vena cava and aorta by the heavy uterus, leading to lowering of maternal cardiac output and underperfusion of the placenta. In addition, the weight of the term uterus can compress the internal and external iliac vessels, resulting in poor perfusion of the uterus and fetal bradycardia. When this occurs, the femoral pulse cannot be palpated on the affected side. This is called the Poseiro effect.

2.   Give oxygen by face mask; this can increase fetal Po_2 by 5 mm Hg.

3.   Stop any oxytocic infusion to exclude uterine hyperstimulation.

4.   Monitor maternal blood pressure to exclude hypotensive episodes that can occur as a consequence of epidural analgesia.

When late decelerations persist for greater than 30 minutes despite the above-mentioned maneuvers, fetal scalp blood pH measurements are indicated. In order to interpret pH values properly, notation should be made by means of an event marker on the fetal monitor indicating the timing of the scalp blood sample.

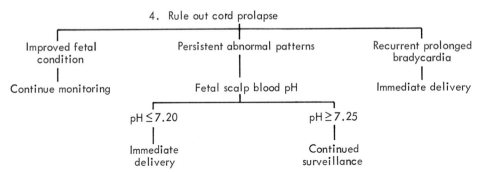

Figure 20–5 Algorithm for the management of an abnormal fetal heart tracing.

Operative delivery for fetal distress is indicated when fetal acidosis is present (pH less than 7.2) or when late decelerations are persistent in early labor and the cervix is insufficiently dilated to allow blood sampling from the presenting part.

Fetal Tachycardia

As a baseline change, tachycardia is not a very good sign of fetal distress. In general, fetal tachycardia occurs to improve placental circulation when the fetus is stressed. Brief periods of tachycardia (15 to 30 minutes) are usually associated with excessive oxytocin (Pitocin) augmentation of labor, after which the heart rate returns to baseline when the augmentation is discontinued. Prolonged periods of tachycardia are usually associated with elevated maternal temperature or an intrauterine infection, which should be ruled out. The acid-base status is usually normal.

MECONIUM

The presence of meconium in the amniotic fluid may be a sign of fetal distress. Classification of meconium into early and late passage facilitates a clearer understanding of its importance. *Early passage* occurs any time prior to rupture of the membranes and is classified as light or heavy, based on its color and viscosity. Light meconium is lightly stained amniotic fluid, yellow or greenish in color. Heavy meconium is dark green or black in color, and usually thick and tenacious. Light passage is not associated with poor outcome. Heavy passage is associated with lower one- and five-minute Apgar scores, and is associated with the risk of meconium aspiration. *Late passage* usually occurs during the second stage of labor, after clear amniotic fluid has been noted earlier. Late passage, which is most often heavy, is usually associated with some event (e.g., umbilical cord compression or uterine hypertonus) late in labor causing fetal distress. Since heavy meconium is associated with poor outcome, aggressive management of these patients is important.

FETAL BLOOD SAMPLING

Fetal scalp blood sampling for pH determination is indicated when fetal distress is suggested by clinical parameters, such as heavy meconium, or by moderate to severely abnormal fetal heart rate patterns. Blood is obtained from the fetus by placing an amnioscope transvaginally against the fetal skull (Fig. 20–6). Cervical mucus is removed with cotton swabs. Silicone grease is applied to the skull for blood bead formation. A 2 × 2-mm lancet is used for a stab incision, and a drop of blood is aspirated into a heparinized glass capillary tube.

Fetal blood pH correctly predicts neonatal outcome 82 percent of the time, as measured by the Apgar score. The false-positive rate is about 8 percent and the false-negative rate

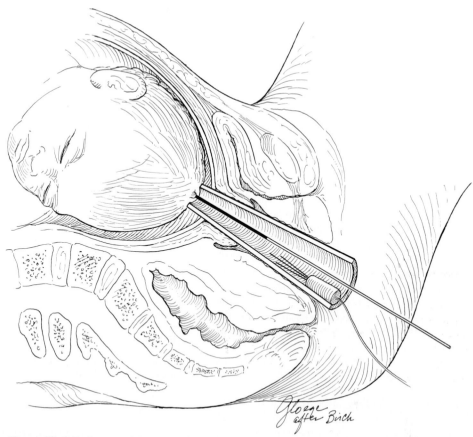

Figure 20–6 Technique of fetal scalp blood sampling via an amnioscope. After making a small stab incision in the fetal scalp, the blood is drawn off through a capillary tube.

about 10 percent. Determination of P_{O_2} and P_{CO_2} from scalp blood is possible, but not particularly useful clinically. A pH value can be obtained from a 7-cm column of blood in a collecting glass capillary tube (0.015 ml). For P_{O_2} and P_{CO_2} determinations, a 25-cm blood column is necessary. This requires a longer sampling time and often leads to clotting within the tube during collection. Clotted blood cannot be aspirated into the gas analyzer. Furthermore, P_{O_2} and P_{CO_2} do not correlate as well as pH with the Apgar score.

It is good clinical practice to doubly clamp the umbilical cord after delivery to allow blood gas analysis from the umbilical artery and vein in order to evaluate the fetal condition at birth. This is particularly true in cases of fetal distress that lead to operative

TABLE 20–3   NORMAL RANGES FOR FETAL SCALP AND CORD BLOOD INDICES

BLOOD	pH	P_{CO_2} (mm Hg)	P_{O_2} (mm Hg)	BASE DEFICIT (mEq/L)
Scalp Blood				
Early labor	7.34–7.38	43–57	20–24	(−0.2)–(0.4)
Active phase	7.34–7.40	36–54	20–24	(−2.0)–(0.0)
Complete cervical dilatation	7.26–7.42	36–60	20–24	(−3.3)–(−0.3)
Cord Blood				
Artery	7.22–7.34	32–64	14–22	(−7.8)–(−2.2)
Vein	7.29–7.41	25–53	23–35	(−6.2)–(−1.8)

Modified with permission from Hobel CJ: Intrapartum clinical assessment of fetal distress. Am J Obstet Gynecol 110:336, 1971.

delivery. Evaluation of pH, P_{O_2}, P_{CO_2}, and base deficit in the cord blood, in addition to Apgar scores, gives valuable information to the pediatrician who assumes responsibility for the newborn. The normal range for these indices is given in Table 20–3.

COMPLICATIONS OF FETAL MONITORING

The introduction of a catheter into the uterine cavity and application of a scalp electrode may cause a slight increase in the incidence of maternal infection, but length of labor, rupture of the membranes, and the number of vaginal examinations are of much greater importance in this regard. The incidence of fetal scalp abscesses and soft tissue injuries from electrode applications is less than 5 percent. Scalp abscesses are managed by opening the intradermal vesicle to allow for drainage. These small abscesses heal without the need for antibiotic therapy. Spread of the infection into adjacent tissues is rare.

The incidence of scalp abscesses from microblood sampling is less frequent than infection from electrode application. After fetal scalp blood sampling, a cotton swab should always be applied throughout the next uterine contraction and the puncture site inspected for hemostasis during the second contraction. If these precautions are followed, hemorrhage does not occur with scalp blood sampling.

SUGGESTED READING

Bieniarz J, Maqueda E, Caldeyro-Barcia R: Compression of aorta by the uterus in late human pregnancy. I. Variations between femoral and brachial artery pressure with changes from hypertension to hypotension. Am J Obstet Gynecol 95:795, 1966.

Hobel CJ: Intrapartum clinical assessment of fetal distress. Am J Obstet Gynecol 110:336, 1971.

Hobel CJ, Hyvarinen MA, Oh W: Abnormal fetal heart rate patterns and fetal acid-base balance in low birth weight infants in relation to respiratory distress syndrome. Obstet Gynecol 39:83, 1972.

Hobel CJ, Hyvarinen MA, Okada DM, et al: Prenatal and intrapartum high-risk screening. I. Prediction of the high-risk neonate. Am J Obstet Gynecol 117:1, 1973.

Hon EH: Atlas of Fetal Heart Rate Patterns. New Haven, CT, Harty Press Inc, 1968.

Kubli FW: Observations on heart rate and pH in the human fetus during labor. Am J Obstet Gynecol 104:1190, 1969.

Lauerson NG: Acid-base fetal monitoring. In Modern Management of High-Risk Pregnancy. New York, Plenum Medical Book Co, 1983, p 482.

Martin CB: Physiology and clinical use of fetal heart rate variability. Clin Perinatol 9:339, 1982.

Meis PJ, Hall M III, Marshall JR, et al: Meconium passage: A new classification for risk assessment during labor. Am J Obstet Gynecol 131:509, 1978.

Modanlou H, Yeh S, Hon EH, et al: Umbilical cord pH, P_{O_2}, P_{CO_2} associated with Apgar scores greater than 6 at 5 minutes. Am J Obstet Gynecol 117:943, 1973.

Parer JT: Fetal heart rate. In Creasy RK, Resnik R (eds): Maternal Fetal Medicine. Philadelphia, WB Saunders Co, 1984, p 292.

Saling E: Foetal and Neonatal Hypoxia. Baltimore, Williams and Wilkins, 1968.

Chapter Twenty-One

DYSTOCIA

RICHARD A. BASHORE

Although the definition of dystocia is "difficult childbirth," it is used interchangeably with "dysfunctional labor," and characterizes labor that does not progress normally. The problem may be caused by (1) ineffective uterine expulsive forces; (2) an abnormal lie, presentation, position, or fetal structure; or (3) disproportion between the size of the fetus and pelvis, resulting in mechanical interference with the passage of the fetus through the birth canal. It is important that the cause or causes of abnormal labor be determined as accurately as possible so that an effective and safe management plan may be developed.

The early part or latent phase of labor is involved with softening and effacement of the cervix, but minimal dilatation. This is followed by a more rapid rate of cervical dilatation known as the active phase of labor, which is further divided into acceleration, maximum slope, and deceleration phases. The descent of the fetal presenting part usually begins during the active phase of labor, then progresses at a more rapid rate toward the end of the active phase, and continues after the cervix is completely dilated. A useful method for assessing the progress of labor and detecting abnormalities in a timely manner is to plot the rate of cervical dilatation and descent of the fetal presenting part (Fig. 21-1).

Normal cervical dilatation and descent of the fetus take place in a progressive manner and occur within a well-defined time period. Dysfunctional labor occurs when rates of dilatation and descent exceed these time limits. The phase of labor when the abnormality occurs and the configuration of the abnormal labor curve may indicate the potential causes of the abnormal labor. Although the management of abnormal labor is not dictated by the appearance of the labor curve, an appreciation of the underlying cause of the problem should suggest rational management plans.

ABNORMALITIES OF THE LATENT PHASE OF LABOR

The normal limits of the latent phase of labor extend up to 20 hours for nulliparous patients and to 14 hours for multiparas. A latent phase that exceeds these limits is considered prolonged (Fig. 21-2) and may be caused by hypertonic uterine contractions, premature or excessive use of sedatives or analgesics, or, less commonly, by hypotonic uterine contractions. Hypertonic contractions are ineffective and painful and are associated with increased uterine tone, while hypotonic contractions are usually less painful and are characterized by an easily indentable uterus during the contraction. Hypotonic contractions occur more frequently during the active phase of labor. A long, closed, firm cervix requires more time to efface and undergo early dilatation than does a soft, partially effaced cervix, but it is doubtful that a cervical factor alone will cause a prolonged latent phase. Some patients who appear to be developing a prolonged latent phase are shown eventually to be in false labor with no progressive dilatation of the cervix.

The identification of the cause or causes of a prolonged latent phase is usually not diffi-

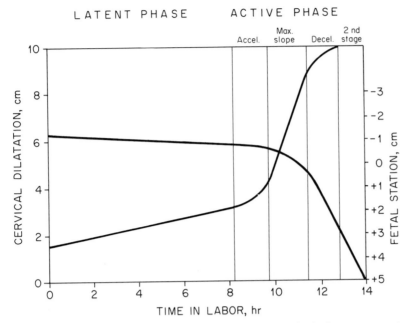

Figure 21–1 Graphic plot of cervical dilatation and descent of the fetal presenting part during labor. (Reproduced with permission from Cohen WR, Friedman EA (eds): Management of Labor. Baltimore, University Park Press, 1983, p 13.)

cult. Palpation or recording of uterine contractions and observation of the patient over a period of time will usually suggest whether uterine activity is hypotonic or hypertonic or whether or not the patient is in false labor. The outcome of a prolonged latent phase is generally favorable for both the mother and fetus, provided no other abnormalities of labor subsequently occur.

Management

The management of a prolonged latent phase depends on the cause. A prolonged latent phase caused by premature or excessive use of sedation or analgesia usually resolves spontaneously after the effects of the medication have disappeared. Hypertonic activity responds erratically to oxytocin but will

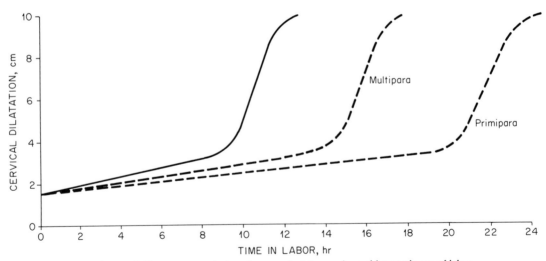

Figure 21–2 Normal cervical dilatation curve (——) and curves depicting prolonged latent phases of labor (---) for multiparous and primiparous patients. (Modified with permission from Friedman EA: Labor: Clinical Evaluation and Management. 2nd ed. New York, Appleton-Century-Crofts, 1978, p 65.)

usually respond to a therapeutic rest with morphine sulfate or an equivalent drug. Hypocontractile dysfunction usually responds well to an intravenous oxytocin infusion. One technique that has been recommended for stimulation of labor involves the addition of 10 units of oxytocin to 1000 ml of intravenous solution for a final concentration of 10 mU of oxytocin to each 1 ml of solution. An infusion of this solution is begun at a rate of between 0.5 to 1.0 mU per minute and is increased at approximately 50 percent increments every 20 to 30 minutes until uterine contractions of the desired frequency and intensity are obtained.

Although for many years clinicians have considered artificial rupture of the membranes an effective method for management of a prolonged latent phase, this approach continues to be controversial. Additionally, this procedure, when undertaken during the latent phase of labor, carries with it the additional risk of intrauterine infection if it does not result in improvement in the labor pattern.

ABNORMALITIES OF THE ACTIVE PHASE OF LABOR

When the cervix reaches a dilatation of approximately 3 to 4 cm, the rate of dilatation progresses more rapidly. Cervical dilatation of less than 1.2 cm per hour in nulliparas and 1.5 cm in multiparas constitutes a *protraction disorder of the active phase of labor*. During the latter part of the active phase, the fetal presenting part also descends more rapidly through the pelvis and continues to descend through the second stage of labor. A rate of descent of the presenting part of less than 1.0 cm per hour in nulliparas and 2.0 cm per hour in multiparas is considered to be a *protraction disorder of descent* (Fig. 21–3). If a period of two hours or more elapses during the active phase of labor without progress in cervical dilatation, an *arrest of dilatation* has occurred; a period of more than one hour without a change in station of the fetal presenting part is defined as an *arrest of descent* (Fig. 21–4).

The appearance of a protraction or an arrest disorder of dilatation or descent during the active phase of labor calls for a careful appraisal of the patient, as either disorder may signal cephalopelvic disproportion or an abnormality of fetal position. In the absence of cephalopelvic disproportion or fetal malposition, protraction or arrest disorders are usually caused by hypotonic uterine contractions, conduction anesthesia, or excessive sedation. With either disorder, the maternal pelvis should be evaluated, although whether or not x-ray pelvimetry is appropriate for this evaluation is controversial and will be discussed later in the section of this chapter on "Dystocia Caused by Maternal Pelvic Abnormalities."

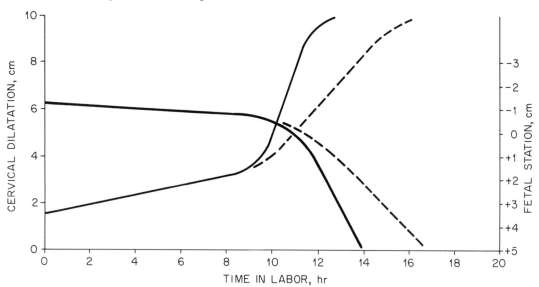

Figure 21–3 Normal dilatation and descent curves of labor (——) and curves depicting protracted dilatation and descent abnormalities of labor (---). (Modified with permission from Friedman EA: Labor: Clinical Evaluation and Management. 2nd ed. New York, Appleton-Century-Crofts, 1978, p 65.)

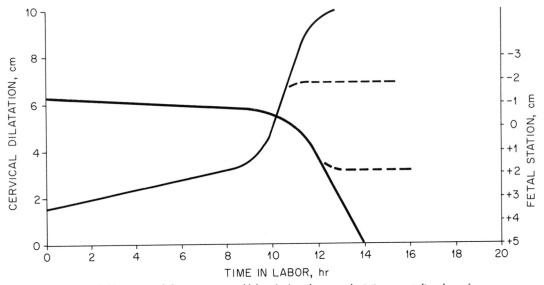

Figure 21–4 Normal dilatation and descent curves of labor (—) and curves depicting arrest disorders of dilatation and descent (---). (Modified with permission from Friedman EA: Labor: Clinical Evaluation and Management. 2nd ed. New York, Appleton-Century-Crofts, 1978, p 66.)

Management

Protraction disorders do *not* respond to oxytocic stimulation, therapeutic rest, or artificial rupture of the membranes. Patients with this disorder should be treated expectantly so long as the fetal heart rate remains satisfactory and labor continues to be progressive. A large percentage of patients with *arrest disorders* unrelated to cephalopelvic disproportion or fetal malposition *do* respond to oxytocic stimulation. If these disorders are related to oversedation, normal labor patterns will resume if the effect of the drug is allowed to wear off.

Dystocia Caused by Abnormal Presentation and Position

Presentations other than vertex and positions other than occipitoanterior are considered to be abnormal in the laboring patient. Disorders of the dilatation and descent phases of labor occur with increased frequency in cases of abnormal presentation or position because of the altered relationship between the presenting part of the fetus and the maternal pelvis. Fetal malpresentations are discussed further in Chapter 18.

Breech Presentation. The average rate of dilatation and descent for frank, complete, and footling breeches does not differ significantly from the average labor curves for a vertex presentation in either nulliparous or multiparous patients. However, patients with a breech presentation experience a greater likelihood of dysfunctional labor than do those with a vertex presentation, most frequently due to the presence of a large fetus.

As previously noted (see Chapter 18), fetuses in a breech presentation estimated to weigh less than 1500 gm or more than 3600 gm are usually delivered by elective cesarean section to reduce the incidence of neonatal morbidity and mortality due to traumatic delivery. The management of patients allowed to labor with a breech presentation who subsequently develop a dysfunctional labor pattern is controversial. If the maternal pelvis is of normal size and configuration on the basis of x-ray pelvimetry, the question of the use of oxytocin arises on the assumption that the abnormal labor is the result of hypotonic uterine activity. Since there is an increase in fetal mortality when oxytocin is used to stimulate dysfunctional labor with a breech presentation, the presence of inadequate contractions may be confirmed with an intrauterine pressure catheter before initiating augmentation of labor. Even though the maternal pelvic measurements may be normal on x-ray pelvimetry, an arrest disorder may indicate fetopelvic disproportion due to the presence of a macrosomic infant whose weight has been underestimated.

Face Presentation. Face presentation occurs when complete deflexion of the fetal head occurs, resulting in substitution of the submentobregmatic diameter for the suboccipitobregmatic diameter as the largest portion of the head presenting to the maternal pelvis. However, since these two diameters are approximately the same length (9.5 cm), progress in early labor for a face presentation is not significantly different from a vertex presentation, provided there is no pelvic contraction. If the mentum is posterior, vaginal delivery of a term-sized fetus is impossible. However, spontaneous rotation of the head to mentum anterior will occur in the majority of cases, but this may require some time to accomplish. Rotation by forceps is not advisable.

Because there is an increased incidence of cephalopelvic disproportion and fetal macrosomia associated with a face presentation, cesarean section, rather than oxytocic stimulation, is the wiser choice in the presence of dysfunctional labor.

Brow Presentation. Brow presentation results from incomplete deflexion of the fetal head with a resulting presentation approximately midway between a vertex and a face. The dilatation phase of labor is usually not significantly different from that for a vertex presentation, but the descent phase is typically prolonged because the brow presentation results in the supraoccipitomental diameter (13.5 cm) presenting to the maternal pelvis. Unless a brow presentation converts spontaneously to a vertex or a face, the head cannot deliver, except when the fetus is unusually small or the pelvis extremely large. It is appropriate to permit a period of observation in the descent phase in the presence of a brow presentation to determine whether or not spontaneous conversion will occur, but a persistent brow should be delivered by cesarean section.

Persistent Occipitotransverse Position. The fetal head normally enters and engages in the maternal pelvis in an occipitotransverse position. It subsequently rotates to an occipitoanterior position or, in a small percentage of cases, to an occipitoposterior position. It is thought that rotation occurs because the head flexes as the leading part of the vertex encounters the pelvic floor and then rotates to accommodate to the shape of the gynecoid pelvis. In a small number of cases, the head fails to flex and rotate and remains in a persistent occipitotransverse position. This position may be caused by cephalopelvic disproportion, altered pelvic architecture, such as in a patient with a platypelloid or android type pelvis, or a relaxed pelvic floor brought about by epidural anesthesia or multiparity.

The diagnosis of a persistent occipitotransverse position may be difficult at times, owing to the obscuring of suture lines and fontanelles by the excessive molding and caput formation that often accompany this abnormal position.

A persistent occipitotransverse position with arrest of descent for a period of one hour or more is known as *transverse arrest*. Arrest occurs because of the deflexion that accompanies the persistent occipitotransverse position, resulting in the larger occipitofrontal diameter (11 cm) becoming the presenting diameter. Until the head undergoes flexion and rotation, further descent cannot take place. Transverse arrest commonly occurs with the vertex at a +2 to +3 station.

The management of transverse arrest at a +2 to +3 station is complex for a number of reasons, among which is the fact that at these stations the widest part of the fetal head is at or above the level of the ischial spines. If the midpelvis is compromised, cesarean section delivery is indicated. If the pelvis is judged to be of normal size, oxytocin stimulation of labor may be appropriate if inadequate uterine contractions are thought to be the cause of the arrest. If the pelvis is of normal size and shape, manual or forceps rotation may be indicated. When the pelvis is of a platypelloid or android type, rotation is not indicated.

Because of the marked degree of molding and caput formation that usually occurs in this position, the bony part of the vertex of the fetal head may be at a +1 station or higher, although the scalp may be visible at the introitus. Thus, what appears to be an uncomplicated low forceps operation may instead become an inadvertent high midforceps procedure. One method for avoiding this mishap involves a clinical evaluation of the relationship between the fetal head and the sacrum. If the fetal head fills the hollow of the sacrum, then the biparietal diameter is usually at or below the spines, and an attempt at forceps delivery is appropriate.

Persistent Occipitoposterior Position. In the majority of cases, the head rotates from occipitotransverse to occipitoanterior in its descent through the maternal pelvis as one of the cardinal movements of labor. Even if the head rotates to an occipitoposterior position, most will eventually rotate spontaneously during labor to occipitoanterior, leaving only a small percentage (5 to 10 percent) of fetuses with a persistent occipitoposterior position.

The course of labor in the presence of a persistent occipitoposterior position is usually normal, except for a tendency for the second stage to be prolonged (greater than two hours) and associated with more discomfort than is usual for the occipitoanterior position. If a normal fetal heart rate is demonstrated by fetal monitoring, observation of a prolonged second stage of labor is appropriate, provided labor continues to be progressive.

Delivery of the head may occur spontaneously in the occipitoposterior position, but if the perineum provides undue resistance to delivery, a forceps-assisted delivery may be required. Forceps rotation of an occipitoposterior to an occipitoanterior position may be performed but should be approached with caution if there is an arrest of descent of the fetal head. As noted in the discussion of the persistent occipitotransverse position, the fetal head may become markedly molded with extensive caput formation, which may cause difficulty in diagnosing its correct station and position. Before performing a forceps rotation, it is important that the pelvis be evaluated, since the size and configuration of the maternal pelvis will influence the outcome of the operation. For instance, an attempt at forceps rotation in the presence of a narrow pelvis would be inadvisable.

Whatever the method chosen for vaginal delivery of the persistent occipitoposterior position, it is important that a wide mediolateral episiotomy be performed to lessen the resistance of the outlet to the delivery of the fetal head.

Dystocia Caused by Abnormalities of Fetal Structure

Macrosomia and Shoulder Dystocia. A fetus weighing 4000 gm or more is above the 90th percentile of fetal weight for term pregnancy and is considered to be of excessive size. Macrosomia may result from genetic determinants, maternal diabetes, multiparity, or post-term gestation. In general, the larger the fetus, the longer the labor and the greater the incidence of midforceps operations and of shoulder dystocia. Also, the more the fetus exceeds 4000 gm, the higher the rate of perinatal mortality and morbidity resulting from shoulder dystocia.

Even with the aid of sonographic techniques for the evaluation of fetal head and body size, an accurate estimate of fetal weight is elusive. Additionally, when the fetus is of excessive size, the occurrence of shoulder dystocia will depend on the size of the maternal pelvis in relationship to the size of the fetus, a clinical correlation that is difficult to make. Although the mean duration of labor is prolonged for excessive-sized fetuses, it is not unusual to encounter unexpected shoulder dystocia after a labor that has been entirely normal up to the moment of delivery.

Since shoulder dystocia may occur unexpectedly, it is necessary to be familiar with methods for dealing with the problem. Shoulder dystocia is not overcome by traction on the fetal head but, instead, by one or more maneuvers designed to displace the anterior shoulder from behind the symphysis pubis. The first maneuver involves downward pressure with the hand over the maternal suprapubic region in an effort to guide the anterior shoulder under the symphysis pubis. If this is not successful, pressure is applied with the operator's fingers against the scapula of the posterior shoulder in an attempt to rotate the posterior shoulder upward until it replaces the anterior shoulder. If this maneuver does not correct the problem, the posterior arm is grasped and pulled across the chest, resulting in delivery of the posterior shoulder and displacement of the anterior shoulder from behind the symphysis pubis. Fracture of the humerus may result from this maneuver, but the bone heals quickly in the neonate. If none of these maneuvers is successful, one or both clavicles are fractured, preferably by pressure on the clavicle directed away from the pleural cavity to prevent traumatic puncture of the lungs. Excessive traction on the head may result in damage to the brachial plexus, with the possibility of a permanent Erb's palsy. However, the maneuvers described above to overcome shoulder dystocia may themselves result in brachial plexus damage.

Developmental Abnormalities. Localized abnormalities of fetal anatomy may lead to dystocia. *Internal hydrocephalus* may cause enlargement of the fetal head to the extent that vaginal delivery is not possible. The diagnosis is usually made by ultrasonography performed because of the clinical suspicion of excessive enlargement of the fetal head, or it may appear as an unexpected finding on an ultrasound performed for other indications.

Several options are available for the delivery of the fetus with hydrocephalus. Excessive cerebrospinal fluid may be removed by inserting a needle directly into the ventricular space through the dilated cervix during labor, or fluid may be removed transabdominally with the aid of ultrasonic visualization of the fetal head prior to or during labor. Alternatively, the fetus may be delivered by cesarean section to avoid the risk of infection, which may result from transvaginal or transabdominal drainage. Intrauterine shunting of the fetal ventricular system into the amniotic fluid compartment is an experimental procedure, and it is unclear at this time whether or not the long-term results justify the procedure.

The accumulation of *ascitic fluid* in the fetal abdomen or *enlargement of fetal organs,* such as the bladder or liver, may result in unexpected dystocia after the fetal head is delivered. Rhesus disease and nonimmune *hydrops* are potential causes of these abnormalities, and, should they be present, careful ultrasonic evaluation before or during labor is indicated to identify excessive enlargement of the fetal abdomen. Ascitic fluid or urine from a massively enlarged bladder may be removed by transabdominal drainage with a needle prior to vaginal delivery. Cesarean section may be indicated if the fetal abdomen cannot be sufficiently decompressed.

A defect in the fetal lumbosacral vertebrae may result in the protrusion of a meningeal sac *(meningocele)* or a sac containing spinal cord *(meningomyelocele)*. These defects are usually detected as a result of abnormal serum or amniotic fluid alpha-fetoprotein values or by ultrasonography. If the sac is large, abdominal delivery is advisable to avoid dystocia or rupture of the sac and potential infection. If the sac is small and covered by fetal skin, as reflected by a normal alpha-fetoprotein value, vaginal delivery is appropriate.

Dystocia Caused by Maternal Pelvic Abnormalities

Cephalopelvic disproportion exists if the maternal bony pelvis is not of sufficient size and of appropriate shape to allow the passage of the fetal head. This problem may occur as a result of contraction of one of the planes of the pelvis. Relative cephalopelvic disproportion may exist if the fetal head is excessively large or if it is in an abnormal position, even though the pelvic measurements are within normal limits. Contraction of the maternal pelvis may occur at the level of the inlet or midpelvis, but contraction of the outlet is extremely unusual unless it is found in association with a midpelvic contraction. Normal and abnormal pelvic architecture are discussed in Chapter 9.

Cephalopelvic disproportion at the level of the pelvic inlet causes a failure of descent of the head, and engagement will not occur. The finding of an unengaged head in a nulliparous patient at the start of labor indicates an increased likelihood of cephalopelvic disproportion at the pelvic inlet, but an unengaged fetal head in a multiparous patient in labor is not an unusual occurrence. However, relative cephalopelvic disproportion can occur in the multiparous patient and should be kept in mind.

The management of a nulliparous patient with an unengaged fetal head in labor should begin with a careful clinical evaluation of the maternal pelvis. If the capacity of the inlet is normal, expectant management with observation of the labor pattern is appropriate. If uterine contractions are ineffective, oxytocic stimulation of labor may be considered.

The occurrence of cephalopelvic disproportion at the level of the midpelvis occurs more frequently than inlet dystocia because the capacity of the midpelvis is smaller than that of the inlet and also because deflection or positional abnormalities of the fetal head resulting in dystocia are more likely to occur at that level. As noted previously in this chapter, the occurrence of bony dystocia at the level of the midpelvis is usually indicated by an arrest of descent of the head at a +2 to +3 station. It has also been noted that with cephalopelvic disproportion and arrest of descent, application of the head to the cervix is poor, resulting in the loss of part of the force needed for cervical distention. Thus, cephalopelvic disproportion may be associated with an abnormal rate of cervical dilatation before an arrest of descent is apparent.

X-ray Pelvimetry. When the question of cephalopelvic disproportion arises, the use of x-ray pelvimetry as a tool for the evaluation of the maternal bony pelvis is controversial. Those opposed to this procedure indicate that the information obtained does not accurately predict which patients will require abdominal delivery because progress in labor with or without oxytocic stimulation is more useful in determining the route of delivery. The opponents also cite the potential hazards that may be associated with radiation exposure of the fetus.

Those favoring the use of x-ray pelvimetry point out that the procedure should be confined to a small group of patients with arrest of descent in whom clinical pelvimetry suggests disproportion and in whom a midpelvic operation is under consideration. They believe that the information obtained will not only provide a precise evaluation of pelvic capacity and architecture, especially the mid-pelvis, but will also indicate the true level of the vertex and allow diagnosis of any deflexion or positional abnormalities of the fetal head. Based upon this information, an ill-advised attempt at midforceps delivery may be avoided. The proponents also indicate that the radiation hazards associated with pelvimetry are more theoretical than real.

SUGGESTED READING

Benedetti TJ, Gatbe SG: Shoulder dystocia: A complication of fetal macrosomia and prolonged second stage of labor with midpelvic delivery. Obstet Gynecol 52:526, 1978.

Brenner WE, Bruce RD, Hendricks CH: The characteristics and perils of breech presentation. Am J Obstet Gynecol 118:700, 1978.

Friedman EA: Labor: Clinical Evaluation and Management. 2nd ed. New York, Appleton-Century-Crofts, 1978.

Laube DW, Varner MW, Cruikshank DP: A prospective evaluation of x-ray pelvimetry. JAMA 246:2187, 1981.

Pritchard JA, MacDonald PC, Gant NF (eds): Williams Obstetrics. 17th ed. Norwalk, CT, Appleton-Century-Crofts, 1985, p 641.

PRETERM LABOR AND PREMATURE RUPTURE OF MEMBRANES

ANNE D. M. GRAHAM

PRETERM LABOR

Preterm labor and delivery are a major cause of perinatal morbidity and mortality. Although less than 10 percent of all infants born in the United States are preterm, their contribution to neonatal morbidity and mortality ranges from 50 to 70 percent. To decrease the medical and economic impact of preterm delivery, a major goal of obstetric care is not only to reduce the incidence of preterm deliveries but also to increase the gestational age of those infants whose preterm births are unavoidable.

Definition and Incidence

Preterm birth is defined as that occurring after 20 weeks and before 37 completed weeks of gestation. Labor occurring between these gestational ages is defined as preterm labor. In older literature, a weight based criterion was used, preterm birth being defined as birth of an infant weighing less than 2500 gm. The advantage of such a parameter is that it is absolute and easily obtained, while determination of gestational age is less precise. However, since birth weight depends not only on the length of gestation but also correlates with other characteristics of the mother and fetus that govern fetal growth, a weight-based criterion does not differentiate between those infants that are merely small

for gestational age and those that are truly preterm.

The true incidence of preterm deliveries is difficult to delineate because of the errors of gestational age assessment and the use of birth weight to define preterm birth in most studies. Although dependent on the population studied, the preterm delivery incidence averages about 7 percent, but varies from a low of 5 percent in some parts of western Europe to a reported 34 percent in India.

Etiology and Risk Factors

The etiologic factors for preterm delivery are outlined in Table 22–1. In most cases, the cause is unknown. A variety of socioeconomic, psychosocial, and medical conditions

TABLE 22–1 ETIOLOGY OF PRETERM LABOR AND DELIVERY

ETIOLOGY	PERCENT OF PRE-TERM LABOR
A. Idiopathic	50
B. Multiple gestation	10–15
C. Medical indications for induction	5–20
D. Uterine anomalies	5–15
E. Miscellaneous (infection polyhydramnios, incompetent cervix)	5

have been found to carry an increased risk of delivering preterm.

Socioeconomic Factors. A higher incidence of preterm births among patients of low socioeconomic status is seen in a number of countries. In the United States, the incidence of preterm deliveries in the black population is twice as high as that in the white population. This factor cannot be viewed as a single entity but probably encompasses other characteristics of the population, such as access to and procurement of antenatal care and information. Other risk factors are shown in Table 6–5.

Medical and Obstetric Factors. When one preterm birth has occurred, the relative risk of preterm delivery in the next pregnancy is 3.9; the risk increases to 6.5 with two previous preterm deliveries. If only one of two previous deliveries was preterm, the relative risk for a subsequent preterm delivery is increased approximately twofold and is greater if the preterm delivery occurred in the second rather than the first pregnancy (2.5 versus 1.3).

Second trimester abortions seem to carry an increased risk for subsequent preterm delivery, especially if a previous preterm birth has also occurred. The risk associated with induced first trimester abortions is controversial. Repeated spontaneous first trimester abortions, however, do increase the risk.

Certain preterm births are unavoidable because of the need for medical intervention for maternal or fetal indications, such as severe pre-eclampsia or uncontrolled third trimester bleeding associated with placenta previa or abruptio placentae. Iatrogenic preterm birth remains a problem because of elective induction of labor or cesarean section in a preterm pregnancy thought to be at term because of incorrect dating. This should decline with physician education and the recent trend toward trial of labor for patients who have had a previous cesarean section.

Other medical and obstetric factors associated with an increased risk of delivering preterm include bleeding in the first trimester, urinary tract infections, multiple gestation, uterine anomalies, polyhydramnios, and incompetent cervix.

Prevention

Steps can be taken to decrease the medical and economic impact of preterm labor and delivery, and these are discussed in Chapter 6.

Diagnosis

The diagnosis of preterm labor should be based on the presence of regular uterine contractions in a preterm gestation associated with the cervical changes of either dilatation or effacement.

Management

The diagnosis of preterm labor necessitates a number of management decisions, such as the appropriateness of labor suppression, the use of glucocorticoids to induce pulmonary maturation, and the optimal conduct of the labor and delivery.

Provided the membranes are not ruptured, an initial cervical examination must be done to ascertain cervical length and dilatation and the station and nature of the presenting part. The patient should be evaluated for the presence of any underlying correctable problem, such as a urinary tract infection. She should be placed in the lateral decubitus position, monitored for the presence and frequency of uterine activity, and re-examined for evidence of cervical change after an appropriate interval. During the period of observation, either oral or parenteral hydration should be carried out.

Once the diagnosis of preterm labor has been made, the following laboratory tests should be obtained: a complete blood count, random blood sugar, serum electrolytes, urinalysis, and urine culture and sensitivity. An ultrasonic examination of the fetus should be performed, especially in a patient who has had no antenatal care and has uncertain dates, in order to document gestational age and to obtain parameters for estimation of fetal weight. In addition, this test may detect the presence of underlying etiologic factors, including twins or uterine anomalies. The increased incidence of congenital malformation in preterm neonates should be kept in mind when performing the ultrasound.

If the patient does not respond to bedrest and hydration, tocolytic therapy is instituted, provided there are no contraindications. Measures implemented at 28 weeks should be more aggressive than those performed at 35 weeks. Similarly, a patient with advanced cervical dilatation requires more aggressive management than one whose cervix is closed and minimally effaced.

Uterine Tocolytic Therapy. The events leading to the initiation of labor are discussed

TABLE 22–2 UTERINE TOCOLYTIC AGENTS

DRUG	DOSAGE

Ritodrine Hydrochloride (Yutopar)	Solution: 150 mg ritodrine in 500 ml 5% dextrose (0.3 mg/ml); IV piggyback
	Parenteral:
	  Initial dose: 0.05–0.1 mg/min
	  Titrating dose: Increase by 0.05 mg q 10 min until contractions cease or unacceptable side effects occur; maximum dose is 0.35 mg/min or maternal pulse of 140 beats/min
	  Maintenance dose: 6 hours at maximum dose
	Oral: 10 mg 1/2 hour prior to discontinuing infusion. 10–20 mg q 2–4 hours; titrate dose and frequency to maintain maternal pulse of > 100

Terbutaline Sulfate (Brethine, Bricanyl)	Solution: 5 mg in 500 ml Ringer's lactate (10 μg/ml)
	Parenteral:
	  Initial dose: 10 μg/min IV piggyback or 0.25 mg SQ
	  Titrating dose: For infusion, increase by 10 μg/min q 20 min or SQ 0.25 mg q 3–6 hours until contractions cease, pulse rate becomes 120–140, or intolerable side effects occur
	  Maintenance dose: One hour at maximum dose with no contractions, then discontinue
	Oral: 2.5–5.0 mg q 4–6 hours; titrate frequency to pulse; begin 1/2 hour prior to discontinuing parenteral therapy

Magnesium Sulfate	Solution: Initial solution contains 6 gm (12 ml of 50% MgSO$_4$) in 100 cc 5% dextrose; maintenance solution contains 10 gm (20 cc of 50% MgSO$_4$) in 500 cc 5% dextrose Initial dose: 6 gm over 15–20 min Titrating dose: 2 gm/hour until contractions cease; follow serum levels (5–7 mg/dl) Maintenance dose: 1 gm/hour for 24–72 hours; may switch to oral β-agonist therapy before discontinuing

in Chapter 45. In the development of tocolytic agents, a number of possible mechanisms can be targeted to be blocked, controlled, or reversed. The pharmacologic agents presently being used all seem to inhibit the availability of calcium ions, but they may also exert a number of other effects. The agents currently utilized and their dosage are presented in Table 22–2.

BETA-ADRENERGIC AGONISTS. Uterine muscle has both α- and β$_2$-adrenergic receptors. Alpha-adrenergic stimulation causes contractions, while stimulation of the β$_2$ receptors initiates myometrial relaxation.

Beta-sympathomimetic agents act by increasing the conversion of adenosine triphosphate (ATP) to cyclic adenosine monophosphate (cAMP). An increase of cAMP within the cell decreases the availability of free calcium ions by increasing their intracellular binding.

Although the β-adrenergic agents are structurally similar to the catecholamines, they are not methylated as readily and thus do not undergo first pass hepatic degradation,

allowing therapeutic levels to be reached with oral administration. They are eliminated by renal excretion, mostly in an unchanged form, although some conjugation occurs.

Parenteral administration achieves quicker therapeutic levels. The drug can be titrated to a dose where uterine contractions cease, maternal pulse reaches 120 to 140 beats per minute, or side effects are poorly tolerated. Dosage is maintained at this level for 6 to 12 hours before weaning to oral therapy 30 minutes before the drug is discontinued. Strict attention must be paid to fluid balance in all patients, and blood glucose and serum potassium levels should be monitored in patients with diabetes or heart disease.

Ritodrine is presently the only agent approved by the Federal Food and Drug Administration (FDA) for the treatment of preterm labor, although clinical trials for another β-agonist, hexoprenaline, are under way. *Terbutaline* and *isoxsuprine* have also been widely used in the United States. In Europe, salbutamol and orciprenaline have been tried. Terbutaline is used similarly to ritodrine. As with all β-agonists, the maternal pulse rate can be used as a guide to effective dosage.

After successful tocolysis, oral therapy is maintained until 36 weeks' gestation. Patients who have preterm labor secondary to a treatable and reversible cause probably do not require continuous therapy.

Although the β-adrenergic tocolytic agents are selected for their β$_2$ specificity, they still possess some β$_1$ activity. The presence of β receptors in a number of organs results in a variety of *side effects*. Cardiovascular side effects are the most common and include an increase in heart rate, a rise in systolic pressure, and a decrease in diastolic pressure. Usually, mean arterial pressure remains the same, but the peripheral vasodilatation produced may cause profound hypotension in some patients. About 1 to 2 percent of patients have chest pain secondary to myocardial ischemia, sometimes associated with arrhythmias or electrocardiographic (EKG) changes.

A rare, more serious side effect is the development of pulmonary edema. A number of factors, both cardiogenic and noncardiogenic, may be involved. Prolonged maternal tachycardia, fluid retention secondary to decreased free water clearance, and increased myocardial work may contribute to cardiac failure. In addition, iatrogenic fluid overload contributes in some cases. Concurrent administration of glucocorticoids for pulmonary maturation may be a risk factor for the development of pulmonary edema.

Beta-adrenergic stimulation causes increased liver and muscle glycogenolysis, resulting in an elevation of plasma glucose, and from muscle, increased lactic acid production. All patients treated with β-sympathomimetic agents are at risk for the development of hyperglycemia, but in a few reported cases, diabetic patients treated with these drugs have developed frank ketoacidosis. Circulating insulin rises secondary to the hyperglycemia, but a direct effect on pancreatic β-adrenergic receptors contributes to the increase. Insulin drives potassium into the cells with resultant hypokalemia. Urinary excretion of potassium remains unchanged, indicating that total body potassium is adequate. Potassium replacement is not needed in otherwise healthy patients, since no adverse effects have been noted, even at levels as low as 2.3 mEq/dl. After several hours of drug administration, serum abnormalities tend to return to normal and are completely reversed by 24 hours.

Placental transfer of β-adrenergic agents does occur, but fetal effects, such as tachycardia, are delayed. At birth, fetal levels are the same or lower than those of maternal plasma. Hypo- and hyperglycemia have been observed in infants born to mothers treated with β-adrenergic agonists.

MAGNESIUM. Parenteral administration of magnesium can be used in the therapy of preterm labor and may be the drug of choice for patients with diabetes mellitus or heart disease. It is thought that magnesium acts at the cellular level by competing with calcium for entry into the cell at the time of depolarization. Successful competition results in an effective decrease of intracellular calcium ions and myometrial relaxation.

Magnesium levels needed for tocolysis are 5 to 7 mg/dl. These can be achieved using the dosage regimen outlined in Table 22–2. After the loading dose is given, a continuous infusion is maintained, and plasma levels should be determined until therapeutic levels are reached. The drug should be continued at therapeutic levels until contractions cease. Since magnesium is excreted by the kidneys, adjustments must be made in those patients with underlying renal disease and an abnormal creatinine clearance. The role of oral magnesium therapy in patients successfully tocolyzed is questionable, and these patients may be switched to an oral β-adrenergic agonist, as this carries less side effects.

A common minor *side effect* of magnesium therapy is a feeling of warmth and flushing upon first administration. Respiratory depression is seen at magnesium levels of 12 to 15 mg/dl, and cardiac conduction defects and arrest are seen at higher levels.

In the fetus, plasma magnesium levels approach those of the mother, and a low plasma calcium may also be demonstrated. The neonate may show some loss of muscle tone and drowsiness resulting in a lower Apgar score. These effects are prolonged in the preterm neonate.

PROSTAGLANDIN SYNTHETASE INHIBITORS. Prostaglandins induce myometrial contractions at all stages of gestation, both *in vivo* and *in vitro*. Because prostaglandins are locally synthesized and possess a relatively short half-life, prevention of their synthesis within the uterus could abort labor. Agents that inhibit prostaglandin synthetase may play a role in the treatment of preterm labor.

Prostaglandin synthetase inhibitors used for treatment of preterm labor include indomethacin (Indocin), aspirin, and flufenamic acid. Indomethacin is the most commonly used and can be administered both orally and rectally with some slight delay in absorption from rectal administration as compared to the oral route. Peak serum levels of indomethacin occur 1.5 to 2 hours after oral administration. Excretion of the intact drug occurs in maternal urine.

Transplacental transfer of the drug to the fetus occurs, and fetal levels approach those of the mother. In addition, about 90 percent of the drug is protein bound in the neonate, which contributes to its prolonged half-life of 15 to 20 hours. An even longer half-life occurs in the preterm infant.

The *side effects* of these agents are related to their effect on the prostaglandin synthetase enzymes in other organ systems. Prostaglandins are important regulators of platelet aggregation, and inhibition of prostaglandin synthetase results in platelet dysfunction. Indomethacin induces a reversible effect that disappears when the drug is eliminated, but the dysfunction induced by aspirin is effective for the life of the platelet. Increased bleeding occurs during delivery and the postpartum period, especially in cases where the drug is chronically administered. In addition, gastric irritation may occur.

During *in utero* existence, the pulmonary circulation is largely bypassed by the ductus arteriosus, which shunts 55 percent of ventricular output to the descending aorta. Major changes in circulatory dynamics occur at the time of birth, during which conversion to a neonatal circulation results in closure of the ductus arteriosus, mediated in part by the high oxygen concentration and alterations in prostaglandin synthesis. It is thought that patency of the ductus during fetal life is maintained by local secretion of prostaglandins, and inhibition of synthesis will result in partial or complete closure of the ductus. Although closure is compatible with *in utero* existence, the resulting increase in blood flow to the pulmonary vasculature may induce hypertrophic changes in the smooth muscle of the pulmonary vessels that subsequently lead to the development of pulmonary hypertension in the neonate with all its coexistent cardiac and respiratory problems.

CALCIUM CHANNEL ANTAGONISTS. Calcium seems to play a pivotal role in the physiology of uterine contractions and the possibility exists of utilizing the calcium channel blockers, such as nifedipine, to abolish uterine contractions. However, these agents are currently under investigation and are not yet used for the management of preterm labor.

EFFICACY OF TOCOLYTIC THERAPY. Although the advent of tocolytic agents has failed to decrease the preterm incidence in large population studies, their use has shifted the distribution of births by gestational age to more prolonged gestations. There has also been an improvement in neonatal survival, a decreased incidence of respiratory distress syndrome (RDS), and an increase in the birth weight of infants treated with these agents. Benefits do not accrue to infants greater than 33 weeks. All the β-sympathomimetic agents have similar efficacy and delay delivery for more than 72 hours in about 80 percent of patients treated.

Magnesium is as effective as ritodrine. The prostaglandin synthetase inhibitors delay delivery in 80 to 90 percent of patients for the 24 hours of treatment.

CONTRAINDICATIONS TO TOCOLYTIC THERAPY. These include severe pre-eclampsia, severe bleeding from placenta previa or abruptio placentae, chorioamnionitis, intrauterine growth retardation, fetal anomalies incompatible with life, and fetal demise. Because of the low success rate, advanced cervical dilatation may also preclude tocolytic therapy, although therapy may delay delivery sufficiently for glucocorticoid administration to accelerate fetal lung maturity.

Use of Corticosteroids. Glucocorticoid administration to the mother at less than 33 weeks' gestation will enhance pulmonary maturation and decrease the incidence of RDS. The benefits derived seem to depend on a number of factors, including fetal sex (female infants benefit more than male infants) and ethnic group (black infants benefit more than white infants). Two glucocorticoids are commonly used to enhance pulmonary maturation—betamethasone, 10 mg, and dexamethasone, 5 mg. Each is given every 24 hours for two doses. Advancement of maturation is seen only if more than 24 hours and less than seven days have elapsed since the onset of therapy. Only about 10 percent of patients in preterm labor qualify for treatment.

Labor and Delivery of the Preterm Infant

A certain number of patients will not respond to tocolytic therapy and will proceed to advanced labor and delivery of a preterm neonate. The goal in these patients is to conduct both labor and delivery in an optimal manner so as not to contribute to the morbidity or mortality of the preterm infant. All parameters for assessing gestational age and fetal weight must be considered in arriving at the best estimate of these parameters. With modern neonatal care, the lower limit of potential viability is 26 weeks or 600 gm.

Fetal heart rate patterns that are relatively innocuous in the term fetus may indicate a more ominous outcome for the preterm fetus. Continuous fetal heart monitoring and prompt attention to abnormal fetal heart rate patterns are extremely important. Acidosis at birth will adversely affect respiratory function by destroying surfactant and delaying its release.

Drugs administered to the mother usually pass to the fetus, and in the preterm fetus, hepatic enzyme degradation and renal excretion are immature, thereby resulting in a more prolonged drug effect.

If the fetus is presenting as a vertex, vaginal delivery is preferred, independent of gestational age, provided fetal acidosis and delivery trauma are avoided. Use of outlet forceps and a large episiotomy to shorten the second stage are advocated.

Approximately 23 percent of infants present as a breech at 28 weeks, compared with about 4 percent at term. This presentation carries an increased risk of cord prolapse or compression. In addition, cervical entrapment of the aftercoming fetal head may occur at delivery because prior to term, the head is proportionally larger than the buttocks. For the breech fetus estimated at less than 1500 gm, neonatal outcome is improved by cesarean section.

PREMATURE RUPTURE OF THE MEMBRANES

Definition and Incidence

Premature rupture of the membranes (PROM) is defined as amniorrhexis prior to the onset of labor at any stage of gestation. It has been suggested that the term "preterm premature rupture of the membranes" (PPRM) should be used to define those patients who are preterm with ruptured membranes, whether or not they have contractions.

Etiology and Risk Factors

The etiology of PROM remains unclear, but a variety of factors are purported to contribute to its occurrence, including vaginal and cervical infections, abnormal membane physiology, incompetent cervix, and nutritional deficiencies of copper or ascorbic acid (Vitamin C). The mechanisms by which these may act are as yet unexplained.

Diagnosis

Diagnosis of PROM is based on the history of vaginal loss of fluid and confirmation of amniotic fluid in the vagina. Episodic urinary incontinence, leukorrhea, or loss of the mucous plug must be ruled out. The patient presenting with this history should have a sterile vaginal speculum examination to confirm the diagnosis, to assess cervical dilatation and length, and to obtain cervical cultures and amniotic fluid samples for pulmonary maturation tests. In the preterm pregnancy, no digital examination should be performed because of the risk of introducing infection.

On examination, pooling of amniotic fluid in the posterior vaginal fornix can usually be seen. A Valsalva maneuver or slight fundal pressure may expel fluid from the cervical os, which is diagnostic of PROM. Confirmation of the diagnosis can be made by (1) testing the fluid with nitrazine paper, which will turn blue in the presence of the alkaline amniotic fluid; and (2) placing a sample on a microscopic slide, air drying, and examining for ferning. False-positive nitrazine tests occur in the presence of alkaline urine, blood, or cervical mucus. As in the case of preterm labor with intact membranes, a complete ultrasonic examination should be carried out to rule out fetal anomalies and to assess gestational age and amniotic fluid volume.

Management

General Considerations. An intact amniotic sac serves as a mechanical barrier to infection, but in addition, amniotic fluid has some bacteriostatic properties that may play a role in preventing chorioamnionitis and fetal infections. Intact membranes are not an absolute barrier to infection, since bacterial colonization occurs in 10 percent of patients in term labor with intact membranes and in up to 25 percent of patients in preterm labor.

For preterm fetuses with PPRM, the risks associated with preterm delivery must be balanced against the risks of infection and sepsis that may make *in utero* existence even more problematic. For the mother, the risks are not only the development of chorioamnionitis, but also the possibility of failed induction in the presence of an unfavorable cervix and subsequent cesarean section.

Oligohydramnios associated with PPRM in the fetus at less than 26 weeks' gestation may lead to the development of pulmonary hypoplasia. In addition, the constraints placed on fetal movements *in utero* can result in a variety of positional skeletal abnormalities, such as talipes equinovarus, although this depends on the duration of ruptured membranes.

If PROM occurs at 36 weeks or later and the cervix is favorable, labor should be induced after four to six hours if no spontaneous contractions occur. In the presence of an unfavorable cervix, it is reasonable to wait 24 hours prior to induction of labor in order to decrease the risk of failed induction and maternal febrile morbidity. The following discussion applies when premature membrane rupture occurs prior to 36 weeks' gestational age.

Laboratory Tests. In addition to those obtained for the patient in preterm labor, tests should include cervical cultures for both group B *Streptococcus* and *Neisseria gonorrhoeae*. Sufficient amniotic fluid can usually be obtained from the vaginal pool for pulmonary maturation studies.

Conservative Expectant Management. This is the term applied to the care of those patients with PPRM who are observed with the expectation of prolonging gestation. Since the risk of infection appears to increase with the duration of membrane rupture, the goal of expectant management is to continue the pregnancy until the lung profile is mature (see Tests of Pulmonary Maturity). Careful surveillance must be maintained in order to diagnose chorioamnionitis at an early enough stage to minimize fetal and maternal risks. In its fulminant state, chorioamnionitis is associated with a high maternal temperature and a tender, sometimes irritable uterus. However, in cases of subclinical infection, diagnosis and treatment may be delayed. A combination of factors should alert the clinician to the possibility of chorioamnionitis, including maternal temperature greater than 100.4°F (38°C) in the absence of any other site of infection, fetal tachycardia, and uterine irritability on nonstress testing.

The presence of bacteria by Gram stain or culture of amniotic fluid obtained at amniocentesis correlates with subsequent maternal infection in about 50 percent of cases and neonatal sepsis in about 25 percent of cases. However, the presence of white blood cells alone in amniotic fluid is unreliable in predicting infection. The decision to perform amniocentesis is based upon the gestational age, the presence of early signs of infection, and the amount of fluid as seen by real-time ultrasound.

Antibiotics should not be used routinely as prophylactic therapy for PROM. They serve to mask maternal infection and may cause the development of resistant organisms. However, if group B streptococci are cultured from the cervix, penicillin G should be given in an attempt to eradicate the organism and lessen the chance of ascending infection, since this is associated with a high fetal mortality rate.

Management of Chorioamnionitis. Once chorioamnionitis is diagnosed, antibiotic therapy should be delayed only until appropriate cultures are taken. Ampicillin is the drug of choice. It is given either alone or in combination with an aminoglycoside, depending on the severity of infection. Good results have also been obtained with third generation cephalosporins. Once antibiotics have been started, labor should be induced. An important indication for immediate abdominal delivery is the presence of active genital herpes in the presence of ruptured membranes.

Tocolytic Therapy. The use of tocolytics to control preterm labor in these patients is controversial. They may mask evidence of maternal infection, such as tachycardia, and contractions associated with PPRM may be indicative of uterine infection. However, preterm labor associated with chorioamnionitis is generally not successfully tocolyzed.

Use of Corticosteroids. There is a decreased incidence of respiratory distress syndrome (RDS) in infants who are born after 16 to 48 hours of ruptured membranes when compared with infants of similar gestational age born without PPRM. Use of corticosteroids is, therefore, not necessary, and the incidence of infection in mothers thus treated is increased.

Outpatient Management. After inpatient observation for a few days without evidence of infection, outpatient management can be considered. The patient so managed should be reliable, fully informed regarding the risks involved, and prepared to participate in her own care. The fetus should be presenting as a vertex, and the cervix should be closed to minimize the chance of cord prolapse. At home, no coital activity should occur, and the patient must monitor her temperature at least four times per day. Instructions should be given to return immediately if the temperature exceeds 100°F (37.8°C).

The patient should be seen weekly, at which time her temperature is taken, nonstress testing is done, and the baseline fetal heart rate is evaluated. Ultrasonic evaluation of fetal growth and amniotic fluid volume should also be done every two weeks.

Labor and Delivery. The same considerations discussed under preterm labor apply to patients with PPRM. The decrease in amniotic fluid that is sometimes seen can result in cord compression and the presence of variable fetal heart decelerations.

TESTS OF PULMONARY MATURITY

By far, the major determinant of successful *ex utero* existence is the ability of the neonate to maintain successful oxygenation. Pulmonary maturation involves changes in pulmonary anatomy in addition to alterations of physiologic and biochemical parameters. Stages of anatomic pulmonary development include (1) an embryonic phase from three to six weeks; (2) a pseudoglandular phase from seven to 17 weeks; (3) a canalicular phase from 18 to 24 weeks, during which capillary plexuses develop around the terminal bronchioles; and (4) the terminal sac phase that occurs at about 24 weeks, during which terminal bronchioles divide into three or four respiratory bronchioles. Type II pneumocytes, important in surfactant synthesis, begin to proliferate during this phase.

Surfactant is required for successful lung function. It is a complex mixture of phospholipids, neutral lipids, proteins, carbohydrates, and salts that is important in decreasing alveolar surface tension, maintaining alveoli open at a low internal alveolar diameter, and decreasing intra-alveolar lung fluid. Synthesis takes place in the type II pneumocytes by incorporation of choline, and there appears to be significant recycling by resorption and secretion.

Initially, the important phospholipid was felt to be phosphatidylcholine (lecithin), but it is apparent that other components, such as phosphatidylinositol (PI) and phosphatidylglycerol (PG), are also important. These substances are produced and secreted in increasing amounts as gestation advances, and the continued egress of tracheal fluid into the amniotic fluid results in their increasing presence near term.

Measurement of these substances in the amniotic fluid obtained by amniocentesis allows prediction of the risk of development of RDS in the neonate. Lecithin levels increase rapidly after 35 weeks' gestation, while sphingomyelin levels remain relatively constant after this gestational age. The lecithin and sphingomyelin concentrations are measured by thin layer or high pressure liquid chromatography and are expressed as the L/S ratio. The presence of blood or meconium in the amniotic fluid will affect the L/S ratio, meconium decreasing it and blood normalizing it to a value of 1.4.

About 2 percent of infants with ratios equal to or greater than 2 develop RDS, compared with 60 percent of infants with ratios less than 2. There is, therefore, a high false-negative rate associated with this test, and in the diabetic patient, a mature L/S ratio is not so reassuring.

The Lung Profile

Using two-dimensional, thin-layer chromatography, both PG and PI can be measured. Along with the L/S ratio, these make up the lung profile. RDS is rare when the L/S ratio is greater than 2 and PG is present, while when the L/S ratio is less than 2 and no PG is present, over 90 percent of infants develop RDS. If the L/S ratio is immature but PG is present, less than 5 percent of infants will develop RDS. The lung profile offers a more reliable predictor of pulmonary maturity, especially in infants of diabetic mothers. Other advantages of using PG are that contamination with vaginal secretions or blood, as occurs in cases of ruptured membranes and vaginal pool sampling, does not interfere with the detection of PG.

The *foam stability test* provides an estimate of the surface-tension lowering capacity of amniotic fluid. Ninety-five percent ethanol is added to amniotic fluid in order to decrease the contribution to bubble formation of other surface-acting components, such as protein and bilirubin. The presence of bubbles is associated with less than a 1 percent incidence of RDS. The *Foam Stability Index* (Beckman) is a commercially available test. In general, it is rapid, and if carried out according to specific directions, it can be used as the first test to assess lung maturity. Its false-positive and negative rates are higher than the L/S ratio and PG determinations.

SUGGESTED READING

Benedetti TJ: Maternal complications of parenteral β-sympathomimetic therapy for premature labor. Am J Obstet Gynecol 145:1, 1983.

Depp R, Boehm JJ, Nosek JA, et al: Antenatal corticosteroids to prevent neonatal respiratory distress syndrome: Risk versus benefit considerations. Am J Obstet Gynecol 137:338, 1980.

Garite TJ, Freeman RK, Linzey EM, et al: Prospective randomized study of corticosteroids in the management of premature rupture of the membranes and the premature gestation. Am J Obstet Gynecol 141:508, 1981.

Gluck L, Kulovich MV, Borer Jr RC, et al: Diagnosis of respiratory distress syndrome by amniocentesis. Am J Obstet Gynecol 109:440, 1971.

Hallman M, Kulovich M, Kirkpatrick E, et al: Phosphatidylinositol and phosphatidylglycerol in amniotic fluid: Indices of lung maturity. Am J Obstet Gynecol 125:613, 1976.

Hobel CJ, Hyvarinen M, Oh W: Abnormal fetal heart rate patterns and fetal acid-base balance in low birth weight infants in relation to respiratory distress syndrome. Obstet Gynecol 39:83, 1972.

Liggins GC, Howie RN: A controlled trial of antepartum glucocorticoid treatment for prevention of the respiratory distress syndrome in premature infants. Pediatrics 50:515, 1972.

Merkatz IR, Peter JB, Barden TP: Ritodrine hydrochloride: A betamimetic agent for use in preterm labor. Obstet Gynecol 56:7, 1980.

Neibyl JR: Prostaglandin synthetase inhibitors. Semin Perinatol 5:274, 1981.

Papiernik E: Prediction of the preterm baby. Clin Obstet Gynecol 11:315, 1984.

Varner MW, Galask RP: Conservative management of premature rupture of the membranes. Am J Obstet Gynecol 140:39, 1981.

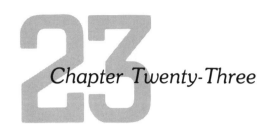

Chapter Twenty-Three

INTRAUTERINE GROWTH RETARDATION, INTRAUTERINE FETAL DEMISE, AND POST-TERM PREGNANCY

LEWIS A. HAMILTON

INTRAUTERINE GROWTH RETARDATION

Intrauterine growth retardation (IUGR) is said to have occurred when the birth weight of a newborn infant is below the tenth percentile for a particular gestational age. This condition is important because it identifies a group of "small-for-dates" infants who are at increased risk for perinatal morbidity and mortality. Growth retarded fetuses are particularly prone to problems such as meconium aspiration, asphyxia, polycythemia, hypoglycemia, and mental retardation. Early recognition of growth retardation offers the opportunity to minimize the adverse effects of many of these complications.

Etiology

The etiologies of IUGR can be grouped into three main categories: maternal, placental, and fetal. Combinations of these are frequently found in pregnancies with IUGR.

Maternal. In this category, inadequate substrate is available. Maternal causes include poor nutritional intake, cigarette smoking, drug abuse, alcoholism, cyanotic heart disease, and pulmonary insufficiency.

Placental. This category is representative of circumstances in which there is inadequate substrate transfer because of placental insufficiency. Conditions that lead to this state include essential hypertension, chronic renal disease, and pregnancy-induced hypertension. If the latter occurs late in pregnancy and is not accompanied by chronic vascular or renal disease, significant IUGR is unlikely to occur.

Fetal. In this case, inadequate substrate is utilized. Examples of fetal causes include intrauterine infection with the "TORCH" agents and congenital anomalies.

Clinical Manifestations

Two types of fetal growth retardation have been described, *symmetric* and *asymmetric*. In fetuses with symmetric growth retardation, there is inadequate growth of both the head and body. The head-abdominal circumference ratio may be normal, but the absolute growth rate is decreased. When asymmetric growth retardation occurs, usually late in pregnancy, the brain is spared so that the head size is proportionally larger than the abdominal size. Symmetric growth retardation is most commonly seen in association with intrauterine infections or congenital fetal anomalies.

Regardless of symmetric versus asymmetric growth retardation, all growth-retarded preg-

214

nancies result in small-for-gestational-age fetuses, usually a smaller placenta, and usually a diminished amount of amniotic fluid.

Diagnosis

IUGR may go undiagnosed unless the obstetrician establishes the correct gestational age of the fetus, identifies high-risk factors from the obstetric data base, and serially assesses fetal growth.

One of the most effective tools in diagnosing IUGR is sonographic evaluation of the fetal parameters. Since repeated sonographic assessments during pregnancy are not feasible in every patient, serial uterine fundal height measurements should serve as the primary screening tool. A more thorough sonographic assessment should be undertaken when (1) the fundal height lags more than 2 cm behind a well-established gestational age or (2) the mother has such high-risk conditions as pre-existing hypertension, chronic renal disease, advanced diabetes with vascular involvement, pre-eclampsia, viral disease, or addiction to nicotine, alcohol, or hard drugs.

At present, sonographic assessment is made primarily through serial determinations of six parameters: (1) fetal biparietal diameter (BPD), (2) head circumference, (3) abdominal circumference (Fig. 23–1), (4) head-body ratio, (5) femur length, and (6) fetal

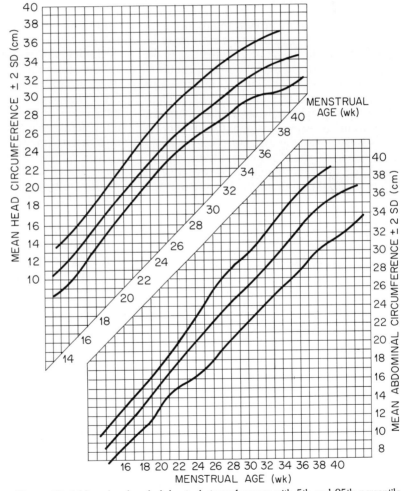

Figure 23–1 Mean head and abdominal circumferences with 5th and 95th percentile confidence limits between 16 and 40 weeks' menstrual age. (Adapted with permission from Campbell S, Griffin D, Roberts A, et al.: Early prenatal diagnosis of abnormalities of the fetal head, spine, limbs, and abdominal organs. In Orlandi C, Polani PE, Bovicelli L (eds): Recent Advances in Prenatal Diagnosis: Proceedings of the First International Symposium on Recent Advances in Prenatal Diagnosis, Bologna, 15th–16th September, 1980. New York, John Wiley and Sons, 1980.)

weight. Quantitating the degree of IUGR is not well established. If the fetal measurements fall within the tenth to twenty-fifth percentile of growth curves, mild IUGR should be considered. When measurements fall below the tenth percentile, the fetus is considered to have moderate IUGR.

During advancing gestation, the head circumference remains greater than the abdominal circumference until approximately 34 weeks, at which point the ratio approaches 1 (Fig. 23–2). Following 34 weeks, the normal pregnancy is associated with an abdominal circumference that is greater than the head circumference. When asymmetric growth retardation occurs, usually late in pregnancy, the BPD is essentially normal, while the ratio of head:abdominal circumference is abnormal. With symmetric growth retardation, the head:abdominal circumference ratio may be normal, but the absolute growth rate is decreased and estimated fetal weight is reduced.

From 50 to 90 percent of infants with manifestations of IUGR at birth can be identified with serial prenatal ultrasonic scans. The accuracy depends upon the quality of the assessments, the criteria used for diagnosis, and the effect of interventions applied when this diagnosis is made. For example, it is not unusual to observe an improvement in

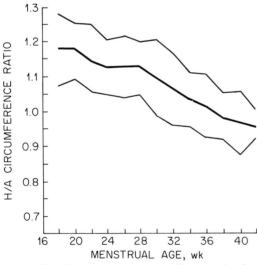

Figure 23–2 Graphic representation of the mean head to abdominal circumference ratios with 5th and 95th percentile confidence limits from 17 to 42 weeks' menstrual age. (Reproduced with permission from Campbell S, Thomas A: Ultrasound measurement of the fetal head to abdominal circumference ratio in the assessment of growth retardation. Br J Obstet Gynaecol 84:165, 1977.)

fetal growth after interventions such as work stoppage, bed rest, dietary modification, and curtailment of the use of tobacco, hard drugs, and alcohol.

Management

Antepartum. Once a fetus has been identified as having decreased growth, the obstetrician should direct his or her efforts toward modifying any associated factors that can be changed. Since poor nutrition and smoking exert their main effects on birth weight in the latter half of pregnancy, cessation of smoking and improved nutrition can have a positive impact. The woman who works becomes fatigued and is more likely to have a low-birth-weight infant. Bedrest in the left lateral position will increase uterine blood flow and has the potential for improving the nutrition of the jeopardized fetus.

The most important clinical decisions revolve around the timing and mode of delivery. The objective is to expedite delivery before the occurrence of fetal asphyxia but after fetal lung maturation. This requires regular fetal monitoring with a nonstress test (NST), biophysical profile, and possible oxytocin challenge test (OCT). With mild IUGR, weekly testing is indicated; with moderate IUGR, biweekly testing is indicated (see Chapter 6).

If the NST is reactive or the OCT is negative and the amniotic fluid volume adequate, the pregnancy is allowed to continue, since there are no data to support early delivery of these infants in the absence of documented fetal distress. Serial ultrasonic evaluations of fetal growth should be done at three-week intervals.

If the NST becomes nonreactive in conjunction with a positive OCT in the presence of mature fetal lungs (lecithin-sphingomyelin ratio greater than 2), interruption of the pregnancy is necessary. In the presence of oligohydramnios, amniocentesis is not safe. Delivery is recommended without assessing lung maturity because these fetuses are at great risk of asphyxia, and the stress associated with IUGR usually accelerates fetal pulmonary maturity.

Labor and Delivery. During labor, these high-risk patients must be electronically monitored in order to detect the earliest evidence of fetal distress (see Chapter 20). The fetoplacental unit in these infants does not have the normal reserve. In the presence of recurrent abnormal fetal heart rate patterns, which are unresponsive to traditional treatment (lateral positioning and oxygen by mask), delivery must be expedited, usually by cesarean section.

A combined obstetric-neonatal team approach to delivery is mandatory because of the likelihood of neonatal asphyxia. Meconium aspiration can often be prevented by suctioning the oropharynx with the delivery of the head and by intubating and suctioning the trachea to clear it after delivery of the trunk (see Chapter 11).

After birth, the infant should be carefully examined to rule out the possibility of congenital anomalies and infections. The monitoring of blood glucose levels is important, since these fetuses do not have adequate hepatic glycogen stores, and hypoglycemia is a common finding. Hypothermia is also prevalent. Respiratory distress syndrome is more common in the presence of fetal distress, since fetal acidosis reduces surfactant synthesis and release.

Prognosis

The long-term prognosis for infants with IUGR must take into account the varied etiologies of the growth retardation. If infants with chromosomal abnormalities, congenital anomalies, and infection are excluded, the outlook for these newborns is generally good.

INTRAUTERINE FETAL DEATH

Intrauterine fetal death (IUFD) is fetal demise after 20 weeks' gestation but prior to the onset of labor. It complicates about 1 percent of pregnancies.

With the development of newer diagnostic and therapeutic modalities over the past two decades, the management of IUFD has shifted from watchful expectancy to a more active intervention.

Etiology

In more than 50 percent of cases, the etiology of antepartum fetal death is not known or cannot be determined. Associated conditions include hypertensive diseases of pregnancy, diabetes mellitus, erythroblastosis

fetalis, umbilical cord accidents, fetal congenital anomalies, fetal or maternal infections, and fetomaternal hemorrhage.

Diagnosis

Clinically, fetal death should be suspected when the patient reports the absence of fetal movements, particularly if the uterus is small-for-dates or if the fetal heart tones are not detected utilizing a Doppler device. Since the placenta may continue to produce hCG for several weeks, a positive pregnancy test does not exclude an intrauterine fetal death.

Diagnostic confirmation has been greatly facilitated since the advent of ultrasonography. Real-time ultrasonography confirms the lack of fetal movement and absence of fetal cardiac activity. With the elapse of sufficient time, collapse of the fetal body is discernible by x-ray or ultrasound. Although rarely indicated at the present time, abdominal x-ray examination will show the following:

1. Gas in the cardiovascular system within three or four days
2. Subsequent overlapping of the fetal skull bones (*Spalding's sign*) due to liquefaction of the brain
3. Marked curvature or angulation of the spine following maceration of the spinous ligaments

Amniocentesis is rarely indicated to confirm the diagnosis of fetal death, but if performed will show dark brown, turbid fluid with markedly elevated levels of creatine phosphokinase.

Management

Fetal demise between 13 and 28 weeks allows for two different approaches.

Watchful Expectancy. About 80 percent of patients will experience the spontaneous onset of labor within two to three weeks of fetal demise. Since the risk of complications is small and the likelihood of spontaneous labor is high, some physicians choose not to intervene for at least three weeks after fetal demise has been confirmed. Unfortunately, the patient's feeling of personal loss and guilt may create such anxiety that this conservative approach may prove unacceptable.

Induction of Labor. Some physicians choose to induce labor as soon as IUFD is confirmed. Justifications for such intervention include the emotional burden on the patient associated with carrying a dead fetus, the increased likelihood of intrauterine infection, and the 10 percent risk of disseminated intravascular coagulation when a dead fetus is retained for more than five weeks.

Vaginal suppositories of prostaglandin E_2 (Prostin) have received the approval of the FDA for use from the twelfth to the twenty-eighth week of gestation. Prostaglandins are very effective drugs with an overall success rate of 97 percent. Although at least 50 percent of patients receiving prostaglandins experience nausea and vomiting and/or diarrhea with temperature elevations, these side effects are transient. There have been reported cases of uterine rupture and cervical lacerations, but with properly selected patients, the drug is safe. The maximum recommended dose is a 20 mg suppository every three hours. Intravenous oxytocin is acceptable for induction of labor if the cervix is favorable.

After 28 weeks' gestation, if the cervix is favorable for induction and there are no contraindications, oxytocin is the drug of choice. The use of prostaglandin E_2 suppositories at this gestational age is associated with an increased risk of uterine rupture, so a smaller dosage should be used. If the cervix is not favorable for induction, expectant observation is appropriate. After three weeks, serial daily controlled infusions of oxytocin may be required to ripen the cervix if induction of labor is attempted.

Monitoring of Coagulopathy. Regardless of the mode of therapy chosen, weekly fibrinogen levels should be monitored during the period of expectant management, along with a hematocrit and platelet count. Even a "normal" fibrinogen level of 300 mg/dl may be an early sign of consumptive coagulopathy in cases of fetal demise. An elevated prothrombin and partial thromboplastin time, the presence of fibrinogen-fibrin degradation products, and a decreased platelet count may clarify the diagnosis.

If laboratory evidence of mild disseminated intravascular coagulation is noted in the absence of bleeding, delivery by the most appropriate means is recommended. If the clotting defect is more severe or if there is evidence of bleeding, blood volume support or use of component therapy (cryoprecipitate or fresh frozen plasma) should be given prior to intervention.

Follow-up

Physician responsibilities do not end with delivery of the fetus. In addition to emotional support of the parents, a search should be undertaken to determine the cause of the intrauterine death. If congenital abnormalities are detected, fetal chromosomal studies and total body x-rays should be done, in addition to a complete autopsy. The autopsy report, when available, must be discussed in detail with both parents. In a stillborn fetus, the best tissue for a chromosomal analysis is the fascia lata, obtained from the lateral aspect of the thigh. The tissue can be stored in saline or Hanks' solution. A significant number of cases of intrauterine fetal demise are the result of fetomaternal hemorrhage, which can be detected by identifying fetal erythrocytes in maternal blood. Subsequent pregnancies occurring in a woman with a history of intrauterine fetal demise must be managed as high-risk cases.

POST-TERM PREGNANCY

The prolonged or post-term pregnancy is one that persists beyond 42 weeks (294 days) from the onset of the last normal menstrual period. Estimates of the incidence of post-term pregnancy range from 6 to 12 percent of all pregnancies.

Perinatal mortality is two to three times higher in these prolonged gestations. Much of the increased risk to the fetus/neonate can be attributed to development of the *fetal postmaturity (dysmaturity) syndrome.* Occurring in 20 to 30 percent of post-term pregnancies, this syndrome is related to the aging and infarction of the placenta, resulting in placental insufficiency with impaired oxygen diffusion and decreased transfer of nutrients to the fetus. If evidence of intrauterine hypoxia is present (such as meconium staining of the umbilical cord, fetal membranes, skin, and nails), perinatal mortality is even further increased.

The fetus with postmaturity syndrome typically has loss of subcutaneous fat, long fingernails, dry peeling skin, and abundant hair.

The 70 to 80 percent of postdate fetuses not affected by placental insufficiency continue to grow *in utero*, many to the point of macrosomia (birth weight greater than 4000 gm). This macrosomia often results in abnormal labor, birth trauma, and an increased incidence of cesarean birth.

Etiology

The initiation of human labor is triggered by a complex of fetal and maternal factors (see Chapter 10). The cause of postdate pregnancy is unknown in most instances. Prolonged gestation is common in association with an anencephalic fetus and is probably linked to the lack of a fetal labor-initiating factor from the fetal adrenals, which are hypoplastic in anencephalics. Prolonged labor may also be rarely associated with placental sulfatase deficiency and extrauterine pregnancy.

Diagnosis

The diagnosis of post-term pregnancy is often difficult. The key to appropriate classification and subsequent successful perinatal management is the accurate dating of gestation. It is estimated that uncertain dates are present in 20 to 30 percent of all pregnancies. The factors to be taken into consideration in attempting to distinguish a postdated pregnancy from a misdated pregnancy are shown in Table 23–1. If there is no concordance between at least two of the criteria listed, the patient is considered to have poor dates.

Management

Antepartum. The appropriate management of prolonged pregnancy revolves around identification of the low percentage of fetuses with postmaturity syndrome who are at risk of intrauterine hypoxia and fetal demise. Now that biophysical and biochemical tests of fetal well-being are available, there has been a movement toward individualization of the time of delivery for each patient. However, if the gestational age is firmly established at 42 weeks, the fetal head is well-fixed in the pelvis, and the cervix is favorable, the patient should generally be induced.

The two main clinical problems that remain are (1) patients with good dates at 42 weeks' gestation with an unripe cervix, and (2) patients with an uncertain gestational age seen for the first time with a possible or probable diagnosis of prolonged pregnancy. In the first group of patients above, antepartum fetal

TABLE 23–1 FACTORS TO BE EVALUATED IN DATING A PREGNANCY

1. The accuracy of the date of the last normal menstrual period
2. The evaluation of uterine size on pelvic examination in the first trimester
3. The evaluation of uterine size in relation to gestational age during subsequent antenatal visits (concordance or size-dates discrepancy)
4. The gestational age when fetal heart tones were first heard utilizing a Doppler ultrasonic device (usually at 12 to 14 weeks)
5. The gestational age when fetal heart tones were first heard with the DeLee stethoscope (generally 18 to 20 weeks)
6. The date of quickening (usually 18 to 20 weeks in a primigravida and 16 to 18 weeks in a multigravida)
7. Sonographic parameters—measurement of the biparietal diameter is most accurate for pregnancy dating between 16 and 20 weeks' gestation

monitoring, as outlined in Figure 6–1, should be undertaken. If the nonstress test is reactive, it should be repeated twice weekly. In the patient at greater than 42 weeks' gestation with a reassuring fetal assessment, labor need not be induced unless the cervix becomes favorable or the fetus is judged to be macrosomic.

At 43 weeks' gestation with firm dates, delivery should be considered by the appropriate route, regardless of other factors, in view of the increasing potential for perinatal morbidity and mortality.

When the patient presents very late in gestation for initial assessment with the label of prolonged pregnancy but the gestational age is in question, an expectant approach is often acceptable. The risk of intervention with delivery of a preterm infant must be considered.

Intrapartum. Continuous electronic fetal monitoring must be utilized during the induction of labor. The patient should be encouraged to stay off her back. The fetal membranes should be ruptured as early as is feasible in the intrapartum period so that internal electrodes can be applied and the color of the amniotic fluid assessed. If electronic fetal monitoring suggests fetal distress, fetal acid-base status should be determined by fetal scalp blood sampling. If fetal acidosis is confirmed (pH less than 7.25), immediate delivery is indicated, usually by the cesarean route (see Chapter 20). If meconium is present, neonatal asphyxia should be anticipated, and the protocol outlined in Chapter 11 should be followed.

SUGGESTED READING

Campbell S: Ultrasound measurement of the fetal head to abdominal circumference ratio in assessment of growth retardation. Br J Obstet Gynaecol 84:165, 1977.

Cetrulo CL, Freeman RF: Bioelectrical evaluation in intrauterine growth retardation. Clin Obstet Gynecol 20:979, 1977.

Creasy RK, Resnik R: Intrauterine fetal growth retardation. In Milunsky A, Friedman EA, and Gluck L (eds): Advances in Perinatal Medicine. New York, Plenum Medical Book Co, 1981.

Evertson LR, Ganthier RJ, Schifrin BS, et al: Antepartum fetal heart rate testing. I. Evolution of the nonstress test. Am J Obstet Gynecol 133:29, 1979.

Fancourt R, Campbell S, Harvey DR, et al: Follow-up study of small-for-dates babies. Br Med J 1:1435, 1976.

Hobbins JC, Berkowitz RL: Ultrasonography in the diagnosis of IUGR. Clin Obstet Gynecol 20:957, 1977.

Lauersen NG, Cederqvist LL, Wilson KH: Management of intrauterine fetal death with prostaglandin E_2 vaginal suppositories. Am J Obstet Gynecol 137:753, 1980.

Liban E, Salzberger M: A prospective clinicopathological study of 1108 cases of antenatal fetal death. Isr J Med Sci 12:34, 1976.

Platt LD, Manning FA, Murata Y, et al: Diagnosis of fetal death *in utero* by real-time ultrasound. Obstet Gynecol 55:191, 1980.

Rozenman D, Kessler I, Lancet M: Third trimester induction of labor with fetal death *in utero*. Surg Gynecol Obstet 151:497, 1980.

Sandler RZ, Knutzen VK, Milano CM, et al: Uterine rupture with the use of vaginal prostaglandin E_2 suppositories. Am J Obstet Gynecol 134:348, 1979.

Southern EM, Gutknecht GD, Mohberg NR, et al: Vaginal prostaglandin E_2 in the management of fetal intrauterine death. Br J Obstet Gynaecol 85:437, 1978.

POSTPARTUM HEMORRHAGE AND PUERPERAL SEPSIS

ROBERT H. HAYASHI

The three most common causes of maternal death are hemorrhage, infection, and hypertensive disease. In this chapter, the postpartum manifestations of two of these problems, hemorrhage and infection, are discussed. Both of these are associated not only with maternal mortality, but also with significant maternal morbidity and prolonged hospitalization.

POSTPARTUM HEMORRHAGE

Postpartum hemorrhage is defined as blood loss in excess of 500 ml at the time of vaginal delivery. There is normally a greater blood loss following delivery by cesarean section; therefore, blood loss in excess of 1000 ml is considered a postpartum hemorrhage in such patients. The excessive blood loss usually occurs in the immediate postpartum period but can occur slowly over the first 24 hours. *Delayed postpartum hemorrhage* can occasionally occur, the excessive bleeding commencing more than 24 hours after delivery. This is usually due to subinvolution of the uterus and disruption of the placental site "scab" several weeks postpartum, or to the retention of placental fragments that separate several days after delivery. Postpartum hemorrhage occurs in about 4 percent of deliveries.

Etiology

Most of the blood loss occurs from the myometrial spiral arterioles and decidual veins that previously supplied and drained the intervillous spaces of the placenta. As the contractions of the partially empty uterus cause placental separation, bleeding occurs and continues until the uterine musculature contracts around the blood vessels and acts as a physiologic-anatomic ligature. Failure of the uterus to contract after placental separation *(uterine atony)* leads to excessive placental site bleeding. Other causes of postpartum hemorrhage are listed in Table 24–1.

Uterine Atony. The majority of postpartum hemorrhages (75 to 80 percent) are due to uterine atony. The factors predisposing to postpartum uterine atony are shown in Table 24–2.

Genital Tract Trauma. Trauma during delivery is the second most common cause of

TABLE 24–1 CAUSES OF POSTPARTUM HEMORRHAGE

1. Uterine atony
2. Genital tract trauma
3. Retained placental tissue
4. Low placental implantation
5. Coagulation disorders
6. Uterine inversion

TABLE 24–2 FACTORS PREDISPOSING TO
POSTPARTUM UTERINE
ATONY

1. Overdistension of the uterus
   a. Multiple gestation
   b. Polyhydramnios
   c. Fetal macrosomia
2. Prolonged labor
3. Oxytocic augmentation of labor
4. Grandmultiparity (a parity of five or more)
5. Precipitous labor (one lasting less than three hours)
6. Magnesium sulfate treatment of pre-eclampsia
7. Chorioamnionitis

postpartum hemorrhage. During vaginal delivery, *lacerations of the cervix and vagina* may occur spontaneously, but are more common following the use of forceps or a vacuum extractor. The vascular beds in the genital tract are engorged during pregnancy, and bleeding can be profuse. Lacerations are particularly prone to occur over the perineal body, in the periurethral area, and over the ischial spines along the posterolateral aspects of the vagina. The cervix may lacerate at the two lateral angles while rapidly dilating in the first stage of labor. Apart from acute postpartum bleeding, neglected lacerations may cause substantial but slow blood loss over many hours. *Uterine rupture* may occasionally occur. At the time of delivery by low transverse cesarean section, an inadvertent lateral extension of the incision can damage the ascending branches of the uterine arteries; an extension inferiorly can damage the cervical branches of the uterine artery.

Retained Placental Tissue. Normally, there is a layer of fibrinoid material called *"Nitabuch's layer"* at the base of the placenta. When the partially empty uterus contracts, the placenta cleanly separates through this layer. However, if the placental anchoring villi grow down into the myometrium disrupting this fibrinoid layer, placental separation will be incomplete or may not occur at all. Extensive growth of placental tissue into the myometrium without an intervening fibrinoid layer is called *placenta accreta.* When the trophoblast penetrates the myometrium to the serosa or beyond, it is called *placenta percreta.* A complete placenta accreta will not cause bleeding because the placenta remains attached, but the partial type may cause profuse bleeding, as the normal part of the placenta separates and the myometrium cannot contract sufficiently to occlude the

placental site vessels. In about half the patients with delayed postpartum hemorrhage, placental fragments are present when uterine curettage is performed.

Low Placental Implantation. Low implantation of the placenta can predispose to postpartum hemorrhage because the relative content of musculature in the uterine wall decreases in the lower uterine segment, which may result in insufficient control of placental site bleeding.

Coagulation Disorders. Peripartal coagulation disorders are high-risk factors for postpartum hemorrhage, but fortunately are quite rare. Patients with coagulation problems, such as occur with thrombotic thrombocytopenic purpura, amniotic fluid embolism, abruptio placentae, idiopathic thrombocytopenic purpura, or von Willebrand's disease, may develop postpartum hemorrhage because of their inability to form a stable blood clot in the placental site.

Patients with *thrombotic thrombocytopenia* have a rare syndrome of unknown etiology characterized by thrombocytopenic purpura, microangiopathic hemolytic anemia, transient and fluctuating neurologic signs, renal dysfunction, and a febrile course. In pregnancy, the disease is usually fatal. An *amniotic fluid embolus* is also rare and is associated with approximately an 80 percent mortality. This syndrome is characterized by a fulminating consumption coagulopathy, intense bronchospasm, and vasomotor collapse. It is triggered by an intravascular infusion of a significant amount of amniotic fluid during a tumultuous or rapid labor in the presence of ruptured membranes. During the process of *placental abruption* (premature separation of the placenta), a small amount of amniotic fluid may leak into the vascular system, and the thromboplastin may trigger a consumption coagulopathy without the other elements of a large amniotic fluid embolus. Patients with *idiopathic thrombocytopenic purpura* have platelets with abnormal function and/or a shortened life span. This causes thrombocytopenia and a bleeding tendency. Circulating antiplatelet antibodies of the IgG type may occasionally cross the placenta and result in fetal and neonatal thrombocytopenia as well. *Von Willebrand's disease* is an inherited coagulopathy characterized by a prolonged bleeding time due to factor VIII deficiency. During pregnancy, these patients are likely to have a decreased bleeding diathesis, since pregnancy elevates factor VIII levels. In the postpartum period, they are susceptible to immediate hemorrhage and also to delayed bleeding as the factor VIII levels fall.

Uterine Inversion. Uterine inversion is the "turning inside out" of the uterus in the third stage of labor. It is quite rare, occurring in only about 1 out of 20,000 pregnancies. Just after the second stage, the uterus is somewhat atonic, the cervix open, and the placenta attached. Improper management of the third stage can cause an iatrogenic uterine inversion. If the inexperienced physician exerts fundal pressure while pulling on the umbilical cord before complete placental separation (particularly with a fundal implantation of the placenta), uterine inversion may occur. As the fundus of the uterus moves through the vagina, the inversion exerts traction on peritoneal structures, which can elicit a profound vasovagal response. The resulting vasodilatation increases bleeding and the risk of hypovolemic shock. If the placenta is completely or partially separated, the uterine atony may cause profuse bleeding, which compounds the vasovagal shock.

OBSTETRIC SHOCK

An occasional patient may develop hypotension without significant external bleeding. This condition is called *obstetric shock*. The causes of obstetric shock include concealed hemorrhage, uterine inversion, and amniotic fluid embolism.

An improperly sutured episiotomy can lead to a concealed postpartum hemorrhage. If the first suture at the vaginal apex of the episiotomy incision does not incorporate the cut and retracted arterioles, they can continue to bleed, creating a hematoma that can dissect cephalad into the retroperitoneal space. This may cause shock, without external evidence of blood loss. A soft tissue hematoma, usually of the vulva, may occur following delivery in the absence of any laceration or episiotomy, and may also contribute to occult blood loss.

Spontaneous uterine rupture during labor is rare (one in every 1900 deliveries), but usually results in significant intraperitoneal bleeding. Uterine rupture can also occur secondary to blunt abdominal trauma at the time of an automobile accident. A predisposing

factor for uterine rupture is a uterine scar, particularly from a previous classic cesarean section.

Differential Diagnosis

Identification of the cause of postpartum hemorrhage or obstetric shock requires a systematic approach. The fundus of the uterus should be palpated through the abdominal wall to determine the presence or absence of uterine atony. In the rare case of uterine inversion, a crater-like depression is felt at the fundus. Next, a quick but thorough inspection of the vagina and cervix should be performed to ascertain whether or not any lacerations may be compounding the bleeding problem. Any uterine inversion or pelvic hematoma should be excluded during the pelvic examination. If the cause of bleeding has not been identified, manual exploration of the uterine cavity should be performed, if necessary under general anesthesia. With fingertips together, a gloved hand is slipped through the open cervix, and the endometrial surface is palpated carefully to identify any retained products of conception, uterine wall lacerations, or partial uterine inversion. If no cause for the bleeding is found, a coagulopathy must be sought.

MANAGEMENT OF POSTPARTUM HEMORRHAGE AND OBSTETRIC SHOCK

The first step toward good management is the identification of patients at risk for postpartum hemorrhage and the institution of prophylactic measures during labor to minimize the possibility of maternal mortality. Patients with any predisposing factors for postpartum hemorrhage, including a past history of a previous postpartum hemorrhage, should be screened for anemia and atypical antibodies to ensure that an adequate supply of type-specific blood is on hand in the blood bank. An intravenous infusion via a large bore catheter should be commenced prior to delivery and blood held in the laboratory for possible cross-matching.

During the diagnostic work-up of an established hemorrhage, the patient's vital signs must be monitored closely. Four units of packed red blood cells must be typed and cross-matched, and intravenous crystalloids (such as normal saline or lactated Ringer's solution) infused to restore intravascular volume.

Uterine Atony

If uterine atony is determined to be the cause of the postpartum hemorrhage, a rapid continuous intravenous infusion of dilute oxytocin (40 to 80 units in one liter of normal saline) should be given to increase uterine tone. If the uterus remains atonic and the placental site bleeding continues during the oxytocic infusion, ergonovine maleate or methylergonovine, 0.2 mg, may be given intramuscularly or as an intravenous bolus. The ergot drugs are contraindicated in patients with hypertension, since the pressor effect of the drug may increase blood pressure to dangerous levels.

Analogues of prostaglandin F2-alpha given intramuscularly are quite effective in controlling postpartum hemorrhage due to uterine atony. The 15-methyl analogue (0.25 mg) has a more potent uterotonic effect and longer duration of action than the parent compound.

Failing these pharmacologic treatments, a bimanual compression and massage of the uterine corpus may control the bleeding and cause the uterus to contract. Although packing the uterine cavity is not widely practiced, it may occasionally control postpartum hemorrhage and obviate the need for surgical intervention. The vital signs, hematocrit, and fundal height should be monitored frequently while the packing is in place, since continued bleeding will not be initially evident through the packing.

Another approach that may be tried if bleeding persists is placement of the patient into an antigravity suit ("G" suit), which will, when inflated, compress the lower extremities and the abdominal cavity. Experience with this device in trauma patients has demonstrated good control of intra-abdominal bleeding. This approach may occasionally be used to temporize while the blood volume is being expanded and preparations are made for more definitive surgery.

Operative intervention is a last resort. If the patient has completed her childbearing, a supracervical abdominal hysterectomy is definitive therapy for intractable postpartum hemorrhage due to uterine atony. If reproductive potential is important to the patient, ligation of the uterine arteries adjacent to the uterus will lower the pulse pressure distal to the ligatures. This procedure is more successful in controlling uterine placental site hemorrhage and easier to perform than bilateral hypogastric artery ligation.

Genital Tract Trauma

When postpartum hemorrhage is related to genital tract trauma, surgical intervention is necessary. Repair of genital tract lacerations requires the implementation of an important principle—the first suture must be placed well above the apex of the laceration to incorporate any bleeding, retracted arterioles into the liagature. Repair of vaginal lacerations requires good light and good exposure, and the tissues should be approximated without dead space. A running lock suture technique is the most hemostatic. Cervical lacerations need not be sutured unless they are actively bleeding. Sponge-holding forceps may be used to pull the cervix down to the introitus to facilitate inspection and suturing (Fig. 24–1). Large expanding hematomas of the genital tract require surgical evacuation of clots and a search for bleeding vessels that can be ligated. Stable hematomas can be observed and treated conservatively. A retroperitoneal hematoma generally begins in the pelvis. If the bleeding cannot be con-

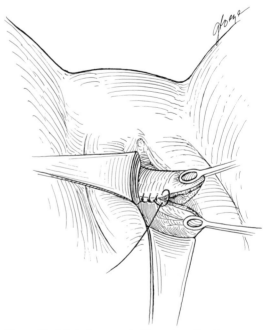

Figure 24–1 Suturing a cervical laceration. The first suture must be placed above the apex of the laceration.

trolled from a vaginal approach, a laparotomy and bilateral hypogastric artery ligation may be necessary.

The intraoperative laceration of the ascending branch of the uterine artery during delivery through a low transverse cesarean section can be easily controlled by the placement of a large suture ligature through the myometrium and broad ligament below the level of the laceration. A uterine rupture usually necessitates subtotal or total abdominal hysterectomy, although small defects may be repaired.

Retained Products of Conception

When the placenta cannot be delivered in the usual manner, manual removal of the placenta is necessary (Fig. 24–2). This should be performed urgently if bleeding is profuse. Otherwise, it is reasonable to delay 30 minutes to await spontaneous separation. General anesthesia may be required. Following manual removal of the placenta or placental remnants, the uterus should be scraped with a large curette. Extensive placenta accreta usually necessitates hysterectomy.

Uterine Inversion

The management of a uterine inversion requires quick thinking. The patient rapidly goes into shock, and immediate intravascular volume expansion with intravenous crystalloids is required. An anesthesiologist should be summoned. When the patient's condition is stable, the partially separated placenta

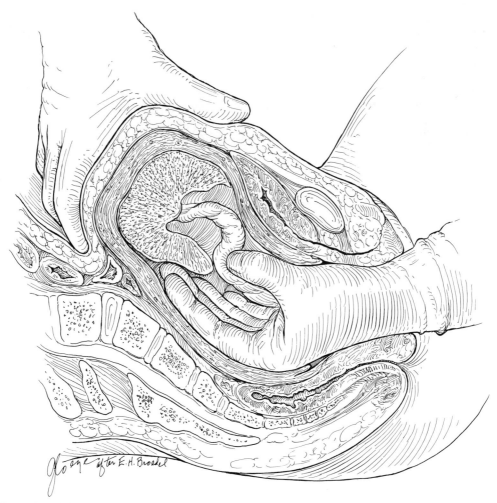

Figure 24–2 Manual removal of the placenta. The abdominal hand provides counterpressure on the uterine fundus against the shearing force of the fingers in the uterus.

should be completely removed and an attempt made to replace the uterus by placing a cupped hand around the fundus and elevating it in the long axis of the vagina. If this is unsuccessful, a further attempt under halothane anesthesia should be made. Once replaced, a dilute oxytocic infusion should be started to cause the uterus to contract before removing the intrauterine hand. Rarely, the uterus cannot be replaced from below, and a surgical procedure may be required. At laparotomy, a vertical incision should be made through the posterior portion of the cervix to incise the constriction ring and allow the fundus to be replaced into the peritoneal cavity. Suturing of the cervical incision will complete this procedure.

Amniotic Fluid Embolus

The principal objectives of treatment for amniotic fluid embolism are to support the respiratory system, correct the shock, and replace the coagulation factors. These necessitate immediate cardiopulmonary resuscitation, usually with mechanical ventilation; rapid volume expansion with an electrolyte solution; placement of a bladder catheter to monitor urine output; correction of the red cell deficit by transfusion with packed red blood cells; and reversal of the coagulopathy with the use of platelets, fibrinogen, and other blood components.

TABLE 24–3   BLOOD PRODUCTS USED TO CORRECT COAGULATION DEFECTS

BLOOD PRODUCT	VOLUME (ML) IN 1 UNIT*	EFFECT OF TRANSFUSION
Platelet concentrate	30–40	Increases platelet count by about 20,000 to 25,000
Cryoprecipitate	15–25	Supplies fibrinogen, factor VIII, and factor XIII (3 to 10 times more concentrated than the equivalent volume of fresh plasma)
Fresh-frozen plasma	200	Supplies all factors except platelets (1 gm fibrinogen)
Packed red blood cells	200	Raises hematocrit 3 to 4 percent

*1 unit = the quantity obtained from 1 unit (500 ml) of fresh whole blood.

Coagulopathy

When postpartum hemorrhage is associated with a coagulopathy, the specific defect should be corrected by the infusion of blood products, as outlined in Table 24–3. Patients with thrombocytopenia require platelet concentrate infusions; those with von Willebrand's disease require fresh frozen plasma. A packed red cell infusion is given to a patient who has bled enough to drop the circulating red cell population sufficiently to compromise the delivery of oxygen to the tissues. Generally, a hematocrit of more than 25 percent will suffice. Massive transfusions (greater than 3 L), especially with whole blood, will aggravate an already disturbed coagulation system by further depleting platelets and factors V and VIII. Thus, one unit of fresh frozen plasma should be given for every two units of blood after six units have been transfused.

PUERPERAL SEPSIS

Prior to the antiseptic and antibiotic era, puerperal sepsis was the overwhelming cause of maternal mortality and morbidity. Nearly 200 years ago, Alexander Gordon in Scotland observed that puerperal fever was transmitted from patient to patient, and about 50 years later, Ignaz Semmelweis in Vienna and Oliver Wendell Holmes in Boston independently concluded that it was the physician who transmitted the disease among puerperae. They proposed that simply washing hands between patient examinations would control the epidemics. Thus began the antiseptic era. Louis Pasteur later identified the hemolytic streptococcus as the pathogen.

Puerperal sepsis still accounts for significant postpartum maternal morbidity and mortality. Patients with a puerperal genital tract infection are susceptible to the development of septic shock, pelvic thrombophlebitis, and pelvic abscess. Possible sequelae include the impairment of future fertility, due to tubal or endometrial damage, or hysterectomy.

Following a vaginal delivery, approximately 6 or 7 percent of puerperae demonstrate febrile morbidity, defined as a temperature of 100.4° F (38° C) or higher, occurring for more than two consecutive days exclusive of the first postpartum day during the first ten postpartum days. Following primary cesarean section, the incidence of febrile morbidity is about twice that following vaginal delivery. The majority of these fevers are caused by endometritis.

Etiology

The pathophysiology of puerperal sepsis is closely related to the various microbial inhabitants of the vagina and cervix. The vaginal flora during gestation resembles that in the nonpregnant state (see Chapter 33), although there is a trend toward isolating more *Mycoplasma genitalis* and anaerobic streptococci in the last trimester. Potentially pathogenic organisms can be cultured from the vagina in approximately 80 percent of pregnant women. These organisms include enterococci, hemolytic and nonhemolytic streptococci, anaerobic streptococci, enteric bacilli, pseudodiphtheria bacteria, and *Neisseria* species other than *N. gonorrhoeae*. Excessive overgrowth of these organisms during pregnancy is inhibited by the acidity of the vagina (pH, 4 to 5), due primarily to the production of lactic acid by the lactobacilli.

The uterine cavity is normally free of bacteria during pregnancy. After parturition, the pH of the vagina changes from acidic to alkaline because of the neutralizing effect of the alkaline amniotic fluid, blood, and lochia, as well as the decreased population of lactobacilli. This change in pH favors an increased growth of aerobic organisms. Approximately 48 hours postpartum, progressive necrosis of the endometrial and placental remnants produces a favorable intrauterine environment for the multiplication of anaerobic bacteria.

About 70 percent of puerperal infections are caused by anaerobic organisms. Most of these are anaerobic cocci *(Peptostreptococcus, Peptococcus,* and *Streptococcus)*, although mixed infections with *Bacteroides fragilis* are encountered in up to one third of cases. Of the aerobic organisms, *Escherichia coli* is the most common pathogen, followed by enterococci. Puerperal infection from clostridia is rare.

During the preantibiotic era, most patients with puerperal sepsis were infected by group A beta-hemolytic streptococci. These organisms are not normal inhabitants of the vaginal flora and originate from an outside source, such as the nasopharynx or skin of a carrier or infected individual. Today, the incidence of this highly contagious and virulent organism is vastly reduced due to antiseptic techniques. Intrauterine infection with beta-hemolytic streptococci rapidly progresses to parametritis, peritonitis, and septicemia. The contagiousness of pyogenic streptococci demands precautionary measures, such as the screening of patients, hospital personnel, and visitors for overt and occult infections in order to avoid contamination of mothers or infants if a case is detected in the neonatal nursery.

Intrauterine staphylococcal infection is rare. This organism is frequently responsible for infection of perineal wounds and abdominal incisions. *Trichomonas vaginalis* and *Candida albicans* are frequent inhabitants of the vagina, but no connection with puerperal sepsis has been established. Recently, mycoplasma organisms have been shown to contribute to puerperal endometritis.

Predisposing Factors

Predisposing factors to the development of a puerperal genital tract infection are shown in Table 24–4.

After delivery, the placental site vessels are clotted off, and there is an exudation of lymph-like fluid along with massive numbers of neutrophils and other white cells to form the lochia. Vaginal microorganisms readily enter the uterine cavity and may become pathogenic at the placental site, depending on such variables as the size of the inoculum, the local pH, and the presence or absence of devitalized tissue. The latter may include tissue incorporated in the suture line of a cesarean section.

The normal body defense mechanisms usually prevent any progressive infection, but a

TABLE 24–4 FACTORS PREDISPOSING TO THE DEVELOPMENT OF PUERPERAL GENITAL TRACT INFECTION

1. Poor nutrition and hygiene
2. Anemia
3. Premature rupture of the membranes
4. Prolonged rupture of the membranes
5. Prolonged labor
6. Frequent vaginal examinations during labor
7. Cesarean section
8. Operative delivery
9. Manual removal of the placenta
10. Retained placental fragments or fetal membranes

breakdown of these defenses will allow the bacteria to invade the myometrium. Further invasion into the lymphatics of the para-metrium can cause a lymphangitis, pelvic cellulitis, and the possibility of widespread infection from septic emboli. An endomy-oparametritis is a potentially life-threatening condition. It commonly begins with retention of secundines that block the normal lochial flow, allowing accumulation of intrauterine lochia that in turn changes the local pH and acts as a culture medium for bacterial growth. Unless normal lochial flow is established, bacterial invasion will progress.

Clinical Features

Puerperal infection manifests as rising fe-ver and increasing uterine tenderness on post-partum day two or three. With the develop-ment of parametritis (pelvic cellulitis), the temperature elevation will be sustained, and the patient may develop signs of pelvic peri-tonitis. Erratic temperature fluctuations and severe chills suggest bacteremia and dissem-ination of septic emboli, with the particular likelihood of spread to the lungs.

When the usual relative pelvic venous stasis is combined with a large inoculum of patho-genic anaerobic bacteria, a pelvic vein throm-bophlebitis is likely to develop, usually on the right side of the pelvis. The clinical pic-ture of *pelvic thrombophlebitis* is character-ized by a persistent spiking fever for seven to ten days after delivery, despite antibiotic therapy.

Diagnosis

Evaluation of a febrile postpartum patient should include a careful history and physical examination. Extrapelvic causes of fever, such as breast engorgement, mastitis, aspir-ation pneumonia, atelectasis, pyelonephritis, thrombophlebitis, or wound infection should be excluded.

Although a pelvic examination is generally not helpful in diagnosing pelvic thrombophle-bitis, occasionally, tender, thrombosed, and edematous ovarian, parauterine, and/or iliac veins may be palpated. However, this diag-nosis is usually made by exclusion and the prompt lysis of fever following commence-ment of heparin anticoagulant therapy.

Before the institution of antibiotic therapy for puerperal endometritis, two aerobic and anaerobic cultures should be obtained from the blood, endocervix, and uterine cavity, and a catheterized urine specimen should be obtained for culture. The antibiotic sensitiv-ities from these cultures may be used to determine appropriate second-line drug ther-apy in the event of failure of the first-line drugs. Antibiotics should commence follow-ing diagnosis rather than waiting for culture results, which may take several days for an-aerobic organisms.

Management

A febrile puerperal patient with cessation of lochial flow should undergo a pelvic ex-amination and removal of any secundines that may be occluding the cervical os.

The antibiotic treatment of puerperal in-fection usually follows two major principles. First, early antibiotic treatment should be instituted to confine, then eliminate, the in-fectious process. Second, the antibiotics should have anaerobic coverage because these organisms are involved in 70 percent of puerperal infections. Antibiotics should be continued for at least six to eight days, even when clinical improvement is obvious. An-aerobic organisms especially require pro-longed chemotherapy for elimination.

Broad-spectrum antibiotics, such as ampi-cillin and the cephalosporins, are effective first-line drugs for mild and moderate cases of puerperal infection. When the infection is moderate to severe, a penicillin-aminoglyco-side combination has traditionally been used as first-line therapy. However, the major pelvic pathogen resistant to this combination is *Bacteroides fragilis*, which is usually sensi-tive to either clindamycin or chlorampheni-col. Therefore, the use of clindamycin with either an aminoglycoside or ampicillin should provide better first-line coverage.

When pelvic thrombophlebitis and/or thromboembolism is suspected or clinically diagnosed, heparin therapy should be insti-tuted to increase the clotting time (Lee-White) or activated prothrombin time two to three times above normal. Only two to three weeks of anticoagulant therapy are needed for uncomplicated pelvic thrombophlebitis. Patients with femoral thrombophlebitis re-quire four to six weeks of heparin therapy followed by the administration of oral anti-coagulants for a few months.

If the patient does not respond to heparin

therapy, and the clinical course is one of unrelenting fever and pelvic tenderness, a diagnosis of pelvic abscess must be entertained. Diagnosis is made by pelvic examination and confirmed by pelvic ultrasound. The finding of a tender, pelvic parametrial mass suggests an abscess. Ultrasound will confirm that the mass is fluid-filled rather than solid. The presence of a pelvic abscess demands surgical drainage.

SUGGESTED READING

Cunningham FG, Hauth JC, Strong JD, et al: Infectious morbidity following cesarean section. Obstet Gynecol 52:656, 1978.

Gibbs CE, Locke WE: Maternal deaths in Texas, 1969 to 1973. Report of 501 consecutive maternal deaths from Texas Medical Association Committee on Maternal Death. Am J Obstet Gynecol 126:687, 1976.

Gibbs RS: Postpartum endometritis. In Monif GR (ed): Infectious Diseases in Obstetrics and Gynecology. 2nd ed. Philadelphia, Harper and Row, 1982, p 377.

Hayashi RH, Castillo MS, Noah ML: Management of severe postpartum hemorrhage due to uterine atony using an analogue of prostaglandin F2 alpha. Obstet Gynecol 58:426, 1981.

Lucas WF: Postpartum hemorrhage. Clin Obstet Gynecol 23:637, 1980.

O'Leary JL, O'Leary JA: Uterine artery ligation for control of postcesarean section hemorrhage. Obstet Gynecol 43:849, 1974.

Schulman H: Use of anticoagulants in suspected pelvic infection. Clin Obstet Gynecol 12:240, 1969.

Sweet RL, Ledger WJ: Puerperal infectious morbidity: A two year review. Am J Obstet Gynecol 117:1093, 1973.

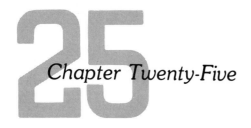

Chapter Twenty-Five

RHESUS ISOIMMUNIZATION

KHALIL TABSH and ROBERT MONOSON

Rhesus (Rh) isoimmunization is an immunologic disorder that occurs in a pregnant, Rh-negative patient carrying an Rh-positive fetus. The immunologic system in the mother is stimulated to produce antibodies to the Rh antigen, which then cross the placenta and destroy fetal red blood cells.

PATHOPHYSIOLOGY

A person who lacks the specific Rh antigen on the surface of the red blood cells is called "Rh-negative," while an individual with the antigen is considered "Rh-positive." A number of antigens make up the Rh complex including C, D, E, c, e, and other variants such as D^u antigen. Over 90 percent of cases of Rh isoimmunization are due to D antigens. Therefore, this chapter will be mainly limited to a discussion of the D antigen, although the same principles apply to any other antigen-antibody combination.

Among black Americans, 8 percent are Rh-negative, while among white Americans, about 13 percent are Rh-negative. When Rh-negative patients are exposed to Rh antigen, they may become sensitized. Two mechanisms are proposed for this sensitization. The most likely mechanism is the occurrence of an undetected fetal to maternal hemorrhage during pregnancy. The other proposed mechanism is the "grandmother" theory. This theory suggests that an Rh-negative woman may have been sensitized from birth by receiving enough Rh-positive cells from her mother during her own delivery to produce an antibody response.

In general, two exposures to the Rh antigen are required to produce any significant sensitization, unless the first exposure is massive. The first exposure leads to primary sensitization, while the second causes an anamnestic response leading to the rapid production of immunoglobulins, which can cause a transfusion reaction or hemolytic disease of the fetus during pregnancy.

The initial response to exposure to Rh antigen is the production of IgM antibodies for a short period of time, followed by the production of IgG antibodies that are capable of crossing the placenta. If the fetus has the Rh antigen, these antibodies will coat the fetal red blood cells and cause hemolysis. If the hemolysis is mild, the fetus can compensate by increasing the rate of erythropoiesis in order to maintain its red cell mass. If the hemolysis is severe, it can lead to profound anemia, resulting in *hydrops fetalis* from congestive cardiac failure and *intrauterine demise*.

The fetal and maternal circulation are normally separated by the *placental "barrier."* However, small hemorrhages can and do occur in either direction across the intact placenta throughout pregnancy. With advancing gestational age, the incidence and size of these *transplacental hemorrhages* increase. Most immunizations occur at the time of delivery, and antibodies appear either during the postpartum period or following exposure to the antigen in the next pregnancy.

If a pattern of mild, moderate, or severe disease has been established with two or more previous pregnancies, the disease tends to be either of the same severity with subsequent pregnancies or to become progressively more severe. It would be unusual for a woman to deliver a mildly affected infant following a previous delivery of a severely affected newborn. If a woman has a history of fetal hydrops with a previous pregnancy, the risk of hydrops with a subsequent pregnancy is about 90 percent. Hydrops usually develops at the same time or earlier than in the previous pregnancy.

INCIDENCE

Although transplacental hemorrhage is very common, the incidence of Rh immunization within six months of delivery of the first Rh-positive ABO-*compatible* infant is only about 8 percent. Also, the incidence of sensitization with the development of a secondary immune response in the next Rh-positive pregnancy is 8 percent. Therefore, the overall risk of immunization following the first full-term Rh-positive ABO-*compatible* pregnancy is about 16 percent. The risk of Rh sensitization following an ABO-*incompatible* Rh-positive pregnancy is only about 2 percent. The protection against immunization in ABO-*incompatible* pregnancies is due to destruction of the ABO incompatible cells in the maternal circulation and the removal of the red blood cell debris by the liver.

Transplacental hemorrhage may occur after spontaneous or induced abortions. The incidence of immunization following spontaneous abortion is 3.5 percent, while that following induced abortion is 5.5 percent. The risk is low in the first eight weeks, but rises to significant levels by 12 weeks' gestation. The risk of immunization following amniocentesis or ectopic pregnancy is less than 1 percent.

RECOGNITION OF THE PREGNANCY AT RISK

A blood sample from every pregnant woman should be sent at the first prenatal visit for determination of the blood group and Rh type and for antibody screening. In Rh-negative patients, the blood group and Rh status of the father of the baby should be determined. If the father is Rh-positive, his Rh genotype and ABO status should be determined. This may be done by testing the

father's red blood cells with the reagents available for the antigens D, E, C, e, and c. If he is homozygous for the D antigen, every fetus he fathers will be Rh-positive and could potentially be affected. If he is heterozygous, only half of his children will be affected. Thus, information regarding the zygosity of the father is only of value in absolutely predicting the presence or absence of the Rh antigen in the fetus if the father is homozygous.

The Rh-negative woman whose partner is Rh-positive and whose initial antibody screen is negative should subsequently have anti-D antibody titers checked at 28 to 30 weeks, and again at 34 to 36 weeks. The risk of transplacental hemorrhage increases at the time of delivery, especially with cesarean section or manual removal of the placenta. At delivery, cord blood must be sent for determination of the fetal blood group, Rh type, and for a direct Coombs' test. If a transplacental hemorrhage of greater than 30 ml of blood is suspected, a Kleihauer-Betke test is helpful in determining the volume of the hemorrhage.

The D antigen is a mosaic and has several alleles. D^u antigen is an incomplete variant that may or may not react with anti-D antibodies. Some Rh-negative patients who are D^u-positive and deliver an Rh-positive (D-positive) infant may become sensitized to the D antigen.

Maternal Rh-Antibody Titer

Anti-D antibody titers generally provide limited information regarding the severity of fetal hemolysis in Rh disease. A relationship between titers and outcome has been observed only in the case of the *first* sensitized pregnancy when the initial antibody screen is *negative*.

Amniotic Fluid Spectrophotometry

Analysis of amniotic fluid remains the most accurate method of gauging the severity of fetal hemolysis. A correlation exists between the amount of biliary pigment in the amniotic fluid and the severity of anemia in the fetus.

The source of bilirubin in the amniotic fluid is controversial. The most likely source is tracheal and pulmonary efflux; however, transudate from the umbilical and placental vessels may contribute. Because the standard biochemical methods for estimation of serum bilirubin are not sensitive enough for the small concentrations found in the amniotic fluid, spectrophotometric analysis is now the most widely used technique for estimating amniotic fluid bilirubin concentration.

Optical density readings are made over the 350 to 700 μ wavelength range, and the values are plotted on a semilogarithmic paper with the wavelength as the linear coordinate and the optical density as the logarithmic coordinate (Fig. 25–1). The optical density deviation (ΔOD) at 450 μ from a baseline drawn between the optical density values at 365 and 550 μ measures the amniotic fluid unconjugated bilirubin level, which in turn correlates with the cord blood hemoglobin of the newborn at birth.

Bilirubin is oxidized to colorless pigments when exposed to light; therefore, the fluid should be protected from light. Heme pigments and meconium may cause falsely high spectrophotometric values.

Bilirubin is normally found in amniotic fluid in a concentration that gradually diminishes toward term. For predictive interpretation, Liley devised a spectrophotometric graph based on the correlation of cord blood hemoglobin concentrations at birth and the amniotic fluid change in optical density at 450 μ. Using this method, Liley was able to establish predictive zones for mild, moderate, and severe disease. The Liley chart (Fig. 25–2) can be used to determine the severity of the disease and the appropriate management at a given gestational age.

Technique of Amniocentesis

Ultrasonically guided amniocentesis carries very little risk to the fetus or mother. An ultrasonic examination is performed to localize a pocket of amniotic fluid far enough away from the fetus and placenta to be safe. A 20-gauge spinal needle is inserted, and 10 ml of fluid is aspirated. The fluid is transferred to a dark tube to prevent deterioration due to light exposure and is sent for assessment of the ΔOD 450.

If ultrasound is not available, a suprapubic amniocentesis may be performed. After the patient empties her bladder, the presenting part is displaced superiorly and the needle is inserted above the symphysis pubis.

DETECTING FETOMATERNAL HEMORRHAGE

The *Kleihauer-Betke test* is dependent on the fact that adult hemoglobin is more readily

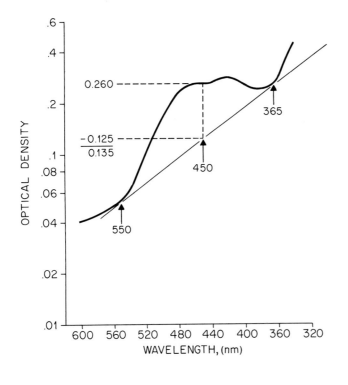

Figure 25–1 Plot of wavelength against optical density.

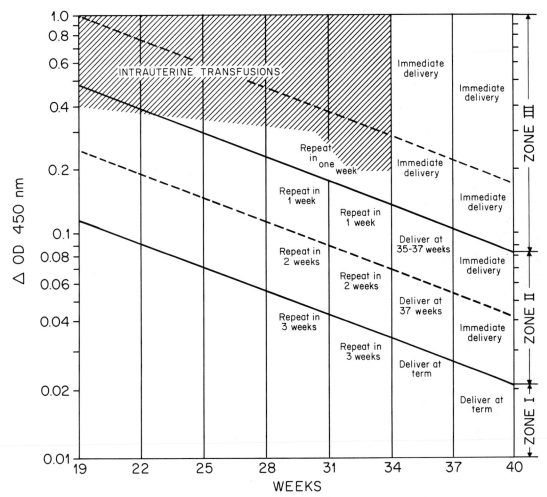

Figure 25–2 Modified Liley chart used to determine the appropriate management of the patient with isoimmunization.

eluted through the cell membrane in the presence of acid than is fetal hemoglobin (HbF). The maternal blood is fixed on a slide with ethanol (80 percent) and treated with a citrate phosphate buffer to remove the adult hemoglobin. After staining with hematoxylin and eosin, the fetal cells can readily be distinguished from the empty maternal cells. All cells are then counted, and an estimate of the extent of the fetal to maternal hemorrhage is made, based on the following equation:

CLINICAL MANAGEMENT OF THE RH SENSITIZED PATIENT

Because single ΔOD 450 values are helpful only if they are very high (zone III) or very low (zone I), serial sampling of amniotic fluid is generally indicated. The severity of hemolytic disease in the prior pregnancy provides an index for the timing of the first amniocentesis (Table 25–1). With serial sampling, one

$$\frac{\text{Number of fetal cells counted}}{\text{Number of maternal cells counted}} = \frac{\times}{\text{Estimated maternal blood volume (in ml)}}$$
$$\times = \text{ml fetomaternal hemorrhage}$$

TABLE 25–1 TIMING OF AMNIOCENTESIS

SEVERITY OF DISEASE IN PREVIOUS PREGNANCIES	TIMING OF FIRST AMNIO-CENTESIS (WEEKS)
No disease	28–30
Mild-moderate: Delivery at 37–40 weeks	26–28
Severe without death: Delivery at 34–37 weeks	24–25
Severely affected neonate with hydrops or stillbirth	22–24

of three trends will emerge. Falling ΔOD 450 values are indicative of a fetus that is either unaffected (e.g., Rh-negative) or very mildly affected. No intervention is indicated in these patients. If the ΔOD 450 is either stable or rising, frequent ΔOD 450 determinations are necessary. If the ΔOD 450 enters zone II or III after 34 weeks, determination of fetal lung maturity and delivery is indicated. However, if this occurs prior to 34 weeks, delivery is best avoided because of the risk of complications from prematurity. In this case, intrauterine transfusion is the treatment of choice if the ΔOD 450 enters zone III. The amniotic fluid L/S ratio and phosphatidylglycerol levels play a key role in determining the optimal timing for delivery.

Intrauterine Transfusion

Intrauterine transfusion was introduced in 1963. This technique has markedly changed the prognosis for severely affected fetuses between 20 and 32 weeks' gestation. The goal is to inject fresh Rh-negative packed red blood cells into the fetal peritoneal cavity, where they are absorbed via the subdiaphragmatic lymphatics and returned via the right lymphatic duct into the fetal intravascular compartment. After transfusion, the absorption of blood may be monitored with serial transverse ultrasonic scans of the fetal abdomen. In nonhydropic fetuses, the blood should be absorbed within seven to nine days. In the presence of hydrops, absorption may be slower but is occasionally quite rapid and may necessitate weekly transfusions with removal of ascitic fluid, if present. Repeat transfusions are generally done at one- to three-week intervals. The final transfusion is performed at 32 weeks' gestation and the fetus delivered at 34 weeks' gestation by cesarean section. Cesarean section is per-

formed because these very anemic fetuses do not tolerate the stress of labor well.

Other Modes of Therapy

Administration of *promethazine hydrochloride* has recently been suggested based on animal studies that have shown that the drug inhibits the ability of fetal macrophages to bind Rh-positive blood cells, therefore decreasing the hemolytic process. The efficacy of this drug in humans is questionable. *Maternal plasmapheresis* may be helpful in severe erythroblastosis when intrauterine transfusions are not successful, but perinatal outcome with this technique has not been impressive. *Phenobarbital* has been used to induce fetal hepatic microsomal glucuronyltransferase activity, thereby increasing uptake and excretion of bilirubin by the liver. Treatment with phenobarbital is initiated two to three weeks prior to delivery.

PREVENTION OF RHESUS ISOIMMUNIZATION

Because Rh isoimmunization occurs in response to exposure of an Rh-negative mother to the Rh antigen, the mainstay for prevention is the avoidance of maternal exposure to the antigen. Rh_o (D) immune globulin (anti-D gamma globulin) diminishes the availability of the Rh antigen to the maternal immune system, although the exact mechanism by which it prevents Rh-isoimmunization is not well understood.

Rh_o (D) immune globulin is prepared from fractionated human plasma obtained from sensitized donors. The plasma is screened for hepatitis B surface antigen and anti $HTLV_3$, the antibody to the AIDS virus. It is available in several dosage forms for intramuscular injection. Since the advent of its use in 1967, Rh-immune globulin has dramatically reduced the incidence of Rh isoimmunization. Between 1970 and 1979, the incidence of hemolytic disease of the newborn in the United States fell 65 percent.

Because the greatest risk for fetal to maternal hemorrhage occurs during labor and delivery, Rh-immune globulin was initially administered only during the immediate postpartum period. However, this resulted in a 1 to 2 percent failure rate, thought to be due to exposure of the mother to fetal red blood cells during the antepartum period. The indications for the use of Rh-immune globulin have, therefore, been broadened to include any antepartum event (such as amniocentesis) that may increase the risk of transplacental hemorrhage. The routine prophylactic administration of Rh-immune globulin at 28 weeks' gestation is also sometimes practiced. This approach is controversial because of concern about its cost-effectiveness and the safety of the volunteers who are used in the commercial production of the vaccine.

Indications for Administration of Rh$_o$ (D) Immune Globulin

The following provides a practical approach to the administration of Rh-immune globulin to an Rh-negative patient with no Rh antibodies.

During a normal pregnancy, 300 μg Rh-immune globulin is administered at 28 weeks' gestation, following testing for sensitization with an indirect Coombs' test. A 300-μg dose is administered following amniocentesis at any gestational age. If a fetomaternal hemorrhage is suspected at any time during the pregnancy, a Kleihauer-Betke test is performed. If positive, Rh-immune globulin is administered in a dose of 10 μg per ml of fetal blood that entered the maternal circulation. Following an uncomplicated delivery, 300 μg Rh-immune globulin is given within 48 hours. If a larger than normal fetal to maternal hemorrhage is suspected, such as may occur in patients with abruptio placentae or those requiring manual removal of the placenta, a Kleihauer-Betke determination should be performed after delivery and the appropriate dose of the Rh-immune globulin determined.

Establishment of fetal circulation occurs at approximately four weeks' gestation, and the presence of the Rh$_o$ (D) antigen has been demonstrated as early as 38 days following conception. Consequently, Rh-isoimmunization can occur at any time during pregnancy, from the early first trimester on. Since fetal erythrocytes can be readily detected in the maternal blood following induced or spontaneous abortion, 50 μg Rh-immune globulin should be given to all Rh-negative women following any type of abortion.

Fetal erythrocytes have been demonstrated in the maternal circulation following rupture of a tubal pregnancy. Consequently, Rh-immune globulin should be given to an Rh-negative woman with an ectopic pregnancy. Since chorionic villi in gestational trophoblastic disease are avascular and devoid of fetal erythrocytes, Rh-immune globulin is probably not necessary following molar pregnancy. However, at least one case of sensitization following a molar pregnancy has been reported.

Whenever maternal exposure to fetal cells seems a possibility, it should be investigated. For example, fetal death of unknown etiology, unexplained newborn anemia, and antepartum bleeding may all be associated with fetal to maternal hemorrhage. If fetal cells are found in the maternal circulation, Rh-immune globulin should be administered in a dose of 10 μg per ml of fetal blood entering the maternal circulation.

IRREGULAR ANTIBODIES

While the prophylactic use of immunoglobulins has led to a decline in the incidence of Rh isoimmunization, hemolytic disease of the newborn due to antibodies produced by other red blood cell antigens (so-called irregular

TABLE 25–2   HEMOLYTIC DISEASE DUE TO IRREGULAR ANTIBODIES

BLOOD GROUP SYSTEM	ANTIGEN	SEVERITY OF HEMOLYTIC DISEASE
Kell	K	Mild to severe (hydrops)
	k	Mild only
Duffy	Fy^a	Mild to severe (hydrops)
Kidd	Jk^a	Mild to severe
	Jk^b	Mild to severe
MNS$_s$	M	Mild to severe
	S	Mild to severe
	U	Mild to severe
Lutheran	Lu^a	Mild
	Lu^b	Mild
Diego	Di^a	Mild to severe
	Di^b	Mild
Public antigens	Yt^a	Moderate to severe
	Ge	Mild
	Co^a	Severe
Private antigens	Becker	Mild
	Biles	Moderate
	Good	Severe
	Heibel	Moderate
	Radin	Moderate
	Wright	Severe

Modified with permission from Weinstein L: Irregular antibodies causing hemolytic disease of the newborn: A continuing problem. Clin Obstet Gynecol 25(2):321, 1982.

antibodies) has increased slightly. This is probably due to the wider use of blood transfusions. Approximately 2 percent of cases of hemolytic disease of the newborn are due to irregular antibodies. The risk to the fetus depends upon both the type of antibody (whether it is IgM or IgG) and the strength of the antibody. For example, the Kell antigen is capable of eliciting a strong IgG response that may cause neonatal disease similar to Rh hemolytic disease.

When an irregular antibody is detected in the maternal blood, the father should be checked for the presence of that antigen. If the father is negative for the antigen in question, no further investigations are necessary. If the father is antigen-positive, the antibody is IgG, and the titer is significant (greater than 1:8), amniotic fluid studies similar to those performed in Rh disease must be carried out. A partial list of the common irregular antibodies that can lead to hemolytic disease of the newborn is shown in Table 25–2.

SUGGESTED READING

Bevis DCA: Blood pigments and hemolytic disease of the newborn. J Obstet Gynaecol Br Emp 63:68, 1956.

Blajachman MA, Maudsley RF, Uchida I, et al: Diagnostic amniocentesis and fetal-maternal bleeding. Lancet 1(864):993, 1974.

Bowman JM: Suppression of Rh-isoimmunization: A review. Obstet Gynecol 52:385, 1978.

Bowman JM: The management of Rh-isoimmunization. Obstet Gynecol 52:1, 1978.

Henry G, Wexler P, Robinson A: Rh-immune globulin after amniocentesis for genetic diagnosis. Obstet Gynecol 48:557, 1976.

Lawrence M: Diagnostic amniocentesis in early pregnancy. Br Med J 2(6080):191, 1977.

Liley AW: Errors in the assessment of hemolytic disease from amniotic fluid. Am J Obstet Gynecol 86:485, 1963.

Liley AW: Liquor amnii analysis in management of pregnancy complicated by rhesus sensitization. Am J Obstet Gynecol 82:1359, 1961.

Queenan JT: Current management of the Rh-sensitized patient. Clin Obstet Gynecol 25:293, 1982.

Queenan JT: Modern Management of the Rh Problem. 2nd ed. Hagerstown, MD, Harper and Row, 1977.

Weinstein L: Irregular antibodies causing hemolytic disease of the newborn: A continuing problem. Clin Obstet Gynecol 25:321, 1982.

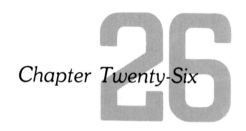

Chapter Twenty-Six

OPERATIVE OBSTETRICS

JOHN NEWNHAM and CALVIN J. HOBEL

In recent years, changing patterns of obstetric care have significantly influenced the methods of operative delivery. During the first 60 years of this century, retreat from a difficult forceps delivery was labeled "obstetric cowardice," and cesarean section was considered the end point of failed obstetric care. In modern obstetric practice, abdominal delivery is readily resorted to when an operative vaginal delivery would be hazardous to mother, child, or both. Widespread improvements in anesthesia, surgical technique, antibiotics, and blood transfusion have decreased the morbidity and mortality from cesarean section, making it a relatively safe option. However, the type and time of operative intervention remain among the most important of the many decisions involved in modern obstetric practice. Current acceptance of the liberal usage of cesarean section in no way obviates the need to acquire a full understanding of the mechanisms of normal child birth and the principles of safe operative vaginal delivery.

CESAREAN SECTION

Cesarean section is defined as delivery of the fetus through incisions in the anterior abdominal and uterine walls. The origin of the term remains a matter of dispute. Claims by legend that Julius Caesar was delivered via this route are unlikely to be true, since his mother lived for many years after his birth in a time when the operation would almost certainly have been fatal. It is possible, however, that the name was derived from the Latin word *caedere,* meaning "to cut"; or, possibly, from the Roman law *lex Caesarea,* whereby abdominal delivery of the fetus from a woman dying in late pregnancy was required in the hope of saving the child.

Survival following cesarean section was a rare event until 1882, when suturing the uterine incision was first suggested. Of the many subsequent milestones that further reduced the operative mortality, perhaps the most notable was the popularization of the transverse lower segment incision in the 1920s. This obviated the need to incise the thick muscular wall of the uterine corpus and excluded the uterine wound from the peritoneal cavity by placing the bladder flap over the lower segment incision.

Epidemiology

The rate of cesarean section deliveries in the United States has increased nearly threefold in recent years, from 5.5 per 100 births in 1970 to 15.2 per 100 births in 1978. The incidence of cesarean section in individual obstetric units is dependent upon the patient population and physicians' attitudes. Currently, the rate ranges from 10 to 40 percent of all births. It is generally agreed that the more liberal use of cesarean section has contributed to a decrease in the perinatal mortality rate.

Indications

The indications for cesarean section, singularly or in combination, are relative rather than absolute and can be classified as shown

TABLE 26–1 INDICATIONS FOR CESAREAN SECTION

TYPE	INDICATION
Maternal/Fetal	Dystocia
	Cephalopelvic disproportion
	Failed induction of labor
	Abnormal uterine action
Maternal	Maternal diseases
	Eclampsia/severe pre-eclampsia
	Diabetes mellitus
	Cardiac disease
	Cervical cancer
	Previous uterine surgery
	Classic cesarean section
	Previous uterine rupture
	Full thickness myomectomy
	Obstruction to the birth canal
	Fibroids
	Ovarian tumors
Fetal	Fetal distress
	Cord prolapse
	Fetal malpresentations
	Breech, transverse lie, brow
Placental	Placenta previa
	Abruptio placentae

in Table 26–1. The most frequent indication for cesarean section is dystocia, which usually presents as "failure to progress" in labor. This problem may result from cephalopelvic disproportion, fetal malpresentation, or failure to induce labor. There are several maternal conditions in which only a short trial of labor is considered safe, including eclampsia, pre-eclampsia, diabetes mellitus, and cardiac disease. Previous classic cesarean section is an absolute indication for a repeat cesarean section. Certain cases of previous lower uterine segment cesarean section and previous myomectomy that did not involve the full thickness of the uterine wall are now considered suitable for a trial of vaginal delivery.

Cesarean section is the appropriate management for fetal distress where vaginal delivery is not imminent. Many fetuses presenting by the breech are best delivered by cesarean section, particularly those in whom the gestation is preterm.

Types of Operation

Classification of the types of cesarean section refers to the uterine incision rather than the skin incision. The operation is generally performed through a *transverse* incision in the *lower segment* of the uterus (Fig. 26–1). The advantages of this approach include a decreased chance of rupture of the scar in a subsequent pregnancy and a reduced risk of bleeding, peritonitis, paralytic ileus, and bowel adhesions.

An alternative approach is the *classic operation* that employs a vertical incision in the *upper segment* of the uterus. A vertical incision may be made in the lower segment, in which case the procedure is referred to as a *low vertical cesarean*, although the incision invariably extends into the upper segment of the uterus (Fig. 26–2).

Several indications for classic and low vertical cesarean section remain and are as follows:

1. When a preterm fetus presents by the breech. In this circumstance, usually at 34 weeks' gestation or less, the lower segment is still poorly formed, and a transverse incision may be too narrow to allow an atraumatic delivery of the fetus.

2. When the fetal lie is transverse at any time during gestation, particularly if the back is inferior and the membranes are ruptured.

3. When access to the lower segment is restricted because of fibroids or, rarely, dense adhesions.

4. When hysterectomy will immediately follow the cesarean section.

5. When a postmortem cesarean section is done to attempt to rescue a live child from a dead mother.

6. When invasive cervical cancer is present.

Morbidity and Mortality

The risk of maternal death from cesarean section is four to six times greater than that from vaginal delivery. Problems related to the anesthetic are currently the major cause of mortality. The overall mortality rate from cesarean section is currently less than one in 1000, although the danger of the procedure itself may be approximately doubled by the medical or obstetric complication that led to the operation.

The maternal complications of cesarean section include those of the normal postpartum period and those of any major surgical procedure. Important complications specific to cesarean section are:

1. *Hemorrhage.* Primary hemorrhage may occur from failure to achieve hemostasis at the site of the uterine incision or from uterine atony, which may follow prolonged labor.

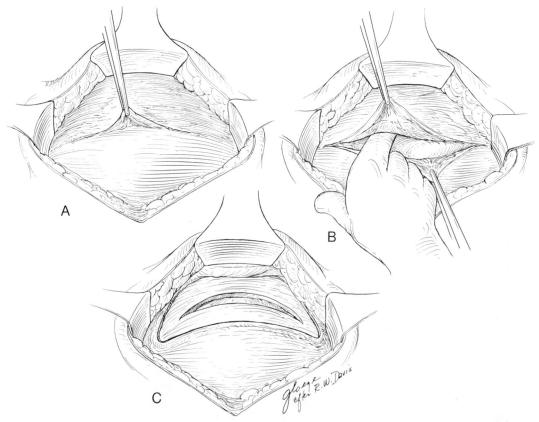

Figure 26–1 Lower transverse cesarean section: *A,* Loose uterovesical fold of peritoneum; *B,* separation of the bladder from the lower uterine segment, after incising the uterovesical fold; *C,* transverse incision through the lower uterine segment exposing the fetal membranes. Note the retraction of the bladder inferiorly.

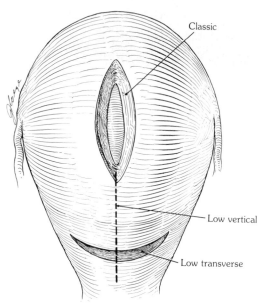

Figure 26–2 Types of cesarean section.

2. *Postoperative sepsis.* The frequency of this complication is significantly greater when cesarean section is performed during labor or in the presence of intrauterine infection. Prophylactic antibiotics for 24 hours significantly reduce the incidence of this problem.

3. *Injury to surrounding structures.* The bowel, bladder, and ureters are particularly liable to injury. Transient hematuria is common and usually results from vigorous use of the retractor in the region of the bladder wall.

Management of Subsequent Pregnancies

The mode of delivery of subsequent pregnancies relates specifically to the risk of uterine rupture. The probability of this complication, if labor is allowed, is about 6 percent for previous classic cesarean sections and about 1 percent for previous transverse lower segment cesarean sections. Rupture of a classic scar can occur prior to the onset of contractions. Whenever the rupture occurs, it may result in a catastrophic hemorrhage, with extrusion of the fetus into the peritoneal cavity.

Lower uterine segment scars are situated mainly in fibrous tissue. Rupture before labor is rare. Moreover, while extension laterally into uterine vessels can occur, dehiscence with only mild to moderate hemorrhage is more common. The dehiscence may not be apparent until manual exploration of the lower segment is performed immediately postpartum.

Because of these considerations, repeat cesarean section prior to the onset of labor is mandatory in the presence of a classic scar. For lower segment scars, the majority of obstetricians in the United States still adhere to the general dictum "once a cesarean, always a cesarean." However, many patients with a history of a transverse lower segment cesarean section are now allowed a trial labor. Contraindications to such a trial include a history of two previous cesarean sections, inadequate pelvic dimensions, the presence of other medical or obstetric complications, and fetal macrosomia.

Cesarean Hysterectomy

On occasion, it may be appropriate to remove the uterus at the time of cesarean section. This option may be lifesaving in cases of postpartum hemorrhage not responsive to more conservative therapy. Relative indications include cervical malignancy and severe damage to the uterus from rupture. Every effort to avoid hysterectomy should be made in those women who wish to retain their fertility.

OBSTETRIC FORCEPS

The obstetric forceps is a tool designed to provide traction, rotation, or both to the fetal head when the unaided expulsive efforts of the mother are insufficient to accomplish safe delivery. The first obstetric forceps was designed and used by the Chamberlen family in England during the seventeenth century. Widespread use of this instrument was not achieved in the United States until the early decades of the twentieth century.

Design of Instrument

The design of the obstetric forceps consists of two blades that are introduced separately into the vagina. The components of each blade are illustrated in Figure 26–3. All varieties of forceps have a *cephalic curve* designed to grasp the fetal head. Conventional forceps used for traction only (for example, Simpson) have in addition a *pelvic curve,* which corresponds to the axis of the birth canal. Forceps designed for rotation of the fetal head, of which Kielland's is the most

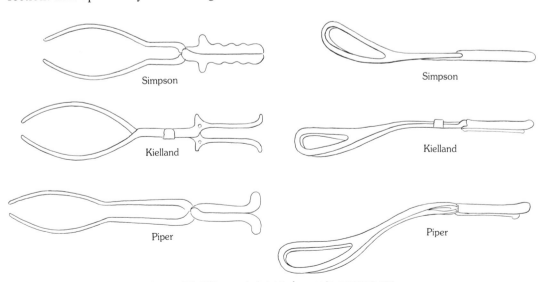

Simpson

Kielland

Piper

Simpson

Kielland

Piper

Figure 26–3 Types of obstetric forceps in common use.

frequently used, are characterized by the absence of a pelvic curve.

Indications

The indications for forceps delivery are best classified as maternal, fetal, or both. The most frequent indication is delay in the second stage of labor, caused by either abnormal uterine action or failure of the head to rotate adequately. Maternal conditions such as hypertension, cardiac disorders, or pulmonary disease, in which strenuous pushing in the second stage of labor is considered hazardous, may be indications for forceps delivery. Fetal distress is a frequent indication, but there is no place for difficult and heroic vaginal procedures when the fetal condition is already compromised. Forceps may also be used to control the aftercoming head in a vaginal breech delivery and to assist delivery of the head at cesarean section.

Types of Forceps Application

Forceps operations may be classified according to the station and position of the presenting part at the time the forceps are applied. The American College of Obstetricians and Gynecologists has proposed the following classification:

1. *Outlet Forceps*—The application of forceps when the scalp is visible at the introitus without separating the labia, the skull has reached the pelvic floor, and the sagittal suture is in the anteroposterior diameter of the pelvis.

2. *Midforceps*—The application of forceps when the head is engaged, but the conditions for outlet forceps have not been met. The sagittal suture is usually in the transverse or one of the oblique diameters of the pelvis.

3. *High Forceps*—The application of forceps at any time prior to full engagement of the fetal head. There is no place for high forceps in modern day obstetrics.

Requirements for Forceps Delivery

To embark on forceps delivery, the following requirements must be fulfilled:

1. Delivery must be mechanically feasible. This is determined by clinical assessment of the level of the presenting part, the presence or absence of molding, and the adequacy of the maternal pelvis. Engagement of the fetal head is mandatory.

2. The presenting part must be suitable. There are only three presentations in which obstetric forceps may be used: vertex, face where the chin is anterior (mentoanterior), and the aftercoming head in a vaginal breech delivery.

3. There must be no doubt regarding the position of the fetal head.

4. Uterine contractions must be present. Second stage uterine atony, fortunately uncommon, should be corrected by an oxytocin infusion prior to forceps delivery, not only because the uterine expulsive efforts are a vital component of delivery, but also because of the grave risk of immediate postpartum hemorrhage if atony persists.

5. The membranes must be ruptured. Intact membranes may retard descent of the presenting part, and their rupture may remove the apparent indication for the forceps.

6. The cervix must be fully dilated.

7. Anesthesia must be adequate. While outlet forceps may be performed with pudendal nerve block and local infiltration, Kielland's forceps rotation usually requires epidural or spinal anesthesia.

8. The bladder must be empty. It is routine to drain the bladder by urinary catheterization prior to forceps delivery.

Complications

Maternal Complications. Forcible rotation or traction may result in trauma to maternal soft tissues, ranging from mild abrasions to severe lacerations. Structures most likely to be injured are the vagina, cervix, and uterus, and bleeding may be profuse. Severe lacerations are most common with a difficult rotation forceps.

Fetal Complications. Inappropriate application of forceps resulting in one blade overlying the fetal face will produce unsightly bruising. This can be expected to disappear within the first few days of life. The use of excessive force for traction or rotation, however, may cause serious injury to the fetal scalp, cranium, or underlying brain. The risk for neurologic damage is greatest when a difficult forceps procedure is used to deliver an already hypoxic fetus.

VACUUM EXTRACTION

The vacuum extractor is an instrument that employs a suction cup applied to the fetal head. Traction is applied to the cup to aid the mother's expulsive efforts. The method has the following advantages over forceps:

1. Unlike forceps, the vacuum extractor cup does not occupy space adjacent to the fetal head. Hence, delivery by this method generally requires a smaller episiotomy than that for a forceps delivery, and in multiparous women, the fetus can often be delivered over an intact perineum, a situation rarely achievable with forceps.

2. Delivery of occipitotransverse and posterior positions does not require forced rotation of the head. Rotation occurs spontaneously at the station best suited to the configuration of the fetal head and maternal pelvis.

3. With correct application of the cup, the vacuum extractor functions to reduce the diameter of the presenting part by flexing the head. The elliptical shape of the deflexed fetal head can be converted to the smaller and more circular diameter of the vertex by traction posteriorly on the head. This is achieved by correctly placing the cup in the midline, over the posterior fontanelle, as displayed in Fig. 26–4.

4. Attempted delivery with the vacuum extractor in the presence of unrecognized disproportion will result in the loss of suction and failure of the procedure. In contrast, forceps will not dislodge during their inappropriate usage, and the unwary operator may proceed to inflict injury to the fetus, mother, or both by forcible and persistent traction.

Requirements for Vacuum Extraction

The requirements for the use of the vacuum extractor are the same as those previously outlined for forceps delivery, with the following exceptions:

1. While generally the cervix should be fully dilated, the vacuum extractor can be used, at times, in multiparous women in whom a small rim of cervix remains, provided the rim will displace easily over the fetal head.

2. The vacuum extractor is contraindicated in preterm delivery, since the fetal head and scalp are prone to injury from the suction cup.

3. The vacuum extractor is suitable for all vertex presentations, but unlike forceps, it must never be used for delivery of fetuses presenting by the face or breech.

Complications

The most frequent complication resulting from the use of the vacuum extractor is

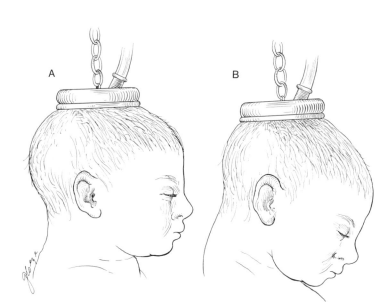

Figure 26–4 Application of the vacuum extractor. *A,* Incorrect application which deflexes the fetal head, thereby increasing the presenting diameter; and *B,* correct application over the posterior fontanelle, which flexes the fetal head.

vaginal laceration from entrapment of vaginal mucosa between the suction cup and fetal head. This problem can be avoided by digital examination of the entire circumference of the suction cup prior to initiation of the vacuum and traction. Fetal scalp injuries, including subaponeurotic hemorrhage and scalp lacerations, may result from prolonged use of the vacuum extractor. As a general rule, if traction on the suction cup during three contractions has not produced encouraging descent of the fetal head, the trial of vaginal delivery by vacuum extractor should be abandoned. If the cup is inadvertently placed on a face presentation, serious eye damage may occur.

CHOICE OF INSTRUMENT

Most obstetricians favor one of the two instruments, forceps or vacuum extractor, based on their experience, training, and general preference. Neither instrument is perfect, and neither is to be condemned. Perhaps of greatest importance is the operator's technical skill and judgment in preoperative evaluation.

SUGGESTED READING

Amirikia H, Zarewych B, Evans TN: Cesarean section: A 15 year review of changing incidence, indications, and risks. Am J Obstet Gynecol 140:81, 1981.

Bird GC: The use of the vacuum extractor. Clin Obstet Gynecol 9:641, 1982.

Bottoms SF, Rosen MG, Sokol RJ: The increase in the cesarean birth rate. N Engl J Med 302:559, 1980.

Cardozo LD, Gibb DMF, Studd JWW, et al: Should we abandon Kielland's forceps? Br Med J 287:315, 1983.

Cesarean Childbirth: Report of a Consensus Development Conference. US Department of Health and Human Services. Bethesda, MD, NIH Publication No. 82-2067, Oct 1981.

Chiswick ML, James DK: Kielland's forceps: Association with neonatal morbidity and mortality. Br Med J 1:7, 1979.

Dyack C: Rotational forceps in midforceps delivery. Obstet Gynecol 56:123, 1980.

Friedman EA: Patterns of labor as indicators of risk. Clin Obstet Gynecol 16:172, 1973.

Friedman EA, Sachtleben MR, Bresky PA: Dysfunctional labor: XII. Long term effects on the infant. Am J Obstet Gynecol 127:779, 1977.

Halme J, Ekbladh L: The vacuum extractor for obstetric delivery. Clin Obstet Gynecol 25:167, 1982.

Lavin JP, Stephens RJ, Miodovnik M, et al: Vaginal delivery in patients with a prior cesarean section. Obstet Gynecol 59:135, 1982.

Schwartz WH, Grolle K: The use of prophylactic antibiotics in cesarean section. A review of the literature. J Reprod Med 26:595, 1981.

Zalar RW, Quilligan EJ: The influence of scalp sampling on the cesarean section rate for fetal distress. Am J Obstet Gynecol 135:239, 1979.

III

GYNECOLOGY

J. George Moore — SUBEDITOR

EMBRYOLOGY AND CONGENITAL ANOMALIES OF THE FEMALE GENITAL SYSTEM

WILLIAM A. GROWDON

A knowledge of the embryology of the female genital tract is critical to the understanding of anomalous development of female genital organs. This chapter discusses the normal embryologic development of the female reproductive system, congenital anomalies, and the clinical features and management of anomalous development.

NORMAL EMBRYOLOGIC DEVELOPMENT OF THE OVARY

The earliest event in gonadogenesis is noted at approximately four weeks' gestational age,* when a thickening of the peritoneal, or coelomic, epithelium on the ventromedial surface of the urogenital ridge occurs. A bulging *genital ridge* is subsequently produced by rapid proliferation of the coelomic epithelium in an area that is medial, but parallel, to the mesonephric ridge. Prior to the fifth week, this indifferent gonad consists of germinal epithelium surrounding the internal blastema, a primordial mesenchymal cel-

---

*Gestational ages are given in weeks from conception, which is approximately two weeks less than menstrual gestational age.

lular mass designated to become the ovarian medulla. After five weeks, projections from the germinal epithelium extend like spokes into the mesenchymal blastema to form *primary sex cords*. Soon thereafter in the seventh week, a testis can be identified histologically if the embryo has a Y chromosome. In the absence of a Y chromosome, definitive ovarian characteristics do not appear until somewhere between the twelfth and sixteenth weeks.

As early as three weeks' gestation, large primordial germ cells appear intermixed with other cells in the endoderm of the yolk sac wall of the primitive hindgut. These germ-cell precursors migrate along the hindgut dorsal mesentery (Fig. 27–1) and are all contained in the mesenchyme of the urogenital ridge by eight weeks' gestation. Subsequent replication of these cells by mitotic division occurs, with maximal mitotic activity noted up to 20 weeks' gestation and cessation noted by term. These oogonia, the end result of this germ-cell proliferation, are incorporated into the cortical sex cords of the genital ridge.

Histologically, the first evidence of follicles is seen at about 20 weeks, with germ cells surrounded by flattened cells derived from the cortical sex cords. These flattened cells are recognizable as *granulosa cells* of coe-

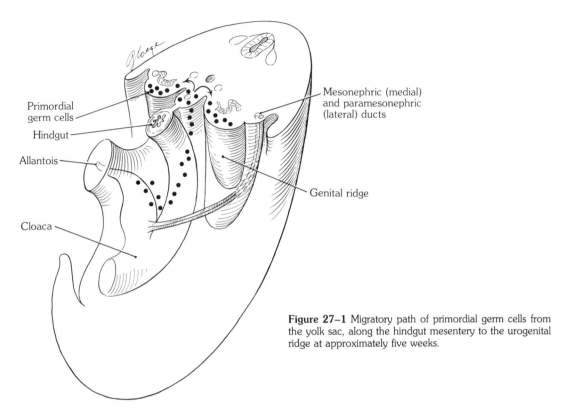

Figure 27–1 Migratory path of primordial germ cells from the yolk sac, along the hindgut mesentery to the urogenital ridge at approximately five weeks.

lomic epithelial origin and *theca cells* of mesenchymal origin. The oogonia enter the prophase of the first meiotic division and are then called *primary oocytes.* It has been estimated that more than two million primary oocytes, or their precursors, are present at 20 weeks' gestation age, but only about 300,000 primordial follicles are present by seven years of age.

Regression of the primary sex cords in the medulla produces the *rete ovarii,* which are found histologically in the hilus of the ovary along with another testicular analogue called *Leydig cells* that are thought to be derived from mesenchyme. Vestiges of the rete ovarii and of the degenerating mesonephros may also be noted, at times, in the mesovarium or mesosalpinx. Structural homologues in males and females are shown in Table 27–1.

INTERNAL GENITAL DEVELOPMENT

The upper vagina, cervix, uterus, and fallopian tubes are formed from the *paramesonephric (müllerian) ducts.* Although human embryos, whether male or female, possess both paired paramesonephric and *mesonephric (wolffian) ducts,* the absence of Y

chromosomal influence leads to the development of the paramesonephric system with total regression of the mesonephric system. With a Y chromosome present, a testis is formed and müllerian inhibiting substance is produced, creating the reverse situation.

Mesonephric duct development occurs in each urogenital ridge between weeks two and four and is thought to influence the growth and development of the paramesonephric ducts. The mesonephric ducts terminate caudally by opening into the urogenital sinus. First evidence of each paramesonephric duct is seen at six weeks' gestation as a groove in the coelomic epithelium of the paired urogenital ridges, lateral to the cranial pole of the mesonephric duct. Each paramesonephric duct opens into the coelomic cavity cranially at a point destined to become a tubal ostium. Coursing caudally at first, parallel to the developing mesonephric duct, the blind distal end of each paramesonephric duct eventually crosses dorsal to the mesonephric duct, and the two ducts approximate in the midline. The two paramesonephric ducts fuse terminally at the urogenital septum, forming the uterovaginal primordium. The distal point of fusion is known as the *müllerian tubercle* (Müller's tubercle) and can be seen protrud-

TABLE 27-1 STRUCTURAL HOMOLOGUES IN MALES AND FEMALES

PRIMORDIA	FEMALE	MALE	MAJOR DETERMINANT FACTORS
Gonadal			
Germ cells	Oogonia	Spermatogonia	Sex chromosomes
Coelomic epithelium	Granulosa cells	Sertoli cells	
Mesenchyme	Theca cells	Leydig cells	
Mesonephros	Rete ovarii	Rete testis	
Ductal			
Paramesonephric (müllerian)	Fallopian tubes Uterus Part of vagina	Testis hydatid	Absence of Y chromosome
Mesonephric (wolffian)	Gartner's duct	Vas deferens Seminal vesicles	Testosterone Müllerian inhibiting factor
Mesonephric tubules	Epoöphoron Paroöphoron	Epididymis Efferent ducts	
External Genitalia			
Urogenital sinus	Vaginal contribution Skene's glands Bartholin's glands	Prostate Bulbourethral glands Prostatic utricle	Presence or absence of testosterone, dehydrotestosterone, and 5-alpha reductase enzyme
Genital tubercle	Clitoris	Penis	
Urogenital folds	Labia minora	Corpora spongiosa	
Genital folds	Labia majora	Scrotum	

ing into the urogenital sinus dorsally in embryos of nine to 10 weeks' gestation (Fig. 27–2). Later dissolution of the septum between the fused paramesonephric ducts leads to the development of a single uterine fundus, cervix, and, according to some investigators, the upper vagina.

Degeneration of the mesonephric ducts is progressive from 10 to 16 weeks in the female fetus, although vestigial remnants of the latter may be noted in the adult (Gartner's duct cyst, paroöphoron, epoöphoron) (Fig. 27–3). While the myometrium and endometrial stroma are derived from adjacent mesen-

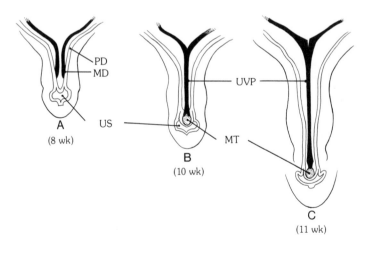

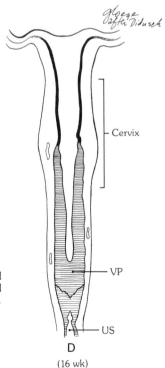

Figure 27–2 Early embryologic development of the genital tract *(A, B, C)* and vaginal plate *(D)*. PD, paramesonephric duct; MD, mesonephric duct; US, urogenital sinus; MT, müllerian tubercle; UVP, uterovaginal primordium; VP, vaginal plate. (Redrawn from Didusch JF, Koff AK: Contrib Embryol Carneg Inst 24:61, 1933.)

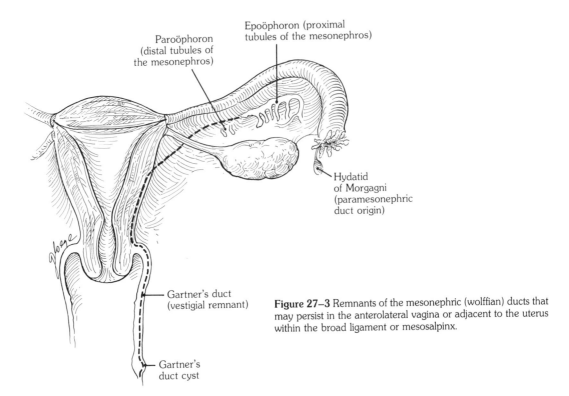

Paroöphoron (distal tubules of the mesonephros)

Epoöphoron (proximal tubules of the mesonephros)

Hydatid of Morgagni (paramesonephric duct origin)

Gartner's duct (vestigial remnant)

Gartner's duct cyst

Figure 27–3 Remnants of the mesonephric (wolffian) ducts that may persist in the anterolateral vagina or adjacent to the uterus within the broad ligament or mesosalpinx.

chyme, the glandular epithelium of the fallopian tubes, uterus, and cervix is derived from the paramesonephric duct.

Solid vaginal plate formation and lengthening occur from the twelfth through the twentieth week, followed by caudad to cephalad canalization, which is usually completed *in utero*. There is controversy surrounding the relative contribution of the urogenital sinus and paramesonephric ducts to the development of the vagina, and it is uncertain whether the whole of the vaginal plate is formed secondary to growth of the endoderm of the urogenital sinus or whether the upper vagina is formed from the paramesonephric ducts.

EXTERNAL GENITAL DEVELOPMENT

Prior to the seventh week of development, the appearance of the external genital area is the same in males and females. Elongation of the genital tubercle into a phallus with a clearly defined terminal glans portion is noted in the seventh week, and gross inspection at this time may lead to faulty sexual identification. Ventrally and caudally, the urogenital

membrane, made up of both endodermal and ectodermal cells, further differentiates into the genital folds laterally and the urogenital folds centrally. The lateral genital folds develop into the labia majora, while the urogenital folds develop subsequently into the labia minora and prepuce of the clitoris.

The external genitalia of the fetus are readily distinguishable as female at approximately 12 weeks (Fig. 27–4). In the male, the urethral ostium is located conspicuously on the elongated phallus by this time and is smaller, due to urogenital fold fusion dorsally, producing a prominent raphe from the anus to the urethral ostium. In the female, the hymen is usually perforated by the time delivery occurs.

ABNORMAL DEVELOPMENT OF THE OVARIES

Abnormal embryologic development of the ovaries is uncommon. Congenital duplication or absence of ovarian tissue may occur, and even ectopic ovarian tissue and supernumerary ovaries have been described. Although rare, the sexual bipotentiality noted in embryologic development can progress without

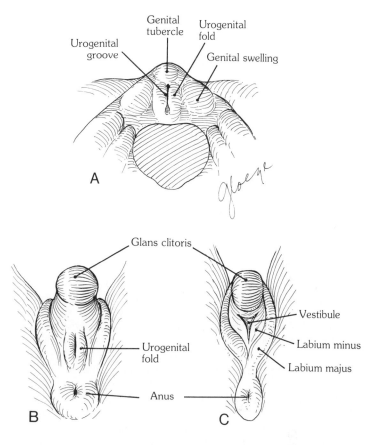

Figure 27–4 Development of the external female genitalia. *A,* Indifferent stage (approximately seven weeks); *B,* approximately 10 weeks; *C,* approximately 12 weeks.

the usual regression of one system, producing an ovotestis with subsequent intersex problems.

Genetic chromosomal disorders, such as Turner's syndrome (45 XO), are associated with a lack of normal gonadal development, as evidenced by the rudimentary streaked ovaries that are a hallmark of the disorder. Whereas this is nature's evidence that two X chromosomes are required for normal ovarian development, testicular predominance occurs with the addition of the Y chromosome, even in the face of multiple X chromosomes. Such predominance is seen in Klinefelter's syndrome (47 XXY) where testicular development occurs embryologically. This is due to the structural gene believed to be contributed by the Y chromosome, which ensures the presence of H-Y histocompatibility *antigen* on all cells containing a Y chromosome. Since both male and female gonadal cells have H-Y *antigen receptors* believed to be contributed by the X chromosome, only the male H-Y antigen contribution will cause testicular development from antigen-receptor interaction.

ANOMALIES OF THE PARAMESONEPHRIC DUCTS AND UROGENITAL SINUS

Anomalies of the fallopian tubes, uterus, cervix, and vagina are uncommon. Although the exact etiology of these malformations is unknown, the three most commonly accepted theories for their occurrence are teratogenesis, genetic inheritance, and multifactorial expression.

Many variations and combinations of anomalies occur. Lack of development (agenesis), incomplete development (hypoplasia), incomplete canalization (atresia), completely separate development, and variations of extent and level of fusion categorize these anomalies.

Fallopian Tube Anomalies

Isolated anomalies of the fallopian tubes, the end result of abnormal development of the proximal unfused portions of the paramesonephric ducts, are rare. Aplasia or atresia, usually of the distal ampullary segment, is most commonly unilateral in the presence of otherwise normal development. Bilateral aplasia is noted in some cases of uterine and vaginal agenesis.

Complete duplication of the fallopian tubes is rarely seen, but distal duplication and accessory ostia are relatively common. Because ovarian development is independent, the ipsilateral ovary of the involved aplastic or atretic side is usually normal in appearance and laterally placed near the pelvic brim.

Anomalies of the Uterine Fundus and Cervix

The most common anomalies are the result of malfusion of the paramesonephric ducts, with lesser or greater degrees of septation. Figure 27–5 shows variations of uterine development and indicates that communications can exist between dual systems at several levels. The genital tract may be obstructed at any level, although minute sinuses exist in some cases despite a lack of an obvious communication.

In *müllerian agenesis,* there is a complete lack of development of the paramesonephric system. Except for the fimbriated end, there is usually incomplete development of fallopian tubes, associated with absence of the uterus, cervix, and most of the vagina (Fig. 27–6). This condition occurs in an otherwise normal karyotypic and phenotypic female.

Vaginal Anomalies

The more common anomalies of the vagina include imperforate hymen, longitudinal and transverse vaginal septa, partial development (vaginal atresia), double vagina, and absence of the vagina.

Imperforate hymen represents the least of these canalization abnormalities, occurring at the site of vaginal plate formation in its contact with the urogenital sinus. After birth, a bulging, membrane-like structure may be noticed in the vestibule, usually blocking egress of mucus (Fig. 27–7). A similar anomaly, the *transverse vaginal septum,* is most commonly found at the junction of the upper and middle third of the vagina. At times, a transverse vaginal septum will have a sinus tract leading to recognition only when intercourse is later impeded. Patients with an imperforate hymen or transverse vaginal septum usually have normal development of the upper paramesonephric system.

Atresia of the vagina generally represents a more substantial lack of canalization at the caudal or cranial end of the vaginal plate. If cranially placed, the upper vagina and cervix may be atretic, with the uterine fundus and fallopian tubes unaffected.

A midline *longitudinal septum* may be present, creating a double vagina. The longitudinal septum may be only partially present at various levels in the upper and middle vagina, either in the midline or deviated to one side. Additionally, a longitudinal septum may attach to the lateral vaginal wall creating a blind vaginal pouch with or without a communicating sinus tract. These septa are usually associated with a double cervix and one of the various duplication anomalies of the uterine fundus, although a normal upper tract may be present.

Vaginal agenesis represents the most extreme case of vaginal anomaly, with total absence of the vagina and usually absence of the uterus and fallopian tubes—that is, *müllerian agenesis* or the *Rokitansky-Kuster-Hauser syndrome.* Isolated complete vaginal atresia with normal uterine and fallopian tube development is rare and is thought to be the end result of isolated vaginal plate malformation.

Concurrent Urinary Anomalies

It is generally accepted that the laterally placed paramesonephric ducts are guided in their development by the mesonephric system. The complex interaction of the three nephric systems and the urogenital sinus is not completely understood. However, it is quite common for an anomaly in one system to be associated with anomalies in the other. Urinary tract abnormalities are uncommon in the face of completely separate but normal development of the paramesonephric ducts, as occurs with uterus didelphys with a double vagina. However, where partial unilateral development occurs, as in the case of a hypoplastic rudimentary horn, a high incidence of unilateral renal anomalies exists, most commonly an absence of the ipsilateral kidney. Uterus didelphys, with one of two vaginas existing as a blind pouch, is associated with renal agenesis on the side of the pouch

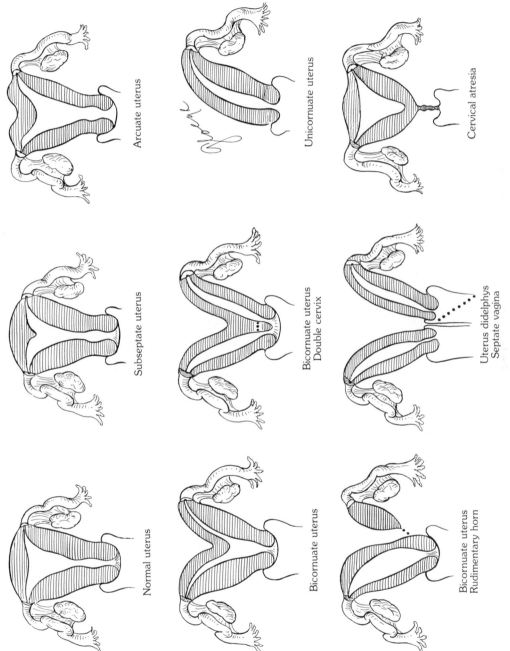

Figure 27–5 Variations in uterine development. The dots (. . . .) represent potential sites of communication or obstruction.

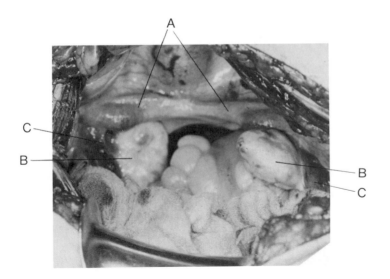

Figure 27–6 Internal genitalia in müllerian agenesis. Note the *(A)* bilateral nonfunctioning fibromuscular cords, *(B)* normal ovaries, and *(C)* fimbriae.

in 100 percent of reported cases. In patients with complete müllerian agenesis, other urinary tract anomalies may be present, such as pelvic kidneys, "horseshoe" kidney, and duplication of the collecting system (Fig. 27–8). In women found to have unilateral renal agenesis, approximately 50 percent have associated genital tract anomalies.

INTERSEXUAL DEVELOPMENT

Problems of sexual identification may be present at birth, or they may not become apparent until later, particularly at puberty.

The conditions may be classified as *female* or *male pseudohermaphroditism* or *true hermaphroditism.*

When ambiguous genitalia are present at birth, the problem of sexual assignment arises. Caution, sensitivity, and the avoidance of hasty decisions and confusing terminology should be the rule when dealing with anxious parents and relatives. Careful physical examination, pelvic ultrasound, hormonal stud-

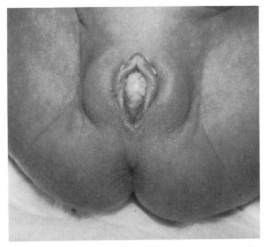

Figure 27–7 Neonate with a bulging introital mass, the tense imperforate hymen blocking the egress of mucus from the vagina (mucocolpos). (Courtesy of Dr. Eric Fonkalsrud, Department of Surgery, UCLA Medical Center, Los Angeles, CA.)

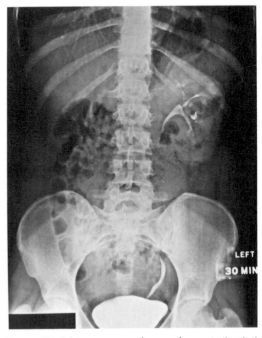

Figure 27–8 Intravenous pyelogram demonstrating ipsilateral renal agenesis in a woman with uterus didelphys and a blind right vaginal pouch.

ies, examination of a buccal smear for sex chromatin, karyotyping, and consultation with colleagues may be necessary before the *sex of rearing* is assigned. The assignment of sex will determine the need for any corrective surgery or hormonal manipulation and the manner in which the parents rear the child. These factors are all critical to the child's proper gender identification.

Female Pseudohermaphroditism

Female pseudohermaphroditism is due to masculinization occurring *in utero,* the infant presenting with ambiguous genitalia. Masculinization of the genetically female fetus occurs secondary to the endogenous hormonal milieu, as in *congenital adrenal hyperplasia,* or as a result of *exogenous hormonal ingestion* by the mother, usually in the form of androgenic progestins. *Tumors of the ovary or adrenal gland,* which produce androgens, may also rarely cause this problem.

Enlargement of the clitoris is the most conspicuous abnormality. There are also various degrees of fusion of the labioscrotal folds, producing a hypospadiac urethral meatus and a malpositioned vaginal orifice (Fig. 27–9). Internal genital development is nor-

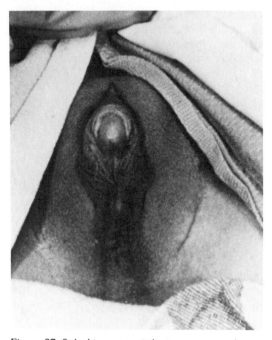

Figure 27–9 Ambiguous genitalia in a patient with congenital adrenal hyperplasia. This female exhibited clitoromegaly, hypospadias, and obscure vaginal orifice.

mal. Congenital adrenal hyperplasia is discussed in Chapter 48.

Male Pseudo-hermaphroditism

When the genetic sex is male (46 XY), there may be complete external phenotypic development along female lines. This occurs in the *testicular feminization syndrome* (androgen insensitivity syndrome), a genetic abnormality most commonly inherited as an X-linked recessive disorder. Secondary sexual characteristics appear at puberty along normal female lines, and the disorder is generally not recognized until menarche has failed to occur. Testes are usually undescended and located in the inguinal canals or labial areas. External genitalia are generally normal on examination, with the exception of scanty or absent pubic hair. Sufficient vaginal development to allow adequate coital activity is present in many cases. The gonads have normal testicular histology, and serum testosterone levels are normal. However, because of a genetic deficiency of androgen receptors, the external genital development is along female lines. Müllerian inhibiting substance is produced, which is the reason for the lack of müllerian duct development.

Male pseudohermaphrodites may occur with varying degrees of virilization and varying degrees of müllerian development. These result most commonly from genetic mosaicism, such as 45 XO/46 XY. Many factors must be taken into account in the determination of gender role in these cases, and a full discussion of this problem is beyond the scope of this book.

True Hermaphroditism

In true hermaphroditism, which is rare, dual gonadal development occurs, either in the form of an ovotestis or as a separate ovary and testis. Although some of these cases represent mosaics of normal female and male chromosomal complement, the usual chromosomal pattern is 46 XX. Most true hermaphrodites have some degree of both female and male development internally and externally. The extent to which masculinization occurs depends on the relative amount of testicular tissue and its relative contribution of testosterone. Confirmation of the diagnosis requires laparotomy.

CLINICAL IMPLICATIONS OF FEMALE GENITAL ANOMALIES

Many anomalies of the female genital tract go unrecognized prior to puberty and, more specifically, menarche. Others, such as unilateral paramesonephric development along normal lines or uterus didelphys, may produce no signs and symptoms and go unrecognized throughout life.

Symptoms

The more usual complaints associated with female genital anomalies are listed in Table 27–2. Many of the anomalies present with symptoms caused by the collection of blood generated by a functioning endometrium. An imperforate hymen may present as a bluish membrane bulging at the vestibule. Cyclic abdominal pain after puberty associated with the presence of a pelvic mass may represent a hematocolpos, hematometra, and/or hematosalpinx. These disorders are produced by the collection of blood above various levels of obstruction resulting from vaginal atresia, longitudinal septa with obstruction, transverse septa with obstruction, or, rarely, isolated cervical atresia. A rudimentary uterine horn with functioning endometrium may produce a hematometra. The symptom complex is quite variable. Some patients may have significant collections of blood in the genital tract with spillage into the peritoneal cavity, yet have minimal signs and symptoms.

TABLE 27–2 SYMPTOMS AND SIGNS ASSOCIATED WITH FEMALE GENITAL ANOMALIES

SYMPTOMS	
Primary amenorrhea	Leakage with tampon in place
Dyspareunia	
Dysmenorrhea	Irregular vaginal bleeding
Cyclic pelvic pain	Habitual abortion
Inability to achieve penile penetration	Spontaneous second trimester abortion
Infertility	Premature labor
	Postpartum hemorrhage
SIGNS	
Vaginal mass (hematocolpos, mucocolpos, Gartner's duct cyst)	Absent uterus/cervix
	Absent/short vagina
	Ambiguous genitalia
Abdominal mass (hematosalpinx, hematometra)	Absent pubic hair
	Fetal malpresentation
	Retained placenta

The extent of vaginal or uterine distension may be sufficient to occlude the ureter, either at the pelvic brim or lower in its retroperitoneal course. Flank pain may then be the most prominent symptom leading to discovery of the abnormality.

If a small sinus tract is present in a vaginal septum, it will allow the egress of a small amount of darkish blood or, if bacterial contamination has occurred, foul odorous vaginal secretions. This may delay the diagnosis by allowing decompression of a noncommunicating vagina. With vaginal agenesis, vaginal atresia, or a noncommunicating transverse vaginal septum, primary amenorrhea will occur. When a communicating double vagina is present, patients may complain of menstrual soiling, despite the placement of one vaginal tampon.

Sexual dysfunction may be the presenting complaint with genital tract anomalies. Inability to achieve penile penetration may lead to the diagnosis of testicular feminization, imperforate hymen, transverse vaginal septum, or vaginal agenesis. With vaginal duplication, there is generally no problem with sexual activity.

Physical Examination

Careful examination of the external genitalia, digital exploration of the vagina, and a bimanual examination through the rectum should be performed. In the case of vaginal agenesis, the gonads may or may not be palpable, but there are usually no palpable midline structures, since the uterus is absent in most cases. The erroneous diagnosis of a vaginal wall cyst, such as a Gartner's duct cyst, may be made in the presence of a noncommunicating lateral vagina. Pelvic masses should not be mistaken for distended internal genital organs due to distal obstruction without excluding the possibility of a pelvic kidney.

Investigations

Many diagnostic tools may be of use in detecting genitourinary anomalies. Sonography may elucidate internal anatomy, although it should be used only as an adjunct to careful history and physical examination, since the information obtained may be nonspecific. An intravenous pyelogram will elucidate unexpected anomalous urinary tract

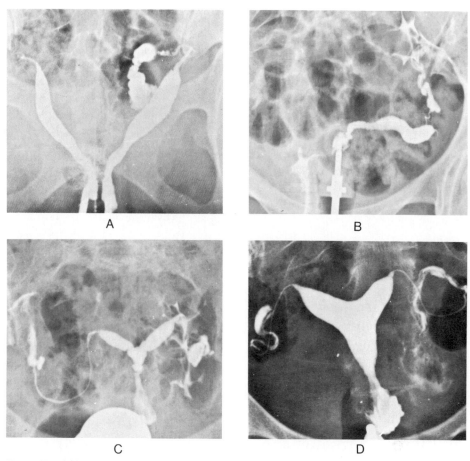

Figure 27–10 Hysterosalpingograms showing *(A)* uterus didelphys, *(B)* unicornuate uterus, *(C)* bicornuate uterus, and *(D)* arcuate uterus. (Courtesy of Dr. Marvin Weiner, Department of Radiological Sciences, UCLA Medical Center, Los Angeles, CA.)

development. A hysterosalpingogram will elucidate uterine and tubal architecture (Fig. 27–10). More recently, hysteroscopy, utilizing low-molecular-weight dextran as a distending medium in the uterus, has been used for the diagnosis and treatment of intrauterine anomalies, such as small septa. In difficult cases, examination under anesthesia combined with laparoscopic visualization of internal anatomy may be helpful, especially in the face of noncommunicating duplication anomalies.

Treatment

Many genital tract anomalies require no treatment. An imperforate hymen or transverse vaginal septum requires excision of the obstructing tissue to remove the obstruction. In a patient with vaginal agenesis, creation of a neovagina using a split thickness skin graft is required. In a patient with a uterine anomaly, the reproductive function should be tested prior to surgical manipulation; however, should a septum in the uterine fundus be identified as a factor contributing to habitual abortion, it may be surgically excised. Favorable pregnancy rates have been noted after some unification procedures, although delivery by cesarean section is necessary to prevent rupture of the uterus. In a phenotypic female with a Y chromosome, localization and removal of the gonadal tissue and subsequent hormonal management are necessary, since neoplastic transformation commonly occurs in these gonads.

SUGGESTED READING

Arey LB: The genital system. In Developmental Anatomy. Philadelphia, W B Saunders Co, 1974, p 315.

Davies J: Human Developmental Anatomy. New York, Ronald Press Co, 1963, p 177.

Gilman J: The development of the gonads in man, with a consideration of the role of fetal endocrines and the histogenesis of ovarian tumors. Contrib Embryol Carneg Inst 32:84, 1948.

Gilsanz V, Cleveland RH, Reid BS: Duplication of the müllerian duct and genitourinary malformation. Radiology 144:793, 1982.

Hamilton WJ, Mossman HW: Urogenital system. In Human Embryology. Baltimore, Williams and Wilkins Co, 1972, p 377.

Jones HW Jr, Scott WW: Genital Anomalies and Related Disorders. Baltimore, Williams and Wilkins Co, 1971.

Koff AK: Development of the vagina in the human fetus. Contrib Embryol Carneg Inst 24:61, 1933.

Rock JA, Jones HW Jr: The double uterus associated with obstructed hemivagina and ipsilateral renal agenesis. Am J Obstet Gynecol 138:339, 1980.

Spaulding MH: The development of the external genitalia in the human embryo. Contrib Embryol Carneg Inst 13:67, 1921.

Speroff L, Glass RH, Kase NG: Normal and abnormal sexual development. In Clinical Gynecologic Endocrinology and Infertility. 3rd ed. Baltimore, Williams and Wilkins Co, 1983, p 335.

Ulfelder H, Robboy S: The embryological development of the human vagina. Am J Obstet Gynecol 126:769, 1976.

Valdes C, Srini M, Malinak LR: Ultrasound evaluation of female genital tract anomalies: A review of 64 cases. Am J Obstet Gynecol 149:285, 1984.

Witschi E: Migration of the germ cells of human embryos from the yolk sac to the primitive gonadal folds. Contrib Embryol Carneg Inst 32:69, 1948.

Chapter Twenty-Eight

DYSMENORRHEA AND PREMENSTRUAL SYNDROME

JOHN E. BUSTER

Dysmenorrhea and premenstrual syndrome (PMS) are the most common afflictions of women of reproductive age. *Primary dysmenorrhea* is painful menstruation with no detectable organic disease; it is generally regarded as a functional disorder. *Secondary*, or *acquired, dysmenorrhea* frequently signals the presence of significant pelvic pathology. *Premenstrual syndrome* is a cluster of physical and psychologic discomforts that commence in varying patterns from 7 to 10 days premenstrually and markedly decrease after the onset of the menses. The premenstrual syndrome includes symptoms such as headache, breast tenderness, abdominal swelling, tiredness, and sweet craving, in addition to coexisting hostility, anxiety, and depression.

Although dysmenorrhea and premenstrual syndrome are separate entities, they can both occur in the same woman. There is a tendency, however, for younger women in their teens and early twenties to describe mostly primary dysmenorrhea-type symptoms, while those in their thirties and forties focus less on pain and more on premenstrual symptoms, such as headaches and depression. These problems are of importance to health care providers because of concern about the possible adverse impact they may have on a woman's productivity and judgment.

DYSMENORRHEA

Primary Dysmenorrhea

Pathophysiology. The uterine contractile pattern of the menstruating woman experiencing primary dysmenorrhea differs from that observed in menstruating normal control subjects. When microtransducer-tipped intrauterine pressure tracings are obtained, measurements from nondysmenorrheic women normally show contractile pressures that last 30 to 90 seconds, are in the 50 to 150 mm H_2O range, and terminate with complete relaxation. In women with dysmenorrhea, the absolute contractile pressure is approximately the same, but the duration of the contraction is longer, and the resting tone frequently does not return to zero.

It is reasonable to assume that the uterine contractions play a central role in the production of the "labor-like" pain experienced by women with primary dysmenorrhea. The reason for the association of pain perception with uterine contractions is not clear. Uterine muscle ischemia is thought to be one factor, but prostaglandin (PG)-mediated sensitization of neuronal endings may be a secondary contributing factor.

The release of prostaglandins as a consequence of endometrial tissue disintegration is a central factor in the pathogenesis of primary dysmenorrhea. Increasing prostaglandin content in menstrual fluid is linearly correlated with an increasing perception of cramping menstrual pain.

The process of uterine contractions begins with corpus luteum lysis and the withdrawal of progesterone, which normally supports endometrial tissues. Lysosomes are labilized and lysed with the release of phospholipases or phospholipid hydrolyzing enzymes. Cell wall phosphatidyl glycerol, an important structural element of cell membranes, is thus hydrolyzed with the release of arachidonic acid. The liberated arachidonic acid is metabolized to form a group of cyclic short-lived prostaglandin precursors that quickly become the classic prostaglandins F_2-alpha (PGF_2-alpha) and E_2 (PGE_2).

Both PGE_2 and PGF_2-alpha induce myometrial contractions *in vitro*. There is a striking similarity between the clinical symptoms of primary dysmenorrhea and similar symptoms induced by intravenous infusion of PGE_2 and PGF_2-alpha. Also, associated symptoms of nausea, vomiting, dizziness, hypotension, and pallor are well known effects of systemic infusion of PGF_2-alpha and PGE_2.

With continued arachidonic acid release, prostaglandin synthesis, increasing myometrial contractility, and increasing arteriolar constriction, the patient perceives painful uterine cramping. Figure 28–1 is a schematic summary of the relationships among endometrial cell-wall breakdown, prostaglandin synthesis, prostaglandin-induced uterine contractions, and menstrual pain.

Clinical Features. The onset of cramping dysmenorrhea usually begins several hours prior to the onset of vaginal bleeding, with symptoms reaching maximum severity on the first day of flow. Cramping may persist only a few hours or may last for two or three days. Symptoms can range from mild cramps to pain severe enough to be incapacitating. The characteristic cramping pain is normally localized to the lower abdomen but may radiate into the lower back and upper thighs. Many women equate the pain to that of intestinal colic. Some describe coexisting symptoms, such as dizziness, hypotension, and pallor.

Symptoms of primary dysmenorrhea begin during the early teenage years and are usually present within six months to a year from the onset of ovulatory cycles. By age 14, nearly half of all teenage girls will have experienced dysmenorrhea. Symptoms normally diminish with advancing age. Although it has long been taught that the first childbirth alleviates dysmenorrhea, this is probably not consistently true and has never been well documented.

Treatment. Nonsteroidal anti-inflamma-

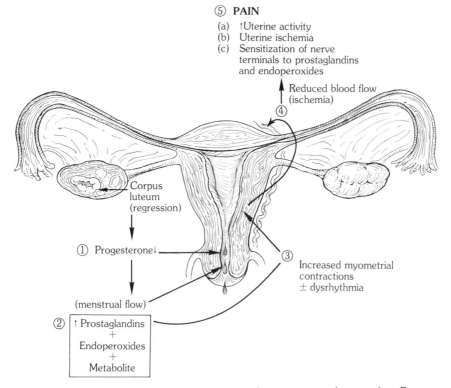

⑤ **PAIN**
(a) ↑Uterine activity
(b) Uterine ischemia
(c) Sensitization of nerve terminals to prostaglandins and endoperoxides

Reduced blood flow (ischemia)
④

Corpus luteum (regression)

① Progesterone↓

③ Increased myometrial contractions ± dysrhythmia

(menstrual flow)

② ↑ Prostaglandins + Endoperoxides + Metabolite

Figure 28–1 Postulated mechanism in the generation of pain in primary dysmenorrhea. Factors affecting central nervous perception of pain are not depicted. (Reprinted with permission from Dawood MY: Hormones, prostaglandins and dysmenorrhea. In Dawood MY (ed): Dysmenorrhea. Baltimore, Williams and Wilkins, 1981.)

tory drugs (NSAID's) are highly effective in the treatment of primary dysmenorrhea. The majority of patients receive nearly total relief from their symptoms. Within 30 minutes of ingestion, there is diminishing magnitude and frequency of uterine contractions and a decreased perception of pain. These drugs markedly decrease the production of endometrial prostaglandins by impeding the conversion of arachidonic acid to prostaglandins and their intermediates. Consequently, the quantity of PGF_2-alpha and PGE_2 released in the menstrual fluid is significantly decreased.

Although aspirin is a classic NSAID, it is not effective for most individuals. Three effective drugs and their doses are ibuprofen (Motrin), 400 mg every 6 hours; naproxen sodium (Anaprox), 275 mg every 6 hours; and diflunisal (Dolobid), 1000 mg loading dose followed by 500 mg every 12 hours.

Secondary Dysmenorrhea

Pathophysiology. The mechanism of pain production in secondary dysmenorrhea is not well understood. While prostaglandins are clearly involved as mediators in primary dysmenorrhea, the pelvic pain of secondary dysmenorrhea is generally associated with various pathologic conditions, such as endometriosis, in which the role of prostaglandins is not understood. Patients with endometriosis do have higher concentrations of PGF_2-alpha in peritoneal lavages done at the time of laparoscopy than do control subjects. Also, intrauterine devices, which trigger an endometrial inflammatory reaction with augmented endometrial prostaglandin release, are commonly associated with secondary dysmenorrhea.

Clinical Features. The clinical features distinguishing primary and secondary dysmenorrhea are shown in Table 28–1.

Differential Diagnosis. The distinction between primary and secondary dysmenorrhea is critical. Secondary dysmenorrhea may be the earliest clue to the presence of significant gynecologic disease. Various conditions are important to consider in the differential diagnosis of a patient with secondary dysmenorrhea.

ENDOMETRIOSIS. Endometriosis is the most common cause of secondary dysmenorrhea. Onset of this disease is normally in the late twenties and early thirties. The history is frequently that of persistent pelvic aching

TABLE 28–1 COMPARISON OF PRIMARY AND SECONDARY DYSMENORRHEA

CHARACTER-ISTIC	PRIMARY	SECONDARY
Time in cycle	Pain slightly before or during menses. Worst pain during menstrual phase.	Pain often not limited to menses. Pain not always worst during menstruation.
Relationship to flow	Pain usually related to first day of flow.	Pain less often related to first day of flow.
Consistency of pain	Pain remains the same each period.	Pain worsens over time.
Age at onset	Teenage years (usually within one or two years of menarche).	Older (20 to 30 for endometriosis; 30 to 40 for adenomyosis), but pain may begin with the first period.
Associated symptoms	Nausea, vomiting, diarrhea, headache, depression.	Infertility, abnormal bleeding, dyspareunia.

between menses with increasingly severe dysmenorrhea. The dysmenorrhea may be associated with rectal pressure and dyspareunia.

SUBMUCOUS FIBROIDS. The classic submucous fibroid history is that of increasing menorrhagia followed by episodes of severe pelvic cramping, occasionally accompanied by peripheral symptoms of hypotension, dizziness, and pallor. This is particularly true when the fibroid has developed above the internal cervical os where it may produce an intermittent ball-valve obstruction. The cramping can be so severe as to be diagnostic on history alone.

INTRAUTERINE DEVICE. Women wearing an intrauterine device (IUD) may experience severe menstrual cramping. The clinical history is normally clear, since the appearance of menstrual cramping occurs with the first menstrual flow following insertion of the IUD.

ANOVULATORY MENORRHAGIA. The passage of blood clots in association with anovulatory menorrhagia may produce labor-like cramping. The pain reaches its peak just as the clot passes through the cervix. Uterine contractions increase in magnitude before the clot has been passed and decrease thereafter.

PELVIC CONGESTION SYNDROME. Pelvic congestion syndrome is a poorly documented functional disorder in which there is a vague pelvic pain in association with a boggy, often retroverted, uterus. In addition to dysmenorrhea, many women describe other symptoms, such as breast tenderness, headache, irritability, and dyspareunia.

Treatment. The treatment for secondary dysmenorrhea is the treatment for the disease that is causing the symptoms. Specific treatment modalities are discussed in the chapters relevant to the various disorders.

PREMENSTRUAL SYNDROME

Pathophysiology

It is difficult to formulate a unified hypothesis that adequately explains the pathophysiology of the premenstrual syndrome (PMS). However, its existence is undeniable to countless women as well as their physicians.

Experimental Findings. A fascinating experiment was reported in 1981 in which the investigators tested the hypothesis that a premenstrual syndrome-dysmenorrhea factor might be present in the blood of symptomatic women. In this experiment, a total of 12 units of blood was collected from 10 women during their symptomatic period. Another unit was obtained at an asymptomatic time. The red cells were removed, and the plasma was stored in a blood bank. The units were then infused blindly back into the women at a time when they were having no symptoms. The symptomatic units produced varying combinations of dysmenorrheic-type pain and/or premenstrual syndrome-type symptoms in 11 out of 12 trials. The asymptomatic units produced symptoms in only 2 out of 10 trials. Seven out of the 10 women underwent hysterectomy shortly after the drawing of the units. They surprisingly had symptoms even in the absence of a uterus. The onset of symptoms following symptomatic transfusions was delayed 4 to 5 hours postinfusion, and the duration of symptoms was from 4 to 10 hours. The circulating factors responsible for these symptoms are unknown. Prostaglandins, once thought to be involved, have a circulating half-life of less than one minute and an almost immediate physiologic effect when infused. Other theories have incriminated autoimmune responses, histamines, and various kinins. This study has not yet been reproduced.

Principal Theories. The three principal theories used to explain premenstrual syndrome are (1) progesterone deficiency, (2) endogenous opiate peptide excess, and (3) pyridoxine deficiency.

PROGESTERONE DEFICIENCY. The possibility that premenstrual syndrome is caused by an insufficiency of progesterone production and a relative excess of estrogen has been widely acclaimed in the popular media. However, there has never been a convincing demonstration of abnormal levels of estradiol and/or progesterone in the circulation of women who suffer from premenstrual syndrome when compared with normal control subjects.

ENDOGENOUS OPIATE PEPTIDE EXCESS. A recent theory proposes that an excessive luteal phase production of endogenous central nervous system endorphins may inhibit the production of neurotransmitter catecholamines. It is suggested that abrupt withdrawal of the endorphin excess may lead to a rebound effect, with excessive catecholamine production just prior to the menses. It is finally suggested that a functional endogenous catecholamine deficiency may account for the depressive-type symptomatology that prevails early in the luteal phase. A functional excess of catecholamines may induce the increasing irritability, aggression, and psychosis that characterize the immediate premenstrual interval. While this hypothesis has more scientific substance than any other currently in vogue, it has yet to be proven.

PYRIDOXINE DEFICIENCY. A deficiency in pyridoxine is one of several theories suggesting that premenstrual syndrome is a nutritional deficiency resulting from dietary habits characteristic of western society. It was initially suggested that a deficiency of pyridoxine led to impaired liver estrogen metabolism and that the relative estrogen excess was responsible for the relative progesterone deficiency. Later, when it was discovered that pyridoxine is a coenzyme in the biosynthesis of dopamine, the theory regained credibility, since a catecholamine deficiency seemed to explain some of the premenstrual syndrome symptoms. However, no well-controlled trial to test the therapeutic effectiveness of pyridoxine in patients with premenstrual syndrome has been reported.

Clinical Features

The premenstrual syndrome encompasses a highly variable cluster of symptoms that appear to occur consistently in the same woman from one episode to the next. Onset may be as late as 2 to 3 days or as early as 10 to 14 days prior to the flow. The only similarity in all cases is the presence of a symptom-free interval shortly after the onset of the menses.

The symptoms change quantitatively and qualitatively as the luteal phase progresses and the onset of menses approaches. The earliest symptoms usually involve varying combinations of fatigue, depression, painful breast swelling, lower abdominal bloating, and constipation. Later symptoms include increasing anxiety, irritability, hostility, craving for sweets, and binge eating. A sensation of fluid retention is frequently experienced during the two to three days before the flow. Weight gain and edema are particularly common and distressing, although rarely is there more than a one- to three-pound gain. Premenstrual acne flair and headaches may precede the flow by one or two days. With flow, there is usually prompt relief from the psychologic disturbances, although some somatic complaints, such as headaches, may persist further for one to three days.

For some women, this monthly experience is devastating. Trivial episodes become major confrontations. Impaired judgment and forgetfulness may be incapacitating. The prevalence of this condition is not clear, but 20 to 40 percent of menstruating women may suffer from at least some discomfort.

Differential Diagnosis

Most patients seeking health care for premenstrual syndrome have already made their own diagnosis. The most consistent feature is the relief of psychologic symptoms with the onset of flow and the relief of physical symptoms shortly thereafter. Women with major psychiatric disorders may be misdiagnosed as having premenstrual syndrome because their symptoms are also influenced by the menstrual cycle.

Treatment

Psychologic Support. There is no documented effective treatment for premenstrual syndrome, but psychologic support for the patient is important. The pathophysiologic mechanism will eventually be understood, so it is important to tell patients that their symptoms are "credible." Taking the time to explain the opiate withdrawal hypothesis and the effects of blindly infusing symptomatic plasma (discussed previously in this chapter) can help to reinforce the "credibility" of the symptoms. Recording symptoms on a calendar may help the patient to predict their occurrence. Physicians should encourage families to provide effective emotional support and to plan discussion of sensitive or important issues at an appropriate time. When symptoms are mild, compassion and reassurance are usually all that is required.

Therapeutic Agents. There is a significant placebo effect from any drug used in this condition. In controlled studies, the placebo effect can account for 30 to 40 percent of the therapeutic effect. Various drugs have been used.

PROGESTERONE. Crystalline progesterone must be administered as an intramuscular injection or as a vaginal suppository because it does not reach the general circulation when taken by mouth. Progesterone proponents recommend doses of 50 to 100 mg intramuscularly daily or 200 to 400 mg vaginally twice daily, beginning with the onset of symptoms and finishing at the expected time of the menses. A rectal liquid is also available. Progesterone treatments are recommended only when more conservative measures have failed. They are not of proven benefit from controlled studies.

DIURETICS. These should be used with caution because they may induce hypokalemia. If a diuretic must be used because of excessive fluid retention during the last week of the cycle, spironolactone, 25 mg two to four times daily, is frequently recommended.

PYRIDOXINE. The usual recommended dose is 25 to 50 mg per day, although some have argued that only doses in the 500-mg range are adequate. Doses exceeding 1000 mg per day have been associated with peripheral nerve toxicity.

BROMOCRIPTINE MESYLATE. Although bromocriptine mesylate (Parlodel) is effective for treating the breast engorgement associated with the premenstrual syndrome in some women, it is expensive, and the side effects can be troublesome.

NONSTEROIDAL ANTI-INFLAMMATORY DRUGS. These agents, which were described earlier in this chapter for the treatment of dysmenorrhea, have been advocated for the symptoms of premenstrual syndrome, but they are of questionable benefit.

SUGGESTED READING

Bergsjo P, Jenessen H, Vellar OD: Dysmenorrhea in industrial workers. Acta Obstet Gynecol Scand 54: 255, 1975.

Chan WY, Fuchs F, Powell AM: Effects of naproxen sodium on menstrual prostaglandins and primary dysmenorrhea. Obstet Gynecol 61:285, 1983.

Dalton K: Premenstrual Syndrome and Progesterone Therapy. London, Heinemann Medical Books, 1977.

Dawood MY: Hormones, prostaglandins and dysmenorrhea. In Dawood MY (ed): Dysmenorrhea. Baltimore, Williams and Wilkins, 1981, p 21.

Irwin J, Morse E, Riddick D: Dysmenorrhea' induced by autologous transfusion. Obstet Gynecol 58:286, 1981.

O'Brien PM, Craven D, Selby C, et al: Treatment of premenstrual syndrome by spironolactone. Br J Obstet Gynaecol 86:142, 1979.

Pickles VR, Hall WJ, Best FA, et al: Prostaglandins in endometrium and menstrual fluid from normal and dysmenorrheic subjects. J Obstet Gynaecol Br Commonw 72:185, 1965.

Reid RL, Yen SSC: Premenstrual syndrome. Am J Obstet Gynecol 139:85, 1981.

Reid RL, Yen SSC: The premenstrual syndrome. Clin Obstet Gynecol 26:710, 1983.

Scommegna A: Secondary dysmenorrhea: Endometriosis. In Dawood MY (ed): Dysmenorrhea. Baltimore, Williams and Wilkins, 1981, p 131.

Speroff L: PMS—Looking for new answers to an old problem. Contemp Obstet Gynecol 22:102, 1983.

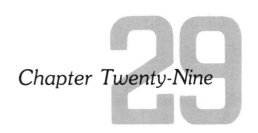

Chapter Twenty-Nine

BENIGN LESIONS OF THE VULVA, VAGINA, AND CERVIX

THOMAS B. LEBHERZ

Vulvovaginal disease is among the ten leading disorders encountered by family practitioners. Diagnosis is often delayed because most lesions produce pruritus and irritation, and there is a tendency for physicians to treat the symptoms without clinical examination. It is important to establish a specific diagnosis before initiating any therapy.

BENIGN VULVAR DISEASE

Medical History

In a patient with vulvar itching or irritation, it is important to inquire about general medical conditions that may have vulvar manifestations, such as diabetes mellitus, Crohn's disease, atopy, and psoriasis or other skin diseases. Urinary incontinence or chronic diarrhea may result in secondary vulvar reactions. Inquiry should be made about the use of soaps, perfumes, deodorants, and nylon or tight-fitting clothing, since these are known to be potential causes of vulvar irritation, especially in a patient with an atopic history. Previous therapeutic measures should be ascertained and the patient's response to such medications determined.

Physical Examination

Careful inspection of the entire vulva under a good light is of utmost importance. Many lesions of the vulva are small and subtle. A simple hand-held magnifying lens, a "poor man's colposcope," aids naked eye inspec-tion. A photograph taken at the initial and subsequent visits can be helpful to follow the natural course of the disease.

Diagnosis

Definitive diagnosis of lower genital tract lesions requires biopsy. In the Navy, there is a saying: "If it doesn't move, paint it." With vulvar and vaginal lesions, a similar statement might be: "If there is a gross lesion, biopsy it." On the vulva, some local anesthesia with 1 percent xylocaine, preferably with the addition of 1 in 200,000 epinephrine, is necessary for biopsy. The Keyes cutaneous biopsy punch or a newer disposable punch biopsy instrument can be used. If the patient complains of vulvar pruritus and there is no discrete vulvar lesion and no evidence of vaginitis, the Collin's test or colposcopy may aid in localizing the best biopsy site. These tests are discussed in Chapter 55.

Classification

Benign lesions of the vulva do not lend themselves to a completely satisfactory classification. Table 29–1 subdivides them into four categories: (1) inflammatory vulvar dermatoses, (2) vulvar dystrophies, (3) benign cysts and tumors, and (4) dermatoses not unique to the vulva.

Inflammatory Vulvar Dermatoses

Intertrigo. This term refers to an inflammatory eruption in body folds brought about

TABLE 29–1 CLASSIFICATION OF BENIGN LESIONS OF THE VULVA

I. Inflammatory vulvar dermatoses
   Intertrigo
   Secondary irritative vulvitis
   Hidradenitis suppurativa
   Fox-Fordyce disease
   Diabetic vulvitis
   Vestibular adenitis
   Behçet's disease
   Crohn's disease
   Bites

II. Vulvar dystrophies
   Hyperplastic dystrophy
   Lichen sclerosus
   Mixed dystrophy

III. Benign cysts and tumors
   Cysts—Bartholin's, sebaceous
   Solid tumors—hidradenoma, nevus, fibroma, hemangioma

IV. Dermatoses not unique to the vulva
   Psoriasis
   Acanthosis nigricans

by apposition of moist skin surfaces with consequent chafing. In the genital area, this problem is commonly seen in the genitocrural folds and inner thighs. Predisposing factors are obesity, occlusive clothing, and sweating. The skin may be fiery red with a malodorous oozing from secondary infection with bacteria or with *Candida albicans*. The affected areas are not sharply defined.

Management consists of correcting the secondary invaders, such as the *Candida albicans*, with an appropriate imidazole preparation. An antiseptic or antibiotic may be helpful for bacterial infection, and a steroid cream is often efficacious for controlling local itching. It is most important to keep the area dry and to educate the patient regarding basic personal hygiene.

Secondary Irritative Vulvitis. This condition presents itself as a nonspecific reddened area with itching and burning. A careful history may reveal the use of a specific irritant, such as deodorant spray or synthetic underclothes.

Physical examination may reveal redness and marked edema. There may be ulceration or even frank necrosis if the condition has been present long enough. Biopsy of these lesions reveals only evidence of chronic inflammatory dermatitis. At the initial visit, it is important to rule out the presence of a diffuse *Candida* infection, which can mimic secondary irritative vulvitis.

Management consists of having the patient stop using all deodorants, perfumes, scented soaps, colored toilet paper, detergents, and clothing softeners. She should be advised to use loose-fitting cotton underclothing. If the condition is severe, she may be advised to refrain from wearing tight pants, to wash in a shower, and to dry the affected area with a hair dryer rather than a towel. The simplest and most effective dusting powder is cornstarch, which causes no allergic response. Topical use of hydrocortisone 1 percent for three to four weeks may be prescribed to help settle the inflammatory response.

Hidradenitis Suppurativa. This is a chronic disease that results from blockage and subsequent infection of the apocrine glands, which are present in the hair-bearing areas of the vulva. The etiology is unknown, and patients may have the same disorder in their axillae. Once the process begins, it usually progresses slowly until all the hair-bearing areas of the vulva are involved. Initially, the patient presents with itching and burning and a skin abscess that opens and drains. Recurrent abscesses develop that coalesce and are extremely painful and tender. Eventually, the vulva becomes a mass of scar tissue, with chronically draining abscesses and sinus tracts. Biopsy allows definitive diagnosis, differentiating it from the chronic granulomatous vulvar infections.

Treatment consists of sitz baths, incision, drainage, and appropriate systemic and topical antibiotics. The patient should be cautioned not to wear tight-fitting underclothing or jeans. The use of oral contraceptives has been suggested to decrease the glandular secretions. Prolonged use of tetracycline can help prevent recurrent infections. If the disease process persists despite local treatment and prolonged antibiotic prophylaxis, partial or total vulvectomy with or without skin grafting may be necessary.

Fox-Fordyce Disease. This disease occurs almost exclusively in women during reproductive years. It may affect the vulva, axilla, or both. It is a disorder in which the apocrine sweat gland openings become plugged with keratin. Intense itching occurs as apocrine secretions leak through the dilated ducts. The skin changes are subtle, consisting of multiple, tiny, flesh-colored papules without erythema or induration. The intensity of itching correlates inversely with the level of estrogen during the menstrual cycle, and remissions are frequently noted in pregnancy. High estrogen oral contraceptives reduce apocrine activity and may produce sustained remissions. Topical medications for acne and topical estrogens may also be helpful.

Diabetic Vulvitis. Diabetic vulvitis (Fig. 29–1) is initiated by an infection with *Candida albicans,* but the distinctive features continue long after the fungus has been eliminated. Diabetics are particularly prone to infection with this organism, so in patients with repeated candidiasis, blood sugar evaluation is indicated.

The symptoms of diabetic vulvitis include chronic pruritus, irritation, burning, dyspareunia, and dysuria. Grossly, the lesion tends to be widespread, involving the inner thighs, perianal area, mons pubis, and the rest of the vulvovaginal tissues. Tissue edema is always present, and the involved skin exhibits a typical livid color variously described as intensely red, beefy, or port wine. White patches representing active *Candida* infections may be seen in the vestibule. Diagnosis can be made by cutaneous scrapings, which, in a potassium hydroxide (KOH) suspension, reveal pseudohyphae. For confirmation, the organism may be cultured using Nickerson's or Sabouraud's medium.

Effective treatment requires strict control of the diabetes. Local measures consist of control of *Candida albicans* with vaginal and vulvar applications of clotrimazole (Gyne-Lotrimin) or miconazole (Monistat). Cutaneous painting with 1 percent aqueous gentian violet weekly for three weeks is helpful. An oral imidazole preparation helps decrease the gastrointestinal reservoir of organisms, which is a source of reinfection. Patients should be advised to use only cotton underclothing, to launder bed sheets daily, to change underclothing frequently, and to rinse the vulva with saline or tap water after voiding.

Vestibular Adenitis. The minor vestibular glands are mucus-secreting glands with a short duct composed of transitional and squamous epithelium that connects the gland with the vestibular skin. The duct openings are difficult to see. There are usually between 2 and 20 such glands. For reasons that are not clear, these glands may become inflamed.

Clinically, these patients present with a complaint of introital discomfort and dyspareunia. The discomfort may be described as burning. Gross examination may be unrewarding, but careful study with a magnifying glass or colposcope reveals tiny erythematous foci with mild edema surrounding the gland openings. Frequently, the hymen is constricted, firm, and tender to palpation. Dysuria is often an associated symptom.

Treatment with topical antibiotic or hormone creams is usually disappointing. Laser therapy may be used to destroy the gland-bearing area to a depth of 1 to 2 mm. Alternatively, the involved vestibular tissue may be excised and the defect primarily repaired.

Behçet's Disease. This is a rare condition characterized by oral and genital ulcerations with associated ocular inflammation. The oral lesions appear like aphthous ulcers, while the genital lesions are more destructive and result in a scarred, fenestrated vulva. The etiology is unknown, but an autoimmune basis has been postulated. Bacterial and viral smears and cultures are negative and biopsy is unrewarding. Diagnosis is made on the basis of the concurrence of oral and ocular involvement, the recurrent nature of the disease, and the exclusion of other specific entities, such as syphilis or Crohn's disease. No specific treatment is known. Remissions may occur with high estrogen oral contraceptives.

Crohn's Disease. While Crohn's disease is considered primarily a disorder of the gastrointestinal tract, vulvar ulcers precede intestinal ulceration in 25 percent of patients. Typically, the ulcers are slit-like with prominent edema. They have been described as "knife-cut" ulcers. Draining sinuses and fistulae may also occur. Biopsy is helpful but not absolutely diagnostic. Steroid therapy is necessary for advanced cases, and occasionally surgical excision of vulvar lesions is required.

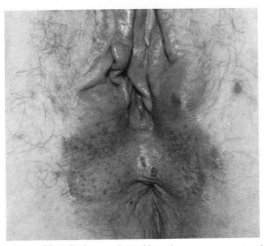

Figure 29–1 Diabetic vulvitis. Note the extensive perineal and perianal involvement.

Insect Bites. Two insects in particular are peculiar to the vulva: *Phthirus pubis,* the crab louse; and *Sarcoptes scabiei,* an itch mite. The organisms are usually transmitted through sexual contact, although they may be acquired by infected bedding and toilet seats.

Pruritus, particularly of the mons, is the most common complaint. Generally, the patient has identified the causative organism and presents for prompt treatment. Diagnosis can be suggested by seeing specks of "ground pepper" (excreta) on the skin. Nits or louse eggs may be attached to the hair shafts. A hand-held magnifying glass or colposcope is most helpful in identifying the organism. Closer identification can be made microscopically.

Treatment of both disorders requires at least two applications of the gamma isomer of benzene hexachloride (Kwell). Proper washing and heat drying of clothing and bed sheets is important. With scabies, all family members should be treated at the same time.

Vulvar Dystrophies

In the past, a variety of terms have been applied to disorders of vulvar epithelial growth and nutrition that produce a number of nonspecific gross changes. Such terms included leukoplakia, lichen sclerosus et atrophicus, sclerotic dermatosis, atrophic and hyperplastic vulvitis, and kraurosis vulvae. The International Society for the Study of Vulvar Diseases has recommended the classification of vulva dystrophies shown in Table 29–1. The malignant potential of the vulvar dystrophies is less than 5 percent, the patient at particular risk being the one with cellular atypia on initial biopsy.

Hyperplastic Dystrophy. This disease is primarily seen in postmenopausal women but may occur during the reproductive years. The most common symptom is pruritus. The surface of the lesion appears thickened and hyperkeratotic, and there may be evidence of scratching. The lesions tend to be discrete but may be symmetrical and multiple. Toluidine-blue-directed biopsies are necessary to make the diagnosis and to evaluate the presence of atypia or even malignancy. This lesion is often seen coexisting with vulvar carcinoma, but in patients followed prospectively, malignancy has developed in less than 2 percent of cases.

Treatment is quite specific, consisting of local applications of a fluorinated corticoster-oid ointment three times a day for six weeks. Typically, the lesion totally disappears. If a new lesion recurs, it must be managed as a new case with repeat biopsy and an additional six weeks of treatment with topical steroids.

Lichen Sclerosus. Lichen sclerosus (Fig. 29–2) is the most common of all white lesions of the vulva. It is characterized by pruritus, dyspareunia, and burning. It may occur at any age, but is most common in postmenopausal women. The lesions characteristically present with a diminution of subepithelial fat such that the vulvar architecture is atrophic, with small, even absent, labia minora, thin labia majora, and sometimes phimosis of the prepuce. The epithelium is pale with a shiny, crinkled surface, often with fissures and excoriation. The changes tend to be symmetrical and often coexist with perianal and perineal lesions that produce a butterfly pattern. Definitive diagnosis can be made only by biopsy, preferably directed by toluidine-blue staining to detect areas of atypia. Malignancy associated with this lesion is rare but has been reported.

Treatment consists of a 2 percent testosterone cream. This should be in a petrolatum base and applied twice daily for three weeks, then once daily for three weeks. A maintenance course of once daily or once every other day is continued, depending upon the patient's needs. The patient must be cautioned concerning absorption of testosterone, which will occur and may produce defeminizing or masculinizing side effects. Treatment must be continued indefinitely, since the tes-

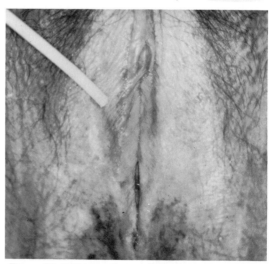

Figure 29–2 Lichen sclerosus. Note the symmetrical distribution of the atrophic changes, the very small labia minora, and flattened labia majora.

tosterone allows the patient to live with the disease rather than curing it. Approximately 80 percent of patients have a satisfactory response. Laser therapy and vulvectomy have been used. Recurrences are common following surgical treatment however, so close follow-up is necessary.

Mixed Dystrophy. As the name suggests, this lesion consists of hypoplastic and hyperplastic areas. It accounts for about 20 percent of vulvar dystrophy cases. Atypia occurs somewhat more frequently in this lesion than in pure hyperplastic dystrophies. Symptoms consist of burning, pruritus, and dyspareunia. The lesion appears as areas of piled-up keratinized white epithelium along with patches of pale, thin, shiny, wrinkled epithelium. Diagnosis requires toluidine-blue-directed biopsy, and multiple biopsies are necessary to exclude focal areas of atypia. Treatment consists of a fluorinated corticosteroid ointment three times daily for six weeks and then 2 percent testosterone ointment, three times daily for six weeks. Testosterone ointment should then be continued indefinitely. Areas of severe atypia may best be treated by local excision.

Cysts

Bartholin's Cyst. A Bartholin's cyst is the most common vulvar tumor. It presents as a swelling posterolaterally in the introitus, usually unilaterally. The cyst is usually about 2 cm in diameter, but may be up to 8 cm. It contains sterile mucus when punctured, and, except for the enlargement, it is usually asymptomatic. Secondary infection sometimes occurs, producing a Bartholin's abscess. Treatment is by marsupialization of the gland to create a fistulous tract between the cyst or duct wall and the skin.

Sebaceous Cysts. These occur at all ages and are especially common in black women. They present as single or multiple firm, yellowish cysts in the vulvar hair-bearing skin. The contents have the typical odor of sebaceous material. No specific treatment is indicated unless infection occurs or a cyst becomes too large.

Solid Tumors

Hidradenoma. This is an unusual lesion, seen mainly in women in their late twenties and thirties, that originates from the apocrine sweat glands. Hidradenomas are usually solitary and start as a small cyst-like lesion on a labium or interlabial sulcus. Initially, the overlying skin may appear umbilicated, but as the tumor enlarges, the covering epithelium becomes necrotic, leaving a central area of ulceration. Diagnosis and treatment are accomplished by excisional biopsy, which can usually be done in the office. The hydradenoma is never malignant, although histologically the papillary nature of the tumor may initially suggest an adenocarcinoma.

Nevus. Pigmented nevi occur on the vulva as they do elsewhere, but junctional activity, which carries a risk for subsequent malignant transformation, is more common in this location (Fig. 29–3). They may appear in a wide variety of colors. Excisional biopsy should be performed on all pigmented lesions on the vulva so that tissue can be sent for pathologic evaluation. These lesions should never be treated by cryosurgery or laser therapy.

Fibroma. Fibromas of the vulva are uncommon and when present are usually fibromyomas or fibrolipomas. They occasionally grow to a huge size. Neurofibromas may develop on the vulva as a manifestation of von Recklinghausen's disease. These lesions should be surgically removed if they cause a problem to the patient.

Hemangioma. The vulva may be the site of congenital hemangiomas. In the adult, three types of hemangiomata occur on the vulva. The small *cherry angiomata* are usually multiple and are less than 2 to 3 mm in size. They begin to appear during the fourth or fifth decade, and are generally asymptomatic, unless bleeding occurs with trauma. As a rule, no treatment is required. *Angiokerato-*

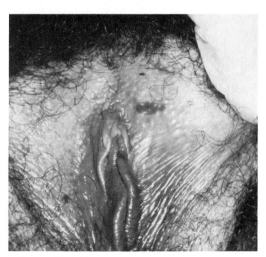

Figure 29–3 Multiple pigmented nevi on the vulva.

mas measure about 5 mm in diameter and are also frequently multiple. *Pyogenic granulomas* usually arise on the labia during pregnancy. They are the largest of the adult vulvar hemangiomas, and although some regression may occur postpartum, wide excision is usually necessary to prevent recurrence.

Dermatoses Not Unique to the Vulva

Psoriasis. Psoriasis often involves the genital area. It is usually evident on the outer aspects of the labia majora and the genitocrural area but can involve the entire vulva. Frequently, there is evidence of psoriasis elsewhere. The silver scaling associated with psoriasis in other areas is rarely present in the sheltered genitocrural area, so clinical diagnosis may be difficult. Biopsy of the lesion allows definitive diagnosis, since the histologic picture is characteristic.

Treatment initially with a fluorinated corticosteroid is usually justified, and the initial response may be satisfactory. However, chronic persistence and recurrence are common. Usually this problem is referred to a dermatologist.

Acanthosis Nigricans. This is a rare dermatologic problem that commonly involves skin folds, such as the axillae and genitocrural areas. Three variants of the disease have been described:

1. A *"malignant" variety,* itself a benign condition, which accompanies an internal adenocarcinoma, most commonly of the gastrointestinal tract. It spontaneously regresses with successful treatment of the bowel cancer.

2. A *"benign" variety* that may occur at birth, but which occurs more often in early childhood and, occasionally, in adulthood. After puberty, the lesion usually regresses.

3. *Pseudoacanthosis nigricans,* which develops most often in darkly pigmented persons and is invariably accompanied by marked obesity. The lesion usually disappears as the patient loses weight.

No specific treatment is available. When the malignant variety is present, a search must be made for an underlying adenocarcinoma.

VAGINA

Inclusion Cysts

These are common lesions that result from an infolding of vaginal epithelium. They are usually associated with lacerations from childbirth or surgery, particularly episiotomy. The cysts are usually asymptomatic and need not be removed.

Endometriosis

Endometriosis may occur in the upper one third of the vagina. It presents as cysts, often steel gray or black, that may bleed slightly at the time of the menses. These lesions are most common in the posterior fornix, where they usually represent an extension of endometriosis from the cul-de-sac peritoneum into the rectovaginal septum. Endometriotic cysts are usually 3 to 10 mm in size and, if punctured, are found to contain a thick, dark chocolate material. Diagnosis is made by biopsy. The lesions can be excised. If other endometriosis exists, it should be treated appropriately (see Chapter 32).

Gartner's Duct Cysts

These are usually benign cysts resulting from remnants of the wolffian duct. Rarely, a primary carcinoma of a Gartner's duct cyst can occur. These cysts may develop anywhere from the top of the broad ligament down to the middle one third of the vagina and are usually situated laterally. The cysts usually produce no symptoms and are diagnosed on routine pelvic examination. Unless the cyst is symptomatic, it should not be removed. Transvaginal excision may be necessary for large, symptomatic cysts.

Urethral Diverticulum

Urethral diverticuli are small sacs that can be palpated adjacent to the urethra. They arise from obstructed, infected periurethral glands that discharge into the urethra. The abscess lining becomes epithelialized, with the ultimate formation of a diverticulum. Diagnosis can usually be made by visualizing the opening into the urethral floor on urethroscopy; however, sometimes the openings are so small they can be missed. A pressure urethrogram is the ideal method of confirming the diagnosis. Urethral diverticuli can cause recurrent urethral infection, dribbling of urine, dyspareunia, and dysuria. Surgical correction is required if they are symptomatic.

CERVIX

Columnar Eversion

Columnar eversion is the most commonly seen lesion on the cervix (Fig. 29–4). Also

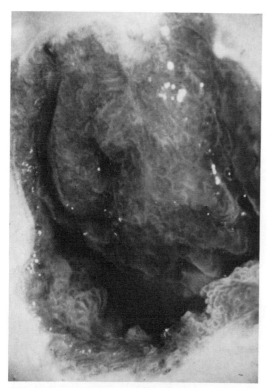

Figure 29–4 Columnar eversion. Note the transverse external os with columnar epithelium extending onto the ectocervix, particularly anteriorly.

erroneously called an "erosion," it represents a protrusion of the endocervical glandular tissue and is a physiologic process, not a disease. It is seen at birth, in patients on the oral contraceptive pill, and during pregnancy. In each of these situations, it is associated with hormonal changes that cause hypertrophy and hyperplasia of the endocervical glands. Because of lack of space in the endocervical canal, the glands must protrude beyond the external os. Columnar eversion may be associated with an increase in nonirritating vaginal discharge (leukorrhea). The diagnosis can be confirmed with colposcopy, and usually no treatment is required. Cessation of pregnancy or discontinuation of the pill is followed by gradual columnar inversion. Any remaining eversion will become covered with squamous epithelium through the process of squamous metaplasia.

Nonspecific Chronic Cervicitis

Nonspecific chronic cervicitis is a common problem. The numerous endocervical glands make the cervix prone to persistent infections, and puerperal lacerations are often a contributing factor in the pathogenesis of the condition. The infection may be caused by any of the organisms found in the vagina, especially staphylococci and streptococci. Chlamydial organisms may also be involved.

Clinically, the most prominent symptom is leukorrhea, which may be whitish or mucopurulent. Lower abdominal discomfort and dyspareunia may also occur. Speculum examination may reveal a chronically infected columnar eversion, and retention cysts of the cervical glands *(nabothian follicles)* may be present. If the usual causes of vaginitis have been ruled out—that is, *Gardnerella vaginalis, Trichomonas hominis,* or *Candida albicans*—further culture or monoclonal immunofluorescent stains for *Chlamydia* should be considered. In all cases, a Pap smear should be performed, and, if the endocervix is red or ulcerated, colposcopy, with or without biopsy, is necessary to exclude malignancy.

If *Chlamydia* is found, appropriate treatment with tetracycline, erythromycin, or trimethoprim should be used. If no specific cause is found, treatment with cryosurgery or electrocautery can be carried out if the symptoms are troublesome.

Cervical Polyp

The cervical polyp is a localized proliferation of cervical mucosa that presents as a soft, red, friable, usually pedunculated lesion. It may occasionally be sessile. It is generally only a few millimeters in diameter, but may reach several centimeters. The vascularity, ulceration, and secondary infection explain the bleeding produced by these small lesions. While the incidence of malignancy is very low, both squamous and adenocarcinoma can develop in these polyps.

Treatment consists of removal in the office, usually by twisting the polyp off and curetting the base. All tissue must be sent for pathologic examination.

SUGGESTED READING

Curth HO, Aschner BM: Genetic studies of acanthosis nigricans. Arch Dermatol 79:55, 1959.

Friedrich EG: Vulvar Diseases. 2nd ed. Philadelphia, W B Saunders Company, 1983.

Hart WR, Norris HH, Helwig EB: Relation of lichen sclerosus et atrophicus to development of carcinoma. Obstet Gynecol 47:122, 1976.

International Society for the Study of Vulvar Diseases: A New Nomenclature for Vulvar Disease. Obstet Gynecol 47:122, 1976.

Woodruff JD, Parmley TH: Infection of the minor vestibular gland. Obstet Gynecol 62:609, 1983.

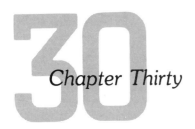

Chapter Thirty

BENIGN DISEASES OF THE UTERUS

J. GEORGE MOORE

Benign diseases of the uterus are commonly encountered in gynecologic practice. In this chapter, uterine leiomyomas, endometrial hyperplasia, and endometrial polyps are discussed.

UTERINE LEIOMYOMA

Uterine leiomyomas ("fibroids") are smooth muscle tumors of the uterus. Twenty percent of women develop uterine fibroids by 40 years of age, and they constitute the most common indication for major surgery in women. They cause serious complications of pregnancy, confuse the management of the menopause, and mask the diagnosis of more serious gynecologic neoplasms. Fibroids have the potential to grow to an enormous size. Their malignant potential is minimal, and the overwhelming majority cause no symptoms and require no treatment other than careful observation.

Pathogenesis

The etiology of uterine leiomyomas remains unclear. Most likely, they develop from uterine smooth muscle cells, although they may be derived from connective tissue cells by a process of metaplasia or from smooth muscle cells of uterine arteries. There is an increased incidence and an increased rate of growth in black women.

Uterine leiomyomas are distinctly estrogen-dependent. They rarely develop before the menarche and seldom develop or enlarge past the menopause, unless stimulated by exogenous estrogens. The neoplasms enlarge with alarming speed and may attain a huge size during pregnancy or when exposed to oral contraceptives containing high doses of estrogen. They occur with increased frequency in conjunction with endometrial hyperplasia, anovulatory states, and granulosa-cell tumors of the ovaries. These conditions are also associated with an increased risk of endometrial cancer. Women with uterine myomas have a fourfold increased risk of developing endometrial cancer.

Although the leiomyoma appears discrete in outline, it does not have a cellular capsule. Compressed smooth muscle cells on the tumor's periphery lead to an increased density of the reticulum in this area, and the layered configuration of the surrounding myometrium gives the false impression of a cellular capsule. Very few blood vessels and lymphatics traverse the pseudocapsule, leading to degenerative changes as the tumors enlarge. The most commonly observed degenerative change is that of *hyaline acellularity,* in which the fibrous and muscle tissues are replaced with hyaline tissue. If the hyaline tissue breaks down from a further reduction in blood supply, *cystic degeneration* may occur. *Calcification* may occur in degenerated fibroids, particularly after the menopause, and is responsible for the term "womb stones." *Fatty degeneration* may also occur, but is rare. During pregnancy, about half of all fibroids undergo *red* or *carneous degener-*

ation caused by hemorrhage into the tumor. *Sarcomatous degeneration* occurs in less than 1 per 1000 fibroids.

Classification

Leiomyomas may occupy various positions in the uterine corpus and are generally described as *submucous, intramural,* and *subserous* (Fig. 30–1). They can also occur in the cervix, between the leaves of the broad ligament (*intraligamentous*), and in the various supporting ligaments of the uterus. As these neoplasms develop, most are intramural (Fig. 30–2); however, they may grow toward the endometrial cavity to occupy a submucous position or grow toward the serous surface of the uterus and become subserous myomas. They may migrate further, eventually protruding through the endometrium or the serosa and becoming *pedunculated.* Occasionally, they become attached to the omentum or the bowel mesentery and lose their connection with the serosal surface of the uterus, develop an omental or mesenteric blood supply, and become *parasitic myomas.* Some submucous leiomyomas become pedunculated in the endometrial cavity, pro-

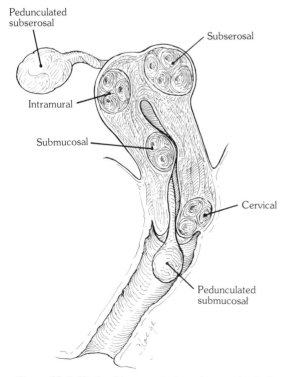

Figure 30–1 Uterine leiomyomata in various anatomical locations, as noted in the text.

Pedunculated subserosal

Subserosal

Intramural

Submucosal

Cervical

Pedunculated submucosal

ject through the cervix, and present as a *leiomyomatous polyp,* usually with an associated endometritis.

Symptoms

The majority of uterine leiomyomas are asymptomatic. Occasionally, the patient may become aware of a lower abdominal mass if it protrudes above the symphysis pubis. Quite often the development of discomfort comes on insidiously, and the symptoms are difficult for a patient to define. She may complain of pelvic pressure, congestion, bloating, or a feeling of heaviness in the lower abdomen. She may note frequency of urination as the bladder and tumor compete for space within the pelvis.

Menorrhagia may be associated with intramural tumors and metrorrhagia may be associated with submucous myomas ulcerating through the endometrial lining. Blood loss occurring over a long period of time may result in anemia, weakness, dypsnea, and even congestive heart failure. The menorrhagia is related to the enlargement of the endometrial cavity and the greater surface area of endometrium, which will slough at the time of menstruation. Also, the presence of large leiomyomas brings about a greater blood supply to the uterus, and the process of menstruation therewith becomes more hemorrhagic.

Pain is generally not a feature, but severe pain associated with red degeneration within a fibroid (acute infarction) is not uncommon during pregnancy. Also, pressure pains may occur in the lower abdomen and pelvis if a myomatous uterus becomes incarcerated within the pelvis. Dyspareunia is also common in this situation. There is a substantially increased incidence of secondary dysmenorrhea in women with uterine myomas.

Although many women with uterine myomas become pregnant and carry their pregnancies to term, these lesions are associated with an increased incidence of infertility. A submucous leiomyoma may interfere with the implantation of the blastocyst or bring about an early abortion. Large leiomyomas may interfere with the growth of the developing fetus, resulting in intrauterine growth retardation. Tumors occurring in the lower uterine segment may cause dystocia and necessitate delivery by cesarean section. However, low-lying uterine myomas usually soften remark-

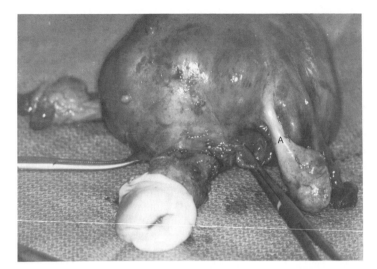

Figure 30–2 Multiple leiomyomata uteri. Note that the right ovarian ligament *(A)* extends from the posterior aspect of the uterine corpus. Clamps are on the uterine arteries and the cervix is parous.

ably and rise from the pelvis as the lower uterine segment elongates during the course of labor, allowing the presenting part to enter the pelvis.

Signs

Very large fibroids can be palpated abdominally. Those smaller than a 12 to 14 week gestation are usually confined to the pelvis. The bladder should be emptied prior to examination to avoid the confusion of urinary retention. Bimanual vaginal examination reveals a firm, irregularly enlarged uterus with smoothly rounded or bosselated protrusions from the uterine wall. The tumors are almost always nontender. Their consistency may vary from rock hard, as in the case of a calcified postmenopausal leiomyoma, to soft or even cystic, as is the case of cystic degeneration of the tumor. Generally, the myomatous masses are in the midline and follow the contour of the uterus. Sometimes a large portion of the tumor lies in the lateral aspect of the pelvis and may be indistinguishable from an adnexal mass. Often the presence of a leiomyoma precludes a proper evaluation of the adnexae. If the mass moves with the cervix, it is suggestive of a leiomyoma.

Multiple large leiomyomas may enlarge the uterus to a size greater than that of a term pregnancy. Such large tumors contain huge reservoirs of blood, which may lead to cardiovascular instability during changes of body position or at the time of operation. Bruits similar to the uterine souffle of pregnancy may be heard and felt over these large masses.

Differential Diagnosis

The most common differential diagnoses are an ovarian neoplasm, a tubo-ovarian inflammatory mass, or a diverticular inflammatory mass. A complete blood count, urinalysis, sedimentation rate, and stool guaiac test may be helpful in this differential diagnosis. A barium enema can exclude diverticular disease. An intravenous pyelogram may exclude the rare pelvic kidney or a retroperitoneal tumor, the latter being suggested by medial displacement of the ureter. A flat film of the abdomen and pelvis or pelvic ultrasonography may reveal characteristic calcification or other patterns suggestive of a leiomyoma. Ultrasonography will delineate the lesions and identify normal ovaries apart from the leiomyomata, thus aiding in the differential diagnosis if there is any uncertainty (Fig. 30–3).

It is occasionally impossible to distinguish between a moderate-sized asymptomatic uterine leiomyoma occupying a lateral pelvic position and a solid ovarian tumor. Often the innocent leiomyoma can be identified at laparoscopy, and laparotomy can be avoided.

In women beyond the age of 35, carcinoma of the endometrium and uterine myomas may coexist and cause abnormal bleeding. In such patients, a fractional curettage is an essential part of the diagnostic work-up.

Treatment

The recommended management for most uterine leiomyomas is prudent observation. If treatment is indicated and future reproduc-

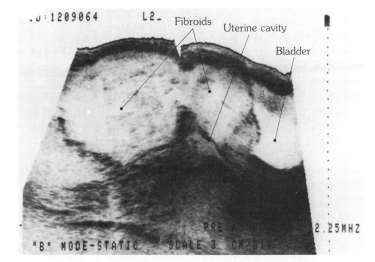

Figure 30–3 Pelvic sonogram showing uterine myomas pressing against the full urinary bladder.

tive capability is desired, *myomectomy* may be performed. *Hysterectomy* is indicated in a symptomatic patient if reproductive capability is not important to the patient. Occasionally, uterine curettage will control menometrorrhagia. The main indications for definitive treatment of a uterine leiomyoma are listed in Table 30–1.

Probably the most common indication for surgical intervention is abnormal uterine bleeding, and it is mandatory that a fractional dilatation and curettage (D & C) be performed initially to rule out endometrial carcinoma. Even when submucous leiomyomata are detected at the time of endometrial curettage, the patient may have no further abnormal uterine bleeding. If the D & C is effective, and if the adnexae can be evaluated sufficiently, the patient can avoid major surgery.

In dealing with moderately sized uterine myomas that are only mildly symptomatic, a relatively young woman is more likely to require surgical treatment (beyond a D & C)

TABLE 30–1 INDICATIONS FOR SURGICAL INTERVENTION IN A PATIENT WITH A UTERINE LEIOMYOMA

1. Abnormal uterine bleeding causing anemia
2. Severe pelvic pain or secondary dysmenorrhea
3. Inability to evaluate the adnexae (usually because fibroid is ≥12 weeks' size)
4. Urinary tract symptoms (frequency or urinary retention)
5. Growth of the myoma following menopause
6. Infertility
7. Rapid increase in size

than a perimenopausal woman. In the latter case, the menopause may soon bring about an abatement of symptoms and shrinkage of the myomatous uterus, whereas the uterine myomas of the young woman will probably continue to grow with the estrogen stimulation of normal ovarian function. If the patient is close to the menopause and represents a very poor surgical risk, irradiation castration may be considered, reluctantly, as definitive therapy if disabling bleeding recurs following a D & C.

Pain may be the single indication for definitive treatment of uterine leiomyomas. Pelvic pain or pressure, low back pain, dyspareunia, secondary dysmenorrhea, or the discomfort associated with a pedunculated leiomyoma coming through the cervical os are all legitimate indications for myomectomy or, in most cases, hysterectomy. In younger women who still desire childbearing, the method of treatment may be a uterine myomectomy, either by the vaginal approach, if it is a pedunculated submucous leiomyoma, or by the abdominal approach, if it is an intramural, subserous, or pedunculated fibroid. There should be a definite reason for myomectomy rather than hysterectomy, since the transabdominal myomectomy is more difficult to manage, results in more blood loss, and has a higher morbidity rate. Also, 20 to 30 percent of patients require a subsequent operation due to recurrence following myomectomy.

Inability to evaluate the adnexae is probably the most important indication for surgery in large asymptomatic leiomyomas. There is no greater tragedy than finding advanced ovarian carcinoma in a patient who has been followed over a period of time for uterine fibroids. When the uterus is greater than the size of a 12-week gestation or when it has been displaced out of the pelvis into the abdomen, palpation of the ovaries on bimanual examination is virtually impossible. It is generally advisable to elect abdominal hysterectomy if the uterus is larger than the size of a 10- to 12-week gestation (three times the normal size). If the patient has a pedunculated submucous leiomyoma projecting through the cervix, a vaginal myomectomy is indicated initially to facilitate the hysterectomy and to avoid contamination of the peritoneal cavity with the infected, pedunculated lesion.

Approximately 5 percent of uterine leiomyomas are characterized by urinary tract abnormalities. Acute or chronic urinary retention, ureteral compression, hydronephrosis, and urgency or frequency of urination are definite indications for surgery. Occasionally, a period of urinary decompression and normalization of blood urea nitrogen levels are necessary prior to surgery.

When not associated with estrogen administration, extremely rapid growth of a uterine myoma during the menstrual years or any growth in a leiomyoma following the menopause represents an important indication for surgery. Although rare, the possibility of a sarcoma developing in a leiomyoma is real under these circumstances, and a hysterectomy and bilateral salpingo-oophorectomy should be carried out.

Although most uterine myomas do not affect fertility, any distortion of the endometrial cavity or compression of the isthmic area of the tube may decrease the fertility potential. If all other features of the fertility study are normal and if a sufficient period of time has elapsed, transabdominal uterine myomectomy for infertility is indicated.

Approximately 10 percent of women who are pregnant with uterine fibroids must be hospitalized for complications relating to the fibroid during pregnancy. Such complications include early abortion, acute infarction of the fibroid, and interference with the proper nutrition of the growing fetus. Surgical intervention should be avoided during pregnancy, but interval myomectomy or hysterectomy following the pregnancy may be necessary.

Prior to any surgical procedure, efforts should be made to suppress menorrhagia with progestogens, and oral iron should be administered. If difficult surgery is expected, as in the case of a large cervical myoma, at least two units of blood should be secured from the patient over a four- to six-week period so that an autologous transfusion of packed red blood cells may be given intraoperatively if necessary.

HYPERPLASIA OF THE ENDOMETRIUM

Endometrial hyperplasia represents an overabundant growth of the endometrium, generally caused by persistently high levels of estrogens, unopposed by progesterone. Endometrial hyperplasia is prone to develop in the years immediately following the menarche and in the years immediately prior to the menopause—periods when ovulation generally is infrequent. It also commonly occurs in association with polycystic sclerotic ovaries and estrogen-producing tumors, such as granulosa-theca cell tumors. Endometrial hyperplasia is also associated with obesity because of the peripheral conversion of androstenedione to estrone in peripheral tissues, especially in postmenopausal women.

Histologic Variants

Cystic Glandular Hyperplasia. The simplest form of endometrial hyperplasia is cystic glandular hyperplasia, which microscopically is referred to as the "Swiss cheese" pattern (Fig. 30–4). Both the epithelial cells lining the glands and the stromal cells participate in the hyperplastic growth, and there are abundant mitotic figures. Cystic glandular hyperplasia may be an early precursor of endometrial cancer. Cystic hyperplasia of the endometrium may be confused with cystic involution of the endometrium, which normally occurs postmenopausally and is not a hyperplastic condition. A variety of microscopic pictures can be seen with cystic hyperplasia, and the hyperplastic areas may be seen only focally. Both secretory and proliferative endometrial patterns can be found.

Adenomatous Hyperplasia. Adenomatous hyperplasia of the endometrium represents a hyperplastic condition in which the glands are not cystic and the stroma does not necessarily participate in the hyperplastic reaction. This

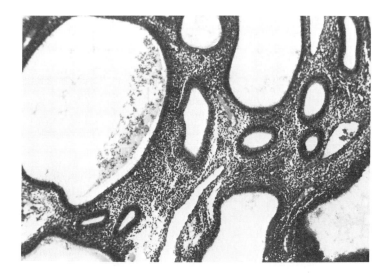

Figure 30–4 Cystic hyperplasia of the endometrium showing dilated cystic glands lined by tall columnar cells and active endometrial stromal proliferation.

condition represents an active proliferation of the glandular epithelium so that the glands are often crowded in a back-to-back manner with no intervening stroma (Fig. 30–5). Adenomatous endometrial hyperplasia represents the next step in the transition toward endometrial cancer, and the two diseases may coexist. When the cellular growth lining the endometrial glands becomes atypical with piling up of the epithelial cells and cellular atypia, the condition is referred to as *adenomatous hyperplasia with cytologic atypia.* This process eventually progresses to carcinoma *in situ.* The more cellular proliferation and cytologic atypia there is in the adenomatous areas, the greater is the chance of endometrial cancer developing. It is estimated that at least 20 percent of patients with adenomatous hyperplasia eventually develop endometrial cancer.

Diagnosis

Generally, the diagnosis of endometrial hyperplasia is suspected on the basis of either postmenopausal bleeding or prolongation or irregularity of menstrual bleeding. Frequently, clots are passed, and the blood loss is sufficient to cause anemia. In the initial stages of estrogen stimulation, there may be a period of amenorrhea, during which endometrial growth takes place, that is eventually followed by prolonged bleeding. Occasionally, the uterus is enlarged, both by the mass of endometrium and also by the growth of the myometrium in response to persistent estrogen stimulation. The diagnosis can be made by endometrial biopsy, but except in a woman under 30 years, dilatation and curettage are usually necessary to exclude endometrial carcinoma.

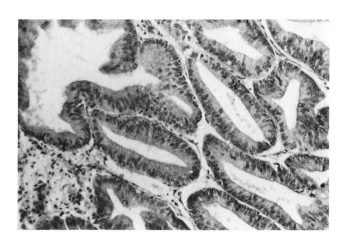

Figure 30–5 Adenomatous hyperplasia of the endometrium showing crowded glands with scanty interglandular stroma. Note the tall columnar cells lining the glands and focal multilayering.

Treatment

The treatment of endometrial hyperplasia depends on the age of the patient and the histologic variety of the lesion. In a young woman with simple cystic hyperplasia, effective treatment involves the use of progestogens on a cyclic basis—usually medroxyprogesterone acetate (Provera), 10 mg daily for ten days each month. Following the cessation of Provera, the hyperplastic endometrium is shed. Occasionally, it may be necessary to add estrogens to the cyclic progestogen therapy to prevent "breakthrough" bleeding. If the bleeding is very heavy, or if the progestogen is unsuccessful, it may be necessary to carry out a D & C for therapeutic purposes.

If cystic hyperplasia is found at dilatation and curettage in an older woman, no further treatment may be necessary. However, if the bleeding recurs, cyclic progestogens or hysterectomy are in order.

If adenomatous hyperplasia is found at any age, especially if there is cellular atypia, there are two alternatives. One is to administer cyclic progestogens for a period of six months and then resample the endometrium. The other alternative is to perform a hysterectomy, probably vaginal, to preclude the later development of an endometrial cancer. The older the patient and the more atypical the adenomatous hyperplasia, the more likely is the subsequent development of endometrial cancer. The constitutional factors that increase the risk for endometrial cancer should also be taken into consideration in deciding whether or not to perform hysterectomy. The nulliparous, obese, diabetic woman in her fifties is at greater risk, so early hysterectomy is indicated.

ENDOMETRIAL POLYPS

Endometrial polyps represent a gross clinical diagnosis. A polyp arising in the area of the endometrium may take the form of a myoma, a carcinoma, a carcinosarcoma, or merely a polypoid endometrial hyperplasia. The pathologic diagnosis can be made only on histologic examination.

Approximately 5 percent of endometrial polyps are associated with malignancy, mostly in postmenopausal women. Most endometrial polyps are made up of benign endometrial tissue and a fair number are asymptomatic. Most, however, are associated with abnormal bleeding (particularly intermenstrual or postmenopausal bleeding), especially if they are large enough to protrude through the cervical os. Both the diagnosis and the treatment take the form of a fractional D & C with the use of endometrial polyp forceps.

SUGGESTED READING

Bartisch EG, Bowe ET, Moore JG: Leiomyosarcoma of the uterus: A 50 year review. Obstet Gynecol 32:101, 1968.

Babaknia A, Rock JA, Jones HW Jr: Pregnancy success following abdominal myomectomy for infertility. Fertil Steril 30:644, 1978.

Corscaden JF, Singh BP: Leiomyosarcoma of the uterus. Am J Obstet Gynecol 75:149, 1958.

Ledger WJ, Sweet RL, Headington JT: Prophylactic cephaloridine in women undergoing hysterectomy. Am J Obstet Gynecol 115:766, 1973.

Miller NF, Ludovici PP: Origin and development of uterine fibroids. Am J Obstet Gynecol 70:720, 1955.

Siddall RS: Leiomyofibroma of the uterus and endometrial cancer. Am J Obstet Gynecol 53:846, 1947.

31

BENIGN TUMORS OF THE OVARIES AND FALLOPIAN TUBES

J. GEORGE MOORE

The human ovary has a striking propensity to develop a wide variety of tumors, the majority of which are benign. Most ovarian lesions are non-neoplastic. As indicated in Table 31–1, ovarian tumors may be functional, inflammatory, metaplastic, or neoplastic. During the menstruating years, 70 percent of non-inflammatory ovarian tumors are functional. The remainder are neoplastic (20 percent) or endometriomas (10 percent).

Ovarian neoplasms have a higher malignancy rate than other pelvic tumors, the overall incidence being about 15 percent. After the menopause, about half of all ovarian tumors are malignant, while during in-

fancy and childhood, 10 percent are malignant. Malignant ovarian tumors are discussed in Chapter 54.

The management of ovarian tumors, whether functional, benign, or malignant, involves difficult decisions that may affect a woman's hormonal status and fertility. Only functional and benign neoplastic tumors are considered in this chapter.

FUNCTIONAL OVARIAN TUMORS

Pathogenesis

If the ovarian follicle fails to rupture in the course of follicular development and ovulation, a *follicular cyst* lined by one or more layers of granulosa cells may develop. Similarly, a *lutein cyst* may develop if the corpus luteum becomes cystic or hemorrhagic (hemorrhagic corpus luteum) and fails to regress normally after 14 days.

Other specific types of lutein cysts may occur with abnormally high serum levels of human chorionic gonadotropin (hCG). *Theca-lutein cysts* may develop in association with the high levels of hCG present in patients with a hydatidiform mole or choriocarcinoma. Patients undergoing ovulation induction with gonadotropins or clomiphene may also develop theca-lutein cysts. These cysts

TABLE 31–1 DIFFERENTIAL DIAGNOSIS OF OVARIAN TUMORS

PATHOGENESIS	SPECIFIC TYPE
Functional	Follicular cysts
	Lutein cysts
	Polycystic sclerotic ovaries
Inflammatory	Neisserian salpingo-oophoritis
	Pyogenic oophoritis— puerperal, abortal, or IUD-related
	Granulomatous oophoritis
Metaplastic	Endometriosis
Neoplastic	Premenarchal years—10% are malignant
	Menstruating years—15% are malignant
	Postmenopausal years—50% are malignant

are usually bilateral, may become quite large (10 to 15 cm), and characteristically regress as the hCG level falls.

A *luteoma of pregnancy* takes the form of extensive luteinization of ovarian theca cells, purportedly from prolonged chorionic gonadotropin stimulation during pregnancy. They may be associated with multiple pregnancy or hydramnios, and they cause maternal virilization, as well as abnormal genitalia, in the female fetus. Although ovarian enlargement may be impressive, surgical resection is not indicated, and regression takes place postpartum.

Polycystic ovarian syndrome, a functional disorder generally associated with oligomenorrhea, anovulation, and elevated testosterone levels, is considered in Chapters 44 and 48.

Clinical Features

An ovarian follicular cyst is usually asymptomatic, unilocular ("simple"), and seldom more than 6 to 8 cm in diameter. It generally regresses during the subsequent menstrual cycle. Generally, a lutein cyst is larger than a follicular cyst, is apt to be more firm or even solid in consistency, and is more likely to cause pain or signs of peritoneal irritation. It is also more likely to cause delay in the upcoming period and some alteration of the next menstrual cycle. Occasionally, a functional ovarian cyst can twist on its pedicle and become infarcted, causing pain, tenderness, and rebound tenderness, as well as a moderate leukocytosis. Rupture of a functional cyst may produce acute lower abdominal pain and tenderness, and, occasionally, a significant hemoperitoneum may occur.

Diagnosis

The presumptive diagnosis of a functional ovarian tumor is usually made when a 4 to 8 cm cystic adnexal mass is noted on bimanual examination; it is confirmed when the lesion regresses following the next menstrual period. Generally, the cyst is mobile, unilateral, and not associated with ascites. On rare occasions, the mass may exceed 8 cm and be quite tender to palpation. Occasionally, hemorrhagic lutein cysts may have a solid rather than a cystic consistency. If the patient has delayed menses, abnormal uterine bleeding, and/or twisting of the cyst on its pedicle with infarction, the differential diagnosis must include ectopic pregnancy, salpingo-oophoritis, or torsion of a neoplastic cyst. Benign cystic teratomas commonly twist and infarct. In these instances, a pregnancy test, erythrocyte sedimentation rate, and ultrasonic evaluation are generally helpful.

Management

If the patient is in her reproductive years and the adnexal cyst is less than 6 cm in diameter, it is appropriate to wait and examine the patient again after her next menses, perhaps with the prescription of an oral contraceptive to suppress gonadotropin levels (Table 31–2). If the cystic mass is between 6 and 8 cm, or if it is fixed or feels solid, a pelvic ultrasound may be obtained to ensure that it is unilocular. If the mass is painful, multilocular, or solid, surgical exploration is in order. When the patient is in her forties, the chances of an ovarian neoplasm are increased, and observational delays must be undertaken with caution.

If the lesion does not fulfill the requirements for observation, surgical exploration may be indicated. Laparoscopy is generally not helpful in differentiating between a functional and a neoplastic ovarian cyst. A laparotomy is necessary to allow resection of the cyst from the ovary (ovarian cystectomy) so that it can be examined histologically.

Table 31–3 demonstrates the outcome of a

TABLE 31–2 MANAGEMENT OF A CYSTIC ADNEXAL MASS

AGE	SIZE OF CYST	MANAGEMENT
Premenarchal	> 2 cm	Exploratory laparotomy
Reproductive age	< 6 cm	Observe for six weeks
	6–8 cm	Observe if unilocular; explore if multilocular or solid on ultrasound
	> 8 cm	Exploratory laparotomy
Postmenopausal	Palpable	Exploratory laparotomy

TABLE 31–3 ADNEXAL CYSTS OBSERVED FOR 6 WEEKS IN 286 PATIENTS AGED 16 TO 48 YEARS*

TYPE OF CYST	NUMBER OF PATIENTS	PERCENTAGE
Regressed under observation	205	72
Required exploratory laparotomy	81	28
Ovarian neoplasms	46	16
Benign epithelial	32	
Benign teratoma	9	
Malignant epithelial	4	
Dysgerminoma	1	
Endometriosis	28	10
Paraovarian cyst	4	1.4
Hydrosalpinx	3	1
Functional cysts	0	0

*Adapted with permission from Spanos WJ: Preoperative hormonal therapy of cystic adnexal masses. Am J Obstet Gynecol 116:551, 1973.

fairly large series of patients with a cystic adnexal mass in their reproductive years who were started on an estrogen-progestogen preparation at the time of diagnosis, then followed for six weeks. Spontaneous regression occurred in approximately 70 percent of patients with cystic ovaries, 16 percent had neoplastic ovarian cysts, and 10 percent had endometriosis. Nine percent of the neoplastic cysts (1.4 percent of the total series) were malignant.

NEOPLASTIC OVARIAN TUMORS

Ovarian neoplasms, as noted in Table 54–3, may be divided by cell type of origin into three main groups: epithelial, stromal, and germ-cell. Taken as a group, the epithelial tumors are by far the most common type, although the single most common benign ovarian neoplasm is the benign cystic teratoma (dermoid cyst), a germ-cell tumor. Mixed tumors, as the name implies, are derived from more than one ovarian cell type. The distribution of the various types of ovarian neoplasms surgically removed in a large metropolitan area is shown in Table 31–4.

Epithelial Ovarian Neoplasms

These tumors are believed to be derived from the mesothelial cells lining the peritoneal cavity; similar tumors occasionally arise

TABLE 31–4 INCIDENCE OF PRIMARY OVARIAN NEOPLASMS IN THE DENVER METROPOLITAN AREA*

TYPE OF OVARIAN NEOPLASM	NUMBER	PERCENTAGE
Benign cystic teratoma	103	26.5
Serous cystadenoma/cystadenofibroma	72	18.5
Mucinous cystadenoma/cystadenofibroma	48	12.5
Fibroma	39	10.0
Serous carcinoma	26	6.7
Endometrioid carcinoma	14	3.6
Mixed carcinoma	12	3.1
Serous borderline tumor	12	3.1
Brenner tumor, benign	11	2.8
Thecoma	11	2.8
Clear cell carcinoma	8	2.1
Mucinous carcinoma	6	1.6
Mucinous borderline tumor	6	1.6
Immature teratoma	3	0.8
Other	18	4.7

*Adapted with permission from Katsube Y, Berg JW, Silverberg SG: Epidemiologic pathology of ovarian tumors: A histopathologic review of primary ovarian neoplasms diagnosed in the Denver Standard metropolitan statistical area, July 1–December 31, 1969 and July 1–December 31, 1979. Int J Gynecol Pathol 1:5, 1982.

from the mesothelium lining the pleural cavity. Since all müllerian structures are derived from the special mesothelium of the gonadal ridge and ultimately differentiate into several different histologic tissues (cervical epithelium, endometrium, ciliated endosalpinx, as well as the serous ovarian surface), it is reasonable to postulate that the ovarian mesothelial cells retain the capability to change by metaplasia into any of these müllerian types of epithelium. Thus, the mucinous ovarian neoplasm cytologically resembles the endocervical epithelium (Fig. 31–1*A*), the endometrioid ovarian neoplasm resembles the endometrium, and, occasionally, ovarian tumors are made up of what appears to be ciliated endosalpingial tissue. The most common ovarian tumors retain their serous cell type and are termed serous cystadenomas (Fig. 31–1*B*).

Each of the epithelial (more accurately, mesothelial) ovarian neoplasms has characteristic clinical and histologic features. The *serous tumors* are bilateral in about 10 percent of cases. Of all serous tumors, about 70 percent are benign, 5 to 10 percent have borderline malignant potential, and 20 to 25 percent are malignant. Serous cystadenomas tend to be multilocular (Fig. 31–2), although small unilocular serous cystomas are not un-

common. Histologically, serous tumors characteristically form psammoma bodies (from the Greek psammos meaning sand), which are calcific, concentric concretions. Psammoma bodies occur occasionally in benign serous neoplasms and frequently in serous cystadenocarcinomas. Papillary patterns are also common.

The *mucinous* (formerly, pseudomucinous) *neoplasms* of the ovary can attain a huge size, often filling the entire pelvis and abdomen (Fig. 31–3). They are often multilocular, and benign mucinous tumors are bilateral in less than 5 percent of cases. About 85 percent of mucinous tumors are benign. Rarely, a benign mucinous tumor may be complicated by *pseudomyxoma peritonei*. Mucinous tumors are sometimes associated with a mucocele of the appendix.

Endometrioid neoplasms are generally malignant (endometrioid carcinoma). Benign endometrial tumors of the ovary most commonly take the form of endometriomas, which are not neoplasms in the strictest sense. Endometriosis is much more common than are benign endometrioid tumors. Benign endometrial neoplasms of the ovary are not associated with endometrial stroma and do not demonstrate the extensive, but generally superficial, invasive characteristics of endo-

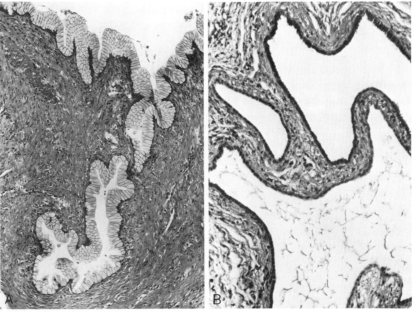

Figure 31–1 Histologic differences between *(A)* a benign mucinous cystadenoma and *(B)* a benign serous cystadenoma. Note the smaller cuboidal cells and focal cilia lining the serous tumor, and the taller columnar cells with basal nuclei and abundant mucin lining the mucinous tumor.

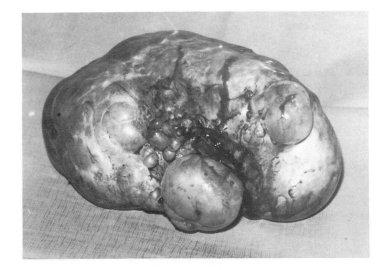

Figure 31–2 Gross appearance of a multilocular serous cystadenoma.

metriosis. The distinction between benign endometrioid neoplasia and endometriosis in the ovary is not conceptually clear.

The *Brenner tumor* is a solid ovarian neoplasm, usually benign, with a large fibrotic component that encases epithelioid cells, which resemble transitional cells. In about one third of cases, they are associated with mucinous epithelial elements.

Sex Cord-Stromal Ovarian Neoplasms

These tumors include *fibromas, granulosa-theca cell tumors,* and *Sertoli-Leydig cell tumors.* Combinations of the latter two types are termed *gynandroblastomas.*

The tumors in this category are derived from the sex cords and specialized stroma of the developing gonad. As noted in Chapter 27, the embryologic origin of granulosa and theca cells, as well as their counterparts in the testes, the Sertoli and Leydig cells, are from cells that make up the specialized gonadal stroma. If the ultimate differentiation of cell types occurring in the tumor is feminine, the neoplasm becomes a granulosa cell tumor, a theca cell tumor, or, as in most instances, a mixed granulosa-theca cell tumor. Those neoplasms containing cells that take on a masculine differentiation (far less common) become Sertoli-Leydig cell tumors. The fibroma represents the stromal cell neoplasm developing from mature fibroblasts in the ovarian stroma.

The *granulosa-theca cell* neoplasms, as well as their androgenic counterparts, are generally referred to as *functioning* (not functional)

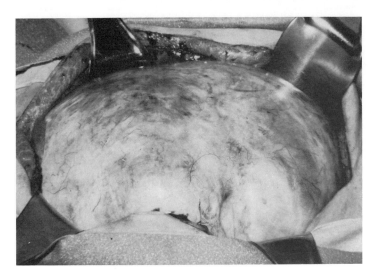

Figure 31–3 Huge mucinous cystadenoma filling the entire pelvis and abdomen.

ovarian tumors. They occur in any age group, from birth on, and their functioning characteristics are responsible for a variety of associated signs and symptoms. The granulosa-theca cell tumors promote feminizing signs and symptoms, such as precocious puberty, precocious thelarche, or premenarchal uterine bleeding during infancy and childhood; menorrhagia (or amenorrhea) and endometrial hyperplasia (or even endometrial cancer), breast tenderness, and fluid retention in the menstruating years; and postmenopausal bleeding in older women. In contrast, the less frequent *Sertoli-Leydig cell tumors* are responsible for virilizing effects, such as hirsutism, recession of the frontal hairline, deepening of the voice, clitoromegaly, and change in body habitus to a muscular build. Fifteen percent of these tumors have no such endocrinologic clinical effects. Except for the pure thecoma, these tumors have malignant potential and are discussed further in Chapter 54.

The ovarian *fibroma* is nonfunctioning, does not secrete steroids, and takes the form of a firm, rounded, smooth-surfaced tumor made up of interlacing bundles of fibrocytes (Fig. 31–4). It is glistening white on cut surface, as opposed to the soft yellow appearance of the granulosa-theca cell or hilus cell tumor. Occasionally, this tumor is associated with ascites. The transudation of this ascitic fluid through the transdiaphragmatic lymphatics into the right pleural cavity may result in *Meigs' syndrome* (ascites and right hydrothorax in association with an ovarian fibroma). The ovarian fibroma may be associated with theca cell elements as a *fibrothecoma*.

Germ-Cell Tumors

Germ-cell neoplasms can occur at any age. They make up about 60 percent of ovarian neoplasms occurring in infants and children.

Benign Cystic Teratoma. As noted previously, the most common ovarian neoplasm is the benign cystic teratoma, a germ-cell tumor that can take on a great variety of forms with virtually all adult tissues being represented. Fifteen to 20 percent are bilateral. The benign cystic teratoma, commonly referred to as a *dermoid cyst* (Fig. 31–5), is composed primarily of skin and the dermal appendages, including sweat and sebaceous glands, hair follicles, and teeth. Because of the oily secretion of the sebaceous glands, the desquamated squamous cells, the presence of hair, and the presence of a dermoid tubercle (of Rokitansky), which often contains a hard, well-formed tooth, the dermoid cyst has a characteristic gross appearance (Figs. 31–6 and 31–7).

Other tissue components commonly found in benign cystic teratomas include brain, bronchus, thyroid, cartilage, intestine, bone, and carcinoid cells. As opposed to similar tissues found in a malignant immature teratoma, the tissues making up the benign (mature) teratoma are all of an adult, well-differentiated form.

Benign cystic teratomas can be found in the retroperitoneal area of the pelvis or upper abdomen, in the mediastinum, and even in the pineal body. Since primary sex (germ) cells originate in early embryonic life near the hindgut in the region of the yolk sac and allantois and migrate along the base of the

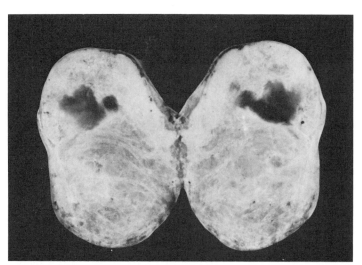

Figure 31–4 Ovarian fibroma that was removed from a patient with ascites and a right pleural effusion (Meigs' syndrome). Note the whorled appearance on the cut section and the area of cystic degenertion.

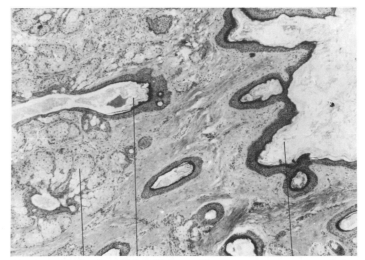

Figure 31–5 Histologic appearance of a dermoid cyst. Note the *(A)* keratinizing squamous epithelium, *(B)* hair follicle, and *(C)* sebaceous glands.

Sebaceous gland   Hair follicle   Keratinizing squamous epithelium

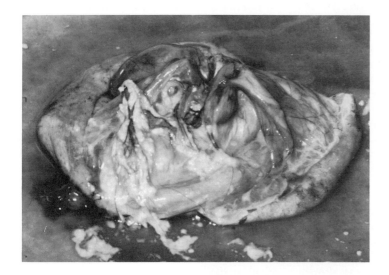

Figure 31–6 Gross appearance of a dermoid cyst cut open. Note the presence of hair and sebaceous material.

Figure 31–7 Pelvic x-ray of a patient with a benign dermoid cyst showing the presence of teeth.

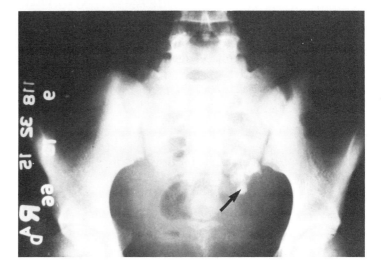

mesentery to the gonadal ridge on either side of the midline (see Chapter 27), it is postulated that some such cells go astray in their migration.

Mixed Ovarian Neoplasms

The most common ovarian tumor in which the neoplastic elements are composed of more than one cell type is the *cystadenofibroma* or the *fibrocystadenoma*. These tumors generally take their characteristics from the epithelial component, although they tend to be more solid than the epithelial ovarian neoplasms.

The *gonadoblastoma* is a benign tumor composed of cells resembling those of a dysgerminoma and others resembling granulosa and Sertoli cells. Characteristically, calcific concretions are a prominent feature of this neoplasm. Almost all patients with a gonadoblastoma have dysgenetic gonads (see Chapter 27), and a Y chromosome has been detected in over 90 percent of cases investigated. Although the gonadoblastoma is initially benign, about half of these tumors may predispose to the development of dysgerminomas or other malignant germ-cell tumors.

Diagnosis of Benign Ovarian Tumors

Symptoms. The clinical features of benign ovarian tumors are often deceptive and nonspecific. Except for the functioning ovarian neoplasms, most benign ovarian tumors are asymptomatic, unless they undergo torsion or rupture. They usually enlarge very slowly, so that an increase in abdominal girth or pressure on surrounding organs is not perceived until the later stages of growth. Any pelvic pain is generally mild and intermittent, unless the tumor twists on its pedicle, when infarction may induce severe pain and tenderness. *Torsion* of an adnexal mass is often associated with "reverse renal colic," the pain originating in the iliac fossa and radiating to the flank. Nausea and vomiting are common. Peritoneal irritation from an infarcted tumor may cause radiation of pain in the distribution of the ilioinguinal and genitofemoral nerves (inguinal area, anterior thigh, and inner portion of the external genitalia).

On rare occasions, an ovarian cyst may *rupture* spontaneously from internal hemorrhage or intracystic pressure, resulting in pain and peritoneal irritation. A cyst may also rupture occasionally during or following a bimanual pelvic examination. Depending on the cystic contents, pain of varying degrees of severity can result. The escape of thin serous fluid without hemorrhage may evoke little pain or tenderness, but the oily contents of a dermoid cyst or the thick mucinous fluid of a mucinous cystadenoma may be irritating to both the parietal and visceral peritoneum, with the development of severe pain and tenderness and the subsequent formation of troublesome intra-abdominal adhesions.

Signs. Bimanual pelvic examination generally indicates the presence of the tumor in the pelvis; if it has risen into the abdomen, however, this examination may be unremarkable. If the tumor is large enough, it may be delineated by abdominal palpation.

In contrast to the findings in a patient with ascites, percussion of the abdomen in a patient with a large ovarian cyst reveals dullness anteriorly with tympany in the flanks as the bowel is displaced laterally by the tumor. Shifting dullness suggests ascites.

If the tumor undergoes torsion and infarcts or ruptures, signs of peritoneal irritation may be present. Occasionally, the patient is initially seen after complete infarction has occurred and the peritoneal irritation has progressed to the point of abdominal rigidity. Paralytic ileus may also be present.

Investigations. Pelvic ultrasound may be helpful if the tumor is indistinguishable from a functional cyst (size 4 to 8 cm, cystic to palpation). The ultrasonic examination may identify a specific calcification, such as a tooth, which is characteristic of a benign cystic teratoma. A lower abdominal or pelvic x-ray will identify calcified structures more clearly or show an encapsulated cyst of low density fluid (Fig. 31–7).

Laparoscopy is helpful in distinguishing between a uterine myoma, a quiescent hydrosalpinx, and an ovarian tumor, but it will not distinguish between a functional cyst, a benign neoplasm, or an encapsulated malignant ovarian neoplasm. Occasionally, laparoscopy may identify endometriosis on the surface of the ovary. However, it cannot identify unequivocally that an ovarian endometrioma is not an ovarian neoplasm. Cystic ovarian tumors should not be biopsied through the laparoscope because of the likelihood of spilling contents around the peritoneal cavity. In general, laparotomy is preferable to laparoscopy in the evaluation of an adnexal mass.

Management of Ovarian Neoplasms

The differentiation between benign and malignant ovarian tumors may be quite difficult. Since the incidence of cancer in ovarian neoplasms is so high, no ovarian neoplasm should be assumed to be benign until proven so by surgical exploration and microscopic examination.

The indications for exploratory laparotomy in a patient with a pelvic mass have been discussed under functional tumors. If laparotomy is indicated, any ascitic fluid should be collected on opening the peritoneal cavity and sent for cystologic examination. Peritoneal washings should be obtained from the pelvis, both paracolic gutters, and both hemidiaphragms (see Chapter 54).

The definitive treatment will depend on the type of neoplasm, the patient's age, and her desire for future childbearing. A frozen section histologic diagnosis should be obtained intraoperatively.

Epithelial Ovarian Neoplasms. Epithelial ovarian neoplasms are generally treated by unilateral salpingo-oophorectomy. The contralateral ovary must be carefully inspected or wedge-biopsied to ensure that it is free of tumor. Because of the possible coexistence of an appendiceal mucocele with a mucinous cystadenoma, appendectomy is also indicated in such patients. If the patient is over 40 years of age, a total abdominal hysterectomy and bilateral salpingo-oophorectomy are ap-

propriate. This is especially true if the tumor is a serous cystadenoma, since the incidence of bilaterality and malignancy are higher in serous tumors.

If the patient is young and nulliparous, the ovarian neoplasm is unilocular, and there are no excrescences within the cyst, an ovarian cystectomy with preservation of the ovary may be performed (Fig. 31–8).

Stromal-Cell Neoplasms. Stromal-cell neoplasms of the ovary are generally treated by salpingo-oophorectomy when future pregnancies are a consideration. Ovarian fibromas, even when associated with ascites and right hydrothorax, are almost always benign and might even be treated by resection from the ovary in a young woman. After 40 years of age, total abdominal hysterectomy and bilateral salpingo-oophorectomy are in order.

Germ-Cell Tumors. Cystic teratomas ("dermoids") can be treated by ovarian cystectomy if future childbearing is desired. Since 15 to 20 percent are bilateral, the contralateral ovary should be carefully evaluated, any cysts resected, and the ovary bivalved if it is enlarged. Bivalve incision or wedge-resection of the opposite ovary is not recommended as a routine procedure, as it may cause adhesions and subsequent infertility. In a patient with a gonadoblastoma, dysgenetic ovaries are usually present, necessitating bilateral salpingo-oophorectomy, particularly in the presence of a Y chromosome. With the possibility of embryo transfer now becoming available to these patients, the uterus should be left *in situ* if future childbearing is desired, even if both ovaries are removed.

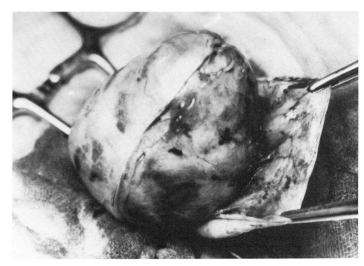

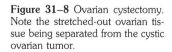
Figure 31–8 Ovarian cystectomy. Note the stretched-out ovarian tissue being separated from the cystic ovarian tumor.

BENIGN TUMORS OF THE FALLOPIAN TUBES

Most benign lesions of the fallopian tubes are inflammatory (hydrosalpinx or pyosalpinx), and benign neoplasms of the oviducts are rare. Although the tubes, uterine corpus, and uterine cervix are from the same müllerian anlage, the tubes, unlike the uterus, have little tendency toward neoplastic transformation.

As might be expected, those tubal neoplasms that do occur are epithelial *adenomas* and *polyps, myomas* from the tubal musculature, *inclusion cysts* from the mesothelium, or *angiomas* from the tubal vasculature.

It is quite difficult to differentiate a tubal neoplasm from other adnexal masses on examination, and, generally, operative exploration is necessary to confirm the diagnosis. Salpingectomy represents the definitive treatment, although if pathologic evaluation confirms the benign nature of the neoplasm, normal portions of the tube may be preserved for fertility reasons in selected instances.

PARAOVARIAN NEOPLASMS

As the name paraovarian implies (beside the ovary), paraovarian neoplasms are generally located within the broad ligament between the tube and the ovary. These tumors are generally small compared with ovarian cysts, measuring less than 8 cm, and, histologically, most appear to be derived from paramesonephric (müllerian) structures or occasionally from mesonephric (wolffian) remnants. Although the malignancy rate is not great (less than 10 percent), it is necessary to resect the cystic mass (generally with the ipsilateral tube) to obtain a pathologic assessment.

SUGGESTED READING

Beck RP, Latour JPA: Review of 1019 benign ovarian neoplasms. Obstet Gynecol 16:479, 1960.

Genadry R, Parmley T, Woodruff JD: The origin and clinical behavior of the paraovarian tumor. Am J Obstet Gynecol 129:873, 1977.

Katsube Y, Berg JW, Silverberg SG: Epidemiologic pathology of ovarian tumors: A histopathologic review of primary ovarian neoplasms diagnosed in the Denver Standard metropolitan statistical area, July 1–December 31, 1969 and July 1–December 31, 1979. Int J Pathol 1:3, 1982.

Limber GK, King RE, Silverberg SG: Pseudomyxoma peritonei: A report of ten cases. Ann Surg 178:587, 1973.

Scully RE: Tumors of the Ovary and Maldeveloped Gonads. Atlas of Tumor Pathology. 2nd series, fasc. 16. Washington, DC, Armed Forces Institute of Pathology, 1979.

Spanos WJ: Preoperative hormonal therapy of cystic adnexal masses. Am J Obstet Gynecol 116:551, 1973.

ENDOMETRIOSIS AND ADENOMYOSIS

J. GEORGE MOORE

Both endometriosis and adenomyosis are benign conditions in which endometrial glands and stroma are found beyond the endometrium.

ENDOMETRIOSIS

Endometriosis is a benign condition in which endometrial glands and stroma are present outside the endometrial cavity, usually in the ovary or on the pelvic peritoneum. It assumes great importance in gynecology because of its frequency, distressing symptomatology, association with infertility, and potential for invasion of adjacent organ systems, such as the gastrointestinal or urinary tracts. In addition, endometriosis often presents a difficult diagnostic problem, and few gynecologic conditions require such difficult surgical dissections.

Incidence

The exact incidence of endometriosis is not known, but it is estimated that more than 15 percent of women have the condition to some degree, and it is noted in about 20 percent of gynecologic laparotomies. It is an unexpected finding in a substantial number of cases.

Characteristically, endometriosis occurs in high-achieving nulliparous women with a type A personality. Less frequently, it is seen in minority ethnic patients on indigent hospital services. Generally, endometriosis is initiated in the third decade of life, becomes clinically apparent in the thirties, and regresses after the menopause. It may, on occasion, occur in infancy, childhood, or adolescence, but at these early ages it is almost always associated with obstructive genital anomalies. Although endometriosis should regress following the menopause if estrogens are not prescribed, the scarifying involution may result in obstructive problems, especially in the gastrointestinal and urinary tracts.

Pathogenesis

Three main theories for the development of endometriosis have been proposed.

1. The *lymphatic spread theory of Halban* suggests that endometrial tissues are taken up into the lymphatics draining the uterus and are transported to the various pelvic sites where the tissue grows ectopically. Endometrial tissue has been found in pelvic lymphatics in up to 20 percent of patients with the disease.

2. The *müllerian metaplasia theory of Meyer* proposes that endometriosis results from the metaplastic transformation of peritoneal mesothelium into endometrium under the influence of certain unidentified stimuli.

3. The *retrograde menstruation theory of Sampson* proposes that endometrial fragments transported through the fallopian tubes at the time of menstruation implant and grow in various intra-abdominal sites. Endometrial tissue normally shed at the time of menstrua-

tion is viable and capable of growth *in vivo* or *in vitro*.

In order to explain some rare examples of endometriosis in distant sites, such as the forehead or axilla, it is necessary to postulate *hematogenous spread*. Quite probably, all of these postulated mechanisms play a role in the development of endometriosis, and no single mechanism explains all cases.

Sites of Occurrence

Endometriosis occurs most commonly in the ovaries; on the broad ligament; on the peritoneal surfaces of the cul-de-sac, including the uterosacral ligaments and posterior cervix; and in the rectovaginal septum (Fig. 32–1). Quite frequently, the rectosigmoid colon is involved, as is the appendix and the vesicouterine fold of peritoneum. Endometriosis is occasionally seen in laparotomy scars, developing especially after cesarean sections or myomectomies when the endometrial cavity has been entered. In spite of the great variety of sites, 60 percent of patients with endometriosis have ovarian involvement.

Pathology

Characteristically, an endometrioma of the ovary forms a small cyst. It is filled with thick, chocolate-colored fluid that sometimes has the black color and tarry consistency of crankcase oil. This characteristic fluid represents aged, hemolyzed blood and desquamated endometrium. Usually, endometrial glands and stroma are present in the cyst wall. Sometimes, however, the pressure of the enclosed fluid destroys the endometrial lining of the endometrioma, leaving only a fibrotic cyst wall infiltrated with large numbers of hemosiderin-laden macrophages. Since corpus luteum cysts can give this same picture, pathologists are sometimes reluctant to diagnose endometriosis in the absence of endometrial glands and stroma in the cyst wall. Instead, they characterize the picture as "consistent with endometriosis."

Most often, the ovarian endometrioma is tightly adherent to the posterior leaf of the broad ligament bound by dense, intractable adhesions. Occasionally, an ovarian endometrioma may reach dimensions as large as 20 cm in diameter. Most instances of ovarian endometriosis are bilateral, and there is usually involvement of parietal and visceral peritoneal surfaces. When endometriosis involves the peritoneal surfaces, it appears as flat, brownish discolorations, often referred to as "powder burns" or, if they are raised and bluish in color, as "mulberry spots." The tissues surrounding these lesions are puckered and scarred as a result of fibrosis. Fre-

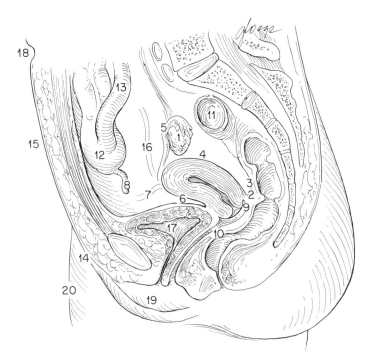

Figure 32–1 Common sites of endometriosis in decreasing order of frequency: (1) ovary, (2) cul-de-sac, (3) uterosacral ligaments, (4) broad ligaments, (5) fallopian tubes, (6) uterovesical fold, (7) round ligaments, (8) vermiform appendix, (9) vagina, (10) rectovaginal septum, (11) rectosigmoid colon, (12) cecum, (13) ileum, (14) inguinal canals, (15) abdominal scars, (16) ureters, (17) urinary bladder, (18) umbilicus, (19) vulva, and (20) peripheral sites.

quently, the rectosigmoid colon becomes tightly bound by dense endometriotic adhesions to the posterior wall of the lower uterine segment and cervix, resulting in fixed retroversion of the uterus.

Staging

Heretofore, the extent of endometriosis has been described anecdotally in each case. Recently, however, the American Fertility Society has employed a staging protocol in an attempt to correlate fertility potential with a quantified stage of endometriosis. The staging is based on the allocation of points depending on the sites and extent of disease (Table 32–1).

Symptoms

The characteristic triad of symptoms associated with endometriosis is dysmenorrhea, dyspareunia, and dyschezia. Generally, *secondary dysmenorrhea* first appears or worsens

in the late twenties or early thirties. If the endometriosis is associated with obstructive genital abnormalities, severe dysmenorrhea may commence at menarche.

Dyspareunia is generally associated with deep penetration and occurs mainly when the cul-de-sac, uterosacral ligaments, and portions of the posterior vaginal fornix are involved. Endometriomata in these sites are usually exquisitely tender to touch.

Dyschezia is experienced with uterosacral, cul-de-sac, and rectosigmoid colon involvement. As the stool passes between the uterosacral ligaments, the characteristic dyschezia is experienced. This symptom is highly characteristic and is much more common with endometriosis than with chronic salpingo-oophoritis, a condition that is often confused with endometriosis.

Pre- and postmenstrual *spotting* is a characteristic symptom of endometriosis. Menorrhagia is uncommon, the amount of menstrual flow usually diminishing with endometriosis. If the ovarian capsule is in-

TABLE 32–1

THE AMERICAN FERTILITY SOCIETY
REVISED CLASSIFICATION OF ENDOMETRIOSIS

Patient's Name _____   Date_____

Stage I (Minimal) - 1-5
Stage II (Mild) - 6-15   Laparoscopy_____ Laparotomy_____ Photography_____
Stage III (Moderate) - 16-40   Recommended Treatment_____
Stage IV (Severe) - >40
Total_____   Prognosis_____

	ENDOMETRIOSIS	<1cm	1-3cm	>3cm
PERITONEUM	Superficial	1	2	4
	Deep	2	4	6
OVARY	R Superficial	1	2	4
	Deep	4	16	20
	L Superficial	1	2	4
	Deep	4	16	20

	POSTERIOR CULDESAC OBLITERATION	Partial	Complete
		4	40

	ADHESIONS	<1/3 Enclosure	1/3-2/3 Enclosure	>2/3 Enclosure
OVARY	R Filmy	1	2	4
	Dense	4	8	16
	L Filmy	1	2	4
	Dense	4	8	16
TUBE	R Filmy	1	2	4
	Dense	4*	8*	16
	L Filmy	1	2	4
	Dense	4*	8*	16

*If the fimbriated end of the fallopian tube is completely enclosed, change the point assignment to 16.

From the American Fertility Society: Revised American Fertility Society Classification of Endometriosis 1985. Fertil Steril 43:351, 1985. Reproduced with permission of the publisher.

volved with endometriosis, *ovulatory pain* and midcycle vaginal bleeding often become a problem. Rarely, as other organ systems are involved, menstrual hematochezia, hematuria, and other forms of vicarious menstruation become evident.

The nature of *pelvic pain* caused by endometriosis is variable. It has been stated that the degree of pain varies inversely with the extent of the disease. Minimal endometriosis in the cul-de-sac is generally much more painful than a huge endometrioma within the ovary that is expanding freely into the abdominal cavity.

Infertility as a symptom of endometriosis is difficult to understand completely and even more difficult to quantify. Whereas approximately 10 percent of "normal" couples are infertile, some 30 to 40 percent of couples are infertile if the female presents with endometriosis. The condition is found in 40 to 50 percent of women who undergo surgery for infertility. Several mechanisms have been postulated to explain the association between endometriosis and infertility, and these are discussed in Chapter 50.

Signs

Endometriosis presents with a wide variety of signs varying from the presence of a small, exquisitely tender nodule in the cul-de-sac or on the uterosacral ligaments to a huge, relatively nontender, cystic abdominal mass. Occasionally, a small tender mulberry spot may be seen in the posterior fornix of the vagina. Characteristically, a tender, fixed adnexal mass is appreciated on bimanual examination. The uterus is retroverted in almost one half of women surgically explored for endometriosis. Frequently, no signs at all are appreciated on physical examination. The characteristic sharp, firm, exquisitely tender "barb" (from barbed wire) felt in the uterosacral ligament is the diagnostic *sine qua non* of endometriosis.

Differential Diagnosis

The main differential diagnoses confused with endometriosis are (1) chronic pelvic inflammatory disease or recurrent acute salpingitis, (2) hemorrhagic corpus luteum, (3) benign or malignant ovarian neoplasm, and, occasionally, (4) ectopic pregnancy.

Diagnosis

The diagnosis of endometriosis should be suspected in an afebrile patient with the characteristic symptom triad of endometriosis, a firm, fixed, tender adnexal mass, and tender nodularity in the cul-de-sac and uterosacral ligaments. This diagnosis is even more likely if the leukocyte count and erythrocyte sedimentation rate are normal. An ultrasonic evaluation may indicate an adnexal mass of complex echogenicity. The definitive diagnosis is generally made by the characteristic gross and histologic findings at laparoscopy or laparotomy.

Management

The management of endometriosis depends on certain key considerations: (1) the certainty of the diagnosis, (2) the severity of the symptoms, (3) the extent of the disease, (4) the desire for future fertility, (5) the age of the patient, and (6) the threat to the gastrointestinal and/or urinary tracts.

Surgical Resection. Large (6 to 20 cm) endometriomata are amenable to surgical resection only. If the patient is in her forties, the preferred treatment is a total abdominal hysterectomy (TAH) and bilateral salpingo-oophorectomy (BSO), even if the disease is resectable. Under such circumstances, the patient is quite likely to develop disconcerting menopausal symptoms, but these may be safely controlled with estrogen therapy without risk of recurrence of the endometriosis. A woman in her middle or late thirties might optimally be treated by resection of the endometriosis from the ovaries and TAH. With reflux menstruation eliminated by the hysterectomy, endometriosis seldom recurs. If fertility is desired, conservative surgery may be considered. Even if removal of the tubes and ovaries are required, leaving the uterus may now be a consideration because embryo transfer to a hormonally prepared uterus has been successfully carried out.

In the late twenties and early thirties, especially with future fertility desired, the patient with fairly extensive endometriosis might well be treated by (1) resecting the endometriomata; (2) lysing tubal adhesions, with or without presacral neurectomy (to relieve dysmenorrhea); (3) suspending the uterus (to preclude the fixed retroversion of the uterine fundus into the cul-de-sac by endometriotic adhesions); (4) and removing the appendix (as the appendix is a likely sight for endometriosis, even when it appears grossly normal). Following the surgical resection of endometriosis, 50 to 60 percent of patients become pregnant, usually in the first two years following surgery. With severe endometriosis, either pre- or postoperative danazol therapy appears to substantially improve the chance of subsequent fertility. Approximately 15 percent of patients treated by such conservative surgery will require reoperation at a later date.

If endometriosis involves the cul-de-sac or uterosacral ligaments, the proximity to the ureter, bladder, and sigmoid colon must be considered. In the course of follow-up, an intravenous pyelogram, colonoscopy, and/or barium enema should be utilized to evaluate the spread to these organ systems. Endometriosis may obstruct the ureter (Fig. 32–2). This is not an entirely benign disease, since 25 percent of kidneys are lost when endometriosis blocks the ureter. Obstruction of the rectosigmoid, and even obstruction of the small intestine, may require resection of the involved intestinal segment. If endometriosis involves the full thickness of the urinary or intestinal tract, TAH and BSO are generally indicated, unless future childbearing is desired.

Electrocautery or *laser treatment* of small foci of endometriosis at the time of laparoscopy is being employed with increasing frequency.

Drug Therapy. If endometriosis is minimal in extent and the symptoms are tolerable, no treatment is necessary, but the patient should be observed at six-month intervals. The use of medroxyprogesterone acetate (Provera) or a combined estrogen/progestin oral contraceptive on a cyclic basis may inhibit the growth of endometriosis, since this treatment effects an "exhaustion atrophy" of the normally placed or ectopic endometrium.

If the disease is minimal and symptoms are incapacitating, or if infertility is a problem, the endometriosis may be treated by a *pseudopregnancy regimen,* utilizing either escalating continuous doses of combined oral contraceptives or progestin only (medroxyprogesterone acetate, 30 mg daily or norethindrone acetate, 5 to 15 mg daily) over a period of six to nine months. Although most cases treated with pseudopregnancy result in temporary relief of symptoms and up to 40 percent may become pregnant following cessation of treatment, this regimen is poorly tolerated by most patients, and the endometriosis generally redevelops following cessation of treatment. Continuous progestin may be more effective than continuous oral contraceptives.

Danazol, an androgen dervative, may also be used in a "pseudomenopause" regimen to suppress symptoms of endometriosis if fertility is not a present concern. It is given over a period of six to nine months, and a dose of 800 mg daily may be necessary to suppress menstruation. Through its weak androgenic properties, danazol decreases the plasma levels of sex-hormine-binding globulin, and the increase of free testosterone can bring about hirsutism and acne. At three years after ces-

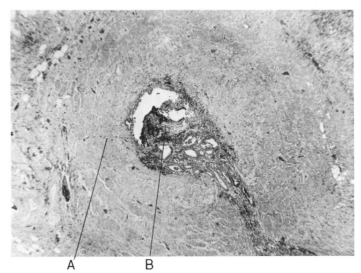

Figure 32–2 Endometriosis obstructing the ureter. Note the disease invading (A) the surrounding ureteric muscle and (B) the lumen of the ureter. This patient had a 2-cm focus of endometriosis confined to the lateral portion of the cardinal ligament with no intraperitoneal involvement.

A   B

sation of therapy, 40 percent of patients have had recurrence. After a full course of danazol therapy, use of a cyclic oral contraceptive may help to delay or prevent recurrence. Whenever a palpable endometrioma is present, the likelihood of a complete response to medical therapy is small.

A relatively recent development in the treatment of endometriosis is the long-term use of a *gonadotropin-releasing hormone (GnRH) agonist* that effects a temporary medical castration, thereby bringing about a marked regression of endometriosis over a period of up to six months. This has not yet been released by the Food and Drug Administration for general clinical use. Also, the long-term effects on endometriosis and its effect on large endometriomas have not been evaluated.

Prevention of Endometriosis

Whenever severe dysmenorrhea occurs in a young patient, the possibility of varying degrees of obstruction to the menstrual flow must be considered. The possibility of a blind uterine horn in a bicornuate uterus or an obstructing uterine or vaginal septum should be kept in mind. In more than half the patients who are noted to develop endometriosis during childhood and adolescence, varying degrees of genital tract obstruction may be found. Cervical dilatation to allow an easier egress of menstrual blood in patients with severe degrees of dysmenorrhea may be helpful in rare instances but is not generally recommended.

Whenever a congenital abnormality of the urinary or intestinal tract is detected, the genital tract should be investigated for an obstructive lesion. Infants with genital tract obstruction have been noted to develop endometriosis even in the first year of life.

ADENOMYOSIS

Adenomyosis is defined as the extension of endometrial glands and stroma into the uterine musculature. It is generally accepted that about 15 percent of women develop adenomyosis in their late thirties and early forties. Originally, adenomyosis was referred to as *endometriosis interna* (as opposed to endometriosis externa), but these terms have become archaic. About 15 percent of patients with adenomyosis have associated endometriosis. The basal layers of the endometrium extend in continuity to sites within the myometrium and generally do not participate in the proliferative and secretory cycles induced by the ovary.

Pathology

Generally, the uterus grossly is diffusely enlarged with a thickened myometrium containing characteristic glandular irregularities (Fig. 32–3). The endometrial cavity is also enlarged, consistent with the increased myometrium. Histologically, the extent of the process varies a great deal from superficial extension into the underlying myometrium to extension throughout the myometrium, occasionally with penetration of the peritoneal surface of the uterus. Occasionally, the adenomyosis may be confined to one portion of the myometrium and take the form of a fairly well circumscribed *adenomyoma*. Contrary to the picture in a uterine myoma, no distinct capsular margin can be detected on cut section between the adenomyoma and the surrounding myometrium. *Stromal adenomyosis* (endometrial stromatosis) is considered to be a variant of adenomyosis in which the endometrium spreading into the myometrium is made up entirely of endometrial stroma without glands.

Symptoms

Typical symptoms of adenomyosis are severe *secondary dysmenorrhea* and *menorrhagia*. The menorrhagia is consistent with the enlarged surface area of the endometrial cavity and the increased volume of sloughed endometrium. The dysmenorrhea is of the colicky type. Some patients may be asymptomatic. In about 30 to 40 percent of patients with adenomyosis, the disease is a surprise pathologic finding in a patient without menorrhagia, dysmenorrhea, or uterine enlargement. Occasionally, in a patient with a large adenomyoma, pressure on the bladder or rectum may create a problem.

Signs

On pelvic examination, the uterus is symmetrically enlarged. Occasionally, it may enlarge asymmetrically and make it impossible to distinguish this condition from that of a myomatous uterus. The consistency of the enlarged adenomyomatous uterus is generally softer than that of a uterine myoma.

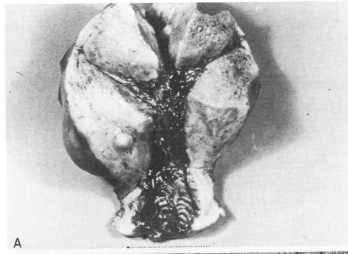

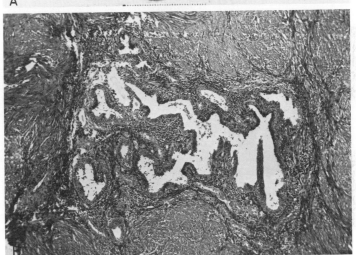

Figure 32–3 *A,* Grossly enlarged uterus with markedly thickened myometrium containing adenomyosis. *B,* Microscopic view of adenomyosis extending deep into the myometrium. Note the presence of both endometrial glands and stroma.

Treatment

The treatment of adenomyosis depends entirely on the symptoms and the possibility of other diagnoses. Any menorrhagia should be investigated by fractional dilatation and curettage (D & C) to rule out endometrial cancer, but if menorrhagia and dysmenorrhea are not a problem, only palliative treatment is indicated. If the menorrhagia is severe and recurrent following a D & C, or if the dysmenorrhea is disabling, total abdominal or vaginal hysterectomy is indicated. The ovaries should be preserved if they are normal, unless the patient is over 45 years.

SUGGESTED READING

ACOG Technical Bulletin. Management of Endometriosis. Washington DC, American College of Obstetricians and Gynecologists, March 1985.

Ansbacher P: Treatment of endometriosis with danazol. Am J Obstet Gynecol 121:283, 1975.

Kistner R: Hormonal treatment of endometriosis. Clin Obstet Gynecol 9:271, 1966.

Meldrum DR, Pardridge WM, Karow WG, et al: Hormonal effects of danazol and medical oophorectomy in endometriosis: Enigmas in diagnosis and management. Obstet Gynecol 62:480, 1983.

Moore JG, Hibbard LT, Growdon WA, et al: Urinary tract endometriosis. Am J Obstet Gynecol 134:162, 1979.

Ranney B: Endometriosis I: Conservative operations. Am J Obstet Gynecol 107:743, 1970.

Ranney B: Endometriosis II: Complete operations. Am J Obstet Gynecol 109:1137, 1971.

Ranney B: The prevention, palliation, and treatment of endometriosis. Am J Obstet Gynecol 123:778, 1975.

Revised Classification of Endometriosis. Birmingham, Alabama, The American Fertility Society, 1984.

Schiffren B, Ereg S, Moore JG: Teenage endometriosis. Am J Obstet Gynecol 116:973, 1973.

Spangler DB, Jones GS, Jones HW Jr: Infertility due to endometriosis: Conservative surgical therapy. Am J Obstet Gynecol 109:850, 1971.

Chapter Thirty-Three

VAGINAL AND VULVAR INFECTIONS

JOHN GUNNING

Vaginal discharge and vulvar irritation are common symptoms, and their evaluation and management form a significant proportion of office gynecologic practice. Some vaginal discharge is always present, although the amount varies with the hormonal status of the patient. This chapter discusses the differentiation between physiologic and pathologic vaginal discharges and outlines the management of patients with a variety of vulvovaginal infections.

NORMAL PHYSIOLOGY AND BACTERIOLOGY OF THE VAGINA

The vagina is lined by nonkeratinized stratified squamous epithelium, and its character is influenced by estrogen and progesterone. At birth, the vagina of the newborn is colonized initially by anaerobic and aerobic bacteria acquired during passage through the birth canal. The epithelium of the vagina at this time is rich in glycogen due to the influence of placental and maternal estrogens. This results in a low pH (3.7 to 6.3), which permits survival and growth of the colonizing organisms. Shortly after birth, available estrogen decreases, and the epithelium becomes thin, atrophic, and largely devoid of glycogen. The pH rises to between 6 and 8. Acidophilic organisms no longer have a selective advantage, and the predominant flora become gram-positive cocci and bacilli.

With the onset of puberty, the vagina be-

comes estrogenized again, and the glycogen content increases. Lactobacilli (Döderlein's bacilli) predominate in the healthy estrogenized vagina and are responsible for the breakdown of glycogen to lactic acid, which results in a vaginal pH of between 3.5 and 4.5. A wide variety of aerobic and anaerobic bacteria can be cultured from the normal vagina (Table 33–1). Most women harbor three to eight types of bacteria at any given time. It is usually under nonphysiologic conditions that organisms colonize in sufficient numbers to produce pathologic states.

TABLE 33–1 PREDOMINANT BACTERIAL FLORA IN THE NORMAL PREMENOPAUSAL VAGINA

BACTERIA	PERCENTAGE RANGE
Aerobes	
Lactobacillus	70–90
Staphylococcus epidermidis	30–60
Diphtheroids	30–60
Alpha-hemolytic *Streptococcus*	15–50
Beta-hemolytic *Streptococcus*	10–20
Non-hemolytic *Streptococcus*	5–30
Group D *Streptococcus*	10–40
Escherichia coli	20–25
Anaerobes	
Bacteroides fragilis	5–15
Bacteroides species	1–40
Peptococcus	5–60
Peptostreptococcus	5–40
Clostridium	5–15
Veillonella	10–15

Physiologic Vaginal Secretions

Vaginal secretions consist of cervical mucus (the major component); endometrial and oviductal fluid; exudates from the sebaceous, sweat, Bartholin's, and Skene's glands; a transudate from the vaginal squamous epithelium together with exfoliated squamous cells; and metabolic products of the microflora. These secretions are composed of proteins, polysaccharides, acids, amino acids, enzymes, enzyme inhibitors, and immunoglobulins. The exact function of these chemicals is poorly understood at the present time. There is a physiologic increase in vaginal secretion during pregnancy and at the midcycle. Postmenopausally, vaginal secretions are markedly decreased, and dyspareunia may result.

Investigation of Vaginal Discharge

Patients with vaginal and/or vulvar infections frequently present complaining of a nonbloody vaginal discharge (*leukorrhea*). The characteristics of the discharge (e.g., color, texture, viscosity, and odor) can often be helpful in making a diagnosis. To evaluate the patient definitively, however, a *wet mount smear preparation* of the discharge must be made. Using a cotton tip applicator, an adequate sample of vaginal discharge is suspended in 2 cc of normal saline. A drop of this solution is placed on a glass slide, covered with a coverslip, and examined under the microscope. To identify mycotic infections, some secretion is placed in a drop of 10 to 20 percent potassium hydroxide (KOH) and examined in the same manner.

CLINICAL CONDITIONS

Trichomonas Vaginitis

Trichomonas vaginitis is caused by the protozoan flagellate *Trichomonas vaginalis*, which is capable of living only in the female vagina and male urethra and is generally transmitted by sexual intercourse.

Clinical Features. Twenty five percent of patients harboring trichomonads are asymptomatic. Symptoms may vary from mild to severe and include vaginal discharge, vaginal and vulvar pruritus and burning, frequency of urination, and dyspareunia. The discharge is thin, bubbly, pale greenish or grayish in color, and has a pH of 5 to 6.5 (Table 33–2). The organism ferments carbohydrates, producing a gas with a rancid odor and causing a frothy appearing discharge. There frequently is erythema and edema of the vulva and vagina. Petechiae or strawberry patches on the vaginal mucosa and cervix are seen in approximately 10 percent of patients harboring trichomonads.

Diagnosis. The diagnosis is made by identifying the organism in a wet mount smear preparation. The organism is pear-shaped

TABLE 33–2 DIFFERENTIAL DIAGNOSIS AND TREATMENT OF VAGINITIS

DESCRIPTION	TRICHOMONIASIS	CANDIDIASIS	GARDNERELLA	HERPES
Discharge				
Amount	2 to 4	0 to 3	2 to 4	0 to 2
Color	yellow-green	white-curdy	gray	mucoid
Odor	1	0	2 to 3	0
Frothy	1	0	1	0
pH	5 to 6.5	4 to 5	5 to 5.5	variable
Symptoms				
Pruritus	0 to 4	2 to 4	0	0 to 1
Burning	0 to 1	1 to 2	0	2 to 4
Physical Examination				
Erythema	1 to 4	2 to 4	0	2 to 4
Edema	1 to 2	2 to 4	0	0 to 3
Petechiae	1	0	0	0
Ulcers	0	0	0	1 to 3
Wet Mount				
Clue Cells	0	0	1	0
Leukocytes	4	2	0 to 1	0 to 2

Key: 0 = none; 4 = severe

and motile, with obvious flagella that propel it through the saline. It is smaller than an epithelial cell and larger than a white cell. Culture techniques confirm the diagnosis, but these are seldom necessary.

Management. The treatment is specific and consists of *oral metronidazole* (Flagyl), in either a single 2 gm dose or a 250 mg dose three times daily for five to seven days. The single 2 gm dose may not be as effective as the longer treatment, but facilitates patient compliance. The side effects of metronidazole include mild nausea, occasional vomiting, and a metallic taste. Since the drug acts like disulfiram (Antabuse), the patient should abstain from alcohol during treatment. Treatment failures are usually related to reinfection and, therefore, the consort should be treated concurrently. Metronidazole should not be given during the first trimester of pregnancy because of possible teratogenicity. During the first trimester, a one week course of clotrimazole (Gyne-Lotrimin) vaginal suppositories or cream applied at bedtime is usually sufficient to alleviate symptoms. Aci-Jel vaginal jelly may also be used for symptomatic relief.

Candida Vulvovaginitis

Candidiasis is caused by the yeast organism *Candida albicans.* High risk factors for developing candidiasis are pregnancy, diabetes mellitus, oral contraceptive use, and recent antibiotic use.

Clinical Features. Approximately 20 per cent of women harboring *Candida albicans* are asymptomatic. Symptoms, which frequently begin in the premenstrual phase of the cycle, include vaginal discharge, vulvar pruritus and burning, and dyspareunia. The discharge has a "cottage cheese" appearance with a pH of 4 to 5. The vagina and vulva may be exquisitely tender with marked erythema and edema.

Diagnosis. The diagnosis is made by identifying the hyphae and buds of *Candida albicans* in a KOH wet mount preparation (Fig. 33–1). When necessary, a culture for diagnosis may be performed using Nickerson's or Sabouraud's medium.

Management. Treatment is with miconazole nitrate (Monistat) vaginal suppositories or cream inserted at bedtime for 7 to 14 days. An alternative is clotrimazole (Gyne-Lotrimin) vaginal suppositories or cream used nightly for 7 to 14 days. Coinfection with *Trichomonas vaginalis* is not unusual, and, if present, treatment for both is recommended.

Gardnerella vaginalis Vaginitis

Gardnerella vaginalis vaginitis (formerly called nonspecific vaginitis) is a sexually transmitted disease caused by a gram-negative bacillus, *Gardnerella* (*Haemophilus*) *vaginalis*, in the presence of anaerobic bacteria, such as *Bacteroides* and *Peptococcus* species. The combination of these bacteria produces the pathologic state.

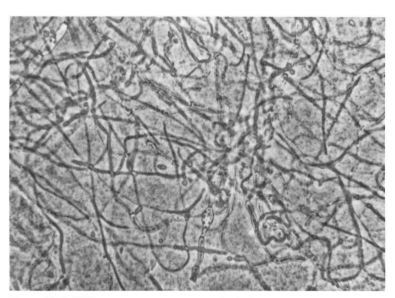

Figure 33–1 KOH wet mount preparation under high power magnification showing fiber-like mycelia of *Candida albicans.*

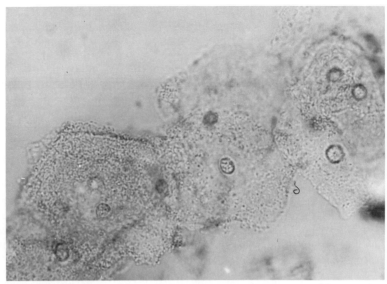

Figure 33–2 Saline wet mount showing clue cells of *Gardnerella vaginalis* vaginitis. Note the clear background.

Clinical Features. The most common symptom is a very profuse malodorous discharge. Itching or burning occurs in less than 20 percent of patients in contrast to trichomoniasis and candidiasis. The discharge is thin and grayish-appearing with a pH of 5.0 to 5.5. It may or may not have a distinctive odor. There is seldom evidence of vaginal or vulvar irritation. The addition of 10 to 20 percent KOH to the discharge releases amines that produce a fishy odor.

Diagnosis. The diagnosis is made by preparing a saline wet mount and identifying characteristic *clue cells,* epithelial cells with numerous bacilli clinging to their surface (Fig. 33–2). There are very few white blood cells present, which also helps distinguish it from trichomoniasis and candidiasis.

Management. *Metronidazole* (Flagyl) is effective against both *Gardnerella vaginalis* and the anaerobic bacteria associated with it. A dose of 500 mg twice daily for seven days is almost 100 percent curative. Alternatives that are not nearly as effective are ampicillin, 500 mg four times daily for seven days, or tetracycline, 500 mg four times daily for seven days. The patient's sexual partner should be treated in the same manner. Treatment for the common types of vaginitis is summarized in Table 33–3.

Condylomata Acuminata

Condylomata acuminata occur as papillomatous lesions on the vulva and may involve the vagina or cervix. The lesions may be small and discrete or large and cauliflower-like. They usually present as multiple small lesions, which have been called "venereal warts," and often occur in association with *Trichomonas vaginitis* and *Gardnerella vaginalis* vaginitis.

The etiologic agent is the human papilloma virus, which is a member of the papovavirus group. It is transmitted by direct contact, usually sexual, and the lesions are much more

TABLE 33–3 TREATMENT OF VAGINITIS

DRUG	TRICHOMONIASIS	CANDIDIASIS	GARDNERELLA
Metronidazole	+	−	+
Miconazole	−	+	−
Clotrimazole	−	+	−
Tetracycline	−	−	±
Ampicillin	−	−	±

Key: + = effective; − = ineffective

profuse in patients who are pregnant, diabetic, on oral contraceptives, or on immunosuppressant therapy. Although the virus of the genital wart and that of the usual skin lesion appear similar under electron microscopy, they are antigenically different, subtypes 6 and 11 being responsible for genital warts.

Management. The first line of treatment for small isolated lesions on the vulva is weekly applications of podophyllin, using a 25 percent suspension in tincture of benzoin. Care must be taken to protect the surrounding normal skin. If after four to six weeks of treatment the lesions persist and/or recur, other forms of desiccation may be used, such as cryosurgery, electrocautery treatment, or laser therapy. Occasionally, surgical extirpation is necessary. If biopsy or surgical excision is performed, the pathologist should be notified if podophyllin has been applied within the last six weeks, since this drug causes metaphase arrest, and its use can result in occasional bizarre mitoses, vacuolar degeneration, cellular necrosis, and an inflammatory response. These changes may be confused with malignancy. Podophyllin treatment should be avoided during pregnancy or if pregnancy is suspected, since maternal death, fetal death, and premature labor have been reported following its use.

In rare instances in which the warts are totally resistant or disseminated, such as seen in immunosuppressed patients, dinitrochlorobenzene (DNCB) sensitization followed by DNCB ointment application may be helpful. Spontaneous regression may occur, particularly if the lesions have appeared and grown rapidly during pregnancy. If the vagina is markedly involved during pregnancy, cesarean section should be entertained as the method of delivery because of the possibility of extensive lacerations and the difficulty of suturing such lesions.

Molluscum Contagiosum

Molluscum contagiosum is an epithelial proliferative process caused by a mildly contagious, growth-stimulating virus. The infection is transmitted by direct and indirect contact. Most patients with this disorder have no symptoms, except occasional mild pruritus. Examination reveals multiple growths varying in size from a pinhead to 1 cm in diameter on the vulva and perineal skin. The typical lesion is a dome-shaped papule with an umbilicated center.

Treatment is to manually express the caseous content from each lesion, followed by an application of carbonic acid, trichloroacetic acid, or silver nitrate. An alternative method of therapy involves removing the papules with a small dermal curette and electrodesiccating the base.

Herpes Genitalis

Herpes genitalis is a venereal disease caused by the herpes simplex virus type II in 90 percent of cases and herpes simplex virus type I in 10 percent of cases. Both are DNA viruses. The symptoms of primary herpes infection usually appear within three to seven days of exposure. The infection may be asymptomatic, since there are a number of patients who have antibodies against type II virus with no prior history of infection. Patients who have had oral herpes (type I virus) may have a degree of protection against subsequent infections with genital herpes (type II virus).

Clinical Features. In patients who become symptomatic, prodromal symptoms, such as mild paresthesia and burning in the perineal area, may be experienced before lesions become visible. The initial lesions may cause severe vulvar pain and exquisite tenderness. If the urethra or bladder mucosa is infected, urination may be extremely painful and occasionally urinary retention occurs. Patients with primary infections usually have inguinal lymphadenopathy, generalized malaise, and a low-grade fever.

Physical findings depend on the stage of the lesions at presentation. The first manifestations are clear vesicles that involve the labia majora, labia minora, perineal skin, and vestibule of the vulva. The vagina and ectocervical mucosa may be involved. Lesions that primarily involve the vagina and ectocervix are usually asymptomatic. The vesicles rupture within one to seven days and form ulcers. The ulcers are shallow, but painful, and each is frequently surrounded by a red areola. Several small lesions may coalesce to form a large ulcer, the surface of which may become secondarily infected and necrotic. The ulcers generally heal in seven to ten days. If superinfection is extensive, they may last for up to six weeks. When healing occurs, there is no residual scarring or ulceration.

Diagnosis. The diagnosis is made by the typical appearance of the vesicles and ulcers and the clinical syndrome. A *cytologic smear* of the ulcer base and cervix can confirm the diagnosis if it shows classic multinucleated cells with acidophilic intranuclear inclusion bodies. The false-negative rate is high, however. The definitive diagnosis is made by *culture* using Hanks' medium. It is important that the culture be taken of fluid from ruptured vesicles or that an ulcer be debrided and material taken from its base. False-negative cultures are frequent unless these precautions are observed.

Recurrence. About 30 percent of patients who have had primary herpes develop recurrences. The virus migrates up nerve fibers to the dorsal root ganglia where it usually remains dormant. A recurrence may be precipitated by an episode of stress, menstruation, or an upper respiratory illness. When recurrence occurs, the virus travels down the nerve fiber to the previously affected area. The resultant lesions are similar to those seen in the primary infection, although usually smaller. Local symptoms are generally of shorter duration, lesser severity, and seldom accompanied by systemic manifestations or inguinal lymphadenopathy.

Pregnancy. Genital infection during pregnancy secondary to herpes simplex virus types I and II is discussed in Chapter 15.

Management. A large number of therapeutic procedures have been recommended for herpes infections, but at the present time no effective treatment is available. Measures such as hot sitz baths and diluted Burow's solution may afford symptomatic relief. A Foley catheter may occasionally be required if voiding is difficult and painful. *Acyclovir* ointment 5 percent, which is an acyclic purine analogue, may shorten the course of the initial attack and shorten the length of viral shedding if applied very early in the infection. However, this regimen does not prevent recurrent infection or have any impact on the time course of recurrent episodes. Parenteral acyclovir is available for patients with severe disease and for immunocompromised patients with life-threatening infections.

Patients should be advised to abstain from sexual contact while lesions are present. If the infection is their first, they should continue to abstain until they become culture-negative, since prolonged viral shedding may occur in such cases. The risk of transmission during the asymptomatic period is unknown.

Syphilis

Syphilis is a sexually transmitted disease caused by *Treponema pallidum,* a motile anaerobic spirochete that invades intact moist mucosa.

Clinical Features. The vulva is the most frequent entry site in the female. About 10 to 60 days after inoculation, a *chancre* appears on the vulva, vagina, or cervix, heralding the stage of *primary syphilis.* The chancre is a firm, completely painless lesion with a punched out base and rolled edges. Painless inguinal lymphadenopathy usually occurs.

Diagnosis. The diagnosis is made by identifying the spirochete on dark-field microscopy of material scraped from the base of the chancre. If untreated, the chancre will heal spontaneously in three to nine weeks. A serologic test for syphilis will be negative at this time but should be obtained for baseline documentation.

About eight weeks after infection, or three to six weeks after the chancre appears, the patient usually develops manifestations of *secondary syphilis,* including such systemic symptoms as malaise, headache, anorexia, and a generalized maculopapular skin rash. At this time, the patient may develop condylomata lata on the vulva and upper thighs; these are broad exophytic excrescences that ulcerate and are highly contagious. Dark-field examination of material from these lesions reveals numerous spirochetes. Serological tests for syphilis are generally positive at this stage.

If primary or secondary syphilis is not treated, the patient is at risk to develop *tertiary syphilis,* which may involve any organ system of the body. A rare manifestation is a *gumma* of the vulva, which appears as a nodule that enlarges, ulcerates, and becomes necrotic.

Management. Treatment of primary and secondary syphilis is benzathine penicillin G, 2.4 million units intramuscularly. An alternative is tetracycline, 500 mg orally four times daily for 15 days. For tertiary syphilis, the penicillin is given weekly for three weeks or the tetracycline is given for 30 days. Erythromycin, 500 mg orally four times daily for 15 days, can be used during pregnancy, if the patient is allergic to penicillin.

Chancroid

Chancroid is a highly contagious, sexually transmitted disease caused by the bacillus *Haemophilus ducreyi*. The disease is seldom seen in the United States and occurs most frequently in tropical and subtropical climates.

Symptoms of vulvar pain and tenderness at the site of a small papule occur three to five days after exposure. The papule rapidly ulcerates and autoinoculation of other areas may occur. The ulcers have a grayish base, a foul odor, and are very painful to the touch. Regional lymphadenopathy and subsequent bubo formation with suppuration frequently occur if the disease is not treated. Massive tissue destruction of the vulva and perineum may also occur if not treated.

The diagnosis is best documented by Gram's stain, culture, and biopsy. All three tests are needed, since the false-negative rate for each individual test is high.

The treatment for this disease is tetracycline, 500 mg orally four times daily for ten days. An alternative is trimethoprim/sulfamethoxazole, 160/800 mg orally twice daily for ten days.

Lymphogranuloma Venereum

Lymphogranuloma venereum is a venereal disease caused by *Chlamydia trachomatis* serotypes L-1, L-2, and L-3. *Chlamydia* organisms are obligatory intracellular parasites that are bacteria-like and definitely not viruses. Other serotypes cause psittacosis, trachoma, inclusion conjunctivitis, nongonococcal urethritis, salpingitis, and pneumonia of newborns. The disease is relatively uncommon in the United States and affects males 20 times more frequently than females.

Clinical Features. One to four weeks after the onset of infection, nonspecific symptoms, such as generalized malaise, headaches, and fever, may accompany the development of a papule, which subsequently develops into a painless vulvovaginal ulcer. This stage may not be clinically apparent but is followed about one month later by adenitis. Inguinal buboes develop frequently in males but are uncommon in females. In females, direct lymphatic spread occurs to the deep nodes around the anus and rectum. Occasionally, lymphatic involvement may be minimal and spontaneous regression may occur. More often there is chronic progressive disease causing ulceration, elephantiasis, sinus tract formation, rectovaginal fistulas, abscesses, and secondary infection of the vulva and rectum. Rectal stenosis secondary to scarring may occur.

Diagnosis. The diagnosis is not easily made on the basis of history and physical examination. Biopsy examination is nonspecific and nondiagnostic. Complement fixation and microimmunofluorescence serologic tests for antibodies to *Chlamydia* are most helpful. Biologic false-positive VDRL tests occur in about 20 percent of patients.

Management. Treatment is tetracycline, 500 mg four times daily for two to three weeks. Alternative drugs are erythromycin, 500 mg four times daily for two to three weeks; doxycycline, 100 mg twice daily for at least two weeks; or sulfamethoxazole, 1 gm twice daily for two to three weeks.

Granuloma Inguinale

Granuloma inguinale is caused by the bacterium *Donovania granulomatis*. It is seldom seen in the United States and occurs predominately in the black population.

Clinical Features. The condition begins with the appearance of a papule on the external genitalia approximately 1 to 12 weeks following initial contact. The papule rapidly ulcerates, and the ulcers are characterized by irregular borders and a beefy red granular base. The beginning papule and ulcer inoculate multiple adjacent sites. Progressively, there may be involvement of the perineum, perianal area, vagina, and cervix. The ulcers are painless. True bubo formation does not occur, although there may be some inguinal lymphadenopathy. As the ulcers become secondarily infected, fibrosis, scarring, depigmentation, and keloid formation characterize the advanced stage of the disease. Progressive fibrosis may lead to vaginal stenosis and elephantiasis, the latter secondary to lymphatic obstruction.

Diagnosis. The diagnosis is made by demonstrating *Donovan bodies* in tissue smears stained with Giemsa or Wright's stain. The Donovan body is an encapsulated bipolar staining bacterium with a reddish color found within the large mononuclear cells.

Management. Treatment is tetracycline in doses of 500 mg every six hours for 10 to 21 days. Healing should be expected within a period of six weeks. In cases that are unresponsive to this regimen, a longer course of treatment may be necessary.

TOXIC SHOCK SYNDROME

Toxic shock syndrome is a rare, potentially fatal, multisystem condition that is associated with strains of staphylococci capable of producing toxins, including an epidermal exfoliative toxin. The syndrome was originally described in children, but has been recognized more recently in women, especially those under 30 years of age who are menstruating and using vaginal tampons. Toxic shock syndrome has also been noted rarely in association with other articles placed vaginally, such as diaphragms, sponges, and cervical caps, and may also be seen rarely in patients with postoperative wound infections, including infections in the postpartum period.

The clinical symptoms include a sudden high fever, flu-like symptoms (sore throat, headache, and especially diarrhea), erythroderma, signs of multisystemic failure, and refractory hypotension. Exfoliation of the palmar and plantar surfaces of the hands and feet as well as other skin surfaces usually occurs one to two weeks after the onset of the illness. Early recognition of the disease is of hallmark importance, for many of the deaths associated with this syndrome have occurred in patients who had been diagnosed incorrectly as having other potentially less dangerous illnesses such as allergic reactions, gastritis, or flu.

Management

Potential sources of infection such as foreign bodies or wound debris should be removed and adequate hydration ensured. Antibiotics specifically directed toward penicillinase-resistant *Staphylococcus aureus* should be used immediately. If steroids are begun within 72 hours, there appears to be a significant reduction in the severity of the overall illness and the duration of fever, but the use of steroids in this disease remains controversial.

Prognosis

If adequate supportive therapy is instituted early, full recovery can usually be expected. Multiple recurrences have been described in individual patients, although usually only one episode is encountered.

Prophylaxis

Tampons should be changed frequently during heavy flow or moderate flow days. Any objects designed for intravaginal use, especially the vaginal sponge, should be used with the knowledge that there is a potential for toxic shock syndrome, so patients should be informed of some of the clinical manifestations. Should any signs or symptoms of toxic shock syndrome occur, the patient should immediately remove the intravaginal product and seek emergency medical attention.

SUGGESTED READING

Bartlett JG, Moon NE, Goldstein PR, et al: Cervical and vaginal bacterial flora: Ecologic niches in the female lower genital tract. Am J Obstet Gynecol 130:658, 1978.

Davis JP, Chesney PJ, Wand PJ, et al: Toxic shock syndrome. N Engl J Med 303:1429, 1980.

Gardner HL: *Haemophilus vaginalis* vaginitis after twenty-five years. Am J Obstet Gynecol 137:385, 1980.

Gardner HL, Kaufman RH: Benign Disease of the Vulva and Vagina. St. Louis, CV Mosby, 1980.

Huggins GR, Preti G: Diagnostic clues from vaginal odors. Contemp Obstet Gynecol 22:199, 1983.

Ledger WJ: Infection in the Female. Philadelphia, Lea & Febiger, 1977.

Mehta P: Vaginal flora: A dynamic ecosystem. J Reprod Med 27:455, 1982.

Pheifer TA, Forsyth PS, Durfee MA, et al: Nonspecific vaginitis. Role of *Haemophilus vaginalis* and treatment with metronidazole. N Engl J Med 298:1429, 1978.

Schachter J: Chlamydial infections. N Engl J Med 298:428, 1978.

Sikat P, Heemstra J, Ranney B, et al: Metronidazole chemotherapy for *Trichomonas vaginalis* infections. JAMA 182:904, 1980.

Spiegel CA, Amsel R, Eschenbach D, et al: Anaerobic bacteria in nonspecific vaginitis. N Engl J Med 303:601, 1980.

Spruance SL, Overall JC, Kern ER, et al: The natural history of recurrent herpes simplex labialis. Implications for antiviral therapy. N Engl J Med 297:69, 1977.

Todd J, Ressman M, Caston S, et al: Corticosteroid therapy for patients with toxic shock syndrome. JAMA 252:3399, 1984.

Toxic shock syndrome update. FDA Drug Bulletin 10(3):17, 1980.

Chapter Thirty-Four

PELVIC INFLAMMATORY DISEASE

LARRY C. FORD, and HUNTER A. HAMMILL

Infections of the female reproductive organs are a major cause of morbidity in gynecologic patients. Fortunately, new concepts regarding etiology and management are evolving. A better understanding of the bacteria involved in these infections is now available, and the proliferation of newer, broader spectrum antibiotics has made successful therapy more feasible, particularly for early infections. In this chapter, pelvic inflammatory disease (PID) occurring in nonpregnant patients is discussed and is divided into salpingo-oophoritis and tubo-ovarian abscess. Postabortal and puerperal genital tract infections are considered in Chapters 24 and 36.

SALPINGO-OOPHORITIS

In the past, salpingo-oophoritis has been classically considered to be either gonococcal or nongonococcal. More recently, it has been shown that many bacterial species may be involved.

Etiology

Apart from *Neisseria gonorrhoeae,* a variety of other microorganisms have been isolated from surgically obtained specimens of patients with acute salpingitis (Table 34–1). Whether these agents are pathogenic or are merely colonizing the tubes is a question that is not completely resolved, but current evidence favors a multibacterial etiology. Sexual activity is responsible for spreading the organisms, and usually numerous bacteria are

transmitted. For example, *N. gonorrhoeae* may be passed, together with *Chlamydia, Mycoplasma,* and *Herpes simplex* Type II virus.

Acute PID sometimes may be exacerbated by menses, sexual intercourse, strenuous physical activity, and even a pelvic examination. The relationship to the menstrual period has been postulated to be due to the breakdown of the antibacterial barrier of cervical mucus, allowing infectious agents present in the lower genital tract to ascend to the upper tract. The possibility that potential pathogens may "cling" to sperm and be carried to the upper genital tract has also been considered.

A special situation is the presence of a

TABLE 34–1 ETIOLOGIC AGENTS IN NONGESTATIONAL ACUTE PELVIC INFLAMMATORY DISEASE

Neisseria gonorrhoeae
Anaerobic bacteria (Bacteroides and gram-positive cocci)
Facultative gram-negative rods (such as *Escherichia coli*)
Chlamydia trachomatis
Mycoplasma hominis
Actinomyces israelii

NOTE: In the individual patient, it is often impossible to differentiate among these agents.

Information obtained from Sexually Transmitted Diseases, Treatment Guidelines: 1982. US Department of Health and Human Services, Centers for Disease Control, Morbidity and Mortality Weekly Report (suppl) 31:335, 1982.

nonvenereally transmitted infection in the presence of an intrauterine device. Such infections may be unilateral, and *Actinomyces israelii* may sometimes be isolated.

Clinical Features

The diagnosis of acute salpingo-oophoritis is made frequently, but often inappropriately. The patient usually presents with lower quadrant pain, which is frequently bilateral. She may have recently started her menses. Occasionally, presenting symptoms may be dysuria and a purulent vaginal discharge. On *physical examination,* the patient is usually febrile and has a tachycardia and a normal blood pressure. There is generalized lower abdominal tenderness without palpable masses. On speculum examination, there may be a purulent cervical discharge. Bimanual examination reveals cervical motion tenderness and bilateral adnexal tenderness, without adnexal masses or induration.

Investigations

A *complete blood count* should be obtained. A neutrophil leukocytosis indicates acute infection. An elevated *erythrocyte sedimentation rate* is also indicative of infection. A *urinalysis* should be carried out to rule out urinary tract infection. A *pregnancy test* may be important if there is a possibility of ectopic pregnancy. A *cervical culture* should be obtained. The presence of gram-negative intracellular diplococci (*N. gonorrhoeae*) on a cervical smear is helpful in making the diagnosis.

Secondary diagnostic tests include *culdocentesis* and *pelvic ultrasound*. Culdocentesis involves inserting an 18- or 20-gauge needle through the posterior vaginal fornix into the *cul-de-sac*. A mass in the *cul-de-sac* is a *contraindication* to the procedure. If purulent or serous material is obtained, it should be Gram stained and cultures for aerobes, anaerobes, and *Neisseria gonorrhoeae* obtained. A pelvic ultrasound is useful to define an adnexal mass, especially if an ectopic pregnancy is being considered.

The Infectious Disease Society for Obstetrics and Gynecology has suggested that certain criteria be present before the diagnosis of acute salpingo-oophoritis is made. These are shown in Table 34–2.

TABLE 34–2 CRITERIA FOR DIAGNOSIS OF ACUTE SALPINGO-OOPHORITIS*

1. Abdominal tenderness
2. Cervical motion tenderness
3. Adnexal tenderness

These should be accompanied by at least one of the following:

1. Elevated erythrocyte sedimentation rate
2. Leukocytosis
3. Purulent cervical discharge (defined as greater than 6 WBC/hpf)†
4. Purulent fluid obtained at culdocentesis
5. Oral temperature greater than 100.4°F (38°C)

*As outlined by the Infectious Disease Society for Obstetrics and Gynecology.
†WBC—white blood cells
hpf—high-power field

Differential Diagnosis

The differential diagnosis must include acute appendicitis, urinary tract infection, adnexal torsion, endometriosis, bleeding corpus luteum, and ectopic pregnancy.

The only definitive method of establishing the diagnosis of acute salpingo-oophoritis is by laparoscopy or laparotomy. Although not necessary for most patients, *laparoscopy* is strongly advised in those in whom the diagnosis is not clinically apparent or in whom the response to antibiotic therapy is inappropriate.

Treatment

Drug Therapy. A variety of chemotherapeutic agents are used in the management of patients with PID, and the choice of agents is somewhat empirical (Table 34–3). An ov-

TABLE 34–3 RATIONALE FOR SELECTION OF ANTIMICROBIALS FOR ACUTE PID

1. Treatment of choice is not established.
2. No single agent is active against the entire spectrum of pathogens.
3. Several antimicrobial combinations provide a broad spectrum of activity against the major pathogens *in vitro*, but many have not been adequately evaluated for clinical efficacy in PID.

Information obtained from Sexually Transmitted Diseases, Treatment Guidelines: 1982. US Department of Health and Human Services, Centers for Disease Control, Morbidity and Mortality Weekly Report (suppl) 31:335, 1982.

erview of the agents that are of most value follows.

PENICILLINS. When penicillin first became available, most organisms, including the enteric and anaerobic organisms, were sensitive to it. However, the use and abuse of penicillin and other antibiotics have resulted in many organisms becoming resistant to drugs to which they were once sensitive. Because penicillin was among the first antibiotics to be isolated, it has seen the most number of "generations" or derivatives.

Of the *first-generation penicillins*, penicillin G is the model. These first generation drugs are indicated for the therapy of syphilis and most streptococcal infections. In doses greater than 15 million units per day, the drug has some activity against nonpenicillinase-producing anaerobic bacteria. However, most *Proteus* and *Pseudomonas* species, as well as many of the enteric organisms, are now resistant.

Second-generation penicillins, such as ampicillin and amoxicillin, have the advantage of oral as well as parenteral administration. They are also inactivated by penicillinase-producing bacteria. Amoxicillin, the hydroxy derivative of ampicillin, has increased gastrointestinal absorption and causes less gastrointestinal irritation. Second-generation penicillins have greater activity against enteric organisms but less anaerobic coverage, since they are active only in doses greater than 12 gm per day.

Of the *third-generation penicillins,* carbenicillin and ticarcillin are commonly used. Their advantage includes some enhanced anaerobic and enteric coverage. In particular, *Pseudomonas* coverage is enhanced. A disadvantage is the high sodium load, especially with carbenicillin.

Currently, two *fourth-generation penicillins* have been approved by the Food and Drug Administration (FDA) for use in the United States—piperacillin and mezlocillin. Their sodium loads are much lower than those of the third-generation drugs. The anaerobic spectrum is excellent, as is the enteric coverage. For example, piperacillin covers greater than 90 percent of *Clostridium* species and has pseudomonal and enteric coverage comparable to the aminoglycosides, but without eighth cranial nerve toxicity.

CEPHALOSPORINS. The *first generation cephalosporins,* such as cephalothin, cover many strains of the gram-positive cocci and

Escherichia coli. The disadvantage of all first-generation cephalosporins is weak to absent enterococcal and anaerobic coverage.

The *second-generation cephalosporins,* such as cefoxitin and cefamandole, differ in their *in vitro* spectrum. The enteric coverage of cefamandole is better than that of cefoxitin, while the anti-anaerobic activity of cefoxitin is clearly superior to that of cefamandole.

The role of *third-generation cephalosporins,* such as moxalactam, cefoperazone, ceftazidime, and cefotaxime, is limited in obstetrics and gynecology. Their purported advantages include enhanced "*in vitro*" anaerobic coverage over the first-generation cephalosporins and increased *Pseudomonas* coverage. They have, as yet, an unproven role as monotherapy for serious pelvic infections. The addition of a third-generation cephalosporin to a standard therapy combination, such as an aminoglycoside and clindamycin or an aminoglycoside plus a penicillin and chloramphenicol, adds nothing to the bacterial coverage. They also have no proven advantage over cefoxitin for prophylaxis.

METRONIDAZOLE. Metronidazole (Flagyl) covers many anaerobic bacteria but has no aerobic coverage, with the exception of *Gardnerella vaginalis.* Therefore, when used for therapy of serious infections, the drug must always be used in combination with other antibiotics, usually an aminoglycoside and frequently also a penicillin or cephalosporin.

Side effects can include an unpleasant metallic taste in the mouth and, rarely, reversible leukopenia. The drug is related to disulfiram (Antabuse), so there are severe untoward reactions with concomitant ethanol ingestion. Metronidazole has been shown to be mutagenic by the Salmonella Mammalian Microsome (Ames) Test and, therefore, should be avoided during pregnancy.

CLINDAMYCIN. Clindamycin is a member of the macrolide family, which also includes erythromycin. The drug has excellent activity against anaerobic organisms and aerobic gram-positive cocci but weaker activity against enteric bacteria. Therefore, it is usually combined with an aminoglycoside for the treatment of severe infections.

Diarrhea occurs in 5 to 10 percent of patients. Although widely publicized, true *pseudomembranous enterocolitis,* which is caused by *Clostridium difficile,* is rare. In fact, ampicillin, because of its very broad usage, causes more cases per year of pseudomembranous enterocolitis than does clindamycin. If a patient develops diarrhea while taking clindamycin, urgent investigations should include (1) stool cultures for *C. difficile* using selective media that can give results in 12 hours, and (2) serum antibody titers to *C. difficile* toxin. If either result is positive or if these tests cannot be performed rapidly, the clindamycin should be stopped.

Clindamycin combined with an aminoglycoside is a very effective treatment for most patients with severe pelvic infections.

TETRACYCLINE. Tetracyclines have long been used for the outpatient treatment of PID. The advantages of these drugs include oral absorption, reasonable aerobic and anaerobic coverage, and chlamydial coverage. All tetracyclines are absolutely contraindicated in patients who are or might be pregnant because of their damaging effect on the fetal teeth.

There are two generations of tetracyclines. Second-generation drugs, which include minocycline and doxycycline, have some *in vitro* advantages over first-generation tetracyclines—in particular, better anaerobic coverage. The main advantage of the second-generation drugs is their higher compliance rate because of the once or twice daily dosage.

CHLORAMPHENICOL. Chloramphenicol diffuses well into tissues after oral or parenteral administration and has excellent anaerobic and aerobic coverage. A rare side effect is idiosyncratic, irreversible aplastic anemia. The true incidence of this complication is probably less than 1 in 100,000 cases. There is a dose-dependent reversible bone marrow depression, primarily of the leukocyte series. The drug is not used routinely as first-line therapy, mainly for medicolegal reasons. However, if the patient is in septic shock, chloramphenicol should be added to the usual combination of antibiotics.

AMINOGLYCOSIDES. The aminoglycosides, such as gentamicin, amikacin, and tobramycin, have excellent activity against enteric organisms, but they have no anaerobic activity. Therefore, aminoglycosides should never be used as single agents to treat PID.

Renal toxicity is the most common complication of aminoglycoside administration, and particular caution is necessary if the patient has had previous exposure to another nephrotoxin, such as *cis*-platinum. It is important to obtain blood urea nitrogen, serum creatinine, and, sometimes, creatinine clearance levels prior to the administration of aminoglycosides. In addition, therapeutic levels should be maintained by monitoring "peak" and "trough" levels of the drug in the serum. These levels should be attained on the second or third day of therapy and every other day thereafter. Tobramycin appears to have the least renal toxicity, so it should be used if there is any impairment of renal function.

Eighth cranial nerve toxicity, both auditory and vestibular, is also a complication associated with aminoglycosides. However, it is seldom seen in gynecologic infections because treatment courses rarely exceed ten days. Neuromuscular blockade is a rare complication.

Outpatient Management. When the symptoms are mild, particularly with recurrent episodes of PID, outpatient treatment may be sufficient, as shown in Table 34–4. Strict pelvic rest (no sexual activity, no douching, no tampons) is necessary, and bedrest should be advised while there is fever or systemic symptoms.

The second-generation tetracyclines have better gonococcal coverage (including penicillinase-producing gonococci), reasonable aerobic and anaerobic coverage, and chlamydial coverage. Recently, minocycline has been approved by the FDA for both male and female chlamydial infections.

Oral penicillins, including oral penicillin VK, ampicillin, amoxicillin, and carbenicillin,

TABLE 34–4 OUTPATIENT TREATMENT OPTIONS FOR ACUTE PELVIC INFLAMMATORY DISEASE

Cefoxitin, 2 gm IM
OR
Amoxicillin, 3 gm by mouth
OR
Ampicillin, 3.5 gm by mouth
OR
Aqueous procaine penicillin G, 4.8 million units IM, at two sites, each given with probenecid 1 gm by mouth
FOLLOWED BY
Doxycycline, 100 mg by mouth twice daily for 10–14 days
OR
Tetracycline HCl, 500 mg by mouth, 4 times a day for 10–14 days

Information obtained from Sexually Transmitted Diseases, Treatment Guidelines: 1982. US Department of Health and Human Services, Centers for Disease Control, Morbidity and Mortality Weekly Report (suppl) 31:335, 1982.

have poor activity against the mixed infections. In addition, while they have some activity against gonococci if given in high enough dosages, they have no antichlamydial activity. Oral cephalosporins have no antichlamydial or antianaerobic activity. Like the penicillins, they do have antigonococcal coverage.

Sexual partners should be examined and treated promptly with a regimen effective against uncomplicated gonococcal and chlamydial infection. The patient should be reevaluated clinically in 48 to 72 hours, and those not responding well should be hospitalized. A repeat culture should be taken to ensure cure. If the patient has an intrauterine device (IUD) *in situ,* it should be removed soon after antimicrobial therapy has been initiated.

TREATMENT OF UNCOMPLICATED GONORRHEA. The treatment of uncomplicated gonorrhea, which is usually diagnosed on a routine cervical culture or by a history of recently diagnosed gonorrhea in a sexual partner, is complicated by the following: (1) the increasing incidence of penicillinase-producing *N. gonorrhoeae* (PPNG); (2) the emergence of tetracycline-resistant gonococci in some geographic areas; and (3) the high frequency of coexisting chlamydial infection, which has been documented in up to 45' percent of patients with gonorrhea for whom adequate chlamydial cultures have been undertaken. Regimens recommended by the United States Department of Health and Human Services are shown in Table 34–5.

Inpatient Therapy. Patients with acute PID, especially the first episode, generally

TABLE 34–6 INDICATIONS FOR HOSPITALIZATION OF WOMEN WITH ACUTE SALPINGO-OOPHORITIS

1. The diagnosis is uncertain.
2. Surgical emergencies, such as appendicitis and ectopic pregnancy, must be excluded.
3. A pelvic abscess is suspected.
4. Severe illness precludes outpatient management.
5. The patient is pregnant.
6. The patient is unable to follow or tolerate an outpatient regimen.
7. The patient has failed to respond to outpatient therapy.
8. Clinical follow-up after 48–72 hours of antibiotic treatment cannot be arranged.

Information obtained from Sexually Transmitted Diseases, Treatment Guidelines: 1982. US Department of Health and Human Services, Centers for Disease Control, Morbidity and Mortality Weekly Report (suppl) 31:335, 1982.

benefit from early hospitalization and intensive therapy. The indications for hospitalization are shown in Table 34–6.

Empiric therapy, based on probable etiologic agents, should be commenced immediately after the diagnosis is made. Cervical and vaginal cultures are useless as a basis for the selection of antibiotic agents. Even if cultures are obtained at laparoscopy or laparotomy, placed immediately in anaerobic transport devices, and rushed to the laboratory, it takes at least three days for the identification of anaerobic organisms and even longer to obtain antibiotic sensitivities. In view of the spectrum of bacteria known to be involved in the pathogenesis of PID, it is

TABLE 34–5 TREATMENT OF UNCOMPLICATED GONORRHEA IN ADULTS

Tetracycline HCl: 500 mg by mouth, four times daily for seven days
OR
Doxycycline: 100 mg by mouth, twice daily for seven days
OR
Amoxicillin, 3 gm or ampicillin, 3.5 gm: either with 1 gm probenecid by mouth
OR
Aqueous procaine penicillin G: 4.8 million units IM at two sites with 1 gm probenecid by mouth

COMMENT: The penicillin regimens are ineffective against chlamydial infections but have the advantage of single-dose therapy. Theoretically, it may be best to combine one of the single-dose regimens with seven days of tetracycline or doxycyline. Patients with incubating syphilis are likely to be cured by all of the above regimens. Tetracycline or aqueous procaine penicillin G is the preferred therapy for pharyngeal gonococcal infections. Follow-up cultures should be obtained from the infected site(s) four to seven days after completion of treatment. Persistent gonorrhea should be treated with 2 gm of spectinomycin IM.

Information obtained from Sexually Transmitted Diseases, Treatment Guidelines: 1982. US Department of Health and Human Services, Centers for Disease Control, Morbidity and Mortality Weekly Report (suppl) 31:335, 1982.

TABLE 34–7 INPATIENT TREATMENT OPTIONS FOR ACUTE PELVIC INFLAMMATORY DISEASE

Clindamycin: 600 mg IV, four times daily*
PLUS
Gentamicin or tobramycin: 2 mg/kg IV followed by 1.5 mg/kg IV, three times daily in patients with normal renal function.
Continue drugs IV for at least 4 days, and at least 48 hours after patient defervesces. Continue clindamycin, 450 mg by mouth, four times daily, after discharge from hospital to complete 10–14 days of therapy.

Comment:	Optimal for:	Anaerobes Facultative gram-negative rods
	May not be optimal for:	C. trachomatis

Doxycycline: 100 mg IV, twice daily
PLUS
Cefoxitin: 2 gm IV, four times daily.
Continue drugs IV for at least 4 days and at least 48 hours after patient defervesces. Continue doxycycline, 100 mg by mouth, twice daily, after discharge from hospital to complete 10–14 days of therapy.

Comment:	Optimal for:	N. gonorrhoeae, including PPNG C. trachomatis
	May not be optimal for:	Anaerobes Pelvic mass PID associated with an IUD

Doxycycline: 100 mg IV, twice daily
PLUS
Metronidazole: 1 gm IV, twice daily
Continue drugs IV for at least 4 days and at least 48 hours after patient defervesces. Continue both drugs at the same dosage orally to complete 10–14 days of therapy.

Comment:	Excellent for:	Anaerobes C. trachomatis
	Not optimal for:	Some strains of N. gonorrhoeae, including PPNG Some facultative gram-negative rods
		Both drugs can be given orally.

*Current Food and Drug Administration recommendation is clindamycin, 900 mg every 8 hours, instead of 600 mg 4 times daily.

Information obtained from Sexually Transmitted Diseases, Treatment Guidelines: 1982. US Department of Health and Human Services, Centers for Disease Control, Morbidity and Mortality Weekly Report (suppl) 31:335, 1982.

desirable to cover the organisms shown in Table 34–1. Regimens recommended by the United States Department of Health and Human Services are shown in Table 34–7.

TUBO-OVARIAN ABSCESS

Clinical Features

Patients with an acute tubo-ovarian abscess are usually very ill with severe pelvic and lower abdominal pain, high fever, prostration, and possible nausea and vomiting.

Physical examination reveals a rapid pulse and a fever that may be up to 103°F (39.5°C). Abdominal examination reveals marked tenderness, muscular rigidity, occasionally a mass arising from the pelvis, and often rebound tenderness. Speculum examination should be performed to obtain a cervical smear for Gram staining, as well as aerobic, anaerobic, and gonococcal cultures. Digital pelvic examination is usually very difficult because of extreme adnexal tenderness. An adnexal mass may be appreciated. On rectal examination, it is usually easier to feel a pelvic mass, which may be pointing into the *cul-de-sac.*

Differential Diagnosis

In the presence of severe lower abdominal pain, fever, leukocytosis, and a tender adnexal mass, the differential diagnosis must include a number of disorders.

Septic Incomplete Abortion. Although illegal abortions are now much less common than in earlier years, this possibility should be kept in mind, particularly as virulent organisms such as *Clostridium perfringens* may be involved.

Acute Appendicitis. The pain of acute appendicitis typically commences in the periumbilical region and subsequently localizes to the right lower quadrant. If the appendix perforates, with resultant peritonitis or appendiceal abscess formation, differentiation may be impossible without a laparotomy.

Diverticular Abscess. Particularly if the mass is on the left side of the pelvis, diverticular abscess should be considered. Usually the patient will have a history of previous episodes of diverticulitis, and a barium enema will reveal the typical features.

Adnexal Torsion. This problem is more likely if an ovarian cyst or hydrosalpinx is present. It may cause necrosis and rupture closely simulating a tubo-ovarian abscess clinically. Fever and leukocytosis are usually much less impressive, but laparotomy is required if torsion appears likely.

Treatment

Patients with tubo-ovarian abscess should be treated with bedrest in the hospital, adequate oral and intravenous fluids, analgesics, and systemic antibiotics. Clindamycin plus an aminoglycoside are usually used. Even large abscesses may resolve without the need for acute surgical intervention.

The timing of any operative intervention requires clinical judgment. Rupture of the abscess with signs of generalized peritonitis requires urgent laparotomy to remove the infected organs and lavage the peritoneal cavity. Traditionally, total (or subtotal) abdominal hysterectomy and bilateral salpingo-oophorectomy have been performed for ruptured tubo-ovarian abscess. However, unilateral lesions do occur, particularly in women who have used intrauterine contraceptive devices. For such patients, unilateral salpingo-oophorectomy may be appropriate.

If the abscess is soft and fluctuant and is pointing into the *cul-de-sac,* as indicated by heat and edema of the posterior fornix, posterior colpotomy to allow drainage usually produces dramatic results. When the patient fails to respond to approximately 72 hours of multiagent broad-spectrum chemotherapy, with persistently spiking fever and pelvic and abdominal tenderness, laparotomy with extraperitoneal drainage is indicated if the abscess is not accessible to drainage through the vagina.

CHRONIC PELVIC INFLAMMATORY DISEASE

Clinical Features

Long-term sequelae of PID may include chronic pelvic pain, menometrorrhagia, dyspareunia, infertility, and ectopic pregnancy. Sterile hydrosalpinges or pyosalpinges, with multiple pelvic adhesions, may result, particularly if proper antibiotic therapy was not instituted early in the course of the acute episode of infection.

On *physical examination,* there is usually some lower abdominal tenderness. Pelvic examination may reveal tenderness in both adnexal regions, or there may be palpable masses and induration from hydrosalpinges or chronic abscesses. Hydrosalpinges may occasionally be quite large and mistaken for ovarian cysts. In long-standing cases, progressive adhesion formation may produce the so-called "frozen pelvis," in which internal genital organs are fixed to the pelvic side walls by the indurated supporting ligaments. The uterus may be deviated from the midline or fixed in the *cul-de-sac.*

Differential Diagnosis

The most common problem clinically is to differentiate chronic pelvic inflammatory disease from endometriosis, particularly if there is no well-documented history of acute infection. A normal sedimentation rate favors endometriosis. However, a number of conditions may be confused with chronic PID, including pelvic pain syndrome, pelvic tuberculosis, inflammatory bowel diseases, and pelvic malignancies. Often, diagnosis cannot be made without laparoscopy or laparotomy.

Treatment

In patients with less severe involvement who wish to become pregnant, various types of tuboplasties may be undertaken. For patients with more severe disease, medical management of large hydrosalpinges is disappointing, and, frequently, control of pelvic pain will necessitate total abdominal hysterectomy and bilateral salpingo-oophorectomy. Replacement hormonal therapy must then be administered to control hot flashes and prevent osteoporosis.

SUGGESTED READING

Bearn AG (ed): Antibiotics in the Management of Infections: Outlook for the 1980's. Merck Sharp & Dohme International Medical Advisory Council. Paris, France, June 14–15, 1982. Raven Press, New York, 1982.

Eschenbach DA, Buchanan TM, Pollock HM, et al: Polymicrobial etiology of acute pelvic inflammatory disease. N Engl J Med 293:166, 1975.

Goodrich J: Pelvic inflammatory disease: Considerations of therapy. Rev Infect Dis 45:S778, 1982.

Landers D, Sweet R: Tubo-ovarian abscess: Contemporary approach to management. Rev Infect Dis 5:876, 1983.

Marier RL, Sanders CV, Faro S, et al: Piperacillin vs carbenicillin in the therapy for serious infections. Arch Intern Med 142:2000, 1984.

Mickal A, Sellman A, Beek J: Ruptured tubo-ovarian abscess. Am J Obstet Gynecol 100:435, 1968.

Sexually Transmitted Diseases, Treatment Guidelines: 1982. US Department of Health and Human Services. J Reprod Med 28:727, 1983.

Toth A: Alternative causes of pelvic inflammatory disease. J Reprod Med 28:699, 1983.

Westrum L: Incidence, prevalence and trends of acute pelvic inflammatory disease and its consequences in industrialized countries. Am J Obstet Gynecol 138:881, 1980.

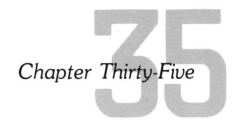

Chapter Thirty-Five

PELVIC RELAXATION AND URINARY PROBLEMS

NARENDER N. BHATIA

The pelvic organs, including the vagina, uterus, bladder, and rectum, are maintained in position by supporting ligaments, fascia, and pelvic floor muscles. The cardinal and uterosacral ligaments assist in maintaining the uterus in an anteflexed position, and in preventing its descensus through the urogenital diaphragm. When these supports become damaged, one or more of the pelvic organs may prolapse within and, occasionally, protrude outside the vagina.

PROLAPSE

There are several types of genital prolapses. They may occur singly, but are more commonly combined.

Uterine Prolapse

Though vaginal prolapse can occur without uterine prolapse, the uterus cannot descend without carrying the upper vagina with it. When the cervix remains within the vagina, it is called a *first-degree prolapse*. When the cervix protrudes beyond the introitus, it becomes a *second-degree prolapse*. A *third-degree prolapse*, or *complete procidentia*, implies descent of the entire uterus outside the vulva (Fig. 35–1).

Complete procidentia represents failure of all the genital supports. Hypertrophy, elongation, congestion, and edema of the cervix may sometimes cause a large protrusion of tissue beyond the introitus, which may be mistaken for a procidentia.

Vaginal Prolapse

The bulging or descent of the bladder into the upper anterior vaginal wall is called a *cystocele* (Fig. 35–2). It represents a weakness in the investing fascia of the vagina (pubocervical fascia). The bulging of the urethra into the lower anterior vaginal wall should be called *urethral displacement*. Older terminology would depict this as a urethrocele; however, there is no dilatation of the urethra in this condition.

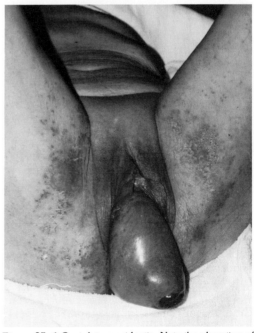

Figure 35–1 Complete procidentia. Note the ulceration of the cervix.

311

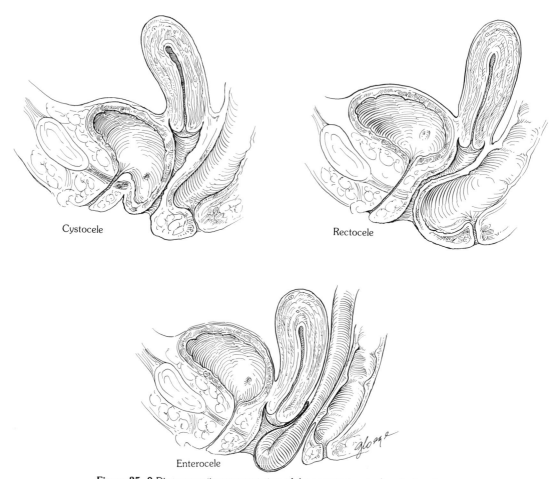

Cystocele

Rectocele

Enterocele

Figure 35–2 Diagrammatic representation of the various types of vaginal prolapse.

Upper posterior vaginal wall prolapse is nearly always associated with herniation of the pouch of Douglas, and, since this is likely to contain loops of bowel, it is called an *enterocele.* Lower posterior vaginal wall prolapse is called a *rectocele.*

Vaginal *vault prolapse* or inversion of the vagina may be seen after vaginal or abdominal hysterectomy and represents failure of the supports around the upper vagina.

Etiology of Prolapse

The pelvic fascia, ligaments, and muscles may become attenuated from excessive stretching during vaginal delivery. However, prolapse often follows easy rather than difficult labor and may occasionally occur in women who have never had children, indicating a congenital or developmental weakness of the pelvic connective tissues.

Increased intra-abdominal pressure result-ing from a chronic cough, ascites, repeated lifting of heavy weights, or habitual straining due to constipation may predispose to prolapse. Atrophy of the supporting tissues with aging, especially after menopause, also plays an important part in the initiation or worsening of pelvic relaxation.

Symptoms

The amount of discomfort and inconvenience experienced by a patient with prolapse is extremely variable. Often there is a feeling of heaviness or fullness in the pelvis. Patients may describe "something falling out" or a bearing down discomfort. Some patients may complain of backache at the level of the sacrum. The characteristic of nearly all symptoms is that they are worse after prolonged standing and immediately and completely relieved by lying down.

When the prolapse is extreme, the patient

may experience difficulty in walking because of the exposed positions of the uterus, bladder, and rectum. Neglected cases of procidentia may be complicated by excessive purulent discharge, decubitus ulceration, bleeding, and, rarely, carcinoma of the cervix.

Symptoms of urinary frequency and urgency, urinary incontinence, and, occasionally, urinary retention may be seen in patients with anterior vaginal wall prolapse. Patients with a rectocele may have difficulty emptying the rectum. Many of them learn to splint the posterior vaginal wall by placing two fingers along it to keep the rectocele from protruding during a bowel movement.

Diagnosis

Vaginal examination should be performed by using a Sim's speculum or by taking a standard Grave's speculum and removing the anterior blade. While depressing the posterior vaginal wall, the patient is asked to strain down. This will demonstrate the descent of the anterior vaginal wall consistent with cystocele and urethral displacement. Similarly, retraction of the anterior vaginal wall during straining demonstrates an enterocele and rectocele. Rectal examination is often useful to demonstrate a rectocele and to distinguish it from an enterocele.

Minor degrees of uterine prolapse may only be recognized by feeling descent of the cervix when the patient is straining. Occasionally, it is necessary to test for uterine prolapse by pulling on the cervix with a tenaculum. If there is doubt about the presence of prolapse, the patient may be asked to stand or walk for some time before the examination.

Treatment

Although treatment of pelvic relaxation is primarily surgical, nonoperative approaches may be used initially. The patient's age, marital status, desire for further childbearing, sexual activity, degree of prolapse, and presence or absence of associated pathologic conditions should be taken into consideration prior to institution of treatment. If it is difficult to be certain whether or not the prolapse is responsible for the symptoms, a trial of pessary may be undertaken.

Nonsurgical Treatment. When there is only a mild degree of pelvic relaxation, *perineal exercises* may improve the tone of the pelvic floor musculature. Their effect is limited, however, because they do not enhance support from the fascia and ligaments.

Pessaries may be used to correct prolapse in the following situations: (1) if the patient is medically unfit for surgery, (2) during pregnancy and the postpartum period, and (3) to promote healing of a decubitus ulcer prior to surgery. Pessaries require a great deal of care to avoid vaginal infection and leukorrhea. A variety of pessaries are shown in Figure 35–3.

Surgical Treatment. Surgical repair is the most satisfactory therapy, and the results are very good. Many surgical procedures have been proposed to correct the pelvic support defects.

ANTERIOR COLPORRHAPHY. This is used to correct a cystocele and urethral displacement. It involves plication of the pubocervical fascia to support the bladder and urethra.

POSTERIOR COLPORRHAPHY. This is the equivalent operation on the posterior vaginal wall. The endopelvic fascia and the perineal muscles are approximated in the midline to support the rectum and perineum.

REPAIR OF ENTEROCELE. The repair of an enterocele follows the general principles of hernia repair. The contents are reduced, the neck of the peritoneal sac is ligated, and the defect is repaired by approximating the uterosacral ligaments and levator-ani muscles.

MANCHESTER OPERATION. This operation combines anterior colporrhaphy, amputation of the cervix, posterior colpoperineorrhaphy, and suturing of the cardinal ligaments in front of the cervical stump to antevert the uterus. It is a low morbidity operation, and the uterus is preserved.

VAGINAL HYSTERECTOMY. This may be performed alone or in conjunction with anterior and posterior colporrhaphy. It may be used for any degree of uterine descent but is especially useful for procidentia.

LEFORT'S PARTIAL COLPOCLEISIS. This operation may be performed in elderly patients with substantial uterine prolapse. It involves suturing the partially denuded anterior and posterior vaginal walls together in such a way that the uterus is supported above the partially occluded vagina.

VAGINAL VAULT SUSPENSION. When vaginal prolapse occurs following hysterectomy, it can be repaired by suspending the vaginal

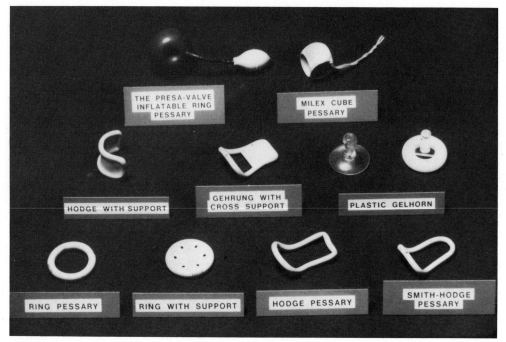

Figure 35–3 Vaginal pessaries.

vault from the sacrum or sacrospinous ligaments. The procedure can be approached either vaginally or abdominally.

COMPLETE COLPOCLEISIS. This procedure may be performed for vaginal inversion after hysterectomy in older patients who are no longer sexually active. It involves total obliteration of the vagina.

URINARY INCONTINENCE

There are four common types of urinary incontinence: (1) stress incontinence, (2) total incontinence, (3) urge incontinence, and (4) overflow incontinence.

Anatomy and Physiology of the Lower Urinary Tract

The bladder *detrusor* is a smooth muscle appearing as a meshwork of fibers that are recognizable only at the bladder outlet as three distinct layers—the outer longitudinal, the middle circular, and the inner longitudinal.

In the adult female, the *urethra* is a muscular tube, 3 to 4 cm in length, lined proximally with transitional epithelium and distally with stratified squamous epithelium. It is surrounded mainly by smooth muscle. The striated muscle *urethral sphincter,* which sur-

rounds the middle one third of the urethra, contributes about 50 percent of the total urethral resistance and serves as a secondary defense against incontinence. It is also responsible for the interruption of urine flow at the end of micturition.

The two *posterior pubourethral ligaments* provide a strong suspensory mechanism for the urethra and serve to hold it forward and in close proximity to the pubis under conditions of stress. They extend from the lower part of the pubic bone to the urethra at the junction of its middle and distal third.

Innervation

The lower urinary tract is under the control of both parasympathetic and sympathetic nerves. The parasympathetic fibers originate in the sacral spinal cord segments S2 through S4. Stimulation of the pelvic parasympathetic nerves and administration of cholinergic drugs cause the detrusor muscle to contract. Anticholinergic drugs reduce the vesicle pressure and increase the bladder capacity.

The sympathetic fibers originate from thoracolumbar segments (T10 through L2) of the spinal cord. The sympathetic system has alpha and beta adrenergic components. The beta fibers terminate primarily in the detrusor muscle, while the alpha fibers terminate primarily in the urethra. Alpha adrenergic stimulation contracts the bladder neck and urethra and relaxes the detrusor. Beta adrenergic stimulation relaxes the urethra and detrusor muscle. The pudendal nerve (S2 through S4) provides motor innervation to the striated urethral sphincter.

Factors Influencing Bladder Behavior

Sensory Innervation. Afferent impulses from the bladder, trigone, and proximal urethra pass to S2 through S4 levels of the spinal cord by means of the pelvic hypogastric nerves. The sensitivity of these nerve endings may be enhanced by acute infection, interstitial cystitis, radiation cystitis, and increased intravesical pressure. The latter may occur in the standing position, when bending forward, or in association with obesity, pregnancy, or pelvic tumors.

Inhibitory impulses, probably relayed by the pudendal nerve, also pass through S2 through S4 following mechanical stimulation of the perineum and anal canal. Their passage may explain why pain in this region can cause urinary retention.

Central Nervous System. In infancy, the storage and expulsion of urine is automatic and controlled at the level of the sacral reflex arc. Later, connections to the higher centers become established and, by training and conditioning, this spinal reflex becomes socially influenced so that voiding can be voluntarily accomplished. Although organic neurologic diseases may interrupt the influence of the higher centers on the spinal reflex arc, micturition patterns may also be profoundly altered by mental, environmental, and sociologic disturbances.

Continence Control

The normal bladder holds urine because the intraurethral pressure exceeds the intravesical pressure. The pubourethral ligaments and surrounding fascia support the urethra so that abrupt increases in intra-abdominal pressure are transmitted equally to the bladder and proximal one-third of the urethra, thus maintaining a pressure gradient between the two. In addition, a reflex contraction of the levator ani compresses the mid-urethra.

Involuntary escape of urine is common.

Approximately 50 percent of young, healthy females occasionally experience some degree of urinary incontinence. The incidence of urinary incontinence increases with age and with increasing degrees of pelvic relaxation.

STRESS INCONTINENCE

Stress incontinence is the involuntary loss of urine through an intact urethra, secondary to a sudden increase in intra-abdominal pressure and in the absence of a bladder contraction. Based upon the severity of the incontinence, the following gradation has been found to be of clinical value:

Grade I   Incontinence only with severe stress, such as coughing, sneezing, or jogging.

Grade II   Incontinence with moderate stress, such as rapid movement or walking up and down stairs.

Grade III   Incontinence with mild stress, such as standing. The patient is continent in the supine position.

Etiology

Most patients with clinically significant stress incontinence are multiparous. Pregnancy, labor, and delivery may damage the normal supports of the bladder neck and proximal urethra. In addition, continence deteriorates with increasing age, even in women who have not borne children, since intraurethral pressure decreases after the menopause.

The most commonly accepted theory for the pathogenesis of stress urinary incontinence is that the proximal urethra drops below the pelvic floor because of pelvic relaxation defects. Therefore, the increase in intra-abdominal pressure induced by coughing is not transmitted equally to the bladder and proximal urethra. The urethral resistance is overcome by the increased bladder pressure, and leakage of urine results.

Symptoms

When the sole complaint is of involuntary loss of urine on coughing or straining, urinary stress incontinence is the likely diagnosis. Frequently, the symptoms of stress and urge incontinence occur concurrently. The use of protective underwear is some guide to the severity of incontinence. Gradual onset of stress incontinence after bilateral oophorectomy or menopause may indicate estrogen deficiency. The past history should include details of any neurologic diseases, vaginal repair, or bladder neck surgery.

Pelvic Examination

Inspection of the vaginal walls should be performed with a Sims' speculum, which allows optimal visualization of the anterior vaginal wall and urethrovesical junction. Scarring, tenderness, and rigidity of the urethra from previous vaginal surgeries or pelvic trauma may be reflected by a scarred anterior vaginal wall. Since the distal urethra is estrogen-dependent, the patient with atrophic vaginitis also has atrophic urethritis.

Diagnostic Tests

Stress Test. This test objectively demonstrates urinary incontinence. The patient is examined with a full bladder in the lithotomy position. While the physician observes the urethral meatus, the patient is asked to cough. Stress urinary incontinence is suggested if short spurts of urine escape simultaneously with each cough. A delayed leakage, or loss of large volumes of urine, suggests uninhibited bladder contractions. If loss of urine is not demonstrated in the lithotomy position, the test should be repeated with the patient in a standing position.

In patients with demonstrated stress urinary incontinence, elevation of the bladder neck with one finger on either side of the urethra (*Bonney test*) or a partially opened Allis clamp (*Marshall-Marchetti test*) should prevent leakage of urine on coughing. If urine loss stops, the test is considered positive and suggests that bladder neck suspension should control the incontinence. Both of these tests may occlude the urethra while elevating the bladder neck and, therefore, should not be relied upon. Recently, a *pessary test* that does not cause urethral occlusion has been found to be reliable for the diagnosis of stress urinary incontinence.

Cotton-Tip Applicator Test. This test determines the mobility and descent of the urethrovesical junction on straining. With the patient in the lithotomy position, the exam-

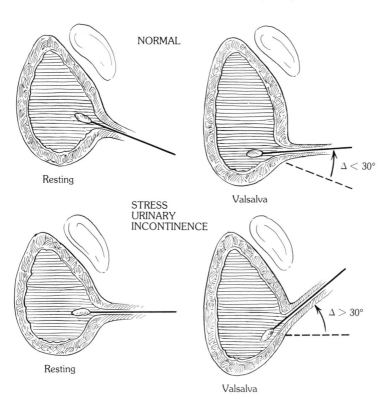

NORMAL

Resting

Valsalva

$\Delta < 30°$

STRESS URINARY INCONTINENCE

Resting

Valsalva

$\Delta > 30°$

Figure 35–4 Diagrammatic representation of the Q-tip test showing mobility of the urethrovesical junction in a continent patient, and a patient with stress urinary incontinence.

iner inserts a lubricated Q-tip into the urethra to the level of the urethrovesical junction and measures the angle between the Q-tip and the horizontal. The patient then strains maximally, which produces descent of the urethrovesical junction. Along with the descent, the Q-tip moves, producing a new angle with the horizontal. The normal change in angle is up to 30 degrees. In patients with pelvic relaxation and stress urinary incontinence, the change in Q-tip angle is in the range of 50 to 60 degrees or more (Fig. 35–4).

Urethrocystoscopy. Urethrocystoscopy allows the physician to examine the urethra, urethrovesical junction, bladder walls, and ureteral orifices. Either water or carbon dioxide may be employed as filling media. Ideally, urethrocystoscopy should be performed prior to any surgery on the urethra or bladder. The following observations should be made:

1. The amount of residual urine
2. The bladder capacity (normal capacity is 400 to 500 ml of water)
3. The appearance of the urethral and bladder urothelium, noting any inflammation, diverticulae, or trabeculation
4. The mobility of the urethrovesical junction in response to commands of rectal squeeze, urine hold, cough, and Valsalva. In a normal patient, the internal urethral orifice closes in response to these commands. Prior vaginal surgery may result in restricted urethral mobility (frozen urethra or drain-pipe urethra), which may also cause stress urinary incontinence.

Cystometrogram. Cystometry consists of distending the bladder with known volumes of water or carbon dioxide and observing pressure changes in the bladder during filling (Fig. 35–5). During the test, the patient is asked about the sensation of bladder fullness. The presence or absence of a detrusor reflex associated with a strong desire to void is noted. The most important observation is the presence of a detrusor reflex and the patient's ability to control or inhibit this reflex.

The ability of the patient to perceive the filling of the bladder indicates that sensory innervation of the bladder is intact. The first sensation of bladder filling should occur at volumes of 150 to 200 ml. The volume threshold for the detrusor reflex is a measure of the functional capacity of the bladder muscle. This critical volume (400 to 500 ml) is the

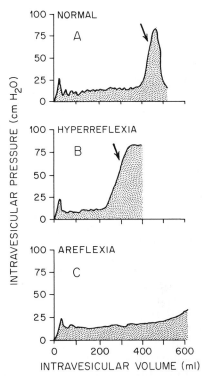

Figure 35–5 Water cystometrogram in (A) a normal patient, (B) a patient with detrusor hyperreflexia, and (C) a patient with detrusor areflexia (hypotonic bladder).

capacity that the bladder musculature tolerates before the patient experiences a strong desire to urinate. At this point, if the patient is asked to void, a terminal contraction may appear and is seen as a sudden rise in intravesical pressure. At the peak of the contraction, the patient is instructed to inhibit this reflex (indicated by arrows in Figs. 35–5A and B). A normal person should be able to inhibit this detrusor reflex and bring down intravesical pressure (Fig. 35–5A). In a urologically or neurologically abnormal patient, the detrusor reflex may appear without the specific instruction to void, and the patient cannot inhibit it (Fig. 35–5B); this observation is referred to as an uninhibited detrusor contraction. Other terms for this disorder include detrusor dysenergia, detrusor hyperreflexia, irritable bladder, hypertonic bladder, unstable bladder, and uninhibited neurogenic bladder.

These cystometric procedures allow differentiation between those patients who are incontinent as a result of uninhibited detrusor contraction and those who have stress urinary incontinence. Conversely, the hypotonic bladder accommodates excessive amounts of gas or water with little increase in intravesical pressure, and there is absence of the terminal detrusor contraction when the patient is asked to void (Fig. 35–5C).

Urethral Pressure Measurements. A low urethral pressure may be found in patients with stress urinary incontinence, while an abnormally high urethral closing pressure may be associated with voiding difficulties, hesitancy, and urinary retention.

The *urethral closing pressure profile* (UCPP) is a graphic record of pressure along the length of the urethra obtained by means of a pressure-sensitive recording catheter, which is slowly and progressively withdrawn through the urethra. The resulting bell-shaped curve provides a measurement of the urethral closing pressure (intraurethral minus intravesical pressure) and the functional length of the urethra (the length of the urethra along which urethral pressure exceeds bladder pressure). The urethral closing pressure normally varies between 50 and 100 cm water and the functional length between 3 and 5 cm. A normal continent woman responds to the stress of bladder filling, postural change, coughing, sneezing, or jolting by increasing the urethral closing pressure and urethral length. Patients with stress urinary incontinence characteristically demonstrate decreases in urethral closing pressure.

Uroflowmetry. Uroflowmetry records rates of urine flow through the urethra when the patient is asked to void spontaneously while sitting on a uroflow chair. From the flow rate curve, the physician relates the voided volume to the maximum flow rate and the time for urine flow. The normal female voids by the *"rule of twenties"*—that is, the bladder is emptied in less than 20 seconds at a rate of 20 ml per second. For a flow rate to be significant, at least 200 ml of urine should be voided.

Uroflowmetry is indicated in patients complaining of difficulty or hesitancy in voiding, incomplete bladder emptying, poor stream, urinary retention, and in the assessment of patients for incontinence surgery.

Simultaneous Urethrocystometry. This technique employs simultaneous recording of the pressure in the urethra and bladder, and allows the pressure changes during voiding to be recorded. Normally, urethral relaxation precedes bladder contraction. An observation of lack of bladder contraction and the use of abdominal straining during voiding

may indicate a need for prolonged postoperative bladder drainage following incontinence surgery.

Voiding Cystourethrogram (VCUG). In this radiologic investigation, fluoroscopy is used to observe bladder filling, the mobility of the urethra and bladder base, and the anatomic changes during voiding. The procedure provides valuable information regarding bladder size and the competence of the bladder neck during coughing. It may detect any bladder trabeculation, vesicoureteral reflux during voiding, funnelling of the bladder neck, bladder and/or urethral diverticula, and outflow obstruction.

Bead-Chain Cystourethrogram. This static cystourethrogram involves the introduction of a metallic bead-chain into the bladder transurethrally. A lateral x-ray provides information regarding the location of the bladder and urethra in relation to the symphysis pubis and the urethrovesical anatomic configuration during rest and straining. On the basis of a static cystourethrogram, two basic types of anatomic disturbances have been described in patients with stress urinary incontinence (Fig. 35–6). Patients with a type 1 deformity have incomplete or complete loss of the posterior-urethrovesical angle (normal 90 to 100 degrees). Patients with a type 2 deformity have an increased angle of urethral axis inclination to the vertical (normal is less than 30 degrees), in addition to loss of the posterior urethrovesical angle. Patients with a type 2 deformity have a more severe variety of stress urinary incontinence. This classification has been used to select the type of surgical approach—that is, anterior vaginal repair for patients with a type 1 deformity and an abdominal approach for patients with a type 2 deformity. With better understanding of the pathophysiology of urinary incontinence and increased utilization of urodynamic studies, the role of the static cystourethrogram has come under increasing criticism and is presently infrequently employed in the diagnostic work-up of stress urinary incontinence.

Ultrasound. Employing real-time or sector ultrasonography, information can be obtained about the inclination of the urethra, flatness of the bladder base, and mobility and funnelling of the urethrovesical junction, both at rest and with a Valsalva's maneuver. In addition, any bladder or urethral diverticula may be identified.

Summary. For about 90 percent of patients

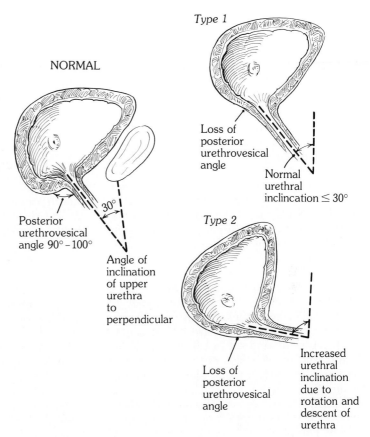

STRESS INCONTINENCE

Type 1

NORMAL

Loss of
posterior
urethrovesical
angle

Normal
urethral
inclincation ≤ 30°

Figure 35–6 Anatomic deformities associated with type 1 and type 2 stress urinary incontinence.

Posterior
urethrovesical
angle 90° – 100°

30°

Type 2

Angle of
inclination
of upper
urethra
to
perpendicular

Loss of
posterior
urethrovesical
angle

Increased
urethral
inclination
due to
rotation and
descent of
urethra

with stress urinary incontinence, a good history and physical examination, uroflowmetry, cystourethroscopy, the Q-tip test, the stress test, the pessary test, and the cystometrogram will be adequate investigations. Additional urodynamic, electromyographic, neurologic, and radiologic procedures may be necessary in patients with a history of multiple previous surgeries for urinary incontinence and for patients with associated neurologic disease.

Treatment

Medical Therapy. After the menopause, atrophic changes occur in the lower urinary tract. Estrogens improve urethral closing pressure, mucosal thickness and vascularity, and possibly reflex urethral functions. Alpha adrenergic stimulants, such as phenylpropanolamine (Propadrine) or pseudoephedrine, may enhance urethral closure and improve continence.

Physical Therapy. Pelvic diaphragm exercises (Kegel exercises) are known to improve or cure mild forms of stress incontinence. Since the entire pelvic floor exerts sphincteric action on the urethra, an increase in resting and active muscle tone will increase urethral closing pressure. To employ the exercises, the patient must be asked to learn to interrupt urine flow during voiding. Kegel exercises require diligence and willingness to practice at home and at work. Many women find them difficult, fatiguing, or time consuming. Kegel exercises before and after delivery may help patients with postpartum urinary incontinence.

Intravaginal Devices. Large pelvic diaphragms, tampons, and various types of vaginal pessaries have been used to elevate and support the bladder neck and urethra. The pessary may provide an acceptable alternative for patients unfit for surgery. They must be regularly cleansed and replaced.

Surgical Therapy. Surgery is the most commonly employed treatment of stress urinary incontinence. The aim of all the surgical procedures is to correct the pelvic relaxation defect and to stabilize and restore the normal intra-abdominal position of the proximal urethra. The approach may be vaginal, abdominal, or combined abdominovaginal.

VAGINAL APPROACH. Anterior vaginal repair (Kelly's operation) is an excellent procedure for correction of cystocele, but less useful for correction of stress incontinence. It may be difficult to place the urethra high enough in the pelvis, thereby reducing the short- and long-term success rate.

In patients with large cystoceles, overcorrection of the cystocele may result in postoperative stress incontinence in a previously continent patient. Such patients may require prophylactic retropubic urethropexy in addition to anterior colporrhaphy.

ABDOMINAL APPROACH. The retropubic approach to urethrovesical elevation has a long-term success rate of approximately 85 percent. The retropubic urethropexy is performed extraperitoneally (in the space of Retzius) by placing sutures in the fascia lateral to and on each side of the bladder neck and proximal urethra, and elevating the vesicourethral junction by attaching the sutures to the symphysis pubis (*Marshall-Marchetti-Kranz, MMK procedure*) or to Cooper's ligament (*Burch procedure*). This restores the normal intra-abdominal position of the urethra. Care must be taken to correct any associated cystocele.

Postoperatively, a transurethral or suprapubic catheter is left in the bladder for continuous bladder drainage for 48 to 72 hours prior to instituting spontaneous voiding. Some patients (20 to 30 percent) may need prolonged postoperative bladder drainage (more than seven days). An occasional patient may develop osteitis pubis after the MMK procedure.

COMBINED ABDOMINOVAGINAL PROCEDURES. The *modified Pereyra procedure* is being increasingly employed because of its simplicity and short postoperative recovery period. The principle of the Pereyra technique is suspension of the vesical neck, as in the retropubic procedures, but the operation is primarily done via the vagina. Monofilament nylon sutures are placed in the endopelvic fascia on either side of the urethra, through a vaginal incision at the level of the bladder neck. The sutures are threaded through the space of Retzius with a special needle and are tied to the anterior rectus fascia through a small suprapubic incision.

In the *Stamey procedure,* a 1-cm sleeve of 5 mm Dacron is threaded under the urethra at the bladder neck to provide additional support. Postoperative voiding difficulties and a need for prolonged postoperative bladder drainage or intermittent self-catheterization represent the main drawbacks of this procedure.

Comparison of Vaginal and Abdominal Procedures

Anterior colporrhaphy with plication of the vesical neck has been standard therapy for mild or moderate stress incontinence for decades. It is a convenient approach, especially when concomitant vaginal procedures are being performed, and avoids the necessity of an abdominal incision. Success rates are better in patients with mild incontinence, but not as good in the more severe forms. Long-term success rates are 55 to 65 percent.

The Pereyra and Stamey procedures, with their several modifications, have about an 80 to 90 percent success rate, which is comparable to open retropubic techniques. Some surgeons use these procedures routinely and achieve good results, even in cases of previous surgical failure. They require a relatively short amount of time to perform, and a wide abdominal incision is not required. An area of concern is the inability to precisely control the amount of elevation of the bladder neck. Avoidance of this problem comes only with experience with the technique.

Special Procedures

If conventional surgical procedures fail, special, more complicated operations may be performed. These include *sling procedures, neourethra construction, implantation of an artificial urinary sphincter,* and *urinary diversion.* The latter is the final solution for intractable incontinence.

It is important to recognize that the critical operation for urinary stress incontinence is the first one, and the cure rate declines more or less proportionately to the number of subsequent operations performed. Every effort should be made to utilize all necessary resources for a proper preoperative evaluation of patients before embarking on any kind of surgical procedure for incontinence.

TOTAL INCONTINENCE— URINARY FISTULA

Pelvic surgery, irradiation, or both now account for 95 percent of the vesicovaginal fistulas in the United States. More than 50 percent occur following simple abdominal or vaginal hysterectomy. Obstetric injuries, once the leading cause for urinary fistulas, have almost disappeared in the United States, Canada, and Western Europe. They usually result from operative deliveries (e.g., forceps) rather than from neglected labor and pressure necrosis. One or 2 percent of radical hysterectomies are followed in 10 to 21 days by a urinary fistula, usually ureterovaginal. These fistulas are usually due to devascularization of the ureter, rather than to direct injury.

Urethrovaginal fistulas generally occur as complications of surgery for urethral diverticula, anterior vaginal wall prolapse, and/or stress urinary incontinence.

Diagnosis of Fistulas

The usual history of painless and continuous vaginal leakage of urine soon after pelvic surgery is strongly suggestive of this problem. Installation of methylene blue dye into the bladder will discolor a vaginal pack if a vesicovaginal fistula is present. Intravenous indigo-carmine is excreted in the urine and will discolor a vaginal pack in the presence of a vesicovaginal or ureterovaginal fistula. In addition, cystourethroscopy should be performed to determine the site and number of fistulas. The majority of posthysterectomy vesicovaginal fistulas are located just anterior to the vaginal vault. An intravenous pyelogram and retrograde pyelogram should be undertaken to localize a ureterovaginal fistula.

Fistula Repair

Most of the obstetric fistulas can be repaired immediately upon detection. For postsurgical fistulas, it is usual to wait three to six months to allow the inflammation to settle and the tissues to obtain good vascularity and pliability. During this waiting period, urinary tract infection should be treated and estrogen therapy instituted in postmenopausal women. Steroids have been advocated to hasten resolution of inflammatory changes and allow early surgical intervention. Their use in this circumstance is controversial.

In repairing urinary fistulas, the following principles must be observed:

1. All involved organs should be widely mobilized.
2. All scar tissue should be excised.
3. Nontraumatic instruments should be used.
4. Adequate hemostasis must be achieved.
5. A layer by layer closure should be used, without tension.
6. Minimal tissue necrosis should occur by nonstrangulating suture placement.
7. All dead space should be obliterated.
8. The bladder must be drained postoperatively.

Vesicovaginal Fistula. The vaginal approach (*Latzko's operation*) is suitable for most of these fistulas. After localization of the fistula, an area with a radius of 1.5 to 2 cm around the vaginal opening of the fistula is denuded of vaginal mucosa. Then, multiple layers of interrupted sutures are placed to bring together the denuded areas of anterior and posterior vaginal walls. Postoperatively, the bladder is drained suprapubically for a period of 7 to 14 days. Sexual intercourse is inadvisable for two months. A bulbocavernosus muscle flap (*Martius graft*) may be interposed between the bladder and vagina to provide support, vascularity, and strength to the suture line, especially in patients who have had multiple previous attempted repairs and in those with a postradiation fistula. Large radiation-induced fistulas may necessitate an ileal conduit for urinary diversion.

Ureterovaginal Fistula. Treatment of a ureterovaginal fistula depends on its location. If it is close to the ureterovesical junction, the ureter proximal to the fistula can be implanted into the bladder (*ureteroneocystostomy*). If the fistula is several centimeters from the bladder, a segment of ileum may be interposed between the proximal ureter and the bladder. Occasionally, it may be necessary to remove the kidney on the involved side.

URGE INCONTINENCE

Urge incontinence results from detrusor instability. It is characterized by the presence of involuntary and uninhibited detrusor contractions of 15 cm of water or more during cystometric evaluation.

The incidence of bladder instability in the general population varies from 10 to 15 percent. In most patients, the exact etiology of bladder instability remains unknown. Clinical symptoms may include urinary urgency, frequency, urge incontinence, and nocturia.

Neurologic Examination

Since the innervation to the lower urinary tract is closely related to the innervation of the lower extremities and perineum, neurologic deficits of the bladder and rectum may be reflected in a systematic examination of the deep tendon reflexes and motor and sensory functions. For instance, the presence of hyperactive deep tendon reflexes and an extensor plantar response in a patient with a history of urinary frequency, urgency, and/or urge incontinence is likely to be associated with detrusor instability as a cause for the patient's symptoms. Similarly, in a patient with urinary retention or voiding difficulties, evidence of peripheral neuropathy, autonomic neuropathy, diminished tendon reflexes, or a cauda equina lesion is more likely to be associated with a hypotonic or areflexic bladder.

Reflex contraction of the pelvic floor muscles indicates neuronal integrity of the sacral dermatomes S2, S3, and S4. Stroking the skin lateral to the anus elicits the anal reflex. The bulbocavernosus reflex involves contraction of the bulbo and ischiocavernosus muscles in response to gentle tapping or squeezing of the clitoris. Abnormalities of these reflexes are highly suggestive of peripheral and/or central nervous system disease as a cause for urinary tract problems.

Treatment

A number of therapeutic modalities are available, attesting to the unsatisfactory results with any kind of treatment. In treating urge incontinence, it is important to exclude significant outflow obstruction in order to avoid precipitating acute urinary retention.

Pharmacologic. It is reasonable to try several drugs, increasing the dose up to the maximum tolerated, until the most effective drug for a particular patient is found.

ANTICHOLINERGIC DRUGS. These are the most frequently employed agents. Propantheline (Pro-Banthine), 15 to 30 mg three times daily, and oxybutynin chloride (Ditropan), 5 mg three times daily, act by inhibiting the cholinergically innervated detrusor muscle.

BETA SYMPATHOMIMETIC AGONISTS. The detrusor relaxing action of beta adrenergic receptors forms the basis for the use of drugs like metaproterenol (Alupent), 20 mg twice daily. They enhance the effect of propantheline.

MUSCULOTROPHIC DRUGS. Flavoxate (Urispas), 200 mg three times daily, acts by causing direct relaxation of the detrusor muscle. Diazepam (Valium) acts by a combination of direct smooth muscle relaxation, anticholinergic effect, and central nervous system sedation.

TRICYCLIC ANTIDEPRESSANTS. Imipramine (Tofranil), 25 to 50 mg two to three times a day, relaxes the detrusor muscle by virtue of its anticholinergic action, and it helps to enhance continence by its alpha adrenergic stimulation of the urethra.

DOPAMINE AGONISTS. Bromocriptine (Parlodel), 2.5 mg three times daily, has been shown to be beneficial in detrusor instability, probably as a result of both central and peripheral actions.

Bladder Training. Bladder training represents a behavior modification designed to repeat the process of toilet training. The essential aim is to increase bladder capacity day by day and to prolong the intervals between voiding. Schedules are started at half-hour or one-hour intervals and are changed weekly. No night-time schedule is kept. For some patients, hospital admission for a period of seven to ten days may be advisable. Supportive treatment may be provided by the use of various pharmacologic agents.

Biofeedback. Like bladder training, this is a technique in which an attempt is made to induce cortical control through recognition of physiologic changes using various instrumentation. Results seem to be similar to those from bladder retraining. However, with biofeedback, equipment cost, manpower, and inconvenience are significantly increased. This technique should, therefore, be reserved for resistant and/or complicated cases.

Bladder Denervation Procedures. Even total denervation may not paralyze the bladder. Therapeutic bladder denervation may be attempted at many levels from the bladder wall to the brain.

The vaginal approach is the most commonly employed approach for correction of detrusor instability. Through a U-shaped incision in the anterior vaginal wall, the vesical plexus can be identified on each side and resected unilaterally or bilaterally. This approach has the advantage of being close to the target organ and includes both parasympathetic and sympathetic nerves.

Bladder distension can provide useful rehabilitation of bladder function when other measures have failed. Results are uncertain, and repeated attempts may be required. When successful, it is not necessarily permanent; recurrence rates vary from 6 to 15 percent.

OVERFLOW INCONTINENCE

Urinary retention and overflow incontinence may result from *detrusor areflexia* or hypotonic bladder, as is seen with lower motor neuron disease, spinal cord injuries, or autonomic neuropathy (diabetes mellitus). These patients are best managed by intermittent self-catheterization.

Overflow incontinence may also occur when there is an *outflow obstruction*. Straining to void, poor stream, retention of urine, and incomplete emptying may indicate an obstructive disorder. Overdistension of the bladder because of unrecognized urinary retention may occur in the postoperative period. This is a temporary problem related to postoperative pain and may be managed by continuous bladder drainage for 24 to 48 hours.

URETHRAL SYNDROME

The urethral syndrome occurs in a patient with various lower urinary tract symptoms, in the absence of obvious bladder or urethral abnormality, and with no evidence of urinary tract infection. Any combination of symptoms may be present, the most common being urinary frequency, urgency, dysuria, postvoid fullness, incontinence, and dyspareunia. The true incidence is unknown, although it is estimated to occur in 20 to 30 percent of all adult females.

Possible etiologies include psychogenic factors, atrophic urethritis in perimenopausal or postmenopausal patients, bacterial infection, nonbacterial infection with organisms like *Chlamydia* and *Mycoplasma*, urethral stenosis and spasm, allergy, neurogenic factors, and trauma during sexual intercourse.

Diagnosis is based on a detailed history and physical examination, negative urine cultures, dynamic cystourethroscopy, and urodynamic studies.

Treatment

Because of the diverse and indefinite etiologic factors, numerous forms of treatment are in current use. Serial urethral dilatation and urethral massage are the most commonly employed methods for treating chronic urethritis. The rationale is that stretching and massaging allow effective drainage of inspissated mucus from chronically infected periurethral glands and thereby lead to healing and relief of symptoms. Application of vaginal estrogen cream is effective in patients with atrophic urethritis. Some patients may improve with use of tetracyclines for 10 to 14 days. Internal urethrotomy and urethrolysis have also been employed with variable success. Supportive therapy is helpful in all patients with the urethral syndrome, regardless of cause.

URINARY TRACT INFECTIONS

It is estimated that 15 percent of women will have at least one urinary tract infection (UTI) in their lifetime. Ninety five percent of UTI's are symptomatic, and of these symptomatic episodes, three quarters will have positive urine cultures. Almost all asymptomatic patients will have negative cultures.

Terminology

The terminology surrounding urinary tract infections is rather complex and requires some definition.

Bacteriuria. Bacteriuria literally means the presence of bacteria in the urine and may indicate contamination from the urethra, vaginal vestibule, or perineum if care is not exercised during collection of a urine specimen. Significant bacteriuria is generally accepted as indicating a bacterial colony count of 10^5 or more per milliliter of urine in a properly collected "clean catch" urine specimen. However, a colony count of 10^3 or more from a properly collected urine specimen is an indication for treatment if the patient is symptomatic.

Asymptomatic Bacteriuria. Asymptomatic bacteriuria refers to the presence of a positive urine culture in a patient with no clinical symptoms.

Pyelonephritis. Pyelonephritis indicates bacterial infection of the renal parenchyma and the renal pelvicalyceal system. *Acute pyelonephritis* is commonly associated with fever, flank pain, costovertebral tenderness, urinary frequency, urgency, and dysuria. *Chronic pyelonephritis* denotes histologic changes of patchy interstitial nephritis, destruction of tubules, cellular infiltration, and inflammatory changes in the renal parenchyma. Chronic pyelonephritis is not synonymous with chronic urinary tract infection, which means only prolonged presence of bacteria.

Cystitis. Cystitis implies inflammation of the urinary bladder. Patients with cystitis usually have symptoms of lower urinary tract irritation, such as dysuria (burning on urination), urgency, frequency with small amounts of voided urine, nocturia, suprapubic discomfort, and, at times, urinary incontinence and hematuria.

Persistence of Bacteriuria. This indicates the presence of microorganisms that were isolated at the start of treatment and continue to be isolated while the patient is on therapy. Persistence may be caused by several factors, including the presence of resistant organisms, inadequate drug therapy, and poor patient compliance.

Superinfection. This implies appearance of a different organism while a patient is still on therapy. This new organism may be a different strain or a different serologic type.

Relapse. This implies recurrence of significant bacteriuria with the same species and serologic strain of organism. Relapse usually appears within two to three weeks of completion of therapy and most likely represents perineal colonization by the infecting organism.

Reinfection. This means infection occurring after cessation of therapy with a different strain of microorganism or a different serologic type of the original infecting strain. Typically, reinfection occurs 2 to 12 weeks after a previous episode of infection and indicates a recurrent bladder bacteriuria.

Incidence and Prevalence

After the age of one year and throughout adulthood, females are affected more frequently than males (10:1 ratio). Asymptomatic bacteriuria increases from an incidence in preschool children of 1 to 5 percent to a peak of about 10 percent in the postmenopausal female.

Pathogenesis

Bacteria may gain entry to the urinary tract by three pathways: the ascending route, the descending or hematogenous route, and the lymphatic route.

Ascending Infection. This route, which accounts for the majority of UTI's, is through the urethra into the bladder, and, on occasion, through the ureters into the kidneys. The female is more susceptible because of the short length of the urethra, urethral contamination by rectal pathogens, introital and vestibular colonization by pathogenic bacteria, and the decreased urethral resistance after menopause. Sexual activity is a related factor causing urethrovesical bacterial inoculation, especially in the presence of even minor degrees of hypospadias. Additional sources of infection include vulvovaginitis, urethral diverticula, poor hygiene, and indiscriminate urethral catheterization. Infrequent and incomplete voiding resulting in large bladder volumes increases the susceptibility to chronic urinary infection.

Hematogenous Infection. Urinary infection via the hematogenous route is very uncommon, but it is seen occasionally in elderly, debilitated, or immunosuppressed patients with overwhelming infections, in whom kidney infection is only part of the multisystemic involvement. Renal tuberculosis is almost always acquired via the hematogenous route.

Lymphatic Infection. Experimental evidence suggests the possibility of bacterial infection spreading along lymphatic channels connecting the bowel and the urinary tract.

Host Defense Mechanisms

Entrance of bacteria into the urinary tract does not necessarily result in infection. Natural barriers for invasion, such as the "washout" effect of normal periodic voiding, the antiseptic properties of the bladder's mucosa, and the high concentration of organic acids in normal urine prevent bacterial invasion.

Other factors, such as the pH (below 5.5), urea ammonium, and organic acid content of the urine affect bacterial growth. If invasion takes place, the bacteria may remain in the bladder or may ascend to the kidney. Transient vesicoureteral reflux seen in association with severe lower urinary tract infections may allow the infected urine to reach the kidneys.

Perpetuating Factors

The following factors encourage and perpetuate urinary tract infections:

1. *Mechanical urinary obstruction.* Ureteropelvic junction obstruction, ureteral stricture, urethral stenosis, and caliculi are common to patients with recurrent or chronic urinary tract infections.

2. *Functional urinary obstruction abnormalities.* Incomplete bladder emptying and vesicoureteric reflux also encourage stasis of urine and bacterial growth. Pregnancy produces transient functional ureteral obstruction both mechanically and hormonally.

3. *Systemic factors.* Diabetes mellitus, gout, sickle cell trait, cystic renal disease, and metabolic disorders, such as nephrocalcinosis, chronic potassium deficiency, and renal tubular defects, increase susceptibility to pyelonephritis.

Clinical Classification

From the pathogenetic and management point of view, UTI's in nonpregnant females can be considered to be either uncomplicated or complicated. *Uncomplicated UTI's* account for 95 percent of urinary tract infections in women and seldom produce renal damage. They are either the first episode of infection or an episode far removed in time from a previous urinary infection. Ninety percent of first infections are due to *Escherichia coli.* Seventy five percent of these infective episodes will not recur for at least five years. *Complicated UTI's* occur in patients with neurologic or obstructive abnormalities or in those with underlying parenchymal disease.

Investigations

Urinalysis. Microscopic examination of an uncentrifuged, unstained specimen (a drop of urine on the slide covered with a coverslip) provides better than 90 percent accuracy in detecting significant bacteriuria when one or more bacteria are seen per high power field. A positive Gram's stain almost always correlates with a positive quantitative culture. A negative Gram's stain virtually eliminates significant bacteriuria.

Pyuria is arbitrarily defined as the presence of five or more white blood cells per high power field in the centrifuged specimen. The presence of white blood cells (pyuria) and red blood cells along with bacteriuria suggest infection. Pyuria without significant bacteria may indicate a nonbacterial inflammation or a urinary tract foreign body or tumor. It is a classic finding in urinary tuberculosis. Casts, when present, indicate renal parenchymal disease.

Urine Culture. A quantitative urine culture is the most important laboratory test in the diagnosis and management of complicated or uncomplicated UTI's. *Escherichia coli* is the predominant organism in 80 to 85 percent of patients. The remaining less common organisms are *Klebsiella-Enterobacter, Proteus* species, *Enterococcus, Staphylococcus,* and Group D *Streptococcus.* Anaerobic fecal bacteria do not grow well in urine and are rarely seen in urinary infections. Yeast, such as *Candida albicans,* may be seen in patients with diabetes mellitus or in individuals receiving immunosuppressive therapy, especially in the presence of foreign bodies or indwelling catheters.

There are three techniques for urine collection: (1) the midstream "clean-catch" method, (2) urethral catheterization, and (3) suprapubic aspiration. The *midstream clean-catch method* has an 80 percent reliability, which increases to 95 percent if two consecutive specimens show a colony count of 100,000 or more of the same organism. In routine cases of uncomplicated infections, the presence of two or more species of organisms in the same specimen normally suggests contamination. *Urethral catheterization* provides an optimal urine specimen. A positive culture has a 95 percent accuracy, and false-positive cultures are rare. *Suprapubic aspiration,* although providing the most reliable specimen, is reserved for those in whom contamination is difficult to avoid (e.g., in young children and elderly people).

Radiologic Studies. An *intravenous pyelogram* is critical in the evaluation of patients whose recurrences are due to bacterial persistence (for example, due to stones or infected congenital anomalies), but almost of no value in the 99 percent of patients with reinfections. *Cystography* and *voiding urethrocystography* may help to detect ureteric reflux, diverticuli, or fistulous tracts in patients with persistent bacteriuria.

Endoscopic Studies. Endoscopic studies such as *urethroscopy* and *cystoscopy* may be necessary to detect chronic trigonitis, urethritis, urethral or bladder diverticuli, fistulas, foreign bodies, or bladder wall trabeculation.

Renal Function Tests. Renal function tests are not required in a patient with an initial uncomplicated urinary tract infection. If recurrent episodes occur, a blood urea nitrogen and serum creatinine should be obtained. If renal insufficiency is present, a creatinine clearance is helpful.

Urinary Tract Infection Localization Studies. The clinical presentation does not always allow differentiation between renal infections and lower UTI's. The clinical usefulness of localization lies in planning patient management, since the presence of renal infection usually necessitates a more vigorous and extended therapeutic approach than does the presence of lower urinary tract infection alone.

Indirect methods of localization include (1) special staining of urinary sediment to detect polymorphonuclear leukocytes originating in the kidney ("glitter cell" stain); (2) examination of urinary sediment after intravenous injection of bacterial pyrogen or adrenocorticosteroids; (3) measurement of the excretion of various urinary enzymes; (4) tests of maximal urinary concentrating ability; (5) determination of the immunologic response by estimating serum antibody titers against type-specific organisms in the urine; and (6) urine examination for bacteria that are antibody-coated. The latter test is based on the observation that, unlike bladder bacteriuria, renal infection produces a systemic antibody response.

Direct methods of localization, although invasive, are more accurate and include (1) selective ureteral catheterization via cystoscopy; (2) the bladder washout technique; and (3) examination of renal tissue for bacteria or bacterial antigen by the fluorescent antibody technique.

Management

Unless physical examination and urinalysis (bacteriuria) clearly indicate urinary infection, it is advisable to withhold definite antimicrobial therapy until culture and sensitivity reports are available. As a general rule, bacteriuria should be treated and not pyuria. General measures in the management of urinary tract infections involve the following:

1. Rest and hydration. Hydration promotes dilution of bacterial counts, frequent bladder emptying, and reduction of medullary osmolality, which assists phagocytosis.

2. Acidification of the urine. Ascorbic acid (500 mg twice daily), ammonium chloride (12 gm per day in divided doses), or apricot, plum, prune, or cranberry juices have been employed to increase the antibacterial activity of urine and to inhibit bacterial multiplication. Grapefruit juice and carbonated drinks, particularly those containing citrates, turn the urine alkaline and should be avoided.

3. Urinary analgesics. Agents such as phenazopyridine hydrochloride (Pyridium), 100 mg twice daily for two to three days, are often helpful in relieving dysuria.

Basic Principles of Antimicrobial Therapy. The drug selected should be readily available, of low cost, rapidly absorbed from the upper gastrointestinal tract with minimal irritation, and selectively excreted in the urinary tract. A high serum level of antibiotic is undesirable in the treatment of acute cystitis, since it tends to alter normal bacterial flora. Nitrofurantoin (Macrodantin) produces low serum levels with a half-life of only 19 minutes, thereby minimizing the chances of alteration of intestinal and vaginal bacterial flora. Treatment with nitrofurantoin is effective against all uropathogens except *Proteus.*

On the other hand, for pyelonephritis, an antibiotic should be selected that will attain a significant serum level, since the badly infected renal tissue is poorly perfused. The cephalosporins are more effective and cause fewer side effects and relapses. Cephalosporins (Keflex, Duricef) are slowly and effectively excreted in urine, thereby reducing the frequency of daily drug administration (500 mg to 1000 mg twice daily). Antibiotics such as ampicillin, tetracyclines, and trimethoprim-sulfamethoxazole (Septra, Bactrim) alter the intestinal flora, destroy the normal vaginal and periurethral flora, and may result in a relapse of the UTI.

The high pH of urine associated with *Proteus* infection results from the splitting of urea with the subsequent liberation of ammonia. The urine has a characteristic "fishy" smell. If the urine is very alkaline (pH greater than 8.0), trimethroprim-sulfamethoxazole should be prescribed.

For patients with renal insufficiency, ampicillin, trimethoprim-sulfamethoxazole, and doxycycline have been shown to reach adequate levels in the urine without toxic levels in serum. Nitrofurantoin should be avoided, as high serum levels may lead to peripheral neuropathy. Similarly, tetracycline may lead to severe hepatic damage. Dosages of aminoglycosides should be adjusted in accordance with creatinine clearance, and the serum levels should be monitored.

Antimicrobial agents commonly used in the management of urinary tract infections and their relative effectiveness against various organisms are shown in Table 35–1.

SYMPTOMS WITHOUT BACTERIA. Treatment should be symptomatic, such as increased fluid intake, the administration of Pyridium, and warm sitz baths.

ASYMPTOMATIC BACTERIURIA. Although this condition may be ignored in many patients who have no evidence of mechanical obstruction or renal insufficiency, children and pregnant women should be given aggressive antimicrobial therapy. As many as 40 percent of pregnant women with asymptomatic bacteriuria later develop symptomatic UTI's, usually pyelonephritis.

ACUTE SYMPTOMATIC INFECTIONS. Patients with evidence of bacteremia (e.g., shaking chills) or endotoxemia (e.g., hypotension or respiratory alkalosis) should be hospitalized. Almost always it is prudent to hospitalize the febrile diabetic. In the acutely ill patient with suspected bacteremia, aminoglycosides should be employed. The patient's temperature should be monitored. If the fever persists longer than 72 to 96 hours, a complication of infection, such as perinephric abscess, or of treatment, such as drug fever, should be contemplated and investigated.

For the patient without indications for hospitalization with the first episode of UTI, an inexpensive drug such as sulfonamide, nitrofurantoin, ampicillin, or tetracycline should be given for seven days

Treatment with a single dose of an antimicrobial drug e.g., trimethoprim, 320 mg, sulfamethoxazole, 1600 mg given as Bactrim or Septra in four single-strength or two double-strength tablets; kanamycin, 500 mg intramuscularly; or amoxacillin, 3 gm orally is highly successful for bladder infections. However, single-dose therapy fails in more than 50 percent of patients with an upper tract infection, and as many as 40 percent of women with only lower tract symptoms also have upper tract infections.

Recurrent Urinary Tract Infections

These patients demonstrate abnormal vaginal biologic factors. Colonization of vaginal and urethral mucosa usually precedes bacteriuria. Bacterial adherence to squamous cells and lack of vaginal antibody to *E. coli* probably lead to vaginal colonization. Women

TABLE 35–1 ANTIMICROBIAL AGENTS USED IN THE MANAGEMENT OF URINARY TRACT INFECTIONS AND THEIR USUAL EFFECTIVENESS AGAINST COMMON PATHOGENS

AGENT	SERUM LEVELS	URINE LEVELS	Escherichia coli	Klebsiella	Pseudo-monas	Entero-coccus	Proteus
Trimethoprim-sulfamethoxazole	±	+ +	+ +	+ +	−	−	+ +
Nitrofurantoin	−	+ +	+ +	±	−	±	−
Ampicillin	+	+ +	+ +	−	−	+ +	+ +
Cephalothin	+ +	+ +	+ +	+ +	−	±	+ +
Tetracycline	±	+	±	±	−	+ +	−
Kanamycin	+ +	+ +	+ +	+ +	−	−	+ +
Gentamicin	+ +	+ +	+ +	+ +	+ +	−	+ +
Carbenicillin	+ +	+ +	+ +	−	+ +	−	+ +

+ +Good; + Adequate; ± Occasionally effective; − Not effective.

**TABLE 35–2 PRINCIPLES FOR
BLADDER DRAINAGE**

1. Avoid nonessential catheterization.
2. Remove catheters promptly.
3. Use correct sterile procedure for catheterization to avoid introducing bacteria.
4. Maintain closed drainage.
5. Disconnect the drainage system only when there is an obstruction.
6. Avoid prophylactic antibiotics.
7. Use suprapubic catheterization for prolonged bladder drainage.

resistant to *E. coli* carry specific antibodies to their own *E. coli*.

Recently, the benefit of long-term (6 to 12 months) administration of antimicrobials in women with recurrent UTI's has been demonstrated. Trimethoprim-sulfamethoxazole has been found to be effective and is the only antibacterial agent known to be excreted in vaginal fluid. Sulfonamides, tetracycline, and ampicillin are not effective prophylactically because of the rapid emergence of resistant fecal strains. Recurrent infections tend to occur in clusters. There are often prolonged' remissions between these clusters, and the timing of the clusters cannot be predicted. Prophylactic therapy should be initiated when the patient has had two infections within six months, as she faces a 65 percent chance of another infection within the next six months.

For women who are able to closely relate their frequently recurring infections to sexual activity, a single dose of an antimicrobial drug immediately after coitus has been shown to prevent bacteriuria and symptomatic infection.

Prevention of Hospital-Acquired UTI's in Gynecologic Patients

Sixty percent of hospital-acquired infections in gynecologic patients involve the urinary tract, particularly in association with catheterization. The principles shown in Table 35–2 should be employed in effecting drainage of the urinary bladder.

SUGGESTED READING

Beck RP, McCormick S: Treatment of urinary stress incontinence with anterior colporrhaphy. Obstet Gynecol 59:269, 1983.

Bhatia NN, Bergman A: Pessary test in women with urinary incontinence. Ostet Gynecol 65:220, 1985.

Bhatia NN, Ostergard DR: Urodynamics in women with stress urinary incontinence. Obstet Gynecol 60:552, 1982.

Burch JC: Urethrovaginal fixation to Cooper's ligament for correction of stress incontinence, cystocele, and prolapse. Am J Obstet Gynecol 81:281, 1961.

Green TH: Urinary stress incontinence: Differential diagnosis, pathophysiology, and management. Am J Obstet Gynecol 122:368, 1978.

Kunin CM: Detection, Prevention, and Treatment of Urinary Tract Infections. 2nd ed. Philadelphia, Lee & Febiger, 1974.

Marshall VF, Marchetti AA, Krantz KE: The correction of stress incontinence by simple vesicourethral suspension. Surg Gynecol Obstet 88:590, 1949.

Pereyra AJ, Lebherz TB, Growdon WA, et al: Pubourethral support in perspective: Modified Pereyra procedure for urinary incontinence. Obstet Gynecol 59:643, 1982.

Stamey TA: Endoscopic suspension of the vesical neck for urinary incontinence. Surg Gynecol Obstet 136:547, 1973.

Stamey TA: Pathogenesis and treatment of urinary tract infections. Baltimore, Williams and Wilkins, 1981.

Stanton SL, Cardozo L: A comparison of vaginal and suprapubic surgery in the correction of incontinence. Br J Urol 51:497, 1971.

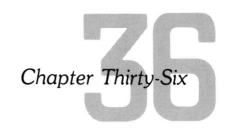

Chapter Thirty-Six

ABORTION

GAUTAM CHAUDHURI

Abortion is defined as the termination of pregnancy before the fetus is sufficiently developed to survive. An abortion may be either *spontaneous* or *induced*. The term "miscarriage" has been applied by lay persons to denote abortion that has occurred spontaneously. Termination of pregnancy before term but after the fetus has achieved some potential for survival is referred to as *preterm or premature delivery*. It is difficult to pinpoint the gestational age at which the fetus, upon delivery, ceases to become an abortus and becomes an infant.

The United States Supreme Court, in its ruling on abortion in 1973, used the term "viability" but did not define it. It stated, "We need not resolve the difficult question of when life begins. When those trained in the respective disciplines of medicine, philosophy and theology are unable to arrive at any consensus, the judiciary, at this point in the development of man's knowledge, is not in a position to speculate as to the answer."

SPONTANEOUS ABORTION

Spontaneous abortion is defined as termination of pregnancy before the end of the twentieth week without voluntary action to effect its interruption on the part of either the pregnant woman or some other person. The fetus should not weigh more than 500 gm and/or have a crown to rump length of more than 16.5 cm. The exact incidence is difficult to determine, but quoted figures range from 10 to 20 percent of all pregnancies.

Etiology

Genetic Factors. Genetic abnormalities are the most common cause of spontaneous abortion. Defective development of the ovum may include defects in the embryo itself or in the placenta. With early abortion, there is commonly an empty amniotic sac present, with absence or degeneration of the fetus. This condition is referred to as a *blighted ovum.*

Of early spontaneous abortions, 50 to 60 percent are associated with a chromosomal anomaly of the conceptus. About half of these chromosomal anomalies are autosomal trisomies. Most of the remainder are triploids, tetraploids, or 45X monosomies.

Endocrine Abnormalities. Adequate progesterone secretion by the corpus luteum is important for both implantation and maintenance of an early pregnancy. A *luteal phase defect* may be due to specific ovarian insufficiency or to a deficiency of progesterone receptors in the endometrium. A specific pituitary dysfunction, such as *hyperprolactinemia,* may occasionally be associated with a luteal phase defect. *Hypothyroidism* may occasionally be responsible for abortions.

Abnormalities of the Reproductive Organs. Uterine septae, submucous myomata, or uterine synechiae may cause abortion, as may cervical incompetence. The latter may be congenital or traumatic, such as following obstetric lacerations or conization of the cervix. Abortions associated with uterine or cervical anomalies usually occur in the second trimester.

Infectious Diseases. Several infectious diseases have been associated with abortions, including viral infections with herpes, rubella, and cytomegalic inclusion disease. Listeriosis, genital mycoplasmosis, toxoplasmosis, and brucellosis have also been implicated.

Systemic Diseases. Chronic diseases may be associated with abortion, although they more commonly cause anovulation. Diseases to consider include nutritional deficiencies, hepatic or renal disorders, diabetes mellitus, and collagen vascular diseases, particularly systemic lupus erythematosus.

Types of Spontaneous Abortion

Threatened Abortion. A threatened abortion is presumed when any bloody discharge appears to come from the pregnant uterus. Approximately 25 percent of pregnant women have vaginal spotting or heavier bleeding during the early months of gestation. Other causes of bleeding in early pregnancy, including ectopic pregnancy and cervical lesions, should be excluded. There may be some associated cramping and lower abdominal pain. About half of these patients actually abort, while spontaneous resolution of symptoms occurs in the others.

TREATMENT. There is no specific treatment for threatened abortion. Bed rest, as well as progesterone administration, has been suggested, but neither has been proven to be beneficial. Abstention from coitus during bleeding, and perhaps for two or more weeks thereafter, is usually recommended, although there is no scientific validation for this advice. Patients should be instructed to inform the physician if the bleeding or cramping pains increase in severity. If blood loss is excessive and affects the patient's well-being, evacuation of the products of conception is desirable.

Inevitable Abortion. The inevitability of an abortion is signaled by the rupture of membranes in the presence of cervical dilatation. Nothing can be done to salvage the pregnancy at this stage.

TREATMENT. Once the diagnosis of inevitable abortion is made, the uterus should be evacuated by uterine curettage in order to decrease blood loss and prevent infection.

Incomplete Abortion. Incomplete abortion implies that some products of conception have been retained in the uterus. The patient usually reports passage of tissue, but an actual fetus is rarely observed. The main danger is profuse bleeding caused by the prevention of myometrial contraction by the partially separated placenta.

TREATMENT. The remaining products of conception should be evacuated from the uterus. Loose fragments of placental tissue can be removed with ring forceps, after which the endometrium is scraped gently with a sharp curette following the administration of intravenous oxytocin (Pitocin) or intramuscular methylergonovine (Methergine). Blood transfusion may be necessary if bleeding is profuse.

Missed Abortion. This term is used when the embryo is not viable but is retained *in utero* for at least six weeks. Subjective symptoms of pregnancy, such as nausea, breast tenderness, and urinary frequency, disappear. There is usually an intermittent brown vaginal discharge. Uterine growth stops and eventually uterine size diminishes. The pregnancy test becomes negative. Occasionally, after prolonged retention of a dead second trimester fetus, disseminated intravascular coagulation may occur, and the patient may note bleeding from the nose, gums, or, especially, sites of trauma. Ultrasonography is diagnostic.

TREATMENT. In most cases of missed abortion, no treatment is required, as ultimately the abortus will be expelled. However, if the patient is particularly anxious and especially if there is constant vaginal bleeding, evacuation of the uterus should be recommended (see also Chapter 23). If it appears that the patient is developing a coagulation defect, a full coagulation profile should be obtained to rule out disseminated intravascular coagulation.

Septic Abortion. A septic abortion is one in which there is infection of the conceptus and upper genital tract. The abortal infection is most often caused by pathogenic organisms from the bowel and vaginal flora. The organisms cultured are both anaerobic and aerobic, *Peptostreptococcus* being the most frequently isolated, followed by *Escherichia coli*. Other organisms that may be involved include *Bacteroides, Clostridium perfringens, Pseudomonas,* beta-hemolytic *Streptococcus,* and *Enterococcus.*

Infection is usually confined to the uterus, but parametritis, peritonitis, and septicemia can occur. Symptoms include fever, pelvic pain, and uterine tenderness. Generalized abdominal tenderness and guarding will be noted if peritonitis is present. Bacterial shock may occur with hypotension and oliguria. Speculum examination often reveals a foul-smelling, purulent discharge from the external os. However, its absence does not exclude the diagnosis.

TREATMENT. Pulse rate, blood pressure, and urine output should be closely monitored. Blood and uterine cultures for both aerobic and anaerobic organisms should be obtained, and a smear for Gram staining should be made from the cervical discharge or products of conception to help identify the organisms present. An intravenous infusion should be commenced and any fluid and electrolyte imbalance corrected. Blood transfusion may be necessary. Intravenous broad spectrum antibiotics should be commenced immediately. Surgical evacuation of the products of conception should be performed after intravenous antibiotics have been given.

If bacterial shock is present, it should be managed aggressively. A Swan-Ganz catheter should be placed to allow accurate monitoring of intravenous fluids, and an indwelling catheter placed to monitor urine output. Corticosteroids should be given if the vital signs do not respond adequately to intravascular volume replacement. Once an adequate dose of antibiotics has been given, the nidus of infection must be removed by performing uterine curettage, and, if necessary, a hysterectomy.

Habitual Abortion. Habitual abortion, which is said to occur when a woman has had three or more consecutive spontaneous abortions, is discussed in Chapter 50.

INDUCED ABORTION

The practice of abortion, or elective termination of pregnancy, has had tremendous social and medicolegal implications in different countries. The United States Supreme Court declared all restrictive abortion laws unconstitutional in 1973, making abortion legal in all states. This resulted in a marked decrease in the number of illegal abortions, and maternal morbidity and mortality from abortions fell dramatically (Fig. 36–1). Table 36–1 shows the incidence of legal abortions per 1000 women 15 to 44 years of age from selected countries.

Table 36–2 gives the death-to-case rate for legal abortions by week of gestation in the United States from 1972 to 1978. It is apparent that the risk of death from abortion increases with gestational age. It is therefore important to have early diagnosis of pregnancy and appropriate counseling to aid in reducing the risk.

Prior to any abortion, the blood group, Rhesus (Rh) type, and antibody status of the patient should be ascertained. Any Rh-negative woman who has no evidence of isoimmunization should be given anti-D gamma globulin (see Chapter 25).

Patient Assessment

Individual patient counseling should be an integral part of the abortion service. The counseling should be carried out to assess the patient's mental status, as well as the social circumstances that prompted her to seek abortion.

If a patient has missed her period, a urine pregnancy test may be used as the first screening procedure. If the urine test is negative and the uterus is small but pregnancy is still suspected, a more sensitive serum pregnancy test (radioreceptor assay or beta hCG immunoassay) should be offered. Alternatively, the patient could be asked to return in one to two weeks for further evaluation.

If the patient is only six weeks or less from her last menstrual period with no symptoms of an ectopic pregnancy and the examiner finds a small uterus, the patient is told that even with a positive pregnancy test, it is advisable to wait one or two weeks because of the possibility of an unsuccessful extraction. If gestation is 12 or more weeks by dates, or the examiner feels that it is more than 12 weeks by size, it may be advisable for the patient to have an ultrasound to assess gestational age accurately. Thus, the appropriate procedure for terminating the pregnancy can be determined.

Indications for Abortion

Elective or Voluntary Abortion. This is the interruption of pregnancy before viability at the request of the woman but not for reasons of maternal health or fetal disease.

Maternal Indications. This is abortion performed where continuation of pregnancy will seriously jeopardize the well-being of the

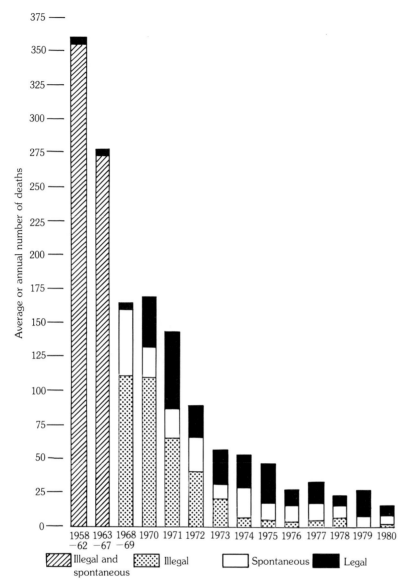

Figure 36–1 Number of deaths associated with abortion by type of abortion—United States, 1958–1980. (Reproduced with permission of the Population Council from Tietze C: Induced Abortion: A World Review, 1983. 5th ed. New York, The Population Council Inc, 1983.)

mother, either because of medical problems in the mother that contraindicate pregnancy or because of psychologic reasons.

Fetal Indications. This is abortion done for a fetal reason, such as a congenital anomaly or exposure to a teratogenic agent.

Techniques for Induced Abortion

First Trimester Abortion. Up to 12 weeks' gestation, there are two methods of perform-

ing an abortion: menstrual extraction and dilatation and suction curettage (D & C).

MENSTRUAL EXTRACTION. This is a low-morbidity procedure used for gestations up to seven weeks. A small, flexible cannula is inserted into the uterus without dilatation of the cervix, and suction is applied from a syringe. The procedure is performed under a paracervical block. The term "menstrual extraction" was originally used to designate an early abortion performed shortly after a missed menstrual period and often before the

TABLE 36–1 LEGAL ABORTIONS PER 1000 WOMEN AGED 15 TO 44 YEARS— SELECTED COUNTRIES, 1977–1981

COUNTRY	YEAR	ABORTION POLICY	ABORTION RATE
Netherlands*	1981	R	6.0
Scotland†	1981	S	9.2
Finland	1981	S	11.9
England and Wales*	1981	S	12.6
Norway	1981	R	16.4
Sweden	1981	R	19.4
Denmark	1981	R	20.7
German Democratic Republic	1977	R	22.5
United States	1980	S	29.3
Czechoslovakia	1981	R	32.1
Hungary	1981	S	35.3
Bulgaria	1979	S	69.6

*Residents only.
†Including residents of Scotland aborted in England.
R, on request; S, social or socio-medical indication.
Reproduced with permission from Tietze C: Induced Abortion: A World Review, 1983. 5th ed. New York, The Population Council Inc, 1983.

diagnosis of pregnancy was verified by a pregnancy test or examination. Nowadays, the procedure is not performed unless a positive pregnancy test is obtained.

There is a high incidence of continued pregnancy when the procedure is performed less than seven weeks from the last menstrual period, and the rate of failure varies with the experience of the person performing the procedure. The increased failure rate in very early pregnancies may outweigh the benefits of the procedure.

SUCTION CURETTAGE. This procedure is appropriate for termination of a pregnancy up to 12 weeks' gestational age. Placement of a *Laminaria* tent from a few hours to one day prior to the procedure aids in slow dilatation of the cervix. *Laminaria* is a sea-grown plant that is compacted into a stick. The most common type currently used in the United States is the *Laminaria japonica*. The *Laminaria* swells gradually after insertion, probably by absorbing fluids from the uterine cervix. Most of the swelling occurs within the first four to six hours after insertion, but it may continue to swell for up to 12 hours. The advantage of the *Laminaria* over the metallic dilator is that it allows more gentle dilatation of the cervix. Because *Laminaria* is sea-grown, it may have residual spore-forming organisms, even after processing with ethylene oxide.

The abortion is performed after undertaking aseptic precautions. After stabilizing the anterior lip of the cervix with a single-toothed tenaculum, a cannula of appropriate size for the length of gestation is inserted to the level of the fundus. The cannula is attached to

TABLE 36–2 DEATH-TO-CASE RATE FOR LEGAL ABORTIONS, BY WEEKS OF GESTATION: UNITED STATES, 1972 TO 1978

WEEKS OF GESTATION	DEATHS*	ABORTIONS†	RATE‡	RELATIVE RISK§
≤ 8	13	2,749,725	0.5	1.0
9 to 10	24	1,705,478	1.4	2.8
11 to 12	20	883,932	2.3	4.6
13 to 15	20	300,186	6.7	13.4
16 to 20	47	338,488	13.9	27.8
≥21	12	68,584	17.5	35.0
Totals	136	6,046,393	2.2	

*Excludes deaths from ectopic pregnancy.
†Based on distribution of 4,292,615 abortions (71 percent) with weeks of gestation known.
‡Deaths per 100,000 abortions.
§Based on index rate for ≤8 menstrual weeks' gestation of 0.5 per 100,000 abortions.
Reproduced with permission from the Centers for Disease Control: Abortion Surveillance, 1978. November 1980.

sterile suction tubing, and, with the aid of negative pressure created by the suction machine, the products of conception are evacuated. The procedure is completed by sharp curettage.

Midtrimester Abortion (from 13 to 24 weeks' gestation). In the early midtrimester (13 to 16 weeks' gestation), there is a limited quantity of amniotic fluid available; during this period, therefore, it is recommended that dilatation and evacuation (D & E) of the uterus be performed. For abortions 17 weeks and beyond, the choices are among D & E, intra-amniotic installation of an abortifacient, or extrauterine administration of an abortifacient. In the past, hysterotomy or hysterectomy was often performed for midtrimester abortion, but these procedures have been abandoned because of the associated high morbidity and mortality.

DILATATION AND EVACUATION (D & E). Midtrimester D & E is an extension of first trimester suction and sharp curettage. The uterus is larger, requiring special instruments for vaginal evacuation, and it is difficult to insert these larger instruments through the cervix without damaging it. Most physicians rely on overnight placement of multiple intracervical *Laminaria* tents to dilate the cervix. Thereafter, the uterus is emptied using a combination of large bore suction equipment, special forceps (Sopher and Bierer), and, finally, a sharp curette.

Complications of surgical evacuation of the uterus include:

1. Incomplete evacuation of the uterus or failure to evacuate an early pregnancy.

2. Perforation of the uterus with or without damage to other pelvic structures, particularly bowel.

TABLE 36–3 ABORTIFACIENT AGENTS

DRUG	DOSE AND ROUTE OF ADMINISTRATION	MEAN INSTALLATION TO ABORTION TIME	SUCCESS RATE (TIME)	SIDE EFFECTS
Prostaglandin F$_2$-alpha	40 mg in a single intra-amniotic dose	20 hours	80% (at 48 hrs)	Diarrhea (15%) Vomiting (50%) Heavy uterine bleeding (5%) Bronchoconstriction (2%) Incomplete abortion (33%) Hypo- and hypertension Transverse rupture of the posterior uterine wall at the cervicoisthmic junction
Prostaglandin F$_2$-alpha, and urea	20 mg PGF$_2$-alpha and 80 gm of urea dissolved in 130 to 150 ml of distilled water. Oxytocin infusion started 24 hrs after installation for failure to abort or 4 hrs after rupture of membranes	13 hours	100% (at 24 hrs)	Nausea and vomiting (60%) Incomplete abortion (45%) Hemorrhage (10%) Diarrhea (1%) Cervical laceration (3%)
Hypertonic saline	200 ml of 20% NaCl injected intra-amniotically	26 hours	80% (at 48 hrs)	Vomiting (20%) Diarrhea (2%) Hypernatremia Heavy uterine bleeding (1%) Disseminated intravascular coagulation (1%) Necrosis of myometrium if injected directly Incomplete abortion (30%)
Prostaglandin E$_2$ suppositories	20 mg intravaginally every 3 to 4 hours for missed abortion or intrauterine fetal death	9 hours	97%	Nausea (60%) Vomiting (60%) Diarrhea (60%) Pyrexia (>38°) (60%) Tachycardia (50%) Tachypnea (20%) Blood loss >500 ml (5%)

3. Hemorrhage requiring transfusion.

4. Septic abortion leading to endotoxic shock.

INTRA-AMNIOTIC INSTALLATION OF AN ABORTIFACIENT AGENT. Intra-amniotic infusion of a hypertonic solution, such as saline or urea, or of a uterotonic agent, such as prostaglandin F_2-alpha, induces myometrial contractility and usually results in expulsion of the products of conception. The agents used, their appropriate dosages, and main side effects are shown in Table 36–3.

In this technique, the patient empties her bladder, after which the lower abdomen is cleansed with an antiseptic. Under local anesthesia, a needle with an obturator (such as a #18 spinal needle) is inserted into the uterus, the obturator is removed, and the needle is adjusted until a free flow of amniotic fluid is obtained. Testing of the fluid for alkalinity with litmus paper usually distinguishes amniotic fluid from urine (which is usually acidic). As approximately 25 percent of women benefit from more than one injection of the abortifacient, many operators place an indwelling catheter through the needle, which is then withdrawn.

The most serious *complications* of a saline abortion are hypernatremia and disseminated intravascular coagulation, while the most serious complication of a prostaglandin-induced abortion is transverse rupture of the posterior uterine wall at the level of the cervicoisthmic junction. Cervical injury is probably the result of strong uterine contractions and is more likely to occur in young nulliparas in the late second trimester of pregnancy. The incidence has been reported to range from 0.3 to 8 percent.

PROSTAGLANDIN SUPPOSITORIES. Prostaglandins administered by the vaginal route are absorbed into the systemic circulation. The main disadvantage peculiar to this route of administration is that early rupture of the membranes may result in leakage of amniotic fluid into the vagina, thus diluting or washing out the drug. Prostaglandin suppositories are used mainly for evacuation of the uterus in patients with a missed abortion or intrauterine fetal death.

Abortion Medications

Postabortion Medications. Methylergonovine maleate, 0.2 mg orally or intramuscularly (IM), is given postabortally for excessive bleeding and uterine atony. This medication contracts the uterus tonically and diminishes bleeding. Intravenous oxytocin infusion may also be used.

Anesthesia and Abortion. Most gynecologists prefer to use local anesthesia, which may be administered in the form of a paracervical block, for both first and second trimester abortions. Under local anesthesia, the patient remains alert, responsive, and communicative during and after the procedure. She is able to report important symptoms that may signal the onset of serious complications. General anesthesia is not preferred, as its use is twice as likely to be associated with uterine perforation and cervical injury.

SUGGESTED READING

Boué J, Boué A, Lazar P: Retrospective and prospective epidemiological studies of 1500 karyotyped spontaneous human abortions. Teratology 12:11, 1975.

Grimes DA, Cates W Jr, Selik RM: Fatal septic abortion in the United States, 1975-1977. Obstet Gynecol 57:739, 1981.

Hertig AT, Livingstone RG: Spontaneous, threatened, and habitual abortion: Its pathogenesis and treatment. N Engl J Med 230:797, 1944.

Karim SMM (ed): Practical Application of Prostaglandins. Baltimore, University Park Press, 1979.

Laros RK, Collins J, Penner JA, et al: Coagulation changes in saline-induced abortion. Am J Obstet Gynecol 116:277, 1973.

Laros RK, Roberts JM: Hemorrhagic and endotoxic shock: A pathophysiologic approach to diagnosis and management. Am J Obstet Gynecol 110:1041, 1971.

Naib ZM, Nahmias AJ, Josey WE, et al: Association of maternal genital herpetic infection with spontaneous abortion. Obstet Gynecol 35:260, 1970.

Singh RP, Carr DH: Anatomic findings in human abortions of known chromosomal constitution. Obstet Gynecol 29:806, 1967.

Warburton D, Fraser FC: Spontaneous abortion risks in man: Data from reproductive histories collected in a medical genetics unit. Am J Hum Genet 16:1, 1964.

Chapter Thirty-Seven

ECTOPIC PREGNANCY

WILLIAM J. DIGNAM

In at least one of every 200 pregnancies, the conceptus implants somewhere other than its usual location in the endometrium. For a variety of reasons, the incidence of this condition has risen sharply in recent years. Currently, ectopic pregnancy accounts for at least 12 percent of maternal mortality in the United States.

The accurate detection of this condition is important for two principal reasons. The first is that ectopic pregnancy may be associated with profuse hemorrhage, and maternal mortality is a distinct possibility. The second is that patients who have had an ectopic pregnancy have a decreased ability to have subsequent children. It is generally estimated that following an ectopic pregnancy, a woman has at best a 50 percent chance of bearing a live infant in the future. This figure may be improved with the increasing availability of *in vitro* fertilization and other similar procedures. Patients with one ectopic pregnancy have at least a 10 percent chance of having a second ectopic pregnancy in the future.

Most ectopic pregnancies are located in one of the fallopian tubes, although a small number are located in the cervix, angular portion of the endometrial cavity, ovary, or elsewhere in the peritoneal cavity. Possible sites of ectopic pregnancies are shown in Figure 37–1.

ETIOLOGY

The cause for ectopic implantation of a pregnancy is not always clear. Many implant in tubes that have been distorted by previous *infection*. This may be due to a venereal infection, such as gonorrhea, or to a tubal infection related to the presence of an intrauterine contraceptive device. The tubes may also be distorted by *endometriosis, previous tubal surgery,* or, rarely, by *congenital anomalies.*

PATHOGENESIS

Ectopic pregnancies implant by the same mechanism as intrauterine pregnancies—that is, by erosion of the tissues. If that erosion takes place at the site of an arteriole, the patient may experience a significant hemorrhage. If the erosion takes place along the mesenteric border of the tube, a broad ligament hematoma may develop, whereas if the erosion takes place elsewhere around the circumference of the tube, the patient may experience a major intraperitoneal hemorrhage with its attendant hypovolemia and shock.

The tube apparently tears at the site of the erosion in some instances because some patients experience very sudden, severe, lancinating pain. Visualization of the tube shows a laceration that may have placental tissue protruding through it.

More common than patients with obvious intraperitoneal hemorrhage are those with some signs of peritoneal irritation but no signs of hypovolemia. In many of these patients, when the tube is visualized, no perforation or laceration is noted, but blood and/or tissue may be seen protruding from the fimbriated end of the tube. These substances

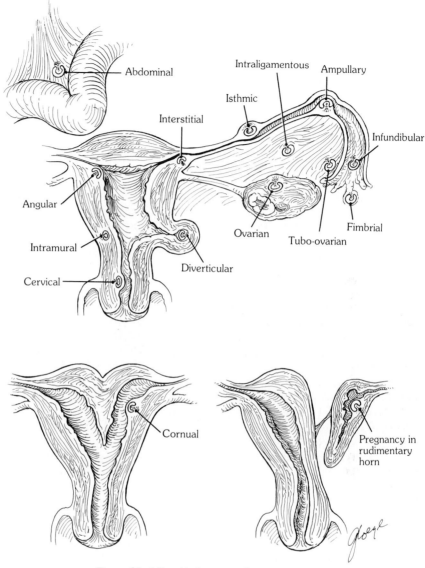

Figure 37–1 Possible locations of ectopic pregnancy.

cause peritoneal irritation and abdominal pain.

CLINICAL MANIFESTATIONS

The clinical manifestations of ectopic pregnancy are variable and partly dependent on the site of implantation. The more distal ampullary portions of the tube are better able to accommodate a developing conceptus. Therefore, symptoms may not develop until several weeks after a missed period. When the conceptus is implanted in the more proximal isthmic portion of the tube, symptoms may occur within two weeks of an expected period or earlier.

The patient with a major intraperitoneal hemorrhage is frequently less of a diagnostic problem than one with only a small amount of intraperitoneal bleeding. The first is obviously critically ill. Typically, she complains of missing an expected period two or three weeks earlier. On the day of admission, there is sudden severe pain in a lower quadrant of the abdomen, often followed by an episode of fainting. If much blood has accumulated in the abdomen, pain might also be experienced on the superior aspect of one or both shoulders due to diaphragmatic irritation from the accumulated blood. There is usually a small amount of vaginal bleeding for a few days prior to the abdominal pain.

For patients who have less dramatic symptoms, the diagnosis is more difficult. Generally speaking, they are several weeks beyond the time of an expected period that was missed and complain of intermittent episodes of lower abdominal pain that may be more prominent on one side. They may or may not have symptoms of pregnancy. There is usually a small amount of intermittent vaginal bleeding. The vaginal bleeding is related to degeneration and desquamation of the endometrial decidua, which is caused by a decrease in placental estrogen and progesterone associated with the disruption of the pregnancy. Occasional patients extrude the entire "decidual cast" intact. This may be associated with tubal abortion and the complete cessation of placental steroid production.

PHYSICAL EXAMINATION

In patients with major bleeding, hypotension and tachycardia will be expected. The abdomen is usually very tender and guarded. It may be quite difficult to palpate the involved fallopian tube, particularly if it has ruptured and expelled the conceptus. If palpable, the tube will frequently be exquisitely tender. It may be possible to palpate accumulated blood and blood clots in the cul-de-sac, particularly if the patient can be placed in a partially upright position for a few minutes before the examination is performed.

In patients with mild symptoms, abdominal examination may not reveal any significant abnormalities. Some patients, however, have definite, although mild, tenderness in one lower quadrant or the other. Pelvic examination should certainly be performed, but the findings may be noncontributory. If a sausage-shaped adnexal mass can be palpated separate from the ovary, it is very suggestive of an ectopic pregnancy. Enlargement and softening of the uterus are not helpful signs because these may be present with either an intrauterine or ectopic pregnancy.

DIFFERENTIAL DIAGNOSIS

Among the diagnoses that must be considered in these patients are amenorrhea for reasons not associated with pregnancy, salpingo-oophoritis, endometriosis, ruptured follicular or corpus luteum cyst, and intrauterine pregnancy with threatened abortion. The last may be very difficult to differentiate from ectopic pregnancy at this early stage.

FURTHER INVESTIGATIONS

When a patient is first seen and ectopic pregnancy is considered to be a possibility, a

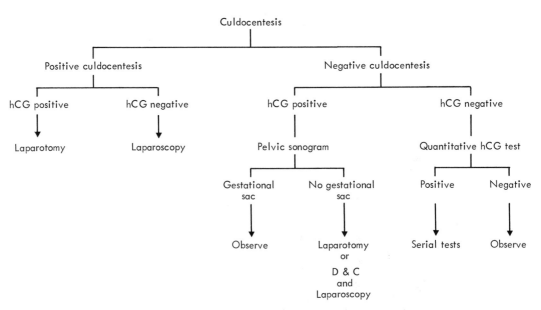

Figure 37–2 Evaluation of a hemodynamically stable patient with a suspected ectopic pregnancy.

complete blood count and urinalysis are ordered, and blood is sent for typing and cross-matching.

A suggested diagnostic work-up for a patient with suspected ectopic pregnancy is depicted in Figure 37–2.

Pregnancy Tests

Establishing an accurate diagnosis of ectopic pregnancy requires a good knowledge of the secretion of chorionic gonadotropin (hCG) during early pregnancy. Chorionic gonadotropin is produced by the conceptus, probably even before implantation occurs,

and it gains access to the maternal circulation very soon after implantation. It increases in amount very rapidly. Therefore, if sensitive assays are employed, hCG may be found in the maternal blood starting eight or nine days after ovulation and fertilization, as depicted in Figure 37–3.

The commonly employed rapid tests for pregnancy—that is, *tests for hCG in urine*—do not differentiate between hCG and luteinizing hormone (LH), which are both glycoproteins with common alpha subunits. Therefore, the sensitivity of these tests (commonly 500 or 1000 international units of hCG per liter of urine) is established by the manufac-

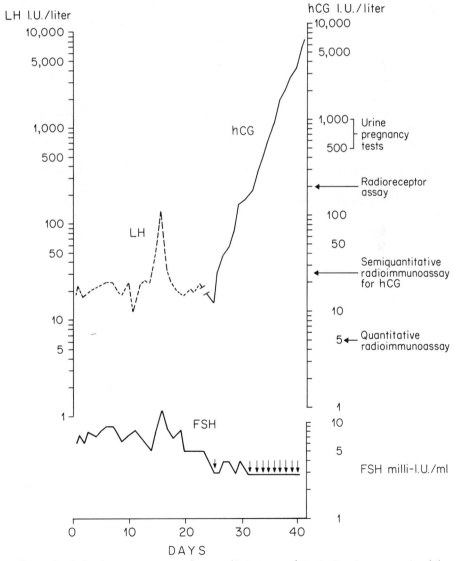

Figure 37–3 Graphic representation of serum chorionic gonadotropin titers in pregnancy and the sensitivities of the various pregnancy tests. Arrows (↓) indicate levels below the sensitivity of the assay.

turers at a point sufficiently high so that LH will not produce a false-positive result. Even the ovulatory peak level of LH would not cause a reaction greater than that caused by 100 units of hCG.

A more sensitive test is the *radioreceptor assay* (RRA), which utilizes the reaction with receptor sites on animal corpora lutea to identify hCG in blood. LH will produce a positive reaction in this test also, so the sensitivity of the test is commonly set at 200 units. This test has the advantage of providing rapid results, usually within two hours of submission of blood to the laboratory.

A more specific test is the *radioimmunoassay for hCG*. This test identifies the beta subunit of hCG and, therefore, avoids cross-reaction with other hormones that have the same alpha subunit, such as LH. The *quantitative radioimmunoassay for hCG* is highly sensitive, and, in most laboratories, as little as 5 mIU of hCG per ml of serum can be identified. This is a complicated test that requires about eight hours to perform and has its major application in the follow-up of patients with gestational trophoblastic disease.

Recently, a modification of this test has been developed. This *semiquantitative radioimmunoassay* takes about two hours to perform because a much shorter incubation period is employed, and only positive and negative controls are used, rather than the quantitative standard. The test has a sensitivity of 25 mIU per ml of serum. It has become the standard pregnancy test in many hospitals and is the pregnancy test that should be utilized for patients with possible ectopic pregnancies.

The relationships among the levels of LH and hCG along with the sensitivities of the commonly available tests are depicted in Figure 37–3. From this figure, it can readily be seen that the semiquantitative hCG should give a positive result by 14 days after ovulation or earlier. If this test is positive, pregnancy is certain, and efforts should be devoted to distinguishing between intrauterine and ectopic pregnancy.

If the semiquantitative assay is negative, the possibility of pregnancy is not excluded, but it is certainly much less likely, and other conditions that may cause these symptoms should be strongly considered. Such patients can be managed safely without hospital admission. When it is available, a quantitative radioimmunoassay for the beta subunit of hCG can be obtained. If that is negative, no further consideration need be given to the possibility of pregnancy. If by chance the patient has a small amount of functioning trophoblastic tissue, as indicated by the detection of hCG in the quantitative assay, it is probable that pregnancy will spontaneously resolve without the need for surgical intervention. Serial hCG titers should be obtained until they become negative.

Culdocentesis

If blood is palpated in the cul-de-sac, or if the presence of an ectopic pregnancy with bleeding is suspected, a culdocentesis should be performed, as illustrated in Figure 37–4. The vagina is comparatively insensitive, and if the examiner is gentle, it is usually possible to introduce a number 18 needle into the cul-de-sac without anesthesia and without undue discomfort for the patient.

From time to time, pure nonclotting blood may be drawn from the cul-de-sac in a patient who has not had very severe symptoms and who does not show evidence of significant blood loss. If the culdocentesis shows clear-cut evidence of a hemoperitoneum, the next step is to identify the source of the bleeding at laparotomy and to control it. It is possible to have a hemoperitoneum with an intrauterine pregnancy, but not at all likely.

If no fluid is obtained at culdocentesis, this test is not helpful because an ectopic pregnancy may still be present while not discharging blood or other fluid into the peritoneal cavity. It is probable that on some occasions the examiner is not successful in reaching the peritoneal cavity with the needle. At times, purulent material is retrieved, suggesting that the symptoms are due to infection. If serosanguineous fluid is obtained, additional diagnostic measures must be carried out in order to reach a final diagnosis.

Pelvic Ultrasonography

A pelvic sonogram may help to distinguish between an intrauterine and an ectopic pregnancy. The ability to visualize a pregnancy in an ectopic location has not yet been well developed. However, an image such as that illustrated in Figure 37–5 may occasionally be seen.

The gestational sac can usually be clearly

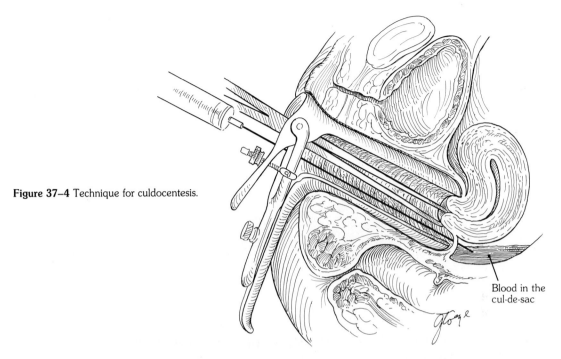

Figure 37–4 Technique for culdocentesis.

Blood in the
cul-de-sac

seen in the uterine cavity by the end of the seventh week of amenorrhea (Fig. 37–6). Therefore, if the presence of a pregnancy has been established by a positive hCG assay, a gestational ring is not visible in the uterine cavity, and the patient is at least five weeks beyond ovulation, it is likely that ectopic pregnancy is present. If sonography demonstrates a gestational sac in the uterus, the diagnosis of threatened abortion is established.

A number of efforts have been made to correlate levels of chorionic gonadotropin with sonographic findings. Gestational sacs are not seen when hCG levels are below 6500 mIU/ml of serum, but are seen in over 90 percent of normal pregnancies with higher hCG levels. Therefore, if the hCG level is 6500 and no gestational sac is present in the uterus, ectopic pregnancy is very likely. The placenta of an ectopic pregnancy is not as productive as that of a normally implanted

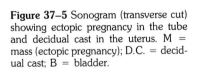

Figure 37–5 Sonogram (transverse cut) showing ectopic pregnancy in the tube and decidual cast in the uterus. M = mass (ectopic pregnancy); D.C. = decidual cast; B = bladder.

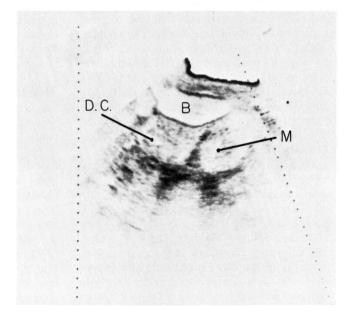

D. C.   B   M

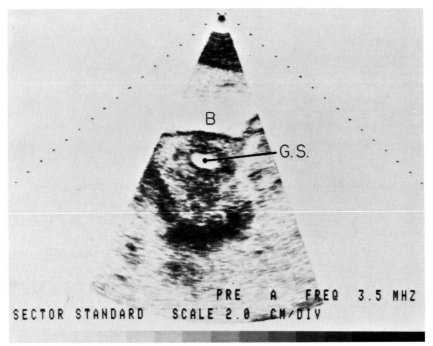

Figure 37–6 Sonogram showing the gestational sac in the uterus. B = bladder; G.S. = gestational sac.

pregnancy, so many patients with ectopic pregnancies have levels of hCG that are well below 6500. It is also true that many of them develop acute problems before the time when a gestational sac might be found in the uterus.

Laparoscopy

If the situation is confusing and the physician continues to suspect that an ectopic pregnancy is present, the matter can usually be resolved by laparoscopy. It is usually, but not always, possible to make a definitive diagnosis at laparoscopy. At times it is difficult to visualize the tubes due to distortion of pelvic anatomy from previous infection or other processes or simply due to technical difficulties.

Laparoscopy may be useful in a patient with a negative pregnancy test but a suggestive history and a positive culdocentesis. Such a patient may have a bleeding corpus luteum, and laparoscopic cautery may prevent laparotomy.

Laparoscopy may also be useful in a patient with a positive pregnancy test and no gestational sac in the uterus. Occasionally, a patient with a missed or incomplete abortion will have sufficient residual placental tissue

to produce a positive semiquantitative hCG assay. If such a condition is suspected, dilatation and curettage should be performed. Placental tissue can usually be identified grossly by the appearance of villi when the tissue is floated in saline. If doubt remains, laparoscopy may be employed.

It is probable that as more experience with the use of the semiquantitative assay for hCG is accumulated, laparoscopy will play a progressively less important role in the diagnostic work-up of these patients.

MANAGEMENT

If the patient has obvious evidence of an acute emergency with hypovolemia and a distended abdomen from a large amount of blood, an intravenous infusion with a large bore catheter should be commenced and a laparotomy performed immediately. On entering the peritoneal cavity, the blood should be rapidly evacuated and the source of bleeding identified and controlled. Apart from a ruptured ectopic pregnancy, other possible reasons for the hemoperitoneum include rupture of an ovarian cyst, spleen, or major intra-abdominal vessel.

It may be helpful to start blood transfusions, but the patient may be bleeding faster intra-abdominally than she can be transfused. Therefore, it may be wiser to perform an immediate laparotomy and control the bleeding quickly than to delay surgery in the hope of stabilizing the patient. A compression suit should be applied to such a patient in the emergency room. The abdominal portion can be released immediately prior to the laparotomy.

Salpingectomy has been the standard treatment for ectopic pregnancy until recent years. However, more attention is presently being directed to the possibility of performing conservative operations, particularly in young patients. The involved tubes are usually abnormal, so it is still customary in many institutions to remove the tube when a patient has her first ectopic pregnancy. However, if the patient has only one remaining tube and that is the site of the ectopic pregnancy, the involved segment of the tube may be removed. Subsequent tubal reanastomosis using microsurgical techniques may restore tubal patency. An alternative approach is to perform a *salpingotomy*. If one of these operations is performed, the tube can usually be left patent at the emergency operation, although subsequent microsurgical revision may be needed if tubal blockage results.

Even when distortion of the tubes is so marked that salpingectomy is carried out for the single remaining tube, the possibility of *in vitro* fertilization remains. More and more clinics are gaining experience with the necessary procedures, and, doubtless, the results will improve as the experience increases.

Patients with ectopic pregnancy do run the risk of Rh sensitization, and, therefore, Rh typing of their blood is important. If the patient is Rh-negative, she should receive 50 micrograms of Rh-D immune globulin.

The overwhelming majority of ectopic pregnancies are located in fallopian tubes, but rarely these pregnancies may be implanted in the cervix, the angular portion of the uterus, or on the abdominal viscera. Each of these locations is associated with the possibility of exsanguinating hemorrhage. Such patients should be managed by experienced experts in facilities equipped for the care of critically ill patients if the diagnosis is established before treatment is initiated.

ABDOMINAL PREGNANCY

Abdominal pregnancy is a very rare occurrence, but because it is a potentially life-threatening condition, it is important to recognize the possibility. Most instances of abdominal pregnancy are probably due to ruptured tubal pregnancies, so these patients may give a suggestive history if questioned closely. There is a very high fetal mortality and a high incidence of congenital anomalies.

An abdominal pregnancy does not cause specific symptoms, so it commonly escapes detection until well advanced. Patients may complain of abdominal pain or gastrointestinal symptoms, but both are so common in normal pregnancy that they may be ignored. On physical examination, the infant may be exceptionally easy to palpate and may be in an abnormal position.

The diagnosis depends upon the identification of the uterine mass separate from the gestational sac and its contents. X-rays or sonograms may occasionally be helpful but are not always definitive.

Laparotomy should be carried out in an institution where a large quantity of blood is available. Commonly, the placenta is attached to structures (such as bowel) that cannot contract to control bleeding, so it is best to deliver the baby and leave the placenta in place, unless the vessels supplying it can be easily visualized and ligated.

SUGGESTED READING

Kadar N, DeVore G, Romero R: Discriminatory hCG zone: Its use in the sonographic evaluation for ectopic pregnancy. Obstet Gynecol 58:156, 1981.

Levi S, Lebicq P: The diagnostic value of ultrasonography in 342 suspected cases of ectopic pregnancy. Acta Obstet Gynecol Scand 59:29, 1980.

McElin TW: Ectopic pregnancy. In Danforth DN (ed): Obstetrics and Gynecology. 3rd ed. Chapter 18. Harper and Row, Hagerstown, MD, 1977.

Rubin GL, Peterson HB, Dorfman SF, et al: Ectopic pregnancy in the United States, 1970 through 1978. JAMA 249:1725, 1983.

Chapter Thirty-Eight

CHRONIC PELVIC PAIN

ANDREA J. RAPKIN

Chronic pelvic pain refers to pain of greater than six months' duration. Although an enigmatic entity, it is one of the most common presenting complaints in a gynecologic practice. As a health problem, it incurs great cost to society in terms of hospital services, loss of productivity, and human misery.

Obviously, not all lower abdominal and low back pains are of gynecologic origin. Careful evaluation is needed to distinguish gynecologic pain from that of orthopedic, gastrointestinal, urologic, neurologic, and psychosomatic origin. The relationship between pelvic pain and the underlying gynecologic pathology is often inexplicable. For example, it is well known that women with severe endometriosis may experience no discomfort, while those with mild to moderate amounts of this disease may have disabling pain. Pelvic adhesions represent another puzzling entity. There is disagreement within the gynecologic community as to whether or not adhesions can cause pelvic pain, and, if so, what types can be implicated. Finally, there are those situations in which no pathology can be found, but pain persists.

The discovery of the role of prostaglandins in primary dysmenorrhea, formerly believed to be a neurotic affectation, calls for caution in making a diagnosis of psychosomatic pelvic pain. There is still much to be learned about the mechanisms involved in the production and perception of pelvic pain.

ANATOMY AND PHYSIOLOGY

The pain fibers to pelvic organs are shown in Table 38–1. Painful impulses that originate

TABLE 38–1 NERVES CARRYING PAINFUL IMPULSES FROM THE PELVIC ORGANS

ORGAN	SPINAL SEGMENTS	NERVES
Perineum, vulva, lower vagina	S2–4	Pudendal Inguinal Genitofemoral Posterofemoral cutaneous
Upper vagina, cervix, lower uterine segment, posterior urethra, bladder trigone, uterosacral and cardinal ligaments, rectosigmoid, lower ureters	S2–4	Pelvic parasympathetics
Uterine fundus, proximal fallopian tubes, broad ligament, upper bladder, cecum, appendix, terminal large bowel	T11–12, L1	Sympathetics via hypogastric plexus
Outer two-thirds fallopian tubes, upper ureter	T9–10	Sympathetics via aortic and superior mesenteric plexes
Ovaries	T9–10	Sympathetics via renal and aortic plexes and celiac and mesenteric ganglia

in the skin, muscles, bones, joints, and parietal peritoneum travel in somatic nerve fibers, while those originating in the internal organs travel in visceral nerves. Visceral pain has a more diffuse localization than that of somatic origin because there is no well-defined projection in the sensory cortex for its identification. Visceral pain is, therefore, usually referred to the skin, which is supplied by the corresponding spinal cord segment (referred pain). For example, the initial pain of appendicitis is referred to the epigastric area, since both structures are innervated by the thoracic cord segments eight, nine, and ten.

The structures of the female genital tract vary in their sensitivity to pain. The skin of the external genitalia is exquisitely sensitive. Pain sensation is variable in the vagina, since the upper segment is somewhat less sensitive than the lower. The cervix is relatively insensitive to small biopsies, but is sensitive to deep incision or to dilatation. The uterus is quite sensitive. The ovaries are insensitive to many stimuli, but they are sensitive to rapid distension of the ovarian capsule or compression during physical examination.

PATIENT EVALUATION

History

The history should include a description of the localization, quality, radiation, intensity, and duration of the pain, together with any aggravating or alleviating factors. The relationship of the pain to the menstrual cycle (including the presence of abnormal bleeding, menorrhagia, or metrorrhagia), bowel movements, urination, sexual intercourse, and physical activity should be noted. A history of similar painful episodes in the past should be sought, as should the presence of other somatic complaints, such as anorexia, weight loss, or gastrointestinal or urologic symptoms. One should establish whether there are solely musculoskeletal complaints, such as low or radicular back pain, or whether these accompany the patient's pelvic pain.

The degree to which the pain disrupts the patient's everyday activities should be ascertained, as should prominent events in the patient's life that may have occurred concurrently with the onset of pain. For example,

the pain may have begun after the placement of an intrauterine device (IUD) (possible infectious etiology), rape (possible psychologic trauma), or after lifting a heavy object (possible hernia). It should be established what pain medications the patient is taking and whether or not there are any compensation or litigation issues pending.

Symptoms of stress (e.g., palpitations, headaches) or depression (e.g., sleep disorders, loss of memory) should be elicited. Other psychologic aspects to be investigated include the attitudes of both the patient and her significant others toward the pain, the illness, and her behavior resulting from the illness. The possibility of secondary gain or other psychologic benefits should be explored, as should concurrent upheavals in the patient's life. Psychologic evaluations should not preclude further diagnostic studies.

Past gynecologic history should include inquiry regarding infertility, pelvic inflammation, usage of an IUD, gonococcal or chlamydial infection, endometriosis, and the time of the last pelvic examination. Details of abortion, childbirth, contraception, and sexual history should be sought. Past surgical history should include all pelvic, orthopedic, urologic, and neurologic procedures. The past medical history should focus on conditions that may impinge on the diagnosis of pelvic pain, such as irritable bowel syndrome, ulcerative colitis, Crohn's disease, and cystitis.

Physical Examination

The examination of the abdomen should be performed gently so as to prevent involuntary guarding, which may obstruct the findings. The patient should be asked to point to the exact location of the pain and its radiation, and an attempt should be made to duplicate the pain by palpation of each abdominal quadrant.

A gentle but thorough pelvic examination should be performed with an attempt to reproduce and localize the patient's pain. The examination may be suggestive of specific pelvic pathology. For example, patients with endometriosis may have a fixed retroverted uterus with tender uterosacral nodularity. Chronic salpingitis may be suggested by bilateral, tender, irregularly enlarged adnexal structures. A prolapsed uterus may account for pelvic pressure, pain, or low backache.

Further Investigations

Psychologic evaluation should be requested if an obviously traumatic event has occurred with the onset of pain or if there is obvious neurosis, psychosis, or secondary gain.

Laboratory studies are of limited utility in the diagnosis of chronic pelvic pain, although a complete blood count, erythrocyte sedimentation rate (ESR), and urinalysis are indicated. The ESR is nonspecific and will be increased in any type of inflammatory condition, such as subacute salpingo-oophoritis, tuberculosis, or inflammatory bowel disease. If bowel or urinary signs and symptoms are present, a barium enema, upper gastrointestinal series, or intravenous pyelogram may be useful. Similarly, if there is clinical evidence of musculoskeletal disease, a lumbosacral x-ray and orthopedic consultation may be in order.

If no obvious cause for the pain is uncovered, a pelvic ultrasound may be helpful, particularly in an obese or uncooperative patient. Diagnostic laparoscopy is the ultimate method of diagnosis for patients with chronic pelvic pain of undetermined etiology. Laparoscopic examination and bimanual examination may differ in 20 to 30 percent of cases.

DIFFERENTIAL DIAGNOSIS

Organic Causes of Chronic Pelvic Pain

If women with chronic pelvic pain are subjected to diagnostic laparoscopy, approximately one third have no apparent pathology, one third have endometriosis, one quarter have adhesions or stigmata of chronic pelvic inflammatory disease, and the remainder have various miscellaneous entities.

Endometriosis. Diagnostic laparoscopy is crucial for the diagnosis of endometriosis, since 30 percent of women with this disease have normal pelvic findings. The size and location of the endometriotic implants do not appear to correlate with the presence of pain, and the reasons for the pain are not understood.

Chronic Pelvic Inflammatory Disease. Chronic pelvic inflammatory disease (PID) may cause pain because of recurrent exacerbations that require active antibiotic therapy, or because of hydrosalpinges and adhesions between the tubes, ovaries, and intestinal structures. Before ascribing symptoms to adhesions, one must have noted adhesions specifically in the area of pain localization, since some patients with extensive pelvic adhesions are asymptomatic.

Ovarian Pain. Ovarian cysts are usually asymptomatic, but pain may occur secondary to rapid distension of the ovarian capsule. An ovary or ovarian remnant may occasionally become retroperitoneal secondary to inflammation or previous surgery, and cyst formation in these circumstances may also be painful. Some women, for unknown reasons, may develop multiple recurrent hemorrhagic ovarian cysts that seem to cause pelvic pain and dyspareunia. Impaired blood supply to the ovaries has been implicated, especially when there has been previous pelvic surgery, such as a partial oophorectomy or hysterectomy.

Uterine Pain. Adenomyosis (or endometriosis interna) may cause dysmenorrhea and menorrhagia, but rarely does it cause chronic intermenstrual pain. Uterine myomata usually do not cause pelvic pain unless they are degenerating, torsing (twisting their pedicles), or compressing pelvic nerves. Occasionally, a submucous leiomyoma may attempt to deliver via the cervix, which may cause considerable pelvic pain akin to childbirth.

Pelvic pain is not likely to be due to variations in uterine position, but deep dyspareunia may occasionally be associated with retroversion. The pain has been ascribed to irritation of pelvic nerves by the stretching of the uterosacral ligaments, as well as to congestion of pelvic veins secondary to retroversion. The dyspareunia is typically worse with the female in the missionary position and improved in the female superior position. If pressure in the posterior fornix reproduces the pain, ventral suspension of the uterus is very likely to be curative. A tender uterus that is in the fixed retroverted position is usually a sign of other intraperitoneal pathology, such as endometriosis or pelvic inflammatory disease, and diagnosis rests on laparoscopic findings. Occasionally, pelvic heaviness and low back pain may be present with advanced degrees of uterine prolapse. Prior to electing hysterectomy, the resolution of these symptoms with uterine replacement may be evaluated with pessary placement.

Gastrointestinal Pain. Chronic pelvic pain may be caused by various nongynecologic conditions. Gastrointestinal sources of chronic pelvic pain include penetrating neoplasms of the gastrointestinal tract, irritable bowel syndrome, partial bowel obstruction, inflammatory bowel disease, diverticulitis, and hernia formation. Since the innervation of the lower intestinal tract is the same as that of the uterus and fallopian tubes, the patient's complaint of pelvic pain may be confused with pain of gynecologic origin.

Neuromuscular Pain. Pain of neuromuscular origin, which is experienced as low back pain, usually increases with activity and stress. Chronic low back pain without lower abdominal pain is seldom of gynecologic etiology. Occasionally, neuromuscular symptoms are accompanied by a pelvic mass, and surgical exploration may reveal a neuroma or bony tumor.

Nonorganic Chronic Pelvic Pain

A pathologic diagnosis is unable to be made in approximately one third of patients with chronic pelvic pain, even after laparoscopy. Historically, various psychologic and physiologic processes have been described to account for this enigmatic occurrence.

Pelvic Congestion Syndrome. The concept of a pelvic congestion syndrome still has many proponents. This entity has been described in multiparous women who have pelvic vein varicosities and congested pelvic organs. The pelvic pain is worse premenstrually and is increased by fatigue, standing, and sexual intercourse. Many women with this condition are noted to have a uterus that is mobile, retroverted, soft, boggy, and slightly enlarged. There may be associated menorrhagia and urinary frequency. Dilated veins may be seen on venographic studies. Factors other than venous congestion may be involved, however, since most women with pelvic varicosities have no pain, and surgery for this condition is not usually beneficial. There have been some noncontrolled observations of similar symptoms of pain and metrorrhagia occurring after tubal ligation, but no prospective studies have been performed.

Psychologic Factors. The finding of chronic pelvic pain without pathology has led to the postulation that psychologic factors may be etiologic. The patients have been assumed to be anxious, neurotic, anorgasmic, and insecure in their roles as women and/or as mothers. When subjected to the Minnesota Multiphasic Personality Inventory (MMPI), these patients have shown a greater degree of anxiety, hypochondriasis, and hysteria than control subjects. However, the profiles are similar in patients who have chronic pain with organic pathology, suggesting that chronic pain *per se* engenders a complex, debilitating, psychologic response. Chronic pain patients with and without pathology tend to feel depressed, helpless, and passive. They withdraw from social and sexual activity and are preoccupied with pain and suffering. There is no scientific evidence to support a preexisting behavioral, personality, or sexual disorder, but no prospective studies have been undertaken.

Pain Perception Factors. More recent theories of the perception of chronic pain suggest that it is characterized by physiologic, emotional, and behavioral responses that are different from those of acute pain. Although both acute and chronic pain consist of a stimulus and a psychic response, for acute pain these may be adaptive and appropriate, while for chronic pain this may not be the case. In fact, the response to chronic pain may be greatly affected by learning. The patient's reaction to pain and the reaction of significant others to the patient and her pain may be so reinforcing that the behavior may persist even after the painful stimulus has resolved. Figure 38–1 illustrates the possible levels of agreement between sensory input, the pain sensation or perception, the patient's suffering, and the patient's pain behavior. In acute pain, the pain perception, suffering, and behavior are usually commensurate with the degree of sensory input. In chronic pain, the suffering and behavioral responses to a given sensory input may be quite exaggerated and may persist even after the stimulus has remitted.

Modulation of Sensation. It is now known that pain impulses are subjected to a large amount of modulation *en route* to the central nervous system. The first synapse in the dorsal horn is an important focus of enhancement, inhibition, or facilitation. Modulation of sensations may also occur within the spinothalamic system, the descending inhibitory neurosystems, and the frontal cortex. Within this context, anxiety and other psychologic states may be considered to be facilitators or

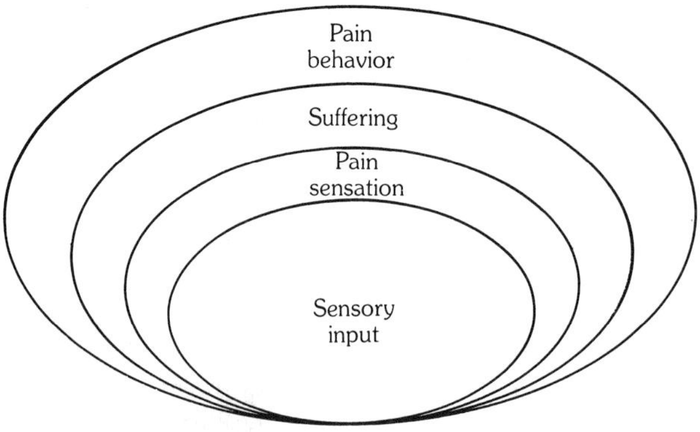

Figure 38–1 A model to illustrate the interplay between pain sensation and experience. (Reprinted with permission from Reading AE: Psychological Aspects of Pregnancy. New York, Longman Press, 1983, p 73.)

inhibitors for neurologic transmission. It is possible that many forms of chronic pelvic pain, in particular those without pathology, may result from modulation of afferent impulses in the dorsal horn, spinal cord, or cerebral cortex.

MANAGEMENT

In dealing with patients with chronic pelvic pain, a therapeutic, supportive, and sympathetic, but structured, physician-patient relationship should be established. The patient should be given regular follow-up appointments and should not be told to call only if the pain persists. This reinforces pain behavior as a means of procuring sympathy and medical attention.

A negative evaluation and laparoscopy, or the finding of pathology not amenable to therapy (for example, dense pelvic adhesions) does not mean that the patient should be discharged from care without therapy directed toward her symptoms. After initial reassurance that there is no serious underlying pathology, symptomatic therapy should be undertaken. The symptoms of pain should be approached with the seriousness and direction afforded to any other condition. The patient should not be placed in the position of "proving that she has pain," or she is apt to withdraw from the therapeutic situation and look for someone who will find out "what is wrong."

Team Management

The most productive strategy for the management of patients with chronic pelvic pain is referral to a multidisciplinary pain clinic. The personnel at such a facility should in-

clude a gynecologist, a psychologist who also has expertise in sexual and marital counseling, an anesthesiologist, and, occasionally, an acupuncturist. It is the role of the psychologist to provide marital and sexual counseling, assertiveness training, and adaptive coping strategies. This aspect of therapy is crucial, since many of these patients have become interpersonally, sexually, and sometimes even occupationally withdrawn. Relaxation, cognitive, and behavioral therapies are utilized to replace the pain behavior and its secondary gain with effective behavioral responses.

Medical and Surgical Management

The gynecologist continues to assess progress, coordinate care, and provide periodic gynecologic examinations. In the initial stages of therapy, a trial of ovulation suppression with the birth control pill may be helpful, especially in patients who have midcycle, premenstrual, or menstrual exacerbation of pain, or in those who have ovarian pathology, such as periovarian adhesions or recurrent functional cyst formation. Nonsteroidal anti-inflammatory analgesics, such as ibuprofen (Motrin) or naproxen (Naprosyn), are also useful.

Surgical procedures that have *not* proven to be effective for chronic pelvic pain without pathology include unilateral adnexectomy for unilateral pain or total abdominal hysterectomy, presacral neurectomy, or uterine suspension for generalized pelvic pain. Lysis of adhesions is usually also nonproductive, unless the site of adhesions visualized by the laparoscope specifically coincides with the localization of pain. It should be kept in mind that pelvic adhesions often recur following surgical lysis.

Anesthesia

Acupuncture, nerve blocks, and trigger-point injections of local anesthetics may provide prolonged pain relief. These therapeutic methods have only recently been directed toward chronic pelvic pain. Acupuncture has been used successfully for dysmenorrhea, and trigger-point injections of local anesthetics have been used successfully for pelvic pain. For pelvic pain, trigger points are either on the lower abdominal wall or in the vaginal and vulvar area. When these areas are subject to pressure, they give rise to pain, both in the area depressed as well as at the site of possible noxious stimulation. Anesthesia of trigger points may abolish pain by lowering the impulses from the area of referred pain, thereby diminishing the afferent impulses reaching the dorsal horn to a level below the threshold for pain transmission.

SUGGESTED READING

Bonica JJ: Neurophysiologic and pathologic aspects of acute and chronic pain. Arch Surg 112:750, 1977.

Elton D, Stanley G, Burrows G: Psychological Control of Pain. New York, Grune and Stratton, 1983.

Fordyce W: Treating chronic pain by contingency management. In Bonica JJ (ed): Advances in Neurology. Vol 4. New York, Raven Press, 1977, p 585.

Renaer M: Chronic Pelvic Pain in Women. New York, Springer-Verlag, 1981.

Slocumb JC: Neurological factors in chronic pelvic pain: Trigger points and the abdominal pelvic pain syndrome. Am J Obstet Gynecol 149:536, 1984.

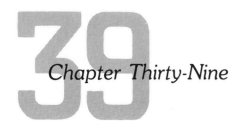

Chapter Thirty-Nine

BREAST DISEASE: A GYNECOLOGIC PERSPECTIVE

NEVILLE F. HACKER

Because gynecologists are often regarded as the primary care physicians for most women, they are frequently the ones to first diagnose breast disease. Therefore, even though the treatment falls under the domain of the surgeon, it is important that gynecologists be expert in breast examination, diligent about screening asymptomatic women for breast cancer, familiar with common benign and malignant disorders of the breast, and conversant with the various therapeutic options.

SCREENING OF THE BREAST IN ASYMPTOMATIC WOMEN

Self-Examination

Self-examination of the breast should be performed monthly by all women after the age of 20. Even though it is a simple and good screening technique for breast disease and is inexpensive, painless, harmless, and convenient, only about two thirds of women practice it at least once a year, and only one third practice it monthly as recommended. Of women performing the technique, only about half perform it correctly. When taught by physicians or nurses, however, more women practice regular breast self examination, and a greater proportion use the correct technique. Since it has been demonstrated that women who regularly practice the technique can discover breast disease at a signif-

icantly earlier stage, it behooves all gynecologists to promote self-examination among their patients.

Breast Self-Examination Technique. The patient should be taught to perform the examination after each menstrual period. She should commence the technique in the upright position, carefully inspecting the breasts initially with her arms by her sides and then raised above her head. She should palpate the supraclavicular and axillary regions for the presence of nodes. The patient should then lie down and systematically palpate each quadrant of the breast against the chest wall, using the flat of the fingers. Finally, she should palpate the areolar areas and then compress the nipples for evidence of secretion.

Breast Examination by Physician

A complete breast examination should be performed by a physician at least annually. The breasts are first inspected with the patient in an upright position. The contour and symmetry are observed, and any skin changes or nipple retraction are noted. Skin retraction because of tethering to an underlying malignancy may be highlighted by having the patient extend her arms over her head.

Palpation of the breast, areola, and nipple is performed with the flat of the hand. If any mass is palpated, its fixation to deep tissues should be determined by asking the patient to place her hands over her hips and contract her pectoral muscles. Each axilla is then carefully examined while the patient's arm is supported. The supraclavicular fossae are also palpated for lymphadenopathy. Following palpation in the upright position, the examination is repeated in the supine position.

Mammography

Radiologic examination of the breast is an important component of the screening process carried out in asymptomatic women and should be performed in conjunction with a thorough physical examination. Densities and fine calcifications constitute suspicious findings, and clinically inapparent malignancies of less than 1 cm in diameter may be detected.

Studies of individuals who survived the atomic bomb, received frequent fluoroscopy for tuberculosis, or underwent breast irradiation for benign disease have indicated that radiation can induce breast cancer. In recent years, there has been a marked improvement in the quality of mammography, with a concomitant decrease in the radiation dose administered to the breasts. Mammograms of high quality can be made with about 0.3 rad or less of radiation, so there is little, if any, risk of this technique causing breast cancer.

In the Breast Cancer Detection Demonstration Project carried out by the American Cancer Society and the National Cancer Institute, 89 percent of 3557 cancers were correctly identified by mammography, 41.6 percent of which were not clinically detectable. The optimal frequency for screening asymptomatic women has not been determined, but the current guidelines of the American Cancer Society are shown in Table 39–1.

Two techniques, film-screen mammography (which produces a regular x-ray film) and xeroradiography (which produces a blue image on paper), are currently available and are equally effective. Xeroradiography is especially good for finding the microcalcifications frequently associated with breast cancer.

Other Imaging Techniques

In addition to x-rays, breast images may also be recorded using heat (thermography), sound (ultrasonography), light (diaphanography), and magnetism (nuclear magnetic resonance). The nonionizing properties of these modalities make them attractive, but there are no reported controlled studies that compare them favorably with the efficacy of x-ray mammography for widespread screening. Ultrasound can differentiate cystic from solid masses and may demonstrate solid tissue that is potentially malignant within or adjacent to a cyst. It is also useful for imaging palpable focal masses in women under 30 years of age, reducing the need for x-ray studies in this population. Further research is needed to define the role that nuclear magnetic resonance may ultimately play in the evaluation of breast disease.

DIAGNOSIS OF BREAST LESIONS

Physiologic nodularity and cyclic tenderness due to the changing hormonal milieu must be distinguished from benign or malignant pathologic changes. Definitive diagnosis of breast neoplasms has traditionally been made by *open breast biopsy,* although recently there has been a revival of interest in *fine-needle* (22-gauge) *aspiration cytology.*

Fine-Needle Biopsy

Fine-needle aspiration biopsy of the palpably suspicious lump in the breast can be performed in the outpatient clinic without anesthesia. Smears are prepared from the aspirate to allow cytologic evaluation. In experienced hands, the test is both sensitive and specific. However, a negative result should never be accepted as definitive when there are clinical or mammographic indications that the lesion may be malignant. In the presence of a palpable lump, fine-needle aspiration cytology should make it possible

TABLE 39–1 AMERICAN CANCER
SOCIETY GUIDELINES
FOR MAMMOGRAPHIC
SCREENING OF
ASYMPTOMATIC WOMEN

1. Baseline mammogram for all women at age 35 to 40 years
2. Mammography at 1- to 2-year intervals from age 40 to 49 years
3. Annual mammograms for women 50 years or older

to diagnose breast cancer without formal excisional biopsy in over 90 percent of cases, allowing the subsequent management of the patient to be discussed prior to operation.

Open Breast Biopsy

Many factors should be considered prior to performing open biopsy, including the risk profile of the patient, the nature of the physical findings, the results of mammography, and the results of the aspiration cytology, if performed. Absolute indications for open breast biopsy are listed in Table 39–2.

Relative indications for breast biopsy include those women with a clinically benign mass but a positive family or personal history of breast cancer, a history of fibrocystic disease with atypia, or an equivocal finding on mammography or cytology. Patients suitable for observation would include those with a clinically benign mass or masses, no risk factors for breast cancer, and no evidence of malignancy on mammography.

Open breast biopsy may be performed as an outpatient procedure under local anesthesia or as an inpatient procedure under general anesthesia. Women with large breasts who have small deeply situated lesions are not good candidates for outpatient biopsies, nor are those who have a nonpalpable lesion detected by mammography.

COMMON BENIGN BREAST DISORDERS

Fibrocystic Disease

Fibrocystic disease is the most common breast disease and is clinically apparent in

TABLE 39–2 ABSOLUTE INDICATIONS FOR OPEN BREAST BIOPSY

1. Clinically suspicious (dominant) mass that persists through a menstrual cycle, regardless of mammographic findings. If fine needle aspiration cytology is unequivocally positive, most surgeons proceed directly to definitive treatment.
2. Cystic mass that does not completely collapse on aspiration (residual solid component) or contains bloody fluid.
3. Spontaneous serous or serosanguineous nipple discharge. In the absence of a mass, a "trigger point" should be demonstrable.
4. Suspicious mammographic abnormalities in the absence of a dominant nodule or discrete thickening.

about 50 percent of women. Histologically, it is characterized by hyperplastic changes that may involve any or all of the breast tissues (lobular epithelium, ductal epithelium, and connective tissue). When the hyperplastic changes are associated with cellular atypia, there is an increased risk for subsequent malignant transformation.

It is postulated that the changes found associated with fibrocystic disease are due to a relative or absolute decrease in production of progesterone or an increase in the amount of estrogen. Estrogen promotes the growth of mammary ducts and the periductal stroma, while progesterone is responsible for the development of lobular and alveolar structures. Prolactin, insulin, corticotropin, thyroxine, and growth hormone are also required for complete functional development. Patients with fibrocystic disease improve dramatically during pregnancy and lactation because of the large amount of progesterone produced by the corpus luteum and placenta and the increased production of estriol, which blocks the hyperplastic changes produced by estradiol and estrone.

Clinically, the lesions are usually multiple and bilateral and are characterized by pain and tenderness, particularly premenstrually. The disease usually occurs in the premenopausal years with a cessation of symptoms postmenopausally, unless exogenous estrogens are administered.

Treatment depends on the age of the patient, the severity of the symptoms, and the relative risk of the development of breast cancer. Women over 25 years of age should undergo baseline mammography to exclude carcinoma. Cysts may be aspirated to relieve pain (Fig. 39–1). If the fluid is clear and the lump disappears, only careful follow-up is indicated. Open biopsy is required if the fluid is bloody or if there is any residual mass following aspiration. An increasing number of subcutaneous mastectomies are being performed, but the only procedure offering complete protection against future breast cancer is bilateral total mastectomy. Although satisfactory breast reconstruction can be performed, no definitive surgery should be considered unless the patient is at high risk to develop breast cancer.

The medical management for fibrocystic disease has not been standardized. *Progesterone,* which can be administered orally as medroxyprogesterone acetate (Provera), 5 to

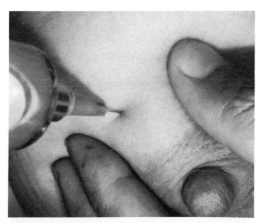

Figure 39–1 Aspiration of a breast cyst. The fluid is clear and there are no other suspicious features in this breast. If the cytology is negative and the lump disappears, only careful follow-up is indicated.

10 mg daily for five to ten days at the end of each month, can be given to patients in whom there is a relative or absolute increase in estrogen. *Tamoxifen,* an antiestrogen that works by bonding to receptor sites, may be taken orally, 10 mg twice daily, and is usually tolerated without side effects. *Bromocriptine* (Parlodel), a potent dopamine receptor agonist that inhibits prolactin secretion, may relieve the mastalgia when taken orally in a dosage of 2.5 mg twice daily. Symptoms related to premenstrual breast edema may be relieved with the administration of diuretics for seven to ten days and a low-salt diet. *Danazol* (Danocrine), an orally active pituitary gonadotropin inhibitory agent, has been effective in ameliorating symptoms in about 80 percent of patients when taken over a period of several months in a dosage of 100 to 400 mg daily. Further studies of the long-term effects of this drug are needed.

Fibroadenoma

Composed of both fibrous and glandular tissue, the fibroadenoma is the most common benign tumor found in the female breast. Clinically, these tumors are sharply circumscribed, freely mobile nodules, which may occur at any age but are more common before the age of 30. They usually are solitary and generally are removed when they reach 2 to 4 cm in diameter, although giant forms up to 15 cm in diameter occasionally occur. Pregnancy may stimulate their growth, and postmenopausally, regression and calcification usually eventuate. These tumors require sur-

gical excision for definitive diagnosis and cure.

Intraductal Papilloma

Papillary neoplastic growths may develop within the ducts of the breast, most commonly just prior to or during the menopause. They are rarely palpable, and usually present because of a bloody, serous, or turbid discharge from the nipple. If a trigger point from which palpation elicits a discharge is clearly identifiable, excisional biopsy of the involved duct should be performed whether or not a mass is palpable. Histologically, there is a spectrum of lesions ranging from those that are clearly benign to those that are anaplastic and give evidence of invasive tendencies. These growths should be differentiated from other causes of benign nipple discharge that do not require surgery. Certain drugs, such as phenothiazines, may cause bilateral nipple discharge as a result of elevated prolactin levels. Mammography and cytologic examination of the fluid are helpful in investigating nipple discharges.

Mammary Duct Ectasia

Mammary duct ectasia (comedomastitis, plasma cell mastitis) is characterized by dilatation of ducts, inspissation of breast secretion, and chronic intraductal and periductal inflammation in which plasma cells predominate. It usually occurs in the fifth decade and is associated with nipple discharge, pain, and tenderness. The ducts, which are dilated and filled with thick, cheesy material, may be palpable through the skin, or the lesion may give the clinical impression of a homogeneous tumor mass. Nipple retraction from the inflammatory scarring and enlarged axillary glands may make the findings indistinguishable from breast cancer. Once the diagnosis is confirmed by breast biopsy, no further treatment is necessary.

Galactocele

A galactocele is a cystic dilatation of a duct that is filled with thick, inspissated, milky fluid. It presents during or shortly after lactation and implies some cause for ductal obstruction, such as inflammation, fibrocystic disease, or neoplasia. Often multiple cysts are present. Secondary infection may produce areas of acute mastitis or abscess formation. Needle aspiration is usually curative. If the fluid is bloody or the mass does not disappear completely, excisional biopsy is required.

BREAST CANCER

Breast cancer is the most common female malignancy, accounting for 26 percent of malignancies in women. Approximately 115,900 new cases were diagnosed in the United States in 1984, and 37,600 women will die from the disease. There is a 1 in 12 chance (8.2 percent) that a woman will develop breast cancer during her lifetime.

Etiology

Little is known about the actual cause of breast cancer. Several risk factors have been identified (Table 39–3), but there is still a substantial number of women who develop the disease in spite of having no apparent increased susceptibility.

The incidence and mortality rates for breast cancer are approximately five times higher in North America and northern Europe than they are in many Asian and African countries. Migrants to the United States from Asia (principally Chinese and Japanese) do not experience a substantial increase in risk, but their first and second generation descendants have rates approaching those of the Caucasian population in the United States. Since age-adjusted mortality rates for breast cancer exhibit a high correlation with *per capita* fat consumption, the difference may be related to dietary customs.

TABLE 39–3   RISK FACTORS FOR
                  BREAST CANCER

TYPE	RISK FACTOR
Genetic	Positive family history
Hormonal	Nulliparity
	Late age at first pregnancy
	Early menarche
	Late menopause
	Age over 40 years
	Prolonged unopposed estrogen usage
Nutritional	High dietary fat intake
Morphologic	Cancer of ovary or endometrium
	Cancer of the other breast
	Fibrocystic disease
Irradiation	Breast irradiation

Unopposed estrogens increase the risk for breast cancer, as is the case for endometrial cancer. However, the breast appears to be less susceptible to the tumor-promoting effects of estrogens than the endometrium, and large amounts of estrogen are required to achieve an observable alteration in the risk of malignancy. Usage of combined oral contraceptives produces no significant alteration of risk. In contrast, oral contraceptive usage significantly decreases the risk for ovarian and endometrial cancer.

Tumor Types

The mammary epithelium gives rise to a wide variety of histologic tumor types. Approximately 90 percent of cases arise in the ducts, and the remainder originate in the lobules. About 80 percent of all breast cancers are nonspecific infiltrating duct carcinomas. These tumors usually induce a significant fibrotic response and are stony hard to clinical palpation. Less common types of ductal cancer include medullary, mucinous, tubular, and papillary. In many tumors, several patterns coexist.

Paget's disease of the breast occurs in about 3 percent of breast cancer patients. It represents a specialized form of intraductal carcinoma that arises in the main excretory ducts of the breasts and extends to involve the skin of the nipple and areola, producing an eczematoid appearance. The underlying carcinoma, although invariably present, can be palpated clinically in only about two thirds of patients.

Inflammatory breast cancer is characterized clinically by warmth and redness of the overlying skin and induration of the surrounding breast tissues. Biopsies of the erythematous areas reveal malignant cells in subdermal lymphatics, causing an obstructive lymphangitis. Inflammatory cells are rarely present. Most patients have signs of advanced cancer at the time of diagnosis, including palpable regional lymph nodes and distant metastases.

Tumor Spread

Breast cancer spreads by local infiltration, as well as by lymphatic or hematogenous routes. Locally, the tumor infiltrates directly into the breast parenchyma, eventually involving the overlying skin or the deep pectoral fascia.

Lymphatic spread is mainly to the axillary nodes, and 40 to 50 percent of patients have involvement of these nodes at the time of diagnosis. Axillary node involvement is directly related to the size of the primary tumor, but not to the location of the tumor within the breast. The second major area for lymph node metastases is the internal mammary node chain. These nodes are most likely to be involved when the primary lesion is medially or centrally situated, but even in these circumstances, axillary node involvement is more common. The supraclavicular nodes are involved only after axillary node involvement.

Hematogenous spread occurs mainly to the lungs and liver, but other common sites of involvement include bone, pleura, adrenals, ovaries, and brain.

Staging

Several systems of staging for cancer of the breast have been recommnended. The one recommended by the American Joint Committee on Cancer is shown in Table 39–4.

Clinical Features

Carcinoma of the breast is usually first discovered by the patient or physician as a breast lump. It is usually painless and may be freely mobile. A serous or bloody nipple discharge may be present. With progressive growth, the tumor may become fixed to the deep fascia. Extension to the skin may cause retraction and dimpling, while ductal involvement may cause nipple retraction. Blockage

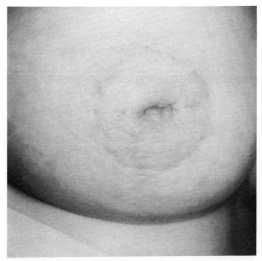

Figure 39–2 Carcinoma of the breast. Note the nipple retraction and the "peau d'orange." (Courtesy of Dr. Guy Juillard, Department of Radiation Oncology, UCLA School of Medicine.)

of skin lymphatics may cause lymphedema and thickening of the skin, a change referred to as "peau d'orange" (Fig. 39–2).

Treatment

With increasing awareness of the likelihood of early hematogenous spread and an increasing number of early lesions being diagnosed, the present trend is toward a more conservative surgical approach to breast cancer in conjunction with adjuvant radiation and, if necessary, chemotherapy.

Surgery. *Radical mastectomy,* as first described in 1894 by Halsted and Meyer, was, until recently, the standard operation for operable breast cancer. The procedure con-

TABLE 39–4   STAGING OF BREAST CANCER*

STAGE	DESCRIPTION
Stage Tis	*In situ* cancer (*in situ* lobular, pure intraductal, and Paget's disease of the nipple without palpable tumor).
Stage I	Tumor 2 cm or less in greatest diameter without evidence of regional or distant spread.
Stage II	Tumor more than 2 cm but not more than 5 cm in greatest diameter with or without movable axillary nodes, but without distant spread.
Stage IIIa	Tumor up to 5 cm in diameter, which may or may not be fixed, with homolateral clinically suspicious regional spread; OR a tumor more than 5 cm in diameter, which may or may not be fixed, with or without clinically suspicious homolateral regional spread. No evidence of distant metastases.
Stage IIIb	Tumor of any dimension with unequivocal homolateral metastatic supraclavicular or infraclavicular nodes or edema of the arm, but without distant metastases.
Stage IV	Tumor of any size with or without regional spread, but with evidence of distant metastases.

*As suggested by the American Joint Committee on Cancer.

sists of an *en bloc* dissection of the entire breast, together with the pectoralis major and minor muscles and the contents of the axilla. Presently, *modified radical mastectomy,* which leaves the pectoralis major intact, has supplanted radical mastectomy as the standard operation. It provides superior functional and cosmetic results, and survival data following both procedures appear to be comparable.

In 1971, a prospective study was initiated in the United States by the National Surgical Adjuvant Breast Project. Its purpose was to compare radical mastectomy with simple mastectomy plus local-regional radiation therapy and with simple mastectomy alone for patients with clinically negative axillary nodes. The latter group underwent subsequent removal of axillary nodes only if they became positive. Ten years later, the survival statistics for all three groups were not significantly different, despite the fact that in those women believed to have clinically negative nodes, 40 percent of the group undergoing radical mastectomy were found to have positive axillary nodes. Being a properly randomized trial, there is no reason to believe that patients in the other two groups did not have a similar incidence of positive nodes. The comparable survival statistics for the three groups indicate that by the time the patient reaches the physician, operable breast cancer is frequently already a systemic disease.

For small primary tumors (≤ 2 cm diameter), *segmental mastectomy* (also called partial mastectomy, quadrantectomy, or lumpectomy) has been advocated by some to improve the cosmetic outcome. This technique is combined with axillary node dissection and postoperative breast irradiation. With the short follow-up presently available, results appear to be comparable to the more radical approaches.

Breast reconstruction after mastectomy is an integral part of the treatment of breast cancer. It should be available to any woman who desires it, provided her general condition allows for operation and her expectation for reconstruction is realistic. The procedure may be performed at the time of the mastectomy or may be delayed for at least three months.

Radiation Therapy. Radiation therapy was initially used postoperatively for patients with positive axillary nodes. Although it significantly decreased local recurrence, it did not improve survival. Currently, there is an increasing use of radiation as initial therapy for relatively small primary tumors. The radiation is given following excision of the primary lesion and axillary node sampling, the latter being undertaken to determine the need for adjuvant chemotherapy or axillary radiation. External beam therapy is used, with 4500 to 5000 rad delivered to the entire breast and the anterior chest wall including the internal mammary chain. The ipsilateral supraclavicular and axillary nodes are treated if lymph node metastases are present. The primary tumor site may be boosted with external irradiation or with interstitial iridium-192. Functional and cosmetic results are improved, and survival does not appear to be compromised, although longer follow-up studies are necessary. Major complications, such as arm edema, arm weakness, radiation pericarditis, and soft tissue necrosis are very uncommon, occurring in about 2 percent of patients.

Chemotherapy. Although many drugs have some activity against breast cancer, the four most commonly used are cyclophosphamide (C), methotrexate (M), 5-fluorouracil (F) and Adriamycin (A). As single agents, each is capable of inducing responses in 25 to 45 percent of patients. Combinations of drugs have been shown to be more effective than single agents. Various combinations have been used, one of the most popular being CMF.

Because it is now clear that breast cancer is a systemic disease in many patients at the time of diagnosis, adjuvant systemic chemotherapy or hormonal therapy is required if cure rates are to improve. Available data suggest that premenopausal women, particularly those with one to three positive nodes, have improved survival (by about 20 per cent) and disease-free interval with the use of adjuvant combination chemotherapy. The advantage is less for patients with four or more positive nodes. Whether or not adjuvant chemotherapy merely prolongs survival without actually increasing the cure rate will be determined by further follow-up studies. At the present time, there is no evidence that adjuvant chemotherapy can benefit patients with negative nodes.

In patients with established metastasis, symptoms may be palliated with combination chemotherapy. Partial responses are obtained in 50 to 75 percent of patients, and complete clinical responses in 5 to 25 percent.

Endocrine Therapy. The response to hormonal therapy of any type is correlated with the incidence of estrogen receptors (ER). Since the synthesis of progesterone receptors is estrogen-dependent, the presence of these receptors may be a better predictor of the response to endocrine treatment than that of estrogen receptors alone. The response rate to hormonal treatment in ER-positive tumors is 50 to 60 percent, while it is less than 10 percent in ER-negative tumors. The response is usually partial and temporary. Progesterone receptors (PR) have been found in about 40 percent of ER-positive tumors. When both receptors are present, the response to hormonal therapy approaches 80 percent. Premenopausal patients have a lower incidence of ER-positive tumors (30 percent) than postmenopausal patients (60 percent).

Antiestrogen therapy with tamoxifen has replaced additive hormones (e.g., diethylstilbestrol), as well as adrenalectomy and hypophysectomy, as first-line hormonal treatment for postmenopausal women. Although less data are presently available, this treatment may replace oophorectomy in premenopausal women.

Prognosis

Although prognosis is related to the stage of the disease and the age of the patient (older patients have a better prognosis), the status of the axillary lymph nodes is the single most important prognosticator. More recently, evidence has indicated that estrogen-receptor status is also of independent prognostic significance, patients with ER-negative tumors having a poorer prognosis.

In the National Surgical Adjuvant Breast Project, patients with negative lymph nodes had an actuarial five-year survival of 83 percent, compared with 73 percent for patients with one to three positive nodes, 45 percent for those with four or more positive nodes, and 28 percent for those with more than 13 positive nodes.

Breast Cancer in Pregnancy

About 3 percent of breast cancers occur during pregnancy, complicating approxi-

mately 1 in every 3000 pregnancies. Diagnosis is usually delayed because small masses are more difficult to palpate in hypertrophied breasts. However, needle aspiration or open biopsy should be performed promptly on any suspicious mass.

The treatment is essentially that of the nonpregnant patient, except that lumpectomy and removal of axillary nodes followed by postoperative irradiation would not be appropriate with a continuing pregnancy. For patients with nodal metastases, abortion is advisable in the first trimester of pregnancy because of the teratogenic risks of the adjuvant chemotherapy. In the third trimester, chemotherapy should be delayed until after delivery, although surgery should occur promptly after diagnosis.

Stage-for-stage prognosis is not much worse than for nonpregnant patients. There is no indication to advise against subsequent pregnancy for those who are without evidence of recurrence.

SUGGESTED READING

American Cancer Society. National Conference on Breast Cancer—1983. Cancer (Supplement) 53:589, 1984.

Baket LH: Breast cancer detection demonstration project: Five year summary report. CA 32(4):194–225, 1982.

Black MM, Barclay THC, Cutler SJ, et al: Association of atypical characteristics of benign breast lesions with subsequent risk of breast cancer. Cancer 29:338, 1972.

Donegan WL: Cancer and pregnancy. CA 33:194, 1983.

Fisher B, Bauer M, Wickerham DL, et al: Relation of number of positive axillary nodes to the prognosis of patients with primary breast cancer. Cancer 52:1551, 1983.

Harris JR, Hellman S: Primary radiation therapy for early breast cancer. Cancer 52:2547, 1983.

Hellman S, Harris JR, Canellos GP, et al: Cancer of the breast. In DeVita VT Jr, Hellman S, Rosenberg SA (eds): Cancer, Principles and Practice of Oncology. Philadelphia, JB Lippincott Company, 1982.

Henderson IC: Chemotherapy of breast cancer. Cancer 51:2553, 1983.

Huguley CM Jr, Brown RL: The value of breast self-examination. Cancer 47:989, 1981.

Kinne DW: Surgical management of primary breast cancer. Cancer 51:2540, 1983.

Veronesi U, Saccozzi R, Del Vecchio M, et al: Comparing radical mastectomy with quadrantectomy, axillary dissection, and radiotherapy in patients with small cancers of the breast. N Engl J Med 305(1):6, 1981.

Winchester DP, Sener S, Immerman S, et al: A systematic approach to the evaluation and management of breast masses. Cancer 51:2535, 1983.

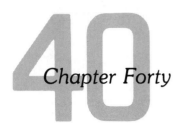

Chapter Forty

CONTRACEPTION AND STERILIZATION

IRVIN M. CUSHNER

In the broadest sense, the term "family planning" could be viewed as a means by which patients are assisted in either achieving or preventing pregnancy. However, family planning is generally defined more narrowly to include only those methods by which couples defer or prevent reproduction. These include temporary contraception, permanent contraception (sterilization), and induced abortion. This chapter is confined to a consideration of the temporary methods of contraception and to female sterilization.

OBJECTIVES OF FAMILY PLANNING

Family planning has broader connotations than the needs of the individual family. Those who are concerned with public health, particularly with maternal and child health, view family planning as an important factor in avoiding the aftermath of unwanted children, preventing excessive parity in high-risk women, and reducing perinatal mortality. Those concerned with stabilizing population growth find family planning a critically important component in these efforts, and they are especially concerned with its availability, accessibility, safety, and utilization. Finally, those concerned with improving the status of women view contraceptive effectiveness and safety as important issues in allowing women to regulate their fertility and to participate in societal activities that have previously been precluded by excessive and frequent pregnancies.

CONTRACEPTIVE COUNSELING, METHOD SELECTION, AND EFFECTIVENESS

There are six types of contraceptive methods: (1) hormonal, (2) intrauterine, (3) barrier, (4) chemical, (5) physiologic, and (6) sterilization. No method is 100 percent effective. Contraceptive counseling is particularly important following a delivery or abortion or at the onset of sexual activity, and the following factors should be considered.

Effectiveness

There are currently two methods being used to study and express the effectiveness of contraceptives. The *life table method* is the preferred and more contemporary method; it expresses contraceptive effectiveness as the percentage of women who are likely to become pregnant within the first year of initiating use of a particular method. The *Pearl rate*, an earlier method, expresses effectiveness as the number of conceptions that will occur among 100 fertile couples utilizing the method for one or more years (that is, the number of conceptions per 100 women-years). The effectiveness of any given method is influenced by a multiplicity of factors: biologic mechanism of action; consistent and correct use; years of use; single or multiple concurrent methods; and method switching. Therefore, published data vary widely and have been subjected to much debate. It does seem clear, however, that unintended pregnancies occur more frequently with some

TABLE 40–1 FAILURE RATES FOR VARIOUS CONTRACEPTIVE METHODS

METHOD	ESTIMATED PREGNANCY RATES (%) IN THE FIRST YEAR OF USE ASSUMING VARIATIONS IN CONSISTENCY OF USE
Vasectomy	<1
Tubal sterilization	<1
Oral contraceptives	2
IUDs	5
Condoms	10
Spermicides alone	15–20
Diaphragm and spermicide	15–20
Natural family planning	20–25
Coitus interruptus	20–25
Postcoital douche	40
No method	90

methods than others. For purposes of patient education, the data in Table 40–1 can be used for counseling in comparative effectiveness. It should be emphasized that consistent and correct use results in significantly fewer failures.

Safety

The most serious complications are related to hormonal, intrauterine, and surgical methods of contraception. Since these methods are also the most effective, they significantly reduce the likelihood of complications from abortion or childbirth.

Availability and Accessibility

Accessibility refers to the patient's personal ability to obtain the method—for example, the ability to pay for the supplies or services, and to secure them at an appropriate time. Some contraceptives, such as condoms and spermicidal agents, can be purchased without a prescription. Others, such as oral contraceptives and intrauterine devices, require the services of a physician.

Coital Dependence

For some couples, methods such as oral contraceptives or the intrauterine device are more acceptable because their use is most removed from the coital experience. For others, this factor is not as important.

Acceptability

Social, cultural, and psychologic factors also influence acceptability. Among these are religion and religiosity, feelings about equality in the sexual relationship and in the responsibilities for contraception, and the value ascribed to "naturalness." In the case of teenage patients, the need for parental consent can strongly influence the selection of a method.

HORMONAL CONTRACEPTIVES

Hormonal contraceptives are the most commonly used of all temporary methods. Among an estimated 36 million sexually active, fertile women in the United States, almost 10 million use hormonal contraceptives. These agents are among the most effective temporary methods of contraception, with a failure rate of only about 2 percent. The vast majority of failures are related to missed pills; ovulatory escape resulting in unintended pregnancies is rare in individuals who use them consistently and correctly.

Injectable, long-acting agents are available in a number of countries, but these have not been approved for contraception in the United States because of unresolved concerns about abnormal bleeding, oncogenesis, and infertility.

Two types of contraceptive tablets are currently in use: combination pills and progestin-only pills.

Combination Pills

There are currently 28 estrogen-progestin products approved for sale in the United States (Table 40–2). They contain one of two estrogens: ethinyl estradiol or mestranol. The

TABLE 40–2 ORAL CONTRACEPTIVES AVAILABLE IN THE UNITED STATES

TRADE NAME	PHARMACEUTICAL COMPANY	ESTROGEN	DOSE (μg)	PROGESTIN	DOSE (mg)
Optimal Doses					
Demulen 1/35	Searle	Ethinyl estradiol	35	Ethynodiol diacetate	1.0
Lo/Ovral	Wyeth	Ethinyl estradiol	30	Norgestrel	0.3
Nordette	Wyeth	Ethinyl estradiol	30	Levonorgestrel	0.15
Norinyl 1 + 35	Syntex	Ethinyl estradiol	35	Norethindrone	1.0
Ortho-Novum 1/35	Ortho	Ethinyl estradiol	35	Norethindrone	1.0
Ortho-Novum 10/11	Ortho	Ethinyl estradiol	35	Norethindrone (10 days)	0.5
		Ethinyl estradiol	35	Norethindrone (11 days)	1.0
Ortho-Novum 7/7/7	Ortho	Ethinyl estradiol	35	Norethindrone (week 1)	0.5
		Ethinyl estradiol	35	Norethindrone (week 2)	0.75
		Ethinyl estradiol	35	Norethindrone (week 3)	1.0
Tri-Norinyl	Syntex	Ethinyl estradiol	35	Norethindrone (7 days)	0.5
		Ethinyl estradiol	35	Norethindrone (9 days)	1.0
		Ethinyl estradiol	35	Norethindrone (5 days)	0.5
Other Combinations					
Brevicon	Syntex	Ethinyl estradiol	35	Norethindrone	0.5
Demulen	Searle	Ethinyl estradiol	50	Ethynodiol diacetate	1.0
Enovid-E	Searle	Mestranol	100	Norethynodrel	2.5
Enovid-5	Searle	Mestranol	75	Norethynodrel	5.0
Enovid-10	Searle	Mestranol	150	Norethynodrel	9.85
Loestrin 1/20	Parke-Davis	Ethinyl estradiol	20	Norethindrone acetate	1.0
Loestrin 1.5/30	Parke-Davis	Ethinyl estradiol	30	Norethindrone acetate	1.5
Modicon	Ortho	Ethinyl estradiol	35	Norethindrone	0.5
Norinyl 1 + 50	Syntex	Mestranol	50	Norethindrone	1.0
Norinyl 1 + 80	Syntex	Mestranol	80	Norethindrone	1.0
Norinyl-2	Syntex	Mestranol	100	Norethindrone	2.0
Norlestrin 1/50	Parke-Davis	Ethinyl estradiol	50	Norethindrone acetate	1.0
Norlestrin 2.5/50	Parke-Davis	Ethinyl estradiol	50	Norethindrone acetate	2.5
Ortho-Novum 1/50	Ortho	Mestranol	50	Norethindrone acetate	1.0
Ortho-Novum 1/80	Ortho	Mestranol	80	Norethindrone acetate	1.0
Ortho-Novum-2	Ortho	Mestranol	100	Norethindrone	2.0
Ovcon-35	Mead Johnson	Ethinyl estradiol	35	Norethindrone	0.4
Ovcon-50	Mead Johnson	Ethinyl estradiol	50	Norethindrone	1.0
Ovral	Wyeth	Ethinyl estradiol	50	Norgestrel	0.5
Ovulen	Searle	Mestranol	100	Ethynodiol diacetate	1.0
Progestin-only					
Micronor	Ortho			Norethindrone	0.35
Nor-Q.D.	Syntex			Norethindrone	0.35
Ovrette	Wyeth			d-1-Norgestrel	0.075

progestational agents currently used are all androgens in which the methyl group is absent at the 19 position. There is an increasing understanding of the relationship between dose, potency, and adverse outcomes. Some consensus has developed that certain agents in certain doses are associated with minimal risks of complications, breakthrough bleeding, and contraceptive failure. These "ideal" agents and appropriate doses are as follows:

Estrogen:
  Ethinyl estradiol: 30 to 35 μg
Progestins:
  Norethindrone: 1.0 mg
  Norethindrone acetate: 0.5 mg
  Ethynodiol diacetate: 1.0 mg
  Norgestrel: 0.3 mg
  Levonorgestrel: 0.15 mg

It should now be common practice, whenever possible, to advise and provide contraceptive pills containing these doses. Table 40–2 designates those products that contain such optimal formulations. Lower doses of estrogens and progestins may be associated with more breakthrough bleeding and higher failure rates. Higher doses are associated with more serious complications. Certain clinical situations will dictate therapeutic trials of other doses for the management of side effects. The wise family planning clinician will advise another method of contraception rather than prescribe or unduly continue a dose considered to be hazardous.

"*Multiphasic*" pills, which have recently become available, contain a constant dose of ethinyl estradiol, but the progestin (norethindrone) dose varies. In the *biphasic* form, the dose is increased at midcycle; in the *triphasic* form, different doses are administered in each of the three weeks. The presumed advantage is a reduction in the total amount of progestin administered in each cycle.

Mechanisms of Action

The contraceptive action of "the pill" is the result of several pathophysiologic changes induced by the synthetic hormones that include (1) suppression of the follicle-stimulating hormone-luteinizing hormone (FSH-LH) sequence from the anterior pituitary; (2) suppression of ovulation; (3) alteration of the cervical mucus, making it less penetrable by spermatozoa; and (4) with less scientific proof, induction of atrophic changes in the endometrium that are not conducive to implantation. Ovulation suppression is the mainstay of this method. However, since ovulatory escapes are known to occur, the remarkably low failure rates are thought to be the "net" result of all of these pathophysiologic changes.

Pharmacologic Considerations

The "potency," or biologic activity, of these agents influences the dose required to achieve the desired action and is thought to be related to some of the side effects and complications associated with oral contraceptives. While the clinical application of this concept is not universally accepted, it is clear that several different types of biologic effects result from these steroids: estrogenic, progestational, androgenic, and endometrial. The first three are measured through the use of animal models; the endometrial response is observed both by the absence of intermenstrual "breakthrough" bleeding and by the regular occurrence of withdrawal bleeding (a "period") following the three weeks of pill-taking. The relative potency of the various progestins is summarized in Table 40–3.

Other pharmacologic aspects of importance are the nonreproductive systemic changes induced by these steroids. Examples of estrogen-induced changes include decreased glucose tolerance, retention of sodium and fluid, and increased renin substrate. Examples of progestin-induced changes are smooth muscle relaxation, increased sebum production, increased facial and body hair, and cholestatic jaundice.

Side Effects

The most common reason for discontinuing the pill is the development of side effects related to the estrogen, progestin, or both. *Estrogenic side effects* include nausea, cyclic weight gain, edema, and headache. *Progestogenic side effects* include depression, acne, and hirsutism. Some clinicians manage these symptoms by revising the estrogen dose or by selecting a progestin whose dominant biologic activity is more appropriate. This is not based on clear scientific proof.

Complications

Women who use oral contraceptives are at higher risk than nonusers for a number of serious and potentially lethal complications.

Cardiovascular Complications. The most serious of these are venous thrombosis, pulmonary embolism, cerebrovascular accidents, and myocardial infarction. The association between these diseases and the use of contraceptive pills has been confirmed through case-control and cohort studies.

The risk of *venous thrombosis* and *pulmonary embolism* among users has been re-

TABLE 40–3 RELATIVE POTENCY OF PROGESTINS USED IN ORAL CONTRACEPTIVES FOR THE FOUR BIOLOGIC EFFECTS

ANDROGENIC	ESTROGENIC	ENDOMETRIAL AND PROGESTATIONAL
1. Norgestrel	1. Ethynodiol diacetate	1. Norgestrel
2. Norethindrone acetate	2. Norethindrone acetate	2. Ethynodiol diacetate
3. Norethindrone	3. Norethindrone	3. Norethindrone acetate
4. Ethynodiol diacetate	4. Norgestrel	4. Norethindrone

1 = most active
4 = least active

ported to be 2 to 11 times greater than among nonusers. This increased risk is thought to be related to estrogen-induced changes in blood clotting mechanisms; it is also dose-related and seems to be associated mostly with estrogen doses of 50 µg and higher. The risk for *stroke* is reported to be 2 to 9 times greater and is apparently related to the progestin component. The risk for *myocardial infarction* is 2 to 14 times greater; this increased risk is, for the most part, confined to women who are over 35 years of age and who smoke. It seems to be related to the elevation of low-density lipoprotein cholesterol and to the reduction of high-density lipoprotein cholesterol, both changes being induced by progestins.

Neoplasia. *Hepatic tumors,* both benign and malignant, have been reported in association with the use of contraceptive pills. They are rare, but the risk increases over time and seems related to pills containing mestranol. The most serious danger of these tumors is related to the risk of sudden, massive intraperitoneal hemorrhage. *Cervical dysplasia* has been reported to occur with increased frequency among women using estrogen-progestin tablets. This may be related to other risk factors related to dysplasia (e.g., early onset of sexual activity, multiple partners, and papilloma virus infections).

Gallbladder Disease. Gallbladder disease is associated with oral contraceptives, primarily in the first year of use, among women who are at high risk or who have pre-existent subclinical disease.

"Postpill" Amenorrhea. The vast majority of those who use oral contraceptives resume normal spontaneous menstruation within three months of discontinuation. However, resumption of normal ovulatory periods can be delayed in a small proportion (less than 3 percent) of these patients. A prepill history of irregular oligo-ovulatory cycles may increase this risk. Some women with postpill amenorrhea notice galactorrhea, and there is some concern about a possible causal relationship between combination pills and pituitary microadenomas. If menstruation has not resumed after six months, an endocrinologic investigation should be carried out.

Contraindications

While the relative risks of some serious complications are increased with these agents, the absolute risk for each of them is much lower than a number of risks taken (and apparently accepted) by most people in their daily activities. In addition, oral contraceptives decrease the risks associated with pregnancy and abortion. The absolute and relative contraindications to oral contraceptives are listed in Table 40–4.

Health Benefits of Oral Contraceptives

Use of oral contraceptives is associated with a significantly reduced risk of hospitalization for ovarian and endometrial cancer, benign breast disease, pelvic inflammatory disease, benign ovarian cysts, and ectopic pregnancy. In addition, there is evidence of a protective effect in relation to rheumatoid arthritis and iron-deficiency anemia.

Progestin-Only Contraceptives

Unlike the combination pills, progestin-only contraceptives are taken daily and continuously, with no cycle. Their use is not as

TABLE 40–4 CONTRAINDICATIONS TO THE USE OF ORAL CONTRACEPTIVES

ABSOLUTE	RELATIVE CONTRAINDICATIONS TO ESTROGEN	OTHER RELATIVE CONTRAINDICATIONS
Venous thrombosis	Uterine fibroids	Anovulation/oligo-ovulation
Pulmonary embolism	Lactation	Depression
Coronary vascular disease	Diabetes mellitus	Severe headaches (especially vascular)
Cerebrovascular accident	Sickle cell disease	Acne
Current pregnancy	Hypertension	Severe varicose veins
Malignant tumor: breast, endometrium, ovary	Age 30+ and cigarette smoking	
Hepatic tumor	Age 40+ and high risk for vascular disease	
Abnormal liver function		

widespread as that of the combination pills because they are associated with a higher risk of failure and with erratic, unpredictable episodes of endometrial bleeding. However, there are some women for whom estrogen is contraindicated but who desire a hormonal contraceptive. In such instances, especially during lactation, the progestin-only pills can be offered (Table 40–2).

Drug Interactions

Reduced efficacy of oral contraceptives may occur when they are taken concurrently with certain other drugs. With rifampin, the mechanism is apparently a significant reduction in the serum levels of the progestin. A similar interaction has been observed with antiepileptic regimens containing phenobarbital and an anticonvulsant; such women will need 50 μg or more of ethinyl estradiol, or they should use another contraceptive method.

INTRAUTERINE DEVICES

Intrauterine contraception is accomplished by the insertion of a plastic device into the endometrial cavity that can remain in place for several years. A filament (or "string") is attached to the lower end. This string protrudes from the cervix into the vagina to confirm the presence of the intrauterine device (IUD) in the uterus and to facilitate its removal.

There are four IUDs in current use (Fig. 40–1):

1. *Lippes Loop:* An unmedicated, double S-shaped device, available in four progressively larger sizes, A to D. The smallest (size A) is recommended for nulliparous women and the largest for multiparous women.

2. *Copper-7:* A medicated device, shaped like the number 7, containing on its vertical arm 89 mg of copper wire. The copper is released continuously within the uterine cavity for three to four years.

3. *Tatum-T (Copper-T):* A medicated, T-shaped device containing 120 mg of copper wire on the vertical arm. The copper is released continuously into the uterine cavity for three to four years.

4. *Progestasert:* A medicated, T-shaped device, the vertical arm of which is tubular and contains 38 mg of progesterone in silicon

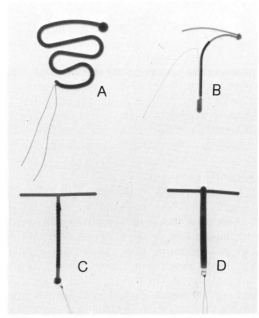

Figure 40–1 Intrauterine devices: *A,* Lippes loop; *B,* Copper-7; *C,* Tatum-T; *D,* Progestasert.

fluid. The progesterone is released into the uterine cavity at a daily rate of 65 μg for one year.

Mechanisms of Action

The precise mechanisms by which IUDs prevent pregnancy are not entirely clear. Animal studies indicate that the insertion of an unmedicated IUD is followed by a marked *inflammatory response,* resulting in inhibition of implantation. Other mechanisms suggested include *increased tubal motility* causing nonimplantation of the immature zygote; *phagocytic destruction* of spermatozoa and blastocytes; *inhibition of sperm transport;* and *interference with implantation* by increased immunoglobulins IgM and IgG. IUDs cause release of prostaglandins by the uterus, which can induce the leukocytic and other responses noted in both animals and humans. The suggested actions of copper include depression and destruction of spermatozoa, interference with glycogen metabolism and cellular DNA activity, reduced estrogen uptake by the endometrium, and induction of embryonic absorption. The presumed action of the progesterone-bearing IUD is that it produces endometrial changes that minimize the chances of implantation.

Effectiveness

In the first year of use, the failure rate for the IUD is about 5 percent. Some of these failures are related to unnoticed expulsion; others occur with the IUD still in place. The estimated lowest failure rate that can be expected is 1.5 percent. In women who do become pregnant, there is about a tenfold increase in the risk of ectopic pregnancy when compared with women without IUDs.

Side Effects and Complications

Abnormal Bleeding. Menorrhagia and metrorrhagia may occur. The etiology of the excessive bleeding is not clear, but may be due to endometrial abrasion, prostaglandin-induced vasodilation and platelet aggregation, or fibrinolysis caused by a plasminogen-plasmin reaction. Prostaglandin synthetase inhibitors have been used to control the bleeding with good results. However, if excessive bleeding persists or secondary anemia results, the device should be removed.

Pain. In some women, the IUD causes severe dysmenorrhea. Others relate the onset of chronic pelvic pain to the insertion of an IUD. The pain may be relieved by analgesics or prostaglandin synthetase inhibitors, but if it continues, the IUD should be removed. A smaller device may be tried if appropriate. The possibility of the pain representing subclinical pelvic inflammatory disease should be considered.

Expulsion. Expulsion of the IUD in the first year occurs in over 5 percent of women. After a first expulsion, the risk of subsequent expulsion is higher. Younger age and lower parity increase the risk of expulsion. Symptoms and findings that suggest expulsion include lengthening of the IUD string, palpation of the lower end of the device, and sudden onset of uterine pain or excessive bleeding. Partially expelled IUDs should be removed.

Pregnancy. A delayed period should be reported early and evaluated promptly. Two potentially serious complications must be considered: *septic abortion* with the IUD in place and *ectopic pregnancy*. Women who conceive with an IUD in place have a significantly increased risk of *spontaneous abortion*—about 25 percent if the IUD is removed and about 50 percent if it is not. In addition, the risk of a septic abortion with possible death is increased by the presence of an IUD. Therefore, if pregnancy is diagnosed, the IUD should be promptly removed, if feasible. If it cannot be found, perforation must be ruled out by ultrasonography.

Uterine Perforation and Myometrial Embedding. Insertion of an IUD can result in perforation of the cervical canal or uterine wall, with or without partial protrusion through the uterine serosa. The incidence is about 40 per 100,000 IUD users. The risk is increased with an inexperienced clinician, uterine malposition, or uterine softening in the postabortal or puerperal period. Perforation or embedding should be suspected when the string is not visible in the cervix/vagina, when the patient is found to have an intrauterine pregnancy, or when a difficult insertion is followed by severe pain and/or bleeding. Localization of a "lost" IUD can be achieved with the hysteroscope, pelvic ultrasound, hysterosalpingogram, or abdominal x-ray with a marker in the uterine cavity. The peritoneal IUD should be removed by laparoscopy, if possible. Alternative approaches are colpotomy or laparotomy. Embedded IUDs can usually be removed by grasping the device with a long alligator-type forceps, which is inserted through the cervix. General anesthesia and cervical dilatation facilitate this procedure and are frequently necessary.

Pelvic Inflammatory Disease. Women using IUDs are at higher risk for pelvic inflammatory disease (PID), such as salpingitis, salpingo-oophoritis, and tubo-ovarian abscess. These infections may be unilateral. The risk is much greater among women who are under 25 years of age and have more than one sexual partner. Infection is most common within a few months after insertion. When PID is found, the device should be removed, and the infection should be treated promptly and aggressively.

Contraindications

The contraindications to IUDs are listed in Table 40–5. Many clinicians now view a desire for future pregnancy as a contraindication to the IUD.

IUD Follow-up and Removal

The patient should be advised to return for evaluation if she cannot feel the string or if

TABLE 40–5 CONTRAINDICATIONS TO THE USE OF AN IUD

Proven or suspected pregnancy
Pelvic infection: current, recent, recurrent, high risk
Menorrhagia/dysmenorrhea
Undiagnosed abnormal bleeding
Abnormal Pap smear
Premalignant/malignant lesion, cervix/endometrium
Uterine fibroids, enlarged cavity
Valvular heart disease
Previous ectopic pregnancy

it has lengthened, if she or her partner experience dyspareunia, or if she develops symptoms suggestive of any of the contraindications to IUD use. If a medicated IUD is used, she must be informed of the need to replace it every three to four years in order to maintain effective contraception.

BARRIER AND CHEMICAL CONTRACEPTIVES

These methods have as their common denominator the intended prevention of viable spermatozoa from gaining access to the endometrial cavity and fallopian tubes. Those currently used are modern versions of some of the oldest principles and historic methods of human contraception. They include condoms, diaphragms, cervical caps, and spermicides in various modalities. In contrast to diaphragms and cervical caps, condoms and spermicides can be employed without any consultation with a physician.

Barrier methods vary in their degree of coital dependence, but generally a motivational factor is involved in their correct use. Thus, the cervical cap and vaginal diaphragm can be used in anticipation of sexual intercourse; spermicides and condoms are utilized during the precoital-coital sequence. Because of their coital dependence, these methods are in a medium range of effectiveness. They are less effective than hormonal and intrauterine methods but more effective than the natural family planning/fertility awareness methods. Except for the risk of unintended pregnancy, there are no serious clinical complications associated with their use.

Condoms

Condoms are sheaths applied over the erect penis prior to ejaculation. Penile sheaths were first suggested in 1564 for the prevention of syphilis, and they were used for contraception in England in the 18th century. Made primarily of rubber or other materials, condoms are sufficiently thin and yet resistant to tearing. Many are packaged with lubricant materials. Recently, some have become available that are prepared with spermicidal agents added to their surface.

If condoms are used correctly with each coital experience, the effectiveness is 98 percent; among couples reporting inconsistent use, the effectiveness is about 90 percent. It is important that there be a "well" at the end of the sheath for collection of the ejaculate and that inadvertent escape of semen be avoided when the penis is withdrawn from the vagina. Except for rather rare cases of penile dermatitis due to hypersensitivity reactions to the rubber or lubricant, there are no associated risks. Some men report erectile dysfunction with their use.

Potential benefits of condoms include their wide availability in pharmacies, markets, and vending machines and the possibility of preventing sexually-transmitted diseases. For those men and couples who place a high value on male responsibility for contraception, condoms are especially well suited.

Spermicidal Agents

Over the centuries, countless chemicals have been used to immobilize and/or destroy spermatozoa. Today, the most widely used spermicidal contraceptives contain one of two agents:

1. nonylphenoxypolyethoxyethanol (nonoxynol 9)
2. *p*-diisobutylphenoxypolyethoxyethanol (octoxynol 9)

These are surface-acting agents that disrupt the cell membrane. They are available in the form of suppositories, creams, foams, and gels and are placed in the vagina about 1 to 30 minutes prior to intercourse. To prevent failures, women should be advised not to use a vaginal douche for about eight hours following coitus. With correct and consistent use, these agents are reported to have an effectiveness rate of 95 percent; with inconsistent use, the effectiveness is 80 percent.

The *contraceptive sponge* is a very recent addition to the spermicidal agents. In premarketing clinical trials, its effectiveness is purported to be about 91 percent. It can be left in the vagina and utilized for 24 hours; however, to avoid the risk of toxic shock syndrome, it should not be left in place for any longer.

Like condoms, these agents are widely available without prescription and are also thought to prevent several sexually transmitted diseases. There is a risk for some women of vaginal and vulvar discomfort, probably due to a hypersensitivity reaction; otherwise, there are no serious complications associated with their use.

Postcoital Douche

A postcoital douche with a weak solution of vinegar or some other presumed spermicidal agent is sometimes used. With a failure rate of 40 percent, it cannot be recommended. However, compared with the risk of pregnancy with no contraceptive method, it offers some degree of protection.

Vaginal Diaphragms

Currently used diaphragms are available with rims measuring 60 to 100 mm in diameter, each size progressively larger by 5 mm. In fitting a woman for diaphragm use, the largest size that can be easily inserted and removed and that is comfortable when correctly placed should be chosen. Most women use sizes 65, 70, 75, or 80. Women should be advised to place a spermicidal agent on both sides of the diaphragm, to insert it prior to intercourse, and to leave it in place for 6 to 8 hours postcoitally. If further intercourse occurs prior to the time of removal, additional spermicide should be added without removing the diaphragm.

When used appropriately with each coital act, the effectiveness rate is 98 percent; with inconsistent use, it is about 80 percent. Postcoital bladder symptoms, including infections, may occur more frequently with this method than with others. Vaginal colonization with *Staphylococcus aureus* has been noted with prolonged retention of the diaphragm. This raises concern about a vulnerability to toxic shock syndrome, which should be preventable by timely removal. Some women cannot use this method because of hypersensitivity to the rubber or spermicide; others have anatomic variations in the vagina that preclude its use (e.g., vaginal relaxation with cystourethrorectocele).

Cervical Caps

At the time of this writing, cervical caps can be obtained in the United States only in certain programs under clinical research protocols approved by the United States Food and Drug Administration. Made of soft rubber, they are fitted over the cervix and held to its circumference by suction and by the flexible rim. Combined with a spermicide, the cap acts as a barrier and chemical contraceptive. For some women, the technique of placement is learned easily, while for others, it is more difficult than diaphragm insertion. Early reports suggest failure rates of about 8 percent. However, with continuation rates of only 30 to 50 percent, it is too early to determine the future role and usefulness of cervical caps.

Combined Use of Vaginal Contraceptives

The effectiveness of vaginal methods is maximized by (1) using them with every act of intercourse and (2) combining mechanical barriers with spermicidal chemicals. For example, the consistent (and concurrent) use of condoms and spermicidal foams is reported to have effectiveness rates that approach those of hormonal contraception. For strongly motivated couples who wish to avoid or defer the use of oral contraceptives or IUDs, this combined approach can be considered.

PHYSIOLOGIC CONTRACEPTION

Physiologic contraception utilizes neither chemical nor mechanical barriers. The methods are natural family planning, fertility awareness, and coitus interruptus.

Natural Family Planning and Fertility Awareness Methods

Mechanisms of Action. During the menstrual cycle, certain physiologic events become manifest, including the *"mittelschmerz"* of ovulation, the thermogenic effect of progesterone, and the cervical mucus changes characteristic of either estrogen or progesterone. These effects, especially in women with regular menstrual cycles, allow for reasonably accurate estimates of those cycle days during which ovulation is most likely to occur. Many couples are able to avoid conception either by cyclic abstinence, by noncoital sexual activity, or by using artificial contraceptive methods during the fertile phase.

Two terms are used to designate this system of contraception. *Natural family planning* is generally meant to indicate cyclic abstinence; its effectiveness is 75 to 80 percent. *Fertility awareness* refers to the use of this system to supplement other methods, such as diaphragms, condoms, and spermicides; data on failure rates are not yet available. Some authors use these terms interchangeably.

Types of Methods. In providing this method, the clinician is engaged primarily in patient education about the physiology of menstruation and conception. Four systems are generally used, and each should be described with particular attention to its effectiveness.

The *calendar method* is based on the usual variations in length of menstrual cycles (in days). The beginning and end of each cycle are recorded over several months. Eighteen days are subtracted from the shortest cycle and 11 days from the longest to determine the phase of the cycle during which ovulation could occur. Thus, a woman whose shortest cycle is 26 days and whose longest is 32 days would consider days 8 through 21 as her fertile phase.

The *basal body temperature (BBT) method* utilizes the progesterone-induced thermogenic response to ascertain that ovulation has already occurred. Women are instructed to take and record their temperature each morning, prior to any physical activity. The postovulatory phase is identified by a rise of about 0.5° F to 1° F, which is maintained for several days. If couples avoid intercourse from the onset of the cycle until after ovulation has been documented, effectiveness is reported to be higher than if the couples also engage in intercourse before ovulation.

With the *mucous method*, women first learn to differentiate between the scant, thick, discolored mucus of the pre- and postovulatory phases and the copious, clear, "stretchable" mucus that appears just prior to and during ovulation. The "safe period" is assumed to commence 72 hours after the last day of ovulatory mucus. As with the BBT method, maximal effectiveness will be attained if intercourse is avoided prior to ovulation. This method is somewhat less effective than the BBT method because observation of mucus is less objective than temperature recording for documenting ovulation.

The *symptothermal method* utilizes both the BBT and mucous methods. It apparently enhances the effectiveness of the natural family planning approach.

Benefits and Risks. The benefits of natural family planning include clinical safety, low cost, and almost singular acceptability among religious groups that do not condone artificial contraception. Its acceptability is also high among women who prefer "naturalness." It also offers a way to increase the effectiveness of barriers and spermicides by identifying the fertile phase when these methods should be used.

The risks of these techniques are primarily associated with the relatively low effectiveness, and, for some, with sexual dissatisfaction resulting from the lack of spontaneity and/or the need to abstain.

Coitus Interruptus (Withdrawal)

Withdrawal of the penis from the vagina just prior to ejaculation has been used for centuries. Failures with this method are related either to the failure to withdraw or to the pre-ejaculatory escape of sperm-laden fluid from the penile urethra. Many couples employ this method under certain circumstances. It should be noted that failure rates are lower than those for postcoital douche.

POSTCOITAL PREGNANCY PREVENTION

A number of situations require a postcoital effort at preventing conception or implantation. These include rape, broken condoms, expelled IUDs, and displaced diaphragms. Two approaches to this problem are in current use.

Postcoital Hormonal Agents

The effectiveness of the oral contraceptive, Ovral, is about 99 percent when two tablets are taken within 72 hours of intercourse and then repeated in 12 hours. If withdrawal bleeding does not occur within five days, pregnancy should be suspected. If unsuccessful in preventing implantation, these agents are associated with a risk of inducing teratogenic or oncogenic changes in the fetus. Women must be warned of this hazard. Some clinicians advise against the use of this technique unless the patient is planning pregnancy termination in the event of failure.

Postcoital IUD Insertion

The insertion of a copper-bearing IUD within five days of unprotected intercourse will usually protect against pregnancy by preventing implantation.

CONTRACEPTION DURING LACTATION

For lactating women, the effect of the contraceptive method on the quantity and quality of milk is a serious consideration. Sterilization, IUDs, and barrier/spermicides have no significant effect on lactation. When combination oral contraceptives are considered, there is concern about potential suppression of lactation, altered composition of the milk, and passage of steroids into the breast milk. Progestin-only pills, taken daily, offer effective contraception without adverse effects on the milk, the infant, or the mother.

STERILIZATION (ELECTIVE PERMANENT CONTRACEPTION)

In recent years, the number of sterilization procedures performed annually has increased dramatically, and the indications have changed to allow for voluntary sterilization on request. Postpartum tubal ligation by inpatient laparotomy has been all but supplanted by interval procedures performed primarily on an outpatient basis, such as laparoscopy or "mini-laparotomy." The use of vasectomy has also increased dramatically in recent years.

Patient Evaluation and Counseling

The intended permanence and the surgical nature of sterilization procedures make adequate evaluation and counseling critical. In 1979, the United States Department of Health and Human Services issued regulations requiring the provision of specific information, as well as a specified consent form to be used for all women whose sterilization services are to be subsidized with federal funds. At the time of this writing, these regulations mandate a 30-day interval between the signing of the consent and the performance of the procedure, with special waivers allowed in the event of premature delivery or emergency abdominal surgery. The patient must fully understand the side effects and complications of the surgery and anesthesia. Both men and women should also understand that sterility cannot be guaranteed.

Mechanisms of Action

Vasectomy results in azospermic semen. Tubal sterilization prevents tubal transportation of the mature ovum beyond the point of occlusion. These are purely mechanical interventions, with no evidence that hormonal changes play any role in the maintenance of the contraceptive state. Following tubal sterilization, levels of FSH, LH, and estrogen remain normal, but there is a slight decrease in levels of serum progesterone. Several studies of men following vasectomy reveal no significant change in spermatogenesis or in the hypothalamic-pituitary-gonadal system.

Types of Procedures

Although most tubal sterilizations are primarily performed in hospital operating rooms as outpatient procedures, a number of family planning programs are now providing these procedures in nonhospital settings. They can be done with either general, conduction, or local infiltration anesthesia. Methods of sterilization are described in Table 40–6.

Laparoscopic Procedures. Using the operating laparoscope, tubal sterilization can be performed through a single incision by *electrocauterization* or the application of a *Hulka clip* to each tube. A second small incision at the suprapubic area is required for the *Falope ring* applicator.

Laparotomy. "Mini-laparotomy" refers to sterilizations performed through a suprapubic incision about 1 to 1.5 inches in length. With a uterine elevator raising the fundus toward the incision, the tubes can be grasped and

TABLE 40–6 METHODS OF TUBAL STERILIZATION

SURGICAL APPROACH	TECHNIQUE	SURGICAL PROCEDURE
Laparotomy	Pomeroy	Ligature around a "knuckle" (or loop) of tube; excision distally
	Madlener	Crushing and ligature of loop of tube
	Irving	Double ligation, excision between; proximal end buried in myometrium; distal end buried in broad ligament
	Uchida	Tubal serosa stripped from muscular coat; tubal segment excised; proximal end ligated and buried in broad ligament
	Fimbriectomy	Ligation of distal end of tube and mesosalpinx; excision of fimbriated end
Laparoscopy	Electrocoagulation	Electrical "burn" of two adjacent segments with/without transection
	Falope ring	Loop of tube drawn into applicator tube; plastic ring placed around both limbs of loop
	Hulka clip	Plastic crushing clip placed across tube (not a loop); kept closed by steel spring
"Mini-laparotomy"	Pomeroy ligation Electrocauterization	
Posterior colpotomy	Falope ring Pomeroy ligation Hulka clip	
Hysteroscopy	Insertion of tubal plug Electrocoagulation Chemical scarification	Cannulation of internal tubal ostia via a transcervical approach
Blind cannulation of tubes via transcervical approach	Chemical scarification	

occluded by the *Pomeroy technique* (Fig. 40–2) or by any of the laparoscopic methods.

Any of the sterilization procedures described can be carried out through a "standard" lower abdominal laparotomy incision. However, such an approach is unnecessary, except when palpable pelvic pathology or other reasons make it necessary to adequately examine the pelvic and upper abdominal viscera.

Vaginal Procedures. An incision through the posterior vaginal fornix gains access to the cul-de-sac, allowing for tubal occlusion by the *Pomeroy technique* or by any of the endoscopic methods. Because of the incidence of postoperative infection and the relative ease of outpatient abdominal procedures, this route is not commonly employed.

Hysteroscopic Sterilization. This approach is still in the investigative stage, but is viewed as having the potential for ultimately becoming a method that, like vasectomy, could be performed in clinics or offices. In the hysteroscopic approach, the internal ostia of the tubes are identified and cannulized under direct vision. The tubal ostia are then occluded by either electrocoagulation, the insertion of tubal plugs, or chemical scarification. For the latter, two chemical agents,

quinacrine and methylcyanoacrylate (MCA), which seem to have minimal side effects, have been clinically tested.

Side Effects and Complications

Immediately following tubal sterilization, most women report mild to moderate discomfort because of incisional pain, tubal ischemia when clips and rings are used, or diaphragmatic irritation and shoulder pain from the pneumoperitoneum. The risk of death from tubal sterilization is about 4 per 100,000 procedures, and the usual causes include complications of general anesthesia, hemorrhage, and infection.

Potentially serious long-term complications include:

1. *Ectopic pregnancy.* This is estimated to occur in about 0.6 per 1000 sterilized women. In any previously sterilized woman who becomes pregnant, the possibility of a tubal pregnancy should be considered.

2. *Dysfunctional uterine bleeding.* This has been reported to be a sequel to tubal sterilization, but the association has never been definitely proven.

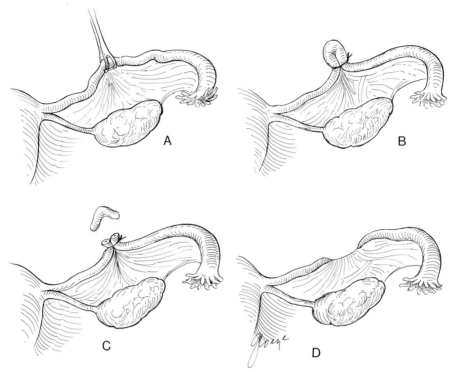

Figure 40–2 Pomeroy method of tubal ligation: *A,* The tube is picked up with Babcock forceps; *B,* the loop is ligated; *C,* the loop is excised; *D,* the fibrosed ends of the tube separate several months later.

3. *Depression and regret.* The literature does not include a clear differentiation between dissatisfaction with sterilization, regret, and desire for reversal. They are three separate sets of feelings, albeit possibly interrelated. The incidence of dissatisfaction seems to be well under 10 percent. Studies of women requesting reversal suggest that those younger than 30 years of age, with fewer than two children, and in unstable relationships at the time of sterilization, are at increased risk of desiring reversal.

Sterilization Reversal

The advent of microsurgical techniques and their application to tubal surgery have significantly increased the possibility of successful reanastomosis of the previously occluded tube. Compared with the success rates of 30 percent using conventional surgical methods, microsurgical techniques are associated with pregnancy rates of 60 to 70 percent. Sterilization techniques that do not result in the loss of large segments of the tube are successfully reversed more often; in addition, the clip and ring methods are more successfully reversed than electrocoagulation. With the advent of *in vitro* fertilization, sterilization reversal is no longer the only option.

SUGGESTED READING

Centers for Disease Control, United States Public Health Service. Oral contraceptive use and the risk of breast cancer in young women. MMWR 33:353, 1984.

Chaudhuri G: Intrauterine device: Possible role of prostaglandin. Lancet 1:480, 1971.

Hatcher RA, Guest F, Stewart F, et al: Contraceptive Technology 1984–1985. New York, Irvington Publishers, Inc, 1984.

Massey FJ, Bernstein GS, O'Fallon WM, et al: Vasectomy and health: Results from a large cohort study. JAMA 252:1023, 1984.

Millen A, Austin F, Bernstein GS: Analysis of 100 cases of missing IUD strings. Contraception 18:485, 1978.

Ory HW, Forrest JD, Lincoln R: Making Choices: Evaluating the Health Risks and Benefits of Birth Control Methods. Washington, DC, The Alan Guttmacher Institute, 1983.

Sciarra JJ, Zatuchni EI, Daly MJ: Gynecology and Obstetrics. Vol 6. Fertility Regulation, Psychosomatic Problems, and Human Sexuality. Philadelphia, Harper & Row, 1984.

Seiler JS: The evolution of tubal sterilization. Obstet Gynecol Surv 39:177, 1984.

Stock RJ: Evaluation of sequelae of tubal ligation. Fertil Steril 29:169, 1978.

Van Lith DAF, Keith LG, van Hall EV (eds): New Trends in Female Sterilization. Chicago, Year Book Medical Publishers, 1983.

Chapter Forty-One

HUMAN SEXUALITY

J. ROBERT BRAGONIER and ANTHONY E. READING

As many as 60 percent of patients seeking a gynecologic consultation have been estimated to have concerns about sexual activity. It is important, therefore, for the gynecologist to become knowledgeable and comfortable with human sexuality.

Early research into uterine activity during orgasm was reported in 1896. Alfred Kinsey in the 1940s and 1950s observed and described sexual activity, but he was hesitant to publish his findings; he apparently considered his epidemiologic studies of sexual behavior that he did publish to be controversial enough for the times. It was not until the pioneering work of Masters and Johnson, published in 1966, that research into the physiology of sex was legitimized. Yet replication of even these studies has been slow.

ANATOMY AND PHYSIOLOGY OF THE FEMALE SEXUAL RESPONSE

Sexual response is mediated through three related, but neurophysiologically discrete, phases: (1) desire (libido), (2) excitement (arousal), and (3) orgasm (climax). Because each of these phases is mediated via different neuronal circuits, sexual dysfunction may affect one or another of them without affecting the others.

Desire Phase

Sexual desire appears to be an appetite similar to hunger, controlled by a dopamine-sensitive excitatory center, in balance with a serotonin (5-hydroxytryptamine)-sensitive inhibitory center. In both males and females, testosterone appears to be the hormone responsible for initially "programming" these centers in prenatal life and for maintaining their threshold of response. Stimulation and ablation experiments in cats and other mammalian species have located these centers within the limbic system, with significant nuclei in the hypothalamic and preoptic regions. These centers, therefore, are part of the archaic organizational system of the brain that is responsible for survival, reproduction, motivation, and emotion.

Desire is modulated by connections between these centers and other parts of the brain. For example, the activity of these centers can be markedly affected by neuro-electric and hormonal interactions with pleasure and pain centers. Connections with memory storage banks enable experience and learning to affect the frequency, direction, intensity, and mode of expression of sexual desire. The net effect of these positive and negative influences modulates genital sexual response via impulses passing down the spinal cord to the spinal reflex centers that govern excitement and orgasm.

Excitement Phase

During the excitement phase, vascular engorgement occurs, mediated primarily by the parasympathetic nervous system. Genital changes include enlargement in the diameter and length of the clitoris; dilatation of perivaginal arterioles with seeping of vascular transudate across the vaginal membrane, re-

TABLE 41–1 NEUROANATOMY OF EXCITEMENT AND ORGASM

REFLEX	MEDIATION	AFFERENT (SENSORY) CONNECTIONS	SPINAL CORD CENTERS	EFFERENT (MOTOR) CONNECTIONS
Excitement	Parasympathetic	From clitoris via the dorsal nerve of clitoris to the pudendal nerve.	S2–S4	Preganglionic fibers travel via the pelvic nerve (nervus erigentes) to the vesical and uterovaginal plexuses.
		From anterior labia via ilioinguinal nerve and the perineal branch of the posterior femoral cutaneous nerve.	T11–L2	Postganglionic fibers travel to the erectile tissue.
Orgasm	Sympathetic	Same	T11–L2	Preganglionic fibers travel via the splanchnic nerve to the inferior mesenteric ganglion and ganglia in the hypogastric, vesical, and pelvic plexuses. Postganglionic fibers pass to genital smooth muscle.
			S3–S4	Pudendal nerve to striated muscle (ischiocavernosus and bulbocavernosus).

sulting in lubrication; and expansion and "tenting" of the upper half of the vagina. Bartholin's glands may secrete several drops of mucoid fluid during the late excitement phase. The neuronal connections for the genital changes of excitement and orgasm are shown in Table 41–1.

Estrogen is the hormone responsible for maintaining the vaginal mucosa and allowing transudation and lubrication to occur. Its deficiency (postsurgically or postmenopausally) is by far the most common cause of excitement phase dysfunction in women.

Extragenital changes during the excitement phase include an increase in heart rate and blood pressure; enhanced muscle tension throughout the body; an increase in breast size, nipple erection, and engorgement of the surrounding areolae; and a sex flush. The latter is an erythematous rash over the chest, neck, and face that occurs to a noticeable degree in 75 percent of women.

Orgasmic Phase

During the orgasmic phase, a series of reflex clonic contractions of the levator sling and related genital musculature occur, mediated primarily via the sympathetic nervous system.

Extragenital reactions during orgasm include contraction of muscle groups throughout the body, maximal intensity of the sex flush, and maximal elevations of heart rate, blood pressure, and respiratory rate.

Excitement and orgasm are reflexes. For the orgasmic reflex to be activated, the stimulus must be applied where the sensory nerve endings are located (primarily in the area of the clitoris), and the stimulation must be of sufficient intensity and duration to reach the threshold for the reflex. For many women, this involves more direct clitoral stimulation than can be achieved from male-superior, penile-vaginal thrusting alone. Many women

TABLE 41–2 CLASSIFICATION OF SEXUAL DYSFUNCTION*

CATEGORY	CHARACTERISTICS	ETIOLOGY
Primary	Sexual expectations have never been met	Usually psychogenic
Secondary	All phases functioned in the past, but one or more no longer do so	May be organic or pharmacologic
Situational	Response cycle functions under some circumstances, but not others	May be psychogenic or relationship-related

*Any of the dysfunctions may involve desire, excitement, or orgasm.

TABLE 41–3 PSYCHOLOGIC CAUSES OF SEXUAL DYSFUNCTION IN WOMEN

A. Intrapersonal
  1. Inadequate self-esteem
  2. Depression
  3. Anxiety
     a. Performance
     b. Irrational fears
     c. Unresolved conflicts
     d. Developmental trauma
  4. Diminished capacity for relationships
  5. Psychosis
B. Interpersonal
  1. Distrust
  2. Resentment
  3. Disillusionment
  4. Dissatisfaction
  5. Poor communication

have discovered that doing Kegel's exercises during sex or voluntarily tensing muscles in other parts of their body may lower the threshold for, or increase the intensity of, orgasm. Women generally experience an increased rate and intensity of organism with self-stimulation.

SEXUAL DYSFUNCTION

Classification

True sexual dysfunction is manifested by failure of one or more phases of the sexual response cycle: desire, excitement, and orgasm. It can be classified according to the earliest phase in which disruption is experienced. Disruption frequently begins with orgasmic disturbance, but if neglected, loss of excitement and, finally, loss of desire may follow.

Sexual dysfunction can also be subdivided into three different categories, depending on

TABLE 41–4 ORGANIC CAUSES OF SEXUAL DYSFUNCTION IN WOMEN

DISORDERS	EXAMPLE
Neurogenic	Central, spinal, peripheral
Vascular	Local and systemic
Endocrine/metabolic	Diabetes mellitus, thyroid, pituitary
Systemic medical	Hepatic, renal, pulmonary
Musculoskeletal	Arthritis
Local pelvic	Genital infections, endometriosis, genital neoplasms, atrophic vaginitis

whether it is *primary* (realistic sexual expectations have never been met under any circumstances), *secondary* (all phases have functioned in the past, but one or more no longer do so), or *situational* (the response cycle functions under some circumstances, but not others).

Etiology

The etiology and classification of sexual dysfunction are summarized in Table 41–2. Most sexual problems are psychologic (Table 41–3), but organic and pharmacologic causes must also be considered (Tables 41–4 and 41–5). Primary problems are predominantly psychogenic and tend to be of longer duration. Secondary problems are often associated with the onset of a disease process or the use of a pharmacologic agent. If such an association cannot be established, a deterioration in the patient's relationship or some other chronologically related change in the patient's life experience should be sought.

The two situational problems of major clinical significance are represented by women who achieve climaxes with petting, oral sex, or self-stimulation, but not with penile thrusting alone (over one-half of all women complaining of orgasmic problems); and men who have erections in the morning, during sleep, or with masturbation, but not when needed for insertion and intercourse. Problems that are situational are noteworthy because they are almost invariably psychogenic or relational and not organic or pharmacologic in origin.

TABLE 41–5 DRUGS THAT CAN DIMINISH SEXUAL FUNCTION IN WOMEN

TYPE OF AGENT	EXAMPLES
Hypnotics	Alcohol, barbiturates
Tranquilizers	Chlordiazepoxide, diazepam
Narcotics	Heroin, methadone
Antipsychotics	Phenothiazines, butyrophenones
Antidepressants	Tricyclics, monoamine oxidase inhibitors
Stimulants	Cocaine, amphetamines
Anorectics	Fenfluramine
Hallucinogens	THC, LSD, PCP, mescaline
Hormones	Progestins, oral contraceptives
Antihypertensives	Reserpine, propranolol, methyldopa
Anticholinergics	Propantheline bromide
Diuretics	Acetazolamide

Factors initiating a problem may be different from those maintaining it. For example, drugs may precipitate a problem, but if anxiety and fear of failure sustain the difficulty, discontinuation of the drug may not rectify it.

SEXUAL ASSESSMENT

Sexual concerns may present as chief complaints or may become apparent during the review of systems. The likelihood of a woman expressing sexual concerns is a direct function of her perception of the clinician's level of comfort in discussing the subject.

Sexual Problem History

The sexual system can be reviewed by asking, "Is your sexual relationship meeting your expectations?" or "Are you experiencing any sexual difficulties?" If no concerns are expressed, no further assessment is warranted.

Once a concern has surfaced, a more detailed sexual history should be obtained by asking appropriate questions in specific problem areas. Questions listed under the following subheadings may be helpful.

Nature of the Problem. What do you perceive as the problem? Does it affect orgasm, excitement, or desire? How long has it been going on? Have things ever been better? Was its onset gradual or sudden? Is the problem intermittent? Is it getting worse, better, or staying about the same? If you have had more than one partner, did the problem occur with each of them? Were there any precipitating events? What does your partner think about the problem? How do you explain its occurrence to yourself? What seems to make the problem better? What makes it worse? What have you previously done to evaluate or treat the problem? What has your partner done to help? Does the problem decrease when you are by yourself (with self-stimulation)?

Earlier Sexual Experience. What were things like when they were the best they have ever been for you? How often were you having intercourse then? Who suggested it? How often did you want to have intercourse? Did you have the right to refuse? Compare and contrast your answers to your current situation.

Sexual Expectations. What do you expect to happen in a sexual encounter? Describe a current, typical sexual encounter. How are your expectations and actual experiences different? Who initiates sex? How much time elapses between initial caressing and entry? How is this decided? Would you ever like foreplay to last longer? Have you ever tried to let your partner know this? How long is the time from insertion until your partner ejaculates? Is this a problem for either of you?

Status of the Relationship. Are you and your partner good friends? What interests do you share? What changes have been occurring in other areas of your relationship?

General Coping Mechanisms. How are you coping with the problem and with life in general? Do you feel creative, successful, and competent in what you do? Do you like yourself? Are you frequently depressed, anxious, or fearful?

General Medical History

The sexual problem history should be accompanied by a general medical history and a physical examination with emphasis on the gynecologic examination. These routine procedures plus standard laboratory evaluation are adequate to rule out nearly all organic causes of sexual dysfunction in women.

MANAGEMENT

General Considerations

The challenge for the gynecologist or other primary care clinician is to (1) characterize the nature of the concern, (2) provide permission, reassurance, or limited information, as necessary, (3) recognize and manage problems caused by organic or pharmacologic factors, and (4) assess the need for referral of those patients with dysfunctions requiring more in-depth psychotherapeutic intervention.

For many patients, reassurance, information, and the opportunity to ventilate concerns and obtain permission and understanding can be extremely helpful. There may be a misfit between expectations and experience or between the expectations of the two partners; counseling might suggest more realistic expectations, more fulfilling practices, or appropriately negotiated compromises.

More serious sexual problems may require behavioral psychotherapy; for some patients referral may be indicated. The approach is aimed at providing conditions conducive for sexual arousal by removing pejorative labels, extinguishing anxiety over performance, replacing avoidance behaviors, and facilitating communication about sexual issues.

Common Conditions

A detailed description of therapeutic techniques is beyond the scope of this chapter. Nonetheless, the principles of management for three common conditions are discussed.

Lack of Orgasm. Women who complain that they are not experiencing orgasm can be separated into four groups: (1) those who have erroneous expectations, (2) those who experience pressure from their partner, (3) those who have lost their orgasmic capacity, and (4) those lacking sufficient stimulation.

A large number of women experience orgasm only with manual or oral stimulation, and not with penile thrusting alone. If they are capable of achieving orgasm with a partner by any means, their problem is primarily one of erroneous expectations. If they are willing to increase direct clitoral stimulation before, during, and/or after penile penetration, they may achieve a wholly satisfactory sexual adaptation.

Some women may enjoy intercourse but be under considerable pressure from partners to experience more intense orgasms. They may be uncertain as to whether or not they are currently experiencing orgasms at all. Exploring their feelings during resolution (euphoria vs. frustration) may clarify this issue. Validation of a woman's current experience may relieve some of the pressure she is experiencing from her partner.

Women who have been orgasmic in the past but have lost that capacity should be carefully screened for organic or pharmacologic causes, and changes in their relationship(s) should be carefully explored.

Most women with primary anorgasm have usually had minimal or no effective stimulation from self or partner. These patients should be encouraged to learn how to achieve orgasm through self-stimulation and then to share this new information with their part-

ners. Increasing the intensity of stimulation should increase the intensity of response.

Vaginismus. With this condition, women experience severe pain on attempted penile penetration or are unable to allow any penetration at all. Examination reveals no organic pathology, but the pubococcygeal muscles are tight, and vaginal penetration by speculum or examining finger is painful and difficult, if not impossible.

Women with vaginismus may or may not remember episodes of sexual trauma, but the important issue is whether or not they are able and motivated to participate with their partners in a stepwise *desensitization* program. This involves the slow, gentle vaginal insertion of dilators of gradually increasing size, under the patient's own control. Once sufficient progress has been made, the partner's fingers and, ultimately, his penis may be substituted for the dilators. Alleviation of the problem is usually accomplished in three to six months. If anxiety precludes her participation, psychotherapeutic intervention may be required.

Secondary Lack of Desire. This complaint, once known as "frigidity," frequently surfaces in women under considerable psychologic stress. It is nearly always due to loss of trust, resentment, or disillusionment with the relationship, although fatigue and boredom may play a role. When interpersonal strife is prominent, referral for therapy is generally necessary. For treatment to be effective, it must be focused on the relationship. If the partner is unwilling to participate in a serious renegotiation of the rules upon which the relationship is based, desire is unlikely to return.

PROGNOSIS

The lack of controlled studies, standard definitions, uniform periods of follow-up, and standard criteria for improvement make more than a few general statements regarding prognosis impossible. As a group, orgasmic difficulties seem to respond to treatment most readily. For example, lack of orgasm in the female and premature ejaculation in the male can be resolved in 80 to 90 percent of cases. Excitement phase dysfunctions do not have such positive outcomes. Although problems in females can nearly always be resolved satisfactorily, erectile difficulties in males respond only 60 to 70 percent of the time. Lack of desire is the most resistant to treatment. Persons with little desire often have little internal motivation to seek more frequent sexual activity, or to seek help. Less than 50 percent of such patients show definite improvement. When the relationship is poor, behavioral approaches directed toward the sexual problem rarely are successful.

SUGGESTED READING

Annon JS: The Behavioral Treatment of Sexual Problems. Brief Therapy, Vol I; Intensive Therapy, Vol II. Honolulu, Enabling Systems, 1974 and 1975.

Barbach LG: For Yourself. Garden City, New York, Doubleday & Co, Inc, 1975.

Barnard M, Clancy B, Krantz, K: Human Sexuality for Health Professionals. Philadelphia, W B Saunders Co, 1978.

Kaplan HS: Disorders of Sexual Desire, and Other New Concepts and Techniques in Sex Therapy. New York, Simon & Schuster, 1979.

Kaplan HS: The Evaluation of Sexual Disorders: Psychological and Medical Aspects. New York, Brunner/Mazel, 1983.

Kaplan HS: The New Sex Therapy. New York, Brunner/Mazel, 1974.

Katchdourian HA, Lunde DT: Fundamentals of Human Sexuality. 2nd ed. New York, Holt, Rinehart and Winston, Inc, 1976.

Kolodny RC, Masters WH, Johnson V: Textbook of Sexual Medicine. Boston, Little, Brown and Co, 1979.

Lief HI (ed): Sexual Problems in Medical Practice. Monroe, Wisconsin, American Medical Association, 1981.

Munjack DJ, Oziel LJ: Sexual Medicine and Counseling in Office Practice. Boston, Little, Brown and Co, 1980.

SEXUAL ASSAULT

ANTHONY E. READING and J. ROBERT BRAGONIER

Rape is the fastest growing violent crime in the United States, with one woman in six likely to be raped in her lifetime. Such figures are undoubtedly underestimates, since many women fail to report their experience. In this chapter, the gynecologic management of cases of sexual assault is discussed.

The medical management of sexual assault cannot be discussed without recognizing the broader social and moral context. In the past, rape was considered to be a sexual experience, and a stigma was attached to the victim. Modern society is increasingly recognizing rape as a violent attack that may or may not stem from the perpetrator's sexual drive or arousal. Research has shown many rapists to be sexually incompetent in the rape setting. Whatever the male intent, rape is definitely not a sexual experience for the victim. During the assault, the victim's predominant feeling is a fear of death or mutilation.

PSYCHOLOGIC SEQUELAE OF SEXUAL ASSAULT

Sexual assault is associated with both immediate and long-term effects on all victims. These effects have been termed the *rape trauma syndrome.* Immediately after the experience, victims frequently appear outwardly calm, although preoccupied and inattentive. As they become more comfortable with the medical personnel, they commonly express shock, disbelief, fear, guilt, and shame. The long-term sequelae include changes in lifestyle, the occurrence of disturbing dreams and nightmares, and the persistence of phobic reactions. Fear persists as the predominant feeling. These reactions often make it difficult for the victim to concentrate effectively on everyday activities and relationships.

The management of the rape victim in the acute phase influences longer term adjustment. Many rape victims may manifest a *posttraumatic stress disorder,* the diagnostic criteria for which are shown in Table 42–1. The likelihood of this disorder developing is high owing to the abrupt nature of the crime, its violence, the passivity and helplessness imposed upon the victim, and the high probability of physical as well as psychologic trauma ensuing.

THE MEDICAL CARE PROCESS

The medical consultation should proceed only after a supportive, caring relationship has been established. Some victims have a need to ventilate their feelings, and it is important to provide sufficient opportunity for them to do this. The woman should be actively involved in the consultation so she may regain a feeling of control over what is happening to her. The purposes of the consultation should be explained, and she should be allowed to dictate the pace of the questioning and the order of the examination.

Medical History

In taking the victim's history, questions regarding the assault should be confined to

TABLE 42–1 DIAGNOSTIC CRITERIA FOR POST-TRAUMATIC STRESS DISORDER

A. Existence of a recognizable stressor that would evoke symptoms of distress in almost everyone
B. Reexperiencing the trauma, as evidenced by at least one of the following:
   1. Recurrent and intrusive recollections of the event
   2. Recurrent dreams of the event
   3. Suddenly acting or feeling as if the traumatic event were recurring because of an association with an environmental or ideational stimulus
C. Numbing of responsiveness to or reduced involvement with the external world, beginning some time after the trauma, as shown by at least one of the following:
   1. Markedly diminished interest in one or more significant activities
   2. Feeling of detachment or estrangement from others
   3. Constricted affect
D. At least two of the following symptoms that were not present before the trauma:
   1. Hyperalertness or exaggerated startle response
   2. Sleep disturbance
   3. Guilt about surviving when others have not or about behavior required for survival
   4. Memory impairment or trouble concentrating
   5. Avoidance of activities that arouse recollection of the traumatic event
   6. Intensification of symptoms by exposure to events that symbolize or resemble the traumatic event

Reprinted with permission from the American Psychiatric Association Committee on Nomenclature and Statistics, Diagnostic and Statistical Manual of Mental Disorders. 3rd ed. Washington, DC, American Psychiatric Association, 1980.

those necessary to determine the need for any acute medical care, and to direct the examination toward the appropriate collection of evidence. Prefacing questions with remarks that certain acts are not uncommon may avoid embarrassment and humiliation. Facts to be determined in the medical history of a rape victim are listed in Table 42–2.

Physical Examination

Separate informed consents must be obtained for examination and collection of evidence. During these procedures, it is important to be gentle and to explain the purpose of everything that is being performed. Steps to be observed in the examination are listed in Table 42–3.

TREATMENT

Medical Treatment

All injuries should be appropriately treated. Tetanus toxoid should be given if injuries are present and no toxoid has been received in the past ten years. Prophylactic treatment for sexually transmitted diseases should be offered; many facilities provide this routinely. Current recommendations are that 4.8 million units of procaine penicillin be administered intramuscularly, following 1 gm of probenecid orally. If the oral route is preferred, ampicillin, 3.5 gm immediately (given with 1 gm of probenecid), followed by tetracycline, 0.5 gm four times a day for seven

TABLE 42–2 HISTORY REQUIRED OF A RAPE VICTIM

1. Date and time of the assault; date and time of the present examination.
2. Physical surroundings and circumstances in which the assault occurred.
3. Nature of the assault and any associated pain experienced.
4. Weapons or foreign objects used and where they were used.
5. The number of assailants.
6. Any acts that were committed, such as coitus, fellatio, cunnilingus, sodomy.
7. Whether or not ejaculation occurred and where; whether or not a condom was used.
8. Whether or not there was vomiting or loss of consciousness.
9. Whether or not the patient washed, wiped, bathed, douched, defecated, brushed her teeth or changed her clothes after the assault.
10. Use of drugs, alcohol, or medications in proximity to the time of the assault; current medication history.
11. Allergies.
12. Date of last tetanus immunization.
13. Date and time of last consensual intercourse.
14. Gravity, parity, and menstrual history.
15. Contraceptive history.
16. General past medical history, as indicated.

TABLE 42–3 PHYSICAL EXAMINATION OF A RAPE VICTIM AND COLLECTION OF EVIDENCE

1. Note and record vital signs.
2. Examine clothing and skin for loose hair, stains, or other debris, and collect as evidence.
3. Inspect fingernails and preserve cleanings.
4. Collect clothing.
5. Comb pubic hair for loose strands and save.
6. Clip and label samples of head and pubic hair for comparison with any loose strands found.
7. Perform and record general physical examination, as indicated, with special attention to evidence of trauma.
8. Carefully inspect the external genitalia for lacerations, abrasions, ecchymoses, or hematomas; give special attention to the posterior fourchette.
9. Gently insert a warmed speculum and carefully inspect for evidence of trauma.
10. Prepare a gonococcal culture and appropriate smears for the detection of spermatozoa.
11. Obtain similar cultures and smears from the throat and anus, as indicated.
12. Collect baseline blood specimens for grouping, syphilis serology, pregnancy testing, and drug or alcohol levels; a reference saliva specimen should be obtained to determine ABO secretor status of the victim.
13. Handle all specimens so as to insure preservation and maintenance of the chain of custody.

days, is effective treatment for incubating syphilis, gonorrhea, and *Chlamydia*. For penicillin-allergic patients, tetracycline, 0.5 gm four times a day for seven days, may be prescribed orally.

If the possibility of pregnancy is likely, alternatives should be discussed, including continuation, first trimester induced abortion if pregnancy ensues, or postcoital drug contraception.

Psychologic Management at the Initial Evaluation

In addition to attending to immediate physical and emotional needs, the initial evaluation provides an opportunity to prepare the victim for the longer term psychologic impact of the experience. This preparation is intended to diminish the long-term consequences and to enable the woman to recognize the common psychosocial sequelae when they occur, thus enabling her to seek professional help at an early stage.

The psychologic problems that may result are varied and may mimic those seen in the aftermath of other kinds of traumatic experiences. Among those expected in the acute phase of adjustment are irritability, tension, anxiety, depression, fatigue, and persistent ruminations. Somatic symptoms of a general nature may occur, such as headaches or irritable bowel syndrome, or symptoms may be more specific to the reproductive system, such as vaginal irritation or discharge. Behavioral problems may also surface, particularly when these have been evident in the

past, such as overeating and alcohol or substance abuse.

Stimuli associated with the rape, such as a similar looking man or similar surroundings, may be associated with *flashbacks*. These are common reactions and relate to the process of classical conditioning, whereby peripheral stimuli associated with an event eliciting a strong emotional response can subsequently elicit an attenuated form of that response. Research on the etiology and maintenance of fears and phobias indicates that avoidance of potentially frightening situations will only strengthen the conditioned emotional reaction and may, in some cases, lead to full-blown phobic avoidance. If the woman continues to engage in normal life experiences rather than trying to avoid such stimuli, the emotional reaction to such innocuous stimuli will extinguish over time. By introducing this principle, the gynecologist may suggest to the woman the most appropriate course of action.

Reactions to the sexual assault may result in problems with sexual behavior and functioning. Loss of libido is a common response to stressful or traumatic circumstances of any kind. Other complaints include vaginismus, impaired vaginal lubrication, and loss of orgasmic capacity. These problems may be even more likely if the assault occurred at home while asleep. Preparing the woman for these eventualities can be extremely helpful in preventing sexual dysfunctions from developing. Giving permission for a lower-than-usual sexual drive during the postassault period may remove some performance anxiety. Explaining how anxiety and stress can inhibit sexual responsiveness and providing ways in which this can be overcome are also important.

After-Care Planning

Whether or not the patient elects to have prophylaxis against sexually transmitted diseases or pregnancy, careful follow-up must be arranged. Tests for gonorrhea should be performed in two weeks and for syphilis in six weeks; if pregnancy is suspected, it should be confirmed or refuted. If any of these tests are positive, appropriate management should be instituted immediately.

Prior to discharging the patient, it is important to ensure that she has a safe place to go and a suitable means of transportation. She should also be given the names, addresses, and phone numbers in writing of resources available in the community to meet medical, legal, and psychosocial needs related to the assault.

SUGGESTED READING

American Psychiatric Association Committee on Nomenclature and Statistics: Diagnostic and Statistical Manual of Mental Disorders. 3rd ed. Washington, DC, American Psychiatric Association, 1980.

Bragonier JR, Nadelson CC: Caring for the rape victim. Interact 1:1, 1977.

Burgess AW, Holstrom LL: Rape trauma syndrome. Am J Psychiatry 131:981, 1974.

Burgess AW, Holstrom LL: Crisis and counselling requests of rape victims. Nurs Res 23:196, 1974.

Ellis L, Beattie C: The feminist explanation for rape: An empirical test. J Sex Res 19:74, 1983.

Marks I: Cure and Care of Neuroses. New York, John Wiley, 1981.

Martin CA, Warfield MC, Braen ER: Physician's management of the psychological aspects of rape. JAMA 249:501, 1983.

Reading AE: The management of anxiety related to vaginal examination. J Psychosom Obstet Gynecol 1:99, 1982.

State of California Department of Health Services: Guidelines for Treatment of Victims of Sexual Assault, 1976.

GYNECOLOGIC OPERATIVE TECHNIQUES

GEORGE S. HARRIS and RONALD S. LEUCHTER

It is not the purpose of this chapter to qualify the reader as a gynecologic surgeon. It is, however, essential that students and junior housestaff become familiar with the basic principles of common gynecologic surgical procedures so that they can properly assist in the operating room.

DILATATION AND CURETTAGE

The most common gynecologic surgical procedure is dilatation of the cervix and curettage of the endometrium. If cancer of the cervix or endometrium is suspected, a *fractional curettage* should be performed. In this procedure, the endocervix is initially curetted, even before sounding the uterine depth. Then the cervix is dilated and the endometrium curetted. The curettings from the endocervix and endometrium are submitted separately.

Indications

Dilatation and curettage may be a *diagnostic* or a *therapeutic* procedure. A *diagnostic dilatation and curettage* is performed for irregular menstrual bleeding, heavy menstrual bleeding, or postmenopausal bleeding, unless an endometrial biopsy has already revealed a diagnosis of malignancy. In patients younger than 35 years with irregular bleeding, hormone manipulation frequently obviates the need for curettage. Irregularities

in the contour of the endometrial cavity, either congenital (e.g., uterine septum) or acquired (e.g., submucous myomata), are frequently determined during the operation.

The dilatation and curettage may have a *therapeutic* effect in patients with heavy or irregular bleeding from endometrial hyperplasia, endometrial polyps, or small, pedunculated submucous myomas. Unwanted first trimester pregnancies are usually evacuated by dilatation and suction curettage.

Technique

The operation is performed with the patient in the dorsal lithotomy position. In the past, dilatation and curettage was considered an inpatient procedure because of the need for general anesthesia. Most curettages are now performed on an outpatient basis. Paracervical blocks and local anesthesia are frequently employed.

A repeat pelvic examination is done under anesthesia, and, after sterile preparation, a weighted speculum is placed in the posterior vagina. The cervix is grasped with a single or double-toothed tenaculum. A Kevorkian curette is used to curette the endocervical canal. The depth of the uterine cavity is determined with a uterine sound, and the cervix is then dilated with a set of graduated dilators. Dilatation to a number 8 Hegar dilator is sufficient for a diagnostic curettage in a premenopausal patient. In postmenopausal women with increasing stenosis of the cervix, extreme caution must be exercised in the dilatation to

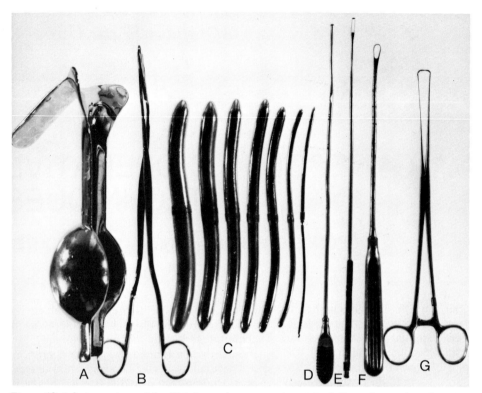

Figure 43–1 Instruments used for dilatation and curettage: *A*, weighted (Auvard) speculum; *B*, polyp forceps; *C*, Hegar dilators; *D*, uterine sound; *E*, Kevorkian curette for endocervical curettage; *F*, sharp uterine curette; and *G*, tenaculum.

avoid lacerating the cervix or perforating the uterus. In such patients, Laminaria tents, either from sea plants or synthetically manufactured, may be inserted some hours preoperatively to enhance cervical dilatation.

A small polyp or ovum forceps is introduced through the dilated cervix and gently rotated to remove any endometrial polyps. A thorough curettage is done with a sharp curette, proceeding with each stroke in either a clockwise or counterclockwise manner to ensure that the entire uterine cavity has been covered. Particular attention must be directed to each cornu. The surgical instruments required for this procedure are shown in Figure 43–1.

Complications

The most common surgical complications of dilatation and curettage are hemorrhage, infection, perforation of the uterus, and laceration of the cervix. Perforation of the uterus, even in experienced hands, is a common complication. As long as no bowel or large blood vessels are injured, careful observation and antibiotics may be all the therapy required. Except in an acute emergency, such as an infected incomplete abortion, no dilatation and curettage should be done in the presence of infection. Any suspicion of infection postoperatively should be vigorously treated with antibiotics. Lacerations of the cervix occurring during the operation must be repaired at the conclusion of the surgery.

CONIZATION OF THE CERVIX

Conization of the cervix is a procedure in which a cone-shaped portion of the cervix is removed for diagnostic or therapeutic purposes. The section of the tissue surrounding the external os represents the base of the removed specimen. The apex is either near or at the internal os.

Indications

Although the use of the colposcope has significantly reduced the need for cone biopsy in the evaluation of an abnormal Pap smear, *diagnostic conization* (Fig. 43–2*A*) is still required under the following circumstances: (1) if the squamocolumnar junction cannot be visualized colposcopically; (2) if the endocervical curettage is positive; (3) if there is a significant discrepancy between the Pap smear and the colposcopically directed cervical biopsy; and (4) if the cervical biopsy reveals microinvasive squamous cell carcinoma.

A *therapeutic conization* may be performed for extensive carcinoma *in situ* of the cervix, particularly in women who have completed childbearing (Fig. 43–2*B*). Provided the surgical margins are free of disease, a diagnostic cone frequently becomes a therapeutic cone once lack of invasion has been established. The amount of tissue excised depends upon the indications for the procedure and the extent of the disease as determined by colposcopy. On rare occasions, the surgery may be employed to eradicate an intractable chronic cervicitis.

Technique

The patient is placed in the dorsal lithotomy position, and a weighted speculum is placed in the vagina. Whenever possible, a colposcopic examination should be performed in the operating room to determine the extent of the dysplastic epithelium on the ectocervix. If colposcopy is not available in the operating room, the cervix is stained with

Lugol's solution (Schiller's test). Dysplastic epithelium, which lacks glycogen, will not stain with iodine and will appear pale (Schiller-positive).

To help control bleeding from the descending branch of the uterine artery, hemostatic sutures are placed at the 3:00 and 9:00 o'clock positions. Some surgeons also inject a saline and epinephrine solution into the cervix to aid hemostasis. A circular incision is made around the external os to incorporate all of the Schiller-positive or colposcopically abnormal areas. The incision is continued into the stroma, angulating toward the canal. The apex is reached just below or at the level of the internal os. After removing the cone, biopsies are taken at the retained apex, and the procedure is completed with a dilatation and curettage. It is usually necessary to place hemostatic sutures in the anterior and posterior lips of the cervix to control bleeding.

The excised cone should be sent fresh to the pathologist. The cone is opened at 12 o'clock, pinned to a cork board, then fixed in formalin (Fig. 43–2*C*). Serial blocks are made, and several sections from each block are examined in a serial manner.

Complications

The most common complication of conization of the cervix is immediate or delayed bleeding. Secondary hemorrhage, which is due to infection, occurs in about 10 percent

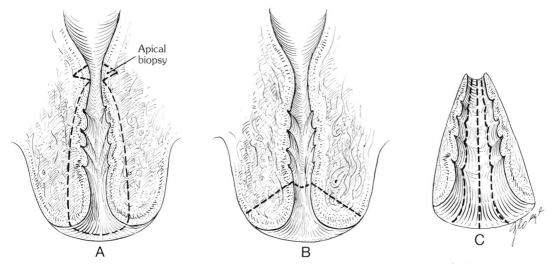

Figure 43–2 Cone biopsy of the cervix: *A*, diagnostic conization performed when transformation zone is not fully visualized colposcopically; *B*, therapeutic conization performed for disease involving ectocervix and distal endocervical canal; and *C*, specimen opened for serial sectioning.

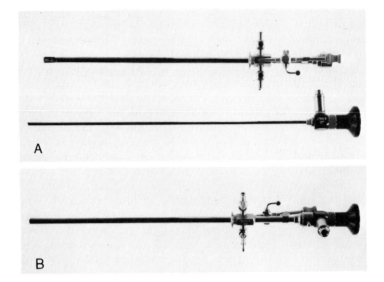

Figure 43–3 Storz operating hysteroscope: *A,* dismantled; *B,* assembled.

of patients. It usually requires antibiotics and vaginal packing but may necessitate resuturing.

HYSTEROSCOPY

With the increasing refinement of fiberoptics, endoscopy has become a valuable adjunct to the practice of gynecology. The hysteroscope, an instrument for viewing the endocervix and endometrial cavity, may be used for diagnosis or therapy. The most common hysteroscopes in use are either the flexible or rigid panoramic instruments (Fig. 43–3).

Indications

Diagnostic indications for hysteroscopy may include primary and secondary infertility, habitual spontaneous abortion, abnormal uterine bleeding, lost intrauterine device, or suspected intrauterine abnormalities. The hysteroscope has also been used to determine the extent of cervical or endometrial malignancies. Biopsies may be obtained via the hysteroscope.

Therapeutic indications include lysis of intrauterine adhesions (synechiae) and the resection of polyps. In some centers, experience is being gained with the use of the hysteroscope for resection of submucous myomata, removal of uterine septa, control of menometrorrhagia with a laser, and sterilization by occlusion of the tubal ostia.

Technique

The procedure is performed with the patient in the dorsal lithotomy position. If the cervical canal is not stenotic, it is possible to perform hysteroscopy as an office procedure under local anesthesia. Otherwise, it is done in the hospital under general anesthesia. A povidone-iodine spray or swab is used on the cervix, and the anterior lip is grasped with a tenaculum. Limited cervical dilatation may be necessary to allow insertion of the hysteroscope. A gas or liquid is circulated to distend the uterus and improve visualization. The most popular media are carbon dioxide or Hyskon hysteroscopy fluid.

Complications

Complications of hysteroscopy include uterine perforation with the scope or instruments, cervical laceration, reactions from the distending medium, and rupture of a hydrosalpinx.

LAPAROSCOPY

The laparoscope is an instrument for viewing the peritoneal cavity (Fig. 43–4). Both pelvic and upper abdominal structures can be

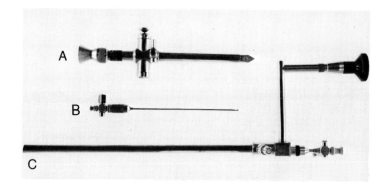

Figure 43–4 Instruments required for single puncture laparoscopy; *A*, trocar and cannula; *B*, Veress needle; and *C*, Wolf laparoscope (10 mm).

inspected. Most laparoscopies are done as outpatient procedures.

Indications and Contraindications

The indications for laparoscopy are both diagnostic and therapeutic. *Diagnostic indications* include the evaluation of infertility, pelvic pain, small pelvic masses, congenital anomalies, and a small hemoperitoneum. The most common indication for *therapeutic laparoscopy* is tubal sterilization. Other therapeutic indications include lysis of adhesions, fulguration of endometriotic implants, aspiration of small cysts, and retrieval of lost intrauterine devices.

Absolute contraindications to laparoscopy include bowel obstruction and large hemoperitoneum. A relative contraindication is obesity. In patients who have had multiple previous laparotomies, a past history of peritonitis, previous bowel surgery, or a lower midline abdominal incision, *open laparoscopy* is preferable. In this procedure, the peritoneal cavity is opened through a small subumbilical incision under direct vision prior to introduction of the trocar and sheath.

Technique

The procedure is performed in a modified dorsal lithotomy position, usually under general anesthesia. An intrauterine manipulator is inserted to help in the visualization of the pelvic organs. A pneumoperitoneum is created by inserting a spring-loaded needle, such as a Veress needle, into the peritoneal cavity via the subumbilical fold. Proper placement of the needle is checked by disappearance of a hanging drop from the needle hub with elevation of the diaphragm or injection of 10 cc of saline and observation of its passage without resistance. The gas line is then connected, and insufflation with either carbon dioxide or nitrous oxide is begun. Between two and four liters of gas are required. The trocar and surrounding sheath are then inserted through a small subumbilical incision, the trocar is withdrawn, and the valve is opened manually. A hiss of escaping gas ensures that the instrument is in the peritoneal cavity.

The lighted telescope is inserted into the sheath and advanced slowly. Visualization of pelvic organs confirms that the peritoneal cavity has been entered. Gas may be added intermittently to maintain a good pneumoperitoneum. To perform a second puncture, which is sometimes necessary, especially in laparoscopic surgical procedures, the abdominal wall is transilluminated, and a 4- or 6-mm trocar and sheath are inserted under laparoscopic guidance through a small incision at the pubic hairline. A probe or other surgical instrument (e.g., Falope ring applicator) is passed through the second sheath (Fig. 43–5).

Upon completion of the procedure, hemostasis is checked, the gas is released from the peritoneal cavity, and the instruments are withdrawn. The small skin incisions are closed with a clip or single suture.

Complications

Insufflation of the abdominal wall may occur from failure to enter the peritoneal cavity with the Veress needle. Perforation of a viscus, especially bowel, may occur at the time of insertion of the trocar and sheath. Once the instruments have been successfully introduced into the peritoneal cavity, lack of proper intraperitoneal hemostasis and coag-

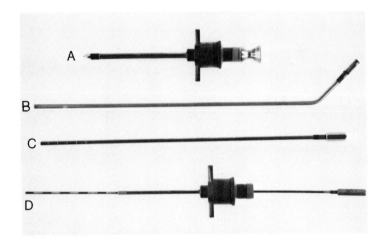

Figure 43–5 Instruments used for second puncture: *A*, 6-mm trocar; *B*, suction catheter; *C*, 6-mm probe; and *D*, 4-mm trocar with secondary probe.

ulation burns of a viscus may occur. A poor pneumoperitoneum increases the risk of these complications.

Bowel burns during fulguration are the most serious complications of laparoscopy, although the most common complications are related to the anesthesia. Bowel burns result either from direct contact with the bowel or from a spark and are usually *not* detected at the time of the procedure. Several days later bowel perforation with peritonitis may occur. The increased use of bipolar instruments has diminished the occurrence of this serious complication.

In addition to the surgical complications, there is an increased risk of anesthetic complications in a patient with a pneumoperitoneum. Both surgical and anesthetic complications are frequently the result of lack of adequate experience with laparoscopy by the relevant physician.

HYSTERECTOMY

Hysterectomy, the most common major gynecologic operation, can be performed abdominally or vaginally. Before performing any hysterectomy, cervical cytology must be evaluated and, if necessary, colposcopy performed to exclude occult cervical cancer.

Abdominal Hysterectomy

Total hysterectomy or panhysterectomy implies removal of both the corpus and the cervix. *Subtotal hysterectomy* implies preservation of the cervix. *Extrafascial hysterectomy* implies removal of the uterus with its outer fascial layer *in toto*. *Intrafascial hysterectomy* implies that the cervix is cored out, and the outer (endopelvic) fascial layer is left attached to the bladder. *Radical hysterectomy* implies removal of the parametrial tissue and uterosacral ligaments in conjunction with the corpus and cervix after dissecting each ureter from its tunnel beneath the uterine artery. Figure 43–6 demonstrates diagrammatically the differences between the various types of hysterectomy.

Indications. The indications for *abdominal hysterectomy* include benign diseases, such as fibroids, endometriosis, chronic pelvic inflammatory disease, persistent dysfunctional uterine bleeding that is unresponsive to conservative medical measures; or malignant diseases, such as Stage I carcinoma of the endometrium, Stage Ia (microinvasive) carcinoma of the cervix, or ovarian cancer. A total extrafascial hysterectomy should normally be performed. A *subtotal hysterectomy* is sometimes performed for disseminated ovarian cancer to prevent tumor growth at the vaginal vault. *Intrafascial hysterectomy* may occasionally be used when it is difficult to dissect the bladder from the front of the cervix, as may occur in patients who have had multiple lower segment cesarean sections. *Radical hysterectomy* is performed for Stage Ib or IIa carcinoma of the cervix and occasionally for Stage II carcinoma of the endometrium.

The question of whether or not to remove the ovaries depends on the individual case. Bilateral salpingo-oophorectomy is routinely performed, along with abdominal hysterectomy, in postmenopausal women. Prior to the menopause, the merits of removing nor-

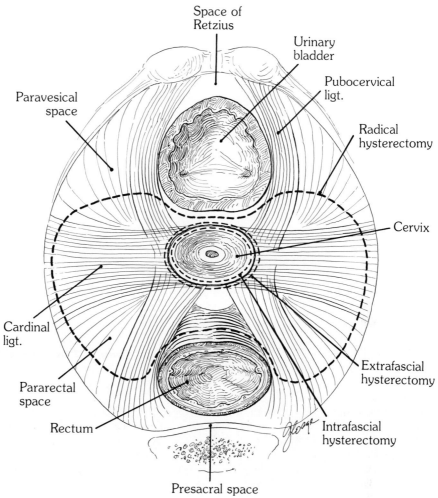

Space of
Retzius

Urinary
bladder

Pubocervical
ligt.

Radical
hysterectomy

Paravesical
space

Cervix

Cardinal
ligt.

Extrafascial
hysterectomy

Pararectal
space

Rectum

Intrafascial
hysterectomy

Presacral space

Figure 43–6 Types of hysterectomy: extrafacial, intrafacial, and radical. Note the extensive amount of parametrial tissue that is removed in a radical hysterectomy.

mal ovaries to prevent subsequent neoplastic disease versus leaving them so that hormonal function can be maintained must be thoroughly discussed with the patient. Prior to age 45 years, the ovaries are generally preserved.

Technique. The operation is performed in the supine position, usually under general anesthesia. The type of skin incision chosen depends on the nature of the disease. In most patients with benign disease, a low transverse (Pfannenstiel's) incision can be used. However, in the presence of proven or suspected malignant disease of the uterus or ovaries, or in cases in which potential complications are anticipated, such as in very obese patients or in those who have had previous surgeries or pelvic inflammatory disease, a vertical lower abdominal incision provides better exposure.

The various lower abdominal incisions are discussed in Chapter 1.

After evaluating the upper abdomen, the abdominal contents are packed out of the pelvis, and the patient is placed in a modified Trendelenburg position. The round ligaments are clamped, cut, and tied (Fig. 43–7*A*). This allows entrance between the leaves of the broad ligament, exposing the retroperitoneal space so that the ureter and pelvic vessels can be identified (Fig. 43–7*B*). The vesico-uterine fold of peritoneum is incised, and the bladder is dissected from the front of the uterus and cervix. If the ovaries are to be removed, each infundibulopelvic ligament is clamped and doubly tied once the ureters have been identified. If the ovaries are to be left behind, each utero-ovarian pedicle, as it attaches to the uterus, is clamped and tied.

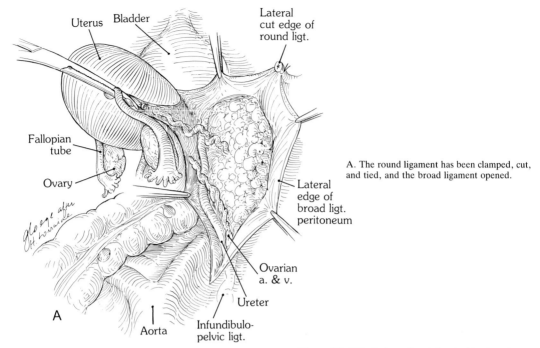

Uterus
Bladder
Lateral cut edge of round ligt.
Fallopian tube
Ovary
Lateral edge of broad ligt. peritoneum
Ovarian a. & v.
Ureter
Aorta
Infundibulo-pelvic ligt.

A

A. The round ligament has been clamped, cut, and tied, and the broad ligament opened.

Figure 43–7 Technique for abdominal hysterectomy.

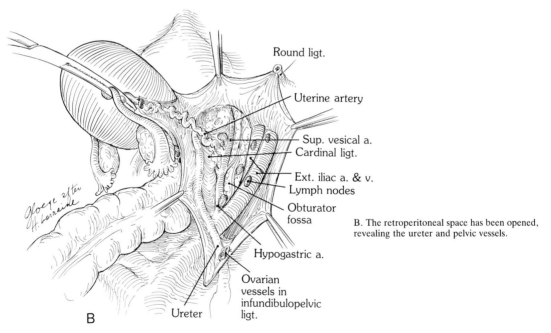

Round ligt.
Uterine artery
Sup. vesical a.
Cardinal ligt.
Ext. iliac a. & v.
Lymph nodes
Obturator fossa
Hypogastric a.
Ovarian vessels in infundibulopelvic ligt.
Ureter

B

B. The retroperitoneal space has been opened, revealing the ureter and pelvic vessels.

The posterior peritoneum between the rectum and the cervix is incised, thereby moving the ureters further down into the pelvis. The uterine vessels are isolated as they come up the side of the uterus at the level of the internal os; they are clamped and doubly tied. The cardinal and uterosacral ligaments are taken down sequentially as they attach to the lateral and posterolateral aspect of the uterus (Fig. 43–7C). This is continued until the cervicovaginal junction is reached, at which point the clamps are placed underneath the cervix across the upper vagina and the specimen is removed (Fig. 43–7D).

The vagina is normally closed, and the cardinal and uterosacral ligaments are incor-

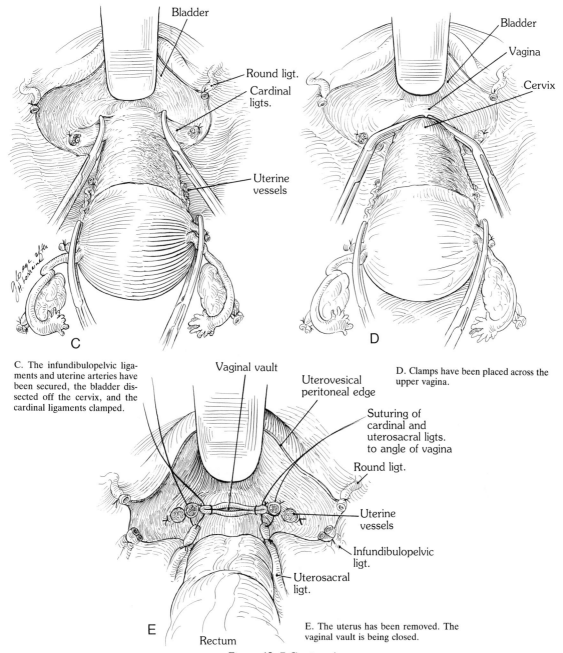

C. The infundibulopelvic ligaments and uterine arteries have been secured, the bladder dissected off the cervix, and the cardinal ligaments clamped.

D. Clamps have been placed across the upper vagina.

E. The uterus has been removed. The vaginal vault is being closed.

Figure 43–7 *Continued*

porated into each angle to prevent vaginal vault prolapse (Fig. 43–7E). The pelvic peritoneum is closed with a running suture after hemostasis has been secured. The uterus, once removed, should be opened in the operating room to exclude unsuspected malignancy, which may necessitate more extensive evaluation and dissection.

Vaginal Hysterectomy

This approach avoids an abdominal scar and is associated with minimal postoperative discomfort.

Indications. Vaginal hysterectomy may be performed provided the uterus is mobile and not larger than ten weeks' gestational size;

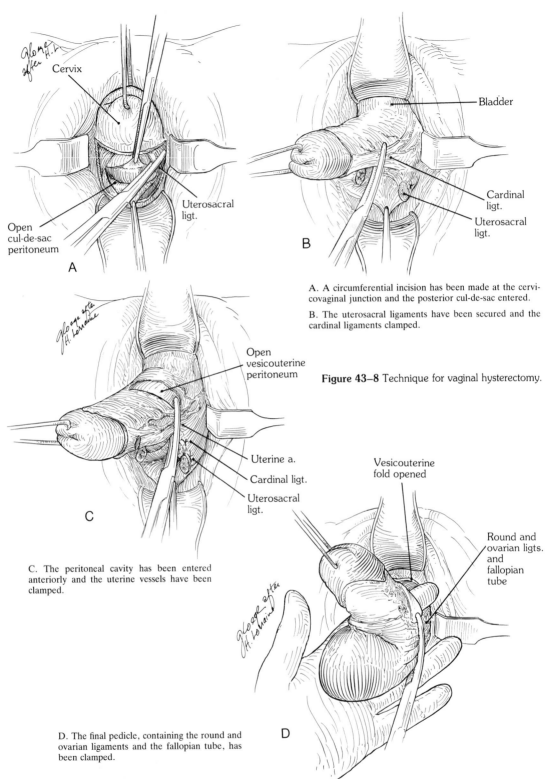

A. A circumferential incision has been made at the cervicovaginal junction and the posterior cul-de-sac entered.

B. The uterosacral ligaments have been secured and the cardinal ligaments clamped.

Figure 43–8 Technique for vaginal hysterectomy.

C. The peritoneal cavity has been entered anteriorly and the uterine vessels have been clamped.

D. The final pedicle, containing the round and ovarian ligaments and the fallopian tube, has been clamped.

there are no adhesions from pelvic inflammatory disease, endometriosis, or multiple laparotomies; and ovarian disease is not suspected. The most common indication for this approach is uterine prolapse, with or without associated cystocele, enterocele, or rectocele.

Other indications include carcinoma *in situ* with positive margins on cone biopsy, or sterilization in the presence of other gynecologic conditions that are amenable to vaginal surgery. The ovaries are not routinely removed through the vaginal approach, since

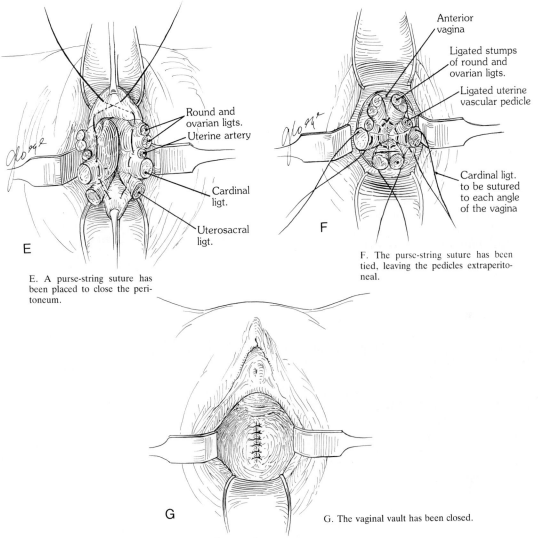

E. A purse-string suture has been placed to close the peritoneum.

F. The purse-string suture has been tied, leaving the pedicles extraperitoneal.

G. The vaginal vault has been closed.

Figure 43–8 *Continued*

this is technically more difficult and occasionally not technically feasible.

Technique. The principles of this operation are similar to those for abdominal hysterectomy, except the ligaments and vessels are clamped and tied in reverse order. The patient is placed in the lithotomy position, and a weighted speculum is placed in the vagina. A tenaculum is placed on the cervix to pull the uterus down into the vagina. A circumferential incision is made at the cervicovaginal junction, and the posterior cul-de-sac is entered (Fig. 43–8*A*). A finger is placed in the cul-de-sac to make sure there are no unsuspected adhesions that would contraindicate proceeding with the surgery vaginally.

The uterosacral ligaments are isolated, clamped, and tied. The cardinal ligaments are isolated, clamped, and tied (Fig. 43–8*B*). Then the bladder is separated from the cervix to expose the anterior peritoneal reflection. The peritoneal cavity is entered anteriorly, and a retractor is placed beneath the bladder. The uterine vessels are secured (Fig. 43–8*C*), and, once this is achieved, the uterus can be brought further down into the vagina, exposing the utero-ovarian pedicles and round ligaments, which are clamped, cut, and tied (Fig. 43–8*D*). The ovaries are inspected, hemostasis is secured, and the peritoneum is then closed in a purse-string fashion (Fig. 43–8*E*).

All pedicles are left extraperitoneally to prevent a hemoperitoneum should secondary bleeding occur. Each cardinal ligament is sutured to the superior angle of the vagina on either side to protect against vaginal vault prolapse, and the uterosacral ligaments are tied in the midline to prevent a subsequent enterocele (Fig. 43–8F). The vaginal cuff is closed with interrupted absorbable sutures (Fig. 43–8G).

Complications of Hysterectomy

General complications associated with any abdominal or pelvic surgery include atelectasis, wound infection, urinary tract infection, thrombophlebitis, and pulmonary embolism. *Atelectasis* occurs most commonly in the first 24 to 48 hours and can be prevented and treated with aggressive pulmonary toilet. *Wound infection* usually occurs about five days postoperatively and is associated with redness, tenderness, swelling, and increased warmth around the wound. Treatment may require systemic antibiotics, opening the incision, draining the discharge, local debridement, and wound care. *Urinary tract infection* can occur at any time in the postoperative period, and urine for microscopy and culture should be obtained on any patient with a postoperative fever. *Thrombophlebitis* (with possible subsequent pulmonary embolism) is manifested by fever and leg swelling or pain; it usually occurs seven to ten days postoperatively. *Pulmonary embolism* may occur, even in the absence of signs of thrombophlebitis. *Wound disruption,* with evisceration of intestine, is generally heralded by a profuse serous discharge from the wound (peritoneal fluid) four to eight days postoperatively. When evisceration is suspected, the wound should be explored in the operating room.

The most common intraoperative complication of abdominal or vaginal hysterectomy is *bleeding,* either from the infundibulopelvic or utero-ovarian pedicle, the uterine pedicle, or the vaginal angle. When postoperative hemorrhage occurs, bleeding from the vaginal angle can sometimes be identified and controlled vaginally. However, if bleeding is sufficient to cause hypotension, laparotomy may be required to tie off the bleeding vascular pedicle.

Infection is common to both procedures and is manifested by fever and lower abdominal pain. Examination often reveals tenderness and induration of the vaginal cuff, indicative of a *pelvic cellulitis.* This can usually be treated with antibiotic therapy. When there has been seroma or hematoma formation, a *pelvic abscess* or *infected pelvic hematoma* can develop. This will be manifested by a hot, tender mass on rectovaginal examination. Such patients require the appropriate drainage of the infected material through the vaginal cuff, in addition to the administration of parenteral antibiotics. Prophylactic cephalosporin intraoperatively and for 24 hours postoperatively has proven beneficial in controlling infection in vaginal hysterectomies done on premenopausal patients.

Injury to the ureter is the most serious complication of hysterectomy and usually occurs during the abdominal procedure, particularly during a difficult dissection for pelvic inflammatory disease, endometriosis, or pelvic cancer. The most common site of injury is just lateral to the cervix; the second most common site is beneath the infundibulopelvic ligament. A suture can be placed through the ureter, or it may be clamped and cut. It is important to identify the ureter before ligating and incising the infundibulopelvic ligament. Postoperatively, the patient will develop a fever and flank pain, and a ureterovaginal fistula or urinoma may occur 5 to 21 days postoperatively. If fluid begins to leak from the vagina, a work-up, including cystoscopy and intravenous pyelography (IVP), is necessary. A ureterovaginal fistula requires reimplantation of the ureter into the bladder, but it is usual to wait several months to allow the inflammatory reaction to settle.

Intraoperative *injury to the bladder* or *intestine* can occur and, if recognized, should be repaired immediately. If a bladder repair is necessary, seven days of postoperative drainage with a Foley catheter is necessary to allow optimal healing.

SUGGESTED READING

Amirikia H, Evans TN: Ten year review of hysterectomies: Trends, indications and risks. Am J Obstet Gynecol 134:431, 1979.

Gray LA: Techniques of abdominal total hysterectomy. Am J Obstet Gynecol 75:334, 1958.

Gray LA: The place of vaginal hysterectomy in gynecological surgery. West J Surg 67:153, 1959.

Pratt JH: Operative and postoperative difficulties of vaginal hysterectomy. Obstet Gynecol 21:220, 1963.

Radman HM, Korman W: Uterine perforation during dilatation and curettage. Obstet Gynecol 21:210, 1963.

Randall CL: Ovarian conservation. Obstet Gynecol 20:880, 1962.

Sigler AM, Kemmann E: Hysteroscopy. Obstet Gynecol Surv 30:567, 1975.

Twombly GH: Hemorrhage in gynecological surgery. Clin Obstet Gynecol 16:135, 1973.

IV

REPRODUCTIVE ENDOCRINOLOGY

John Marshall — SUBEDITOR

PHYSIOLOGY AND BIOCHEMISTRY OF THE NORMAL REPRODUCTIVE CYCLE

JOHN K. H. LU

The female reproductive cycle is a complex endocrinologic event, reflecting the functional integration of the ovary, the pituitary gland, and the central nervous system. During the normal reproductive cycle the ovaries undergo sequential morphologic and functional changes, including follicular development, ovulation, and corpus luteum formation, with consequent changes in steroid production and secretion. These cyclic changes are closely regulated by gonadotropins and, possibly, by prolactin. Circulating ovarian steroid concentrations also modulate the release of gonadotropins through feedback mechanisms.

A normal ovarian cycle can be divided into a follicular phase, a midcycle ovulatory phase, and a luteal phase. During the *follicular phase,* gonadotropins initiate new follicular development and growth and prepare one (or occasionally more than one) follicle for ovulation. At *midcycle,* the neuroendocrine system initiates the preovulatory surge of gonadotropins, resulting in the final maturation of follicle(s) and the induction of ovulation. During the *luteal phase,* the neuroendocrine system prepares the uterine endometrium for implantation of the blastocyst(s) by activating corpus luteum function. Following the luteal phase, menstruation occurs as the result of cessation of corpus luteum function.

This chapter presents the endocrinologic changes in the ovary, the pituitary gland, and the hypothalamus throughout a normal reproductive cycle, and it describes the integrated neuroendocrinologic functions that maintain the cycle's regularity. The first section discusses the relationship between ovarian steroid hormones and the feedback control of gonadotropin secretion; the second section describes the cyclic changes in the histophysiology of the endometrium during the menstrual cycle. The morphologic and functional changes in the ovary during follicular development and ovulation are discussed in Chapter 3.

STEROID SECRETION DURING THE OVARIAN CYCLE

Estrogens

During early follicular development, circulating estradiol levels are relatively low. About one week before ovulation, levels begin to increase—at first slowly, then rapidly. The levels generally reach a maximum one day before the luteinizing hormone (LH) peak. Following this peak and prior to ovulation, there is a marked and precipitous fall. During the luteal phase, estradiol rises to a maximum five to seven days after ovulation

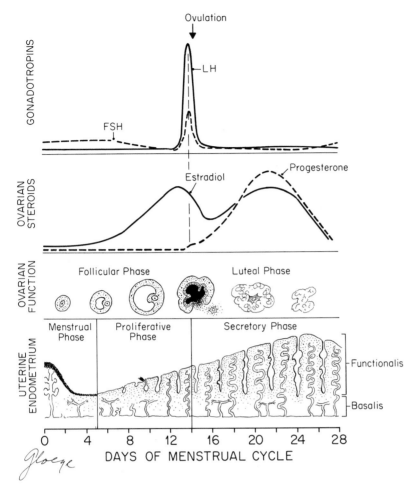

Figure 44–1 Hormone levels during a normal menstrual cycle.

and returns to baseline shortly before menstruation. Estrone secretion by the ovary is considerably less than that of estradiol, but follows a similar pattern (Fig. 44–1). Most of the estrone is derived from the conversion of androstenedione.

Progestins

During follicular development, the ovary secretes only very small amounts of progesterone and 17α-hydroxyprogesterone. The bulk of the progesterone comes from peripheral conversion of adrenal pregnenolone and pregnenolone sulfate. Just before ovulation, the unruptured, but luteinizing, graafian follicle begins to produce some progesterone. At about this same time, there is also a marked increase in 17α-hydroxyprogesterone production. During the luteal phase, the corpus luteum secretes large amounts of progesterone and some 17α-hydroxyprogesterone.

The elevation of basal body temperature is temporarily related to the central effect of progesterone. Similar to estradiol, secretion of progestins by the corpus luteum reaches a maximum five to seven days after ovulation and returns to baseline shortly before menstruation.

Androgens

Both the ovary and the adrenals secrete small amounts of testosterone, but most of the testosterone is derived from the metabolism of androstenedione, which is also secreted by both the ovary and the adrenal gland. The ovary secretes small amounts of dihydrotestosterone (DHT), but the bulk of DHT is derived from the conversions of androstenedione and testosterone. The ovary also secretes some dehydroepiandrosterone (DHEA) and DHEA sulfate (DHEA-S), but the bulk of both of these substances is secreted by the adrenal glands. Near the midcycle, there is an increase in plasma androstenedione, reflecting the secretion from the follicle. During the luteal phase, there is a second rise reflecting secretion by the corpus luteum. The adrenal gland also secretes androstenedione in a diurnal pattern similar to that of cortisol.

Serum Binding Proteins

Circulating estrogens and androgens are mostly bound to specific *steroid hormone-binding globulins* (SHBG) or to serum albumin. The remaining fraction is unbound (free). It is unclear whether or not steroids bound to serum proteins are accessible for tissue uptake and utilization. The synthesis of SHBG in the liver is increased by estrogens and thyroid hormones but decreased by testosterone.

NEUROENDOCRINE CONTROL OF GONADOTROPIN AND PROLACTIN SECRETION

Pituitary Gland

The pituitary gland lies within a bony cavity (sella turcica) at the base of the brain below the hypothalamus. It is separated from the cranial cavity by the diaphragma sellae, a condensation of the dura mater overlying the sella turcica. During embryogenesis, the pituitary develops partly from neural tissue and partly from oral ectoderm. The neural component is known as the *neurohypophysis*, and consists of the *pars nervosa* (or infundibular process or posterior lobe) and the *neural stalk* (or infundibulum) (Fig. 44–2). The neural stalk is composed of the median eminence and stem. These neural tissues are continuous

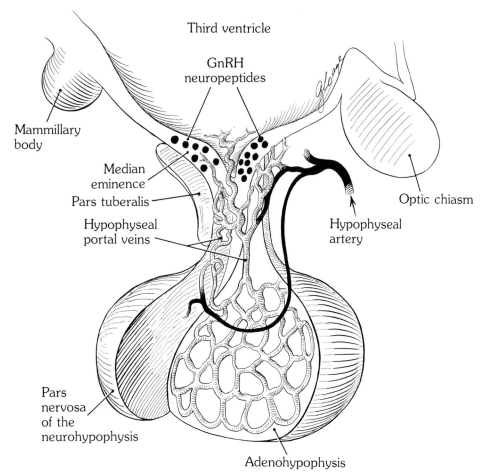

Figure 44–2 Pituitary and hypothalamus.

with the hypothalamus and connect the pituitary with the central nervous system. The part of the pituitary that develops from oral ectoderm is known as the *adenohypophysis,* and it consists of the *pars distalis* (or anterior lobe), the *pars tuberalis* (which surrounds the neural stalk), and the *pars intermedia* (intermediate lobe). Several important nerve tracts (including the tuberoinfundibular dopamine system and the hypothalamo-hypophyseal tract) pass through the neural stalk to influence hormonal secretion from both the posterior and anterior lobes of the pituitary. In addition, arterial blood supply to the neural stalk region forms the *hypophyseal* (or pituitary) *portal system,* which carries neurosecretory substances of hypothalamic origin into the anterior pituitary.

The supraoptic and paraventricular nuclei of the hypothalamus contain neurons that produce oxytocin and vasopressin (or antidiuretic hormone, ADH). These hormones are bound to carrier proteins and transported through the hypothalamo-hypophyseal tract to reach the posterior pituitary, from which they are released into the circulation.

Pituitary Hormones

The anterior pituitary contains different cell types that produce six protein hormones: *follicle-stimulating hormone* (FSH), *luteinizing hormone* (LH), *thyroid-stimulating hormone* (TSH) or thyrotropin, *prolactin, growth hormone* (GH), and *adrenocorticotropic hormone* (ACTH) or corticotropin.

The gonadotropins, FSH and LH, are synthesized and stored in cells called gonadotrophs, while TSH is produced by thyrotrophs. FSH, LH, and TSH are glycoproteins, consisting of alpha and beta subunits. The alpha subunits of FSH, LH, and TSH are identical. This same alpha subunit is also present in human chorionic gonadotropin (hCG). FSH and LH are metabolized mainly in the liver and kidney. The half-life for circulating LH is about 30 minutes, while that of FSH is several hours. This difference in half-life may account for the differential secretion patterns of these two gonadotropins.

Prolactin is secreted by lactotrophs. Unlike other peptide hormones produced by the adenohypophysis, pituitary release of prolactin is under chronic inhibition by the hypothalamus. Both the liver and kidneys are major sites of degradation of prolactin, and the half-life for circulating prolactin is about 20 to 30 minutes. In addition to its lactogenic effect, prolactin may directly or indirectly influence hypothalamic, pituitary, and ovarian functions in relation to the ovulatory cycle, particularly under a chronic state of hyperprolactinemia.

The Hypothalamus

Five different small peptides or biogenic amines that affect the reproductive cycle have been isolated from the hypothalamus. All exert specific effects on the hormonal secretion of the anterior pituitary gland. They are *gonadotropin-releasing hormone* (GnRH), *thyrotropin-releasing hormone* (TRH), *somatotropin release-inhibiting factor* (SRIF) or somatostatin, *corticotropin-releasing factor* (CRF), and *prolactin release-inhibiting factor* (PIF). Only GnRH and PIF are discussed here.

GnRH is a decapeptide that is responsible for the synthesis and release of both LH and FSH. Since it usually causes the release of more LH than FSH, it is commonly called LH-releasing hormone (LH-RH) or LH-releasing factor (LRF). Both FSH and LH appear to be present in two different forms within the pituitary gonadotrophs. One is a releasable form and the other a storage form. GnRH reaches the anterior pituitary via the hypophyseal portal vessels and stimulates the synthesis of both FSH and LH, which are stored within gonadotrophs. Subsequently, GnRH activates and transforms these molecules into releasable forms. GnRH can also induce immediate release of both LH and FSH into the circulation.

GnRH is secreted in a pulsatile fashion that is fundamental to the gonadotropin secretion profile seen during the normal menstrual cycle. In fact, the pulsatile patterns of LH and FSH release from the pituitary are correlated well with the intermittent output of hypothalamic GnRH. Moreover, pulsatile administration of synthetic GnRH can induce ovulation.

The hypothalamus produces PIF, which exerts chronic inhibition of prolactin release from the lactotrophs. A number of pharmacologic agents that affect dopaminergic mechanisms influence prolactin release. Dopamine itself is secreted by hypothalamic neurons into the hypophyseal portal vessels, and it inhibits prolactin release directly within the adenohypophysis. Based on these observations, it has been proposed that hypothalamic dopamine may be the PIF. In addition to the regulation of prolactin release by PIF, the hypothalamus may also produce prolactin-releasing factors (PRF) that can elicit large and rapid increases in prolactin release under different conditions, such as breast stimulation during nursing. Neither PIF nor PRF has been well-characterized biochemically. Very recently, the precursor protein for GnRH has been found to be a potent inhibitor of prolactin secretion and a stimulator of gonadotropin release. These findings suggest that this GnRH-associated peptide may be the physiologic PIF and could explain the inverse relationship between gonadotropin and prolactin secretion seen in many reproductive states. TRH also stimulates prolactin release under experimental conditions.

Feedback Control of Gonadotropin Secretion

A normal ovarian cycle can be divided into a follicular phase, a midcycle ovulatory phase, and a luteal phase. The cycle actually begins in the late luteal phase of the preceding cycle when regression of the corpus luteum causes decreases in circulating estradiol and progesterone, which result in a rise in serum FSH. The *follicular phase* of the ovarian cycle begins with this small but significant rise in serum FSH, which initiates follicular growth. LH begins to increase one to two days later than FSH. About seven days later (or seven to eight days before the midcycle LH surge), ovarian estradiol secretion begins to increase, slowly at first and then rapidly, and reaches a maximum shortly before the midcycle LH surge. The increased estradiol and estrone levels lower serum FSH and cause a small but steady rise in LH.

At this time, the follicle destined to ovulate protects itself from premature atresia by its own secretion of estradiol. The high local concentration of estradiol within the follicular fluid enhances FSH binding to the follicle, thereby increasing follicular sensitivity to FSH stimulation.

During the late follicular phase, the rising estradiol titer initiates the midcycle LH and FSH surges. Estradiol appears to increase hypothalamic secretion of GnRH, which, in turn, enhances pituitary secretion of gonadotropins. Thus, the initiation of the midcycle LH and FSH surges could be due to: (1) an enhanced pituitary gonadotropin responsiveness to hypothalamic GnRH; or (2) increases in hypothalamic GnRH release and in the portal plasma levels of GnRH. Both mechanisms may be operative. As noted previously, the onset of the midcycle LH surge is accompanied by a small but steady increase in progesterone secretion from the preovulatory follicle. This small increase in serum progesterone probably enhances and prolongs the positive feedback effects of estradiol on LH and FSH secretion.

At *midcycle*, the LH surge leads to the final maturation of the preovulatory follicle, and ovulation occurs 16 to 24 hours later. Shortly before the onset of the LH surge and long before the rupture of the follicle, there is a precipitous decrease in estradiol secretion. Although the majority of circulating estradiol during the late follicular phase comes from the single maturing follicle destined to ovulate, the cause for the preovulatory decline in follicular production of estradiol is unknown. A significant fall in circulating estradiol is not a prerequisite for the initiation of the LH surge.

The FSH surge at midcycle follows a similar pattern to that of LH but is smaller in magnitude. The increased serum FSH levels at midcycle may enhance the genesis of LH receptors within the preovulatory follicle, thereby facilitating the processes of LH-mediated ovulation and luteinization.

Following ovulation, both the granulosa cells and theca interna cells undergo *luteinization* in response to LH. The corpus luteum consists of granulosa lutein cells, theca lutein cells, capillaries, and connective tissue. Together they secrete large amounts of progesterone and estradiol.

During the *luteal phase,* both LH and FSH are significantly suppressed through a potent negative feedback effect secondary to elevated circulating estradiol and progesterone levels. This inhibition of gonadotropins persists until near the end of the luteal phase, when the production of both progesterone and estradiol decreases secondary to regression of the corpus luteum. Removal of the steroid negative feedback inhibition then results in a rise in serum FSH, which initiates follicular growth for the subsequent cycle.

Ovarian steroids can either inhibit or stimulate gonadotropin release. Estradiol usually exerts an inhibitory effect on gonadotropin release via a negative feedback mechanism. Estradiol and progesterone in combination exert a very potent negative feedback inhibition on gonadotropins. Of the two gonadotropins, FSH is more sensitive than LH to the negative feedback by estrogens. Thus, there is often a reciprocal relationship between serum levels of estradiol and FSH. It is only under conditions of specific dose levels and duration of exposure that high concentrations of circulating estradiol exert a positive feedback on gonadotropin secretion. Examples are during the late follicular phase of the ovarian cycle and after estradiol administration during the early follicular phase. While the negative feedback of estrogens on gonadotropin release operates within minutes, the positive feedback requires greater than 24 hours of estrogen exposure.

Possible Role of Prolactin in Ovulatory Function

Serum prolactin levels do not change strikingly during the normal menstrual cycle. However, both serum levels of prolactin, as well as prolactin release in response to TRH, are somewhat more elevated during the luteal phase than during the midfollicular phase of the cycle. This suggests that high amounts of circulating estradiol and progesterone may enhance prolactin release. Prolactin release does exhibit a diurnal pattern, with the highest levels occurring during nocturnal sleep.

Prolactin may participate in the control of ovarian steroidogenesis. Prolactin concentrations in follicular fluid change markedly during follicular growth. The highest prolactin concentrations are seen in small follicles during the early follicular phase. Prolactin concentrations in the follicular fluid may be inversely related to the production of progesterone. In addition, hyperprolactinemia may alter gonadotropin secretion. Despite these observations, the physiologic significance of prolactin during the normal menstrual cycle has not been established.

HISTOPHYSIOLOGY OF THE ENDOMETRIUM

The endometrium is uniquely responsive to the circulating progestins, androgens, and estrogens. It is this responsiveness that gives rise to menstruation and makes implantation and pregnancy possible.

Functionally, the endometrium is divided into two zones: (1) the upper portion, or *functionalis,* that undergoes cyclic changes in morphology and function during the menstrual cycle and is sloughed off at menstruation; (2) the lower portion, or *basalis,* that remains relatively unchanged during each menstrual cycle and, after menstruation, provides stem cells for the renewal of the functionalis. Basal arteries are regular blood vessels found in the basalis, whereas spiral arteries are specially coiled blood vessels seen in the functionalis.

The cyclic changes in histophysiology of the endometrium can be divided into three stages: the menstrual phase, the proliferative or estrogenic phase, and the secretory or progestational phase.

Menstrual Phase

Because it is the only portion of the cycle that is visible externally, the first day of menstruation is taken as day one of the menstrual cycle. The first four days of the cycle are defined as the menstrual phase. During this phase, there is disruption and disintegration of the endometrial glands and stroma, leukocyte infiltration, and red blood cell extravasation. In addition to this sloughing of the functionalis, there is a compression of the basalis due to the loss of ground substances. In spite of these degenerative changes, early evidence of renewed tissue growth is usually present at this time within the basalis of the endometrium.

Proliferative Phase

The proliferative phase is characterized by endometrial proliferation or growth secondary to estrogen stimulation. Because the bases of the endometrial glands lie deep within the basalis, these epithelial cells are not destroyed during menstruation. As menstruation ends each month, they provide the source of stem cells that divide and migrate through the stroma to form a new epithelial lining of the endometrium and new endometrial glands.

During this phase of the cycle, the large increase in estrogen secretion causes marked cellular proliferation of the epithelial lining,

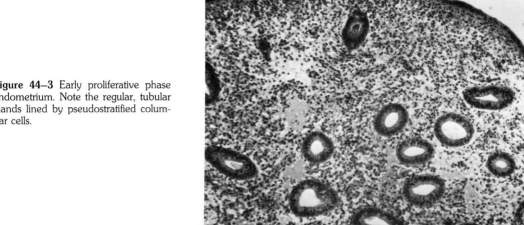

Figure 44–3 Early proliferative phase endometrium. Note the regular, tubular glands lined by pseudostratified columnar cells.

the endometrial glands, and the connective tissues of the stroma (Fig. 44–3). Numerous mitoses are present in these tissues. There is an increase in the length of the spiral arteries, which transgress almost the entire thickness of the endometrium. By the end of the proliferative phase, cellular proliferation and endometrial growth have reached a maximum, the spiral arteries are elongated and convoluted, and the endometrial glands are straight, with narrow lumens containing some glycogen. True secretory function in the glands must await progesterone secretion by the corpus luteum.

Secretory Phase

Following ovulation, progesterone secretion by the corpus luteum stimulates the glandular cells to secrete glycogen, mucus, and other substances. The glands become tortuous, and the lumens are dilated and filled with the secretion. The stroma becomes edematous. Mitoses are rare. The spiral arteries continue to extend into the superficial layer of the endometrium and become convoluted (Fig. 44–4).

The marked changes that occur in endometrial histology during the secretory phase permit relatively precise timing (dating) of secretory endometrium.

If pregnancy does not occur by day 23, the corpus luteum begins to regress, secretion of progesterone and estradiol declines, and the endometrium undergoes involution. About one day prior to the onset of menstruation, there is marked constriction of the spiral arterioles causing ischemia of the endometrium followed by leukocyte infiltration and red blood cell extravasation. It is postulated that this occurs secondary to prostaglandins produced by the endometrium. The resulting

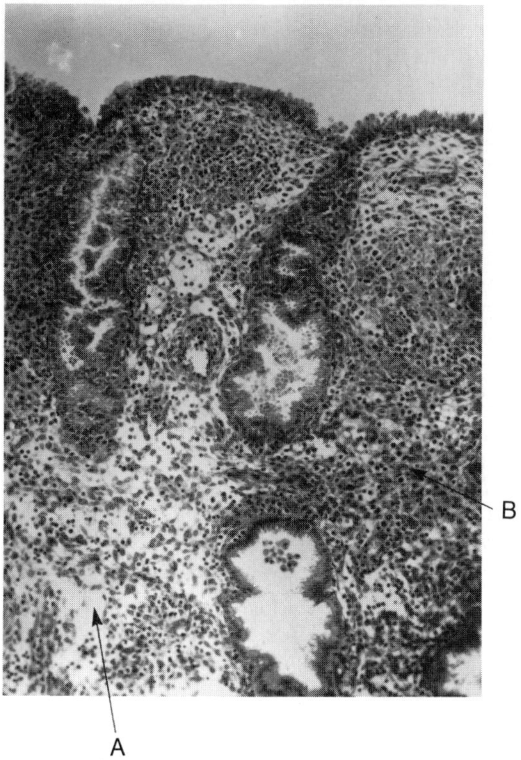

Figure 44–4 Late secretory phase endometrium. Note the tortuous, saw-toothed appearance of the endometrial glands with secretions in the lumen. Edema is seen on the left (A) and decidua (B) on the right.

necrosis causes menstruation or sloughing of the endometrium. Thus, menstruation, which clinically marks the beginning of the menstrual cycle, is actually the terminal event that enables the uterus to prepare itself to receive another conceptus.

SUGGESTED READING

Benirschke K: The endometrium. In Yen SSC, Jaffe RB (eds): Reproductive Endocrinology. Philadelphia, W B Saunders Co, 1978, p 241.

Block E: Quantitative morphological investigations of the follicular system in women: Variations in different phases of the sexual cycle. Acta Endocrinol 8:33, 1951.

Daughaday WH: The adenohypophysis. In Williams RH (ed): Textbook of Endocrinology. Philadelphia, W B Saunders Co, 1981, p 73.

Erickson GF: Normal ovarian function. Clin Obstet Gynecol 21:31, 1978.

McNatty KP: Cyclic changes in antral fluid hormone concentrations in humans. J Clin Endocrinol Metab 7:577, 1978.

Moore RY: Neuroendocrine regulation of reproduction. In Yen SSC, Jaffe RB (eds): Reproductive Endocrinology. Philadelphia, W B Saunders Co, 1978, p 3.

Naftolin F, Tolis G: Neuroendocrine regulation of the menstrual cycle. Clin Obstet Gynecol 21:17, 1978.

Nikolices K, Mason AJ, Szonyi E, et al: A prolactin-inhibiting factor within the precursor for human gonadotropin-releasing hormone. Nature 316:511, 1985.

Noyes RW, Hertig AT, Rock J: Dating the endometrial biopsy. Fertil Steril 1:3, 1950.

Ross GT, Schreiber JR: The ovary. In Yen SSC, Jaffe RB (eds): Reproductive Endocrinology. Philadelphia, W B Saunders Co, 1978, p 63.

Ross GT, Van de Wiele RL: The ovaries. In Williams RH (ed): Textbook of Endocrinology. Philadelphia, W B Saunders Co, 1981, p 355.

Speroff L, Glass RH, Kase NG: Regulation of the menstrual cycle. In Speroff L, Glass RH, Kase NG (eds): Clinical Gynecologic Endocrinology and Infertility. Baltimore, Williams & Wilkins, 1978, p 49.

Yen SSC: The human menstrual cycle. In Yen SSC, Jaffe RB (eds): Reproductive Endocrinology. Philadelphia, W B Saunders Co, 1978, p 126.

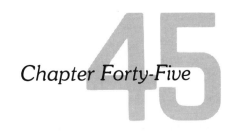

Chapter Forty-Five

ENDOCRINOLOGY OF PREGNANCY AND PARTURITION

MARY E. CARSTEN

Women undergo major endocrinologic and metabolic changes in order to establish, maintain, and terminate pregnancy. The purpose of these changes is the delivery of an infant that can survive outside the uterus. The maturation of the fetus and the adaptation of the mother are regulated by a variety of hormones. This chapter deals with the properties, functions, and interactions of the most important of these hormones as they relate to pregnancy and parturition.

THE FETOPLACENTAL UNIT

The concept of the fetoplacental unit is based on the interactions of a variety of hormones of fetal and maternal origin. The fetoplacental unit largely controls the endocrine events of the pregnancy.

Components of the Unit

Although there is input from the fetus, the placenta, and the mother, the fetus appears to play the most active and controlling role.

The Fetal Adrenal Gland. The adrenal gland is the major fetal endocrine component. In midpregnancy it is larger than the fetal kidney. It consists of an outer definitive or *adult zone* and an inner *fetal zone*. The adult zone later develops into the three components of the adult adrenal cortex—namely, the zona fasciculata, the zona glomerulosa, and the zona reticularis. It secretes mineralocorticoids and glucocorticoids. At term, the fetal zone constitutes 80 percent of the fetal gland. During fetal life, it primarily secretes androgens. It involutes following delivery and completely disappears by the end of the first year of life. The fetal adrenal medulla is poorly developed.

The Placenta. The placenta produces both steroid and peptide hormones in amounts that vary with gestational age. Precursors for progesterone synthesis come from the maternal circulation. Because of a lack of 17α-hydroxylase, the placenta cannot convert progesterone to estrogen but must use androgens, largely from the fetal adrenal, as its source of precursor for estrogen production.

Peptide Hormones

Human Chorionic Gonadotropin (hCG). This hormone maintains pregnancy. It is a glycoprotein with a molecular weight of 40,000 to 45,000 and is secreted by trophoblastic cells of the placenta. It consists of two subunits, alpha (α) and beta (β). The α subunit is shared with luteinizing hormone (LH) and thyroid-stimulating hormone (TSH). The specificity of hCG is related to its β subunit, and a specific β subunit radioimmunoassay allows positive identification of hCG. The presence of hCG at times other than pregnancy signals the presence of an hCG-producing tumor, usually a hydatidiform mole, choriocarcinoma, or embryonal carcinoma.

During pregnancy, hCG begins to rise eight days after ovulation (nine days after the mid-cycle LH peak) and provides the basis for virtually all immunologic or chemical pregnancy tests. With continuing pregnancy, hCG values peak at 60 to 90 days and then decline to a moderate, more constant level. For the first six to eight weeks of pregnancy, hCG maintains the corpus luteum and thereby ensures continued progesterone output until the placenta takes over progesterone production. Titers of hCG are usually abnormally low with ectopic pregnancy and threatened abortion and abnormally high with trophoblastic disease. This hormone may also regulate steroid biosynthesis in the placenta and the fetal adrenal gland and stimulate testosterone production in the fetal testicle. Although immune suppression has been ascribed to hCG, this function cannot be verified using pure preparations.

Human Placental Lactogen (HPL). HPL originates in the placenta and is a single chain polypeptide with a molecular weight of 22,300. It is similar to pituitary growth hormone and to human prolactin. Maternal serum concentrations parallel placental weight, rising throughout gestation to maximum levels in the last four weeks. At term, HPL accounts for 10 percent of all placental protein production. Low values are found with threatened abortion and intrauterine fetal growth retardation. HPL antagonizes the cellular action of insulin and decreases glucose utilization. Therefore, it may play a role in shifting glucose availability toward the fetus.

Prolactin. Prolactin is a peptide from the anterior pituitary with a molecular weight of about 20,000. Normal nonpregnant levels are approximately 10 ng/ml. During pregnancy, maternal prolactin levels rise because of increasing maternal estrogen output, which stimulates the anterior pituitary lactotrophs. Although the decidua is a further source of prolactin production, it contributes little to the plasma pool. Amniotic fluid levels exceed those in the circulation. The main effect of prolactin is stimulation of milk production. In the second half of pregnancy, prolactin secreted by the fetal pituitary may be an important stimulus of fetal adrenal growth. Prolactin may play a role in fluid and electrolyte shifts across the fetal membranes.

Steroid Hormones

Progesterone. Progesterone is the most important human progestogen. In the luteal phase, it induces secretory changes in the endometrium; in pregnancy, higher levels induce decidual changes. Up to the sixth or seventh week of pregnancy, the major source of progesterone is the ovary. Thereafter, the placenta begins to play the major role. Progesterone production by the corpus luteum is essential for continuation of pregnancy up to seven weeks. If the corpus luteum of pregnancy is removed before seven weeks and continuation of the pregnancy is desired, progesterone must be given to prevent spontaneous abortion.

Steroid biochemical pathways are shown in Figure 45–1. Circulating progesterone is mostly bound to carrier proteins (albumin, orosomucoid, transcortin); less than 10 percent is free. Probably only the free progesterone is physiologically active.

Progesterone prevents myometrial contractions and the myometrium receives progesterone directly from the venous blood draining the placenta. Progesterone also probably induces some immune tolerance for the products of conception.

The fetus inactivates progesterone by transformation to corticosteroids or by hydroxylation or conjugation to inert excretory products. However, the placenta can convert these inert materials back to progesterone.

Estrogens. Both fetus and placenta are involved in the biosynthesis of estrone, estradiol, and estriol. Cholesterol is converted to pregnenolone or pregnenolone sulfate in the placenta. These precursors are converted to dehydroepiandrosterone sulfate (DHEA-S) in the fetal and maternal adrenals. The DHEA-S is then converted by the placenta to estrone (E_1) and, via testosterone, to estradiol (E_2). In contrast, estriol (E_3) is synthesized by the placenta largely from 16α-hydroxy DHEA-S, which is produced in the fetal liver from adrenal DHEA-S. Placental sulfatase is required to deconjugate 16-OH-DHEA-S prior to conversion to E_3 (Fig. 45–2). Steroid sulfatase activity in the placenta is high, except in rare cases of sulfatase deficiency.

Anencephalic fetuses lack a hypothalamus and have hypoplastic anterior pituitary and adrenals, so estriol production is only about 10 percent of normal levels. In nonanence-

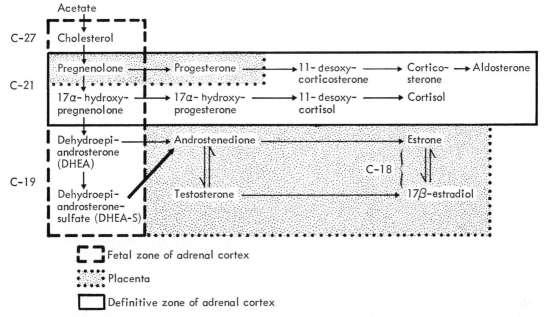

Figure 45–1 Main pathways of steroid hormone biosynthesis. Adrenal DHEA is largely transported as its sulfate, DHEA-S, which can also be formed from steroid sulfates starting with cholesterol sulfate.

phalic fetuses, a sudden fall in estriol may indicate fetal compromise. Although estriol determinations have been used as a means of monitoring fetal well-being, present use is limited, and estriol measurements have generally been replaced by biophysical assessments.

Androgens. During pregnancy, androgens originate mainly in the fetal zone of the fetal adrenal cortex. Androgen secretion is stimulated by adrenocorticotrophic hormone (ACTH) and hCG, the latter being effective primarily in the first half of pregnancy when

it is present in high concentration. The fetal adrenal favors production of DHEA over testosterone and androstenedione, and it sulfurylates almost all steroids. Fetal androgens enter the placental circulation and serve as precursors for estradiol and estriol.

The fetal testis also secretes androgens, particularly testosterone. Testosterone is converted to dihydrotestosterone, which is required for the development of the male external genitalia. The main trophic stimulus appears to be hCG.

Glucocorticoids. Cortisol is derived from

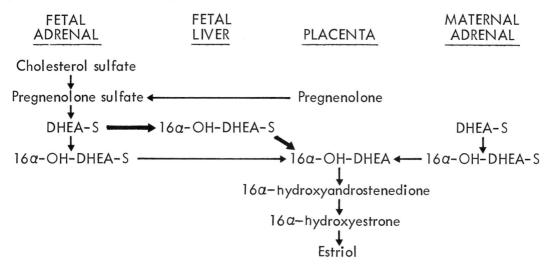

Figure 45–2 Formation of estriol in the fetal placental unit.

circulating cholesterol (Fig. 45–1). Maternal plasma cortisol concentrations rise throughout pregnancy, and the diurnal rhythm of cortisol secretion persists. The plasma level of transcortin rises in pregnancy, probably stimulated by estrogen, and the plasma free cortisol concentration doubles.

The fetal adrenal and the placenta both participate in cortisol metabolism. The fetal adrenal is stimulated by ACTH originating from the fetal pituitary to produce both cortisol and DHEA-S. In contrast to DHEA-S, which is produced in the fetal zone, cortisol originates in the definitive zone.

Cortisol plays an important function in the maturation of the lungs. It promotes differentiation of type II alveolar cells and the biosynthesis and release of surfactant into the alveoli. Surfactant decreases the force required to inflate the lungs. Insufficiency of surfactant leads to respiratory distress, which can cause death.

CHANGES IN MATERNAL METABOLISM

Maternal metabolism adapts to pregnancy through endocrine regulation. The changes in insulin and thyroid hormone metabolism are discussed in Chapter 4.

Angiotensin-Aldosterone

Aldosterone is a mineralocorticoid synthesized in the zona glomerulosa of the adrenal cortex. The fetal adrenal and the placenta do not participate significantly in aldosterone production during pregnancy, although the fetal adrenal is capable of synthesizing aldosterone. Aldosterone secretion is regulated by the renin-angiotensin system. Increased renin formed in the kidney converts angiotensinogen (renin substrate) to angiotensin I, which is converted to angiotensin II, which, in turn, stimulates aldosterone secretion. Aldosterone stimulates the absorption of sodium and the secretion of potassium in the distal tubule of the kidney, thereby maintaining sodium and potassium balance. Renin substrate concentration rises in pregnancy. It is thought that the high concentration of progesterone and estrogen present during pregnancy stimulate renin and renin substrate formation respectively, thus giving rise to

greater aldosterone production. Aldosterone secretion rates decline in toxemic pregnancies and in some cases may fall below nonpregnant levels.

Calcium Metabolism

Although calcium absorption is increased in pregnancy, total maternal serum calcium declines. The fall in total calcium parallels that of serum albumin, since approximately half of the total calcium is bound to albumin. Ionic calcium, the physiologically important calcium fraction, remains essentially constant throughout pregnancy because of increased maternal production of parathyroid hormone. In late pregnancy, increased serum parathyroid hormone enhances both intestinal absorption of calcium and bone resorption. This counteracts the inhibition of bone resorption caused by the increased circulating estrogen. Urinary calcium excretion is decreased.

Calcium ions are actively transported across the placenta, and fetal serum levels of total as well as ionized calcium are higher than maternal levels in late pregnancy. Parathyroid hormone does not cross the placenta. High fetal ionic calcium suppresses fetal parathyroid hormone production and stimulates calcitonin production, thus providing the fetus with ample calcium for calcification of the skeleton. In the first 24 to 48 hours postpartum, the total serum calcium concentration in the neonate usually falls, while the phosphorus concentration rises. Both adjust to adult levels within one week.

Other Hormones and Transmitters

Oxytocin. Oxytocin is an octapeptide that originates in the supraoptic and paraventricular nuclei of the hypothalamus and migrates down the nerve fibers to accumulate at the nerve endings in the posterior pituitary. The release of oxytocin is augmented by several stimuli, such as distension of the birth canal and mammary stimulation. The physiologic role of oxytocin in initiating labor is unclear. Impairment of oxytocin production, as in diabetes insipidus, does not interfere with normal labor. While oxytocin release appears to be inhibited by clinically acceptable levels of ethanol, this is not particularly useful for suppression of labor. Moreover, maternal serum oxytocin levels do not rise prior to labor, although myometrial sensitivity to oxytocin is increased. Administered oxytocin can induce labor only at or near term.

Prostaglandins. Prostaglandins are a family of ubiquitous, biologically active lipids that have many functions. They are not true hormones—for example, they are not synthesized in one gland and transported via the circulating blood to a target organ. Rather, they are synthesized at or near their site of action. Prostaglandin E_2 (PGE_2) and prostaglandin $F_{2\alpha}$ ($PGF_{2\alpha}$) are synthesized in the endometrium and myometrium and cause contraction of the uterus. They can also cause contraction of other smooth muscles, such as those of the intestinal tract. When prostaglandins are used pharmacologically, they may give rise to undesirable side effects such as nausea, vomiting, and diarrhea. PGE_2 and $PGF_{2\alpha}$ amniotic fluid concentrations rise throughout pregnancy and increase further during spontaneous labor. Levels are lower in oxytocin-induced labor than in spontaneous labor. Administration of PGE_2 or $PGF_{2\alpha}$ by various routes induces labor or abortion at any stage of gestation.

Since prostaglandins are believed to be very important in the initiation and control of labor, their synthesis is reviewed in that context. Prostaglandin synthesis begins with the formation of arachidonic acid, an obligatory precursor of the prostaglandins of the "2" series. Free arachidonic acid does not accumulate but is stored in esterified form as glycerophospholipids in the trophoblastic membranes. Labor appears to be accompanied by a cascade of events in the chorion, amnion, and decidua that releases arachidonic acid from its stored form and converts it to active prostaglandin. The initial step is the hydrolysis of glycerophospholipids which is catalyzed by phospholipases A_2 and C. This gives rise to lysoglycerophospholipids and arachidonic acid. Lysoglycerophospholipids are cytolytic agents that cause cell disruption and, consequently, disruption of decidual lysosomes with release of more phospholipase A_2. Phospholipase A_2 preferentially acts on chorionic phosphatidyl ethanolamine to release more arachidonic acid. Progesterone stabilizes cell and lysosomal membranes. This prevents premature release of phospholipase

and the consequent formation of free arachidonic acid. 17β-estradiol stimulates several enzymes active in the synthesis of prostaglandins from arachidonic acid.

Increased phospholipase A_2 activity may lead to premature labor. Endocervical, intrauterine, or urinary tract infections are often associated with premature labor. Many of the organisms producing these infections have phospholipase A_2 activity, which could produce free arachidonic acid, followed by prostaglandin synthesis, which could trigger the labor.

PGE_2 and other prostaglandins play a role in ripening the cervix by inducing changes in the connective tissue. Prostaglandins are clinically useful for cervical ripening prior to induction of labor or abortion.

The Biochemical Basis of Contraction

Contraction of the myometrium is brought about by the sliding of actin and myosin filaments and requires adenosine triphosphate (ATP) and calcium. Unlike skeletal muscle, which requires innervation, smooth muscle contraction depends primarily on hormonal stimuli to regulate calcium movement at the cell membane. Thus, calcium enters the smooth muscle cell through both voltage and receptor-operated channels. Receptors for oxytocin as well as for prostaglandins have been found in the myometrial cell membrane. Recent findings have demonstrated entry of hormones into the cell, and receptors for prostaglandins inside the cell in the sarcoplasmic reticulum. The binding of oxytocin and prostaglandins to the receptors decreases calcium accumulation by the sarcoplasmic reticulum and/or calcium transport out of the cell. The high calcium concentration thus created enables the myofibrils of the myometrium to contract. ATP is subsequently needed for reducing the free calcium to the level of relaxation.

Unlike the heart, where the bundle of His is present, no anatomic structures for synchronization of contractions have been found in the uterus. Instead, contraction spreads as current flows from cell to cell through areas of low resistance. Such areas are associated with gap junctions that become especially prominent at parturition following the decline of circulating progesterone.

PARTURITION

Hormonal Control of Gestational Length and the Initiation of Labor

Gestational length is under hormonal control, and is usually under the hormonal control of the fetus. However, each species has not only a unique gestational interval but also unique mechanisms for controlling the length of the gestation. Thus, although animal models provide important insight, they do not provide specific information concerning the control of the human gestational interval or the mechanisms controlling initiation of labor in the human. Nevertheless, animal models are well worth examining.

Animal Models. In the *sheep,* 17α-hydroxylase in the placenta converts progesterone to estrogen. This conversion is controlled by cortisol. Labor commences when a surge of cortisol from the fetus results in decreased progesterone levels and increased estrogen levels. ACTH, glucocorticoids, or dexamethasone also cause parturition. Removal of the fetal pituitary or adrenal, which are required for the cortisol surge, results in prolonged pregnancy.

In a breed of *Guernsey cows* with a genetic defect resulting in fetal pituitary and adrenal malfunction, pregnancy is prolonged, and normal vaginal delivery does not occur. In the *rabbit*, parturition directly follows a decline in progesterone production secondary to a decline in corpus luteal function. Abortion can be prevented by administration of progesterone.

The Human. In the human, hormonal effects are important in determining gestational length and in initiating labor. Although fetal-maternal interaction occurs, it is largely the fetus that determines the duration of pregnancy. The stimulus for parturition originates in the fetal hypothalamus, but the initiating event is not known.

The current hypothesis is that the fetal hypothalamus stimulates the fetal pituitary to secrete ACTH, and other hormones, which in turn stimulate the fetal adrenal to secrete glucocorticoids and androgens (Fig. 45–3). These are transported to the placenta where the androgens are converted to estrogens. Cortisol stimulates placental estrogen synthesis by direct action on the appropriate enzyme systems and decreases progesterone secretion, thus causing an increase in the estrogen:progesterone ratio. Progesterone decline is followed by (a) the appearance of myometrial gap junctions, which provide areas of low resistance to current flow and increase coordinated uterine contractions; (b) an increase in the concentration of estrogen and oxytocin receptors in the myometrium; and (c) an increase in phospholipase A_2 and C activity, which liberate the prostaglandin precursor arachidonic acid in the fetal mem-

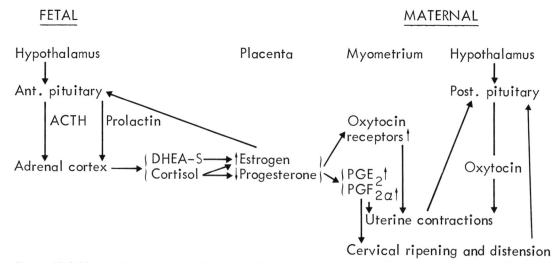

Figure 45–3 Major pathways proposed for hormonal actions in the initiation of human parturition. In addition to myometrial production, PGE_2 and $PGF_{2\alpha}$ are also synthesized in the endometrium and the fetal membranes, and prostacyclin in the cervix. Note the presence of several self-enhancing feedback loops.

branes, thus stimulating PGE_2 and $PGF_{2\alpha}$ synthesis.

Greater production of adrenal androgens provides increased estrogen precursors and results in increased estrogen synthesis. Estrogen appears to have three functions: (a) it stimulates prolactin biosynthesis in the fetal anterior pituitary gland, which, in turn, stimulates fetal adrenal growth; (b) it stimulates prostaglandin biosynthesis in the fetal membranes, decidua, and, probably, in the myometrium by increasing the synthesis and turnover of precursor phospholipid, and activating specific enzymes needed for prostaglandin synthesis; and (c) it enhances uterine responsiveness to oxytocin.

Prostaglandins cause uterine contractions, increase the sensitivity of the uterus to oxytocin, and ripen the cervix. Distension of the cervix stimulates release of more prostaglandin. Distension of the birth canal stimulates release of oxytocin from the maternal posterior pituitary gland via a neural reflex (Ferguson reflex).

For this entire hypothesis to be correct, a functioning fetal hypothalamus, pituitary, and adrenal gland, and a functioning placenta are required. Some clinical experience supports this hypothesis, while some does not. Fetal anencephaly and adrenal hypoplasia frequently cause prolonged pregnancy, which supports the hypothesis. However, infusion of ACTH, glucocorticoids, or dexamethasone does not cause premature labor in the human. A fall in maternal serum progesterone is not always present with the onset of labor, and progesterone injection has not been found helpful in the treatment of premature labor. It is possible that injected progesterone does not reach the myometrial cells in a sufficiently high concentration to inhibit contractions. A precipitous increase in estradiol has not been demonstrated prior to the onset of labor, and administration of estradiol will not induce labor in the human. However, it seems likely that the changes in the estrogen:progesterone ratio play a facilitory role in initiating the onset of human parturition.

Future research should increase our knowledge in this important area, and hopefully improve our ability to prevent premature labor and delivery, which are currently the leading causes of perinatal mortality.

SUGGESTED READING

Carsten ME, Miller JD: Regulation of myometrial contractions. In MacDonald PC, Porter J (eds): Initiation of Parturition: Prevention of Prematurity. Columbus, Ross Laboratories, 1983, p 166.

Hartshorne DJ: Biochemical basis for contraction of vascular smooth muscle. Chest 78:140, 1980.

Jaffe RB: The endocrinology of pregnancy. In Yen SSC, Jaffe RB (eds): Reproductive Endocrinology: Physiology, Pathology and Clinical Management. Philadelphia, W B Saunders Co, 1978, p 521.

Liggins GC: Endocrinology of parturition. In Novy MJ, Resko JA (eds): Fetal Endocrinology. New York, Academic Press Inc, 1981, p 211.

MacDonald PC, Porter JC, Schwarz BE, et al: Initiation of parturition in the human female. Semin Perinatol 2(3):273, 1978.

Pitkin RM: Calcium metabolism in pregnancy and the perinatal period: A review. Am J Obstet Gynecol 151:99, 1985.

Seron-Ferre M, Jaffe RB: The fetal adrenal gland. Ann Rev Physiol 43:141, 1981.

Simpson ER, MacDonald PC: Endocrine physiology of the placenta. Ann Rev Physiol 43:163, 1981.

Small JV: The contractile and cytoskeletal elements of vertebrate smooth muscle. In Casteels R, Godfraind T, Ruegg JC (eds): Excitation-Contraction Coupling in Smooth Muscle. Amsterdam, Elsevier North-Holland Biomedical Press, 1977, p 305.

Szego CM: Parallels in the modes of action of peptide and steroid hormones: Membrane effects and cellular entry. In McKerns KW (ed): Structures and Function of the Gonadotropins. New York, Plenum Publishing Co, 1978, p 431.

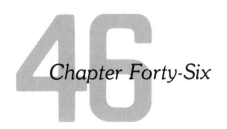

Chapter Forty-Six

PUBERTY AND PRECOCIOUS PUBERTY

MARIA BUSTILLO

Puberty is the period of transition from childhood to adulthood during which reproductive capacity is attained. This transition is associated with many complex physical, endocrinologic, psychologic, and behavioral changes. *Menarche* is the time of occurrence of the first menstrual flow. *Thelarche* is the time of first occurrence of the effects of estrogens, usually manifest by breast development. *Adrenarche* is the time of first occurrence of the effects of androgens, usually manifest by pubic or axillary hair. Puberty is not complete until regular ovulatory cycles and full reproductive capability are established.

In North America, the median age at menarche is approximately 12.8 years. Sexual maturation has accelerated and the age at menarche has declined over the last 100 years. These occurrences have been attributed to improvements in nutrition and general health. In recent years, this trend has not continued.

PHYSICAL CHANGES AT PUBERTY

The significant physical changes of puberty include the acquisition of secondary sexual characteristics, the adolescent growth spurt, changes in body composition, and the commencement of menstruation. The physical changes in breast and pubic hair development have been standardized and are widely utilized for diagnostic purposes.

Secondary Sexual Changes

The first sign of puberty in the female is usually early breast development (thelarche). Breast development is best quantified utilizing Tanner's five stages (Fig. 46–1). The description of these stages is based on anatomic relationships and is independent of breast size. Menarche occurs when breast development has reached Tanner Stage 3 or greater. The average time interval from the onset of breast development to menarche is approximately three years (Fig. 46–2).

Breast development is followed by pubic hair development, which has also been tabulated in Tanner stages from Stage 1, the absence of pubic hair, to Stage 5, the final adult hair pattern (Fig. 46–3). The distribution is in the shape of an inverse triangle (female escutcheon) with some spread to the medial thighs.

Adolescent Growth Spurt

The ultimate adult height is influenced to a major degree by the adolescent growth spurt. The period of most rapid linear growth, referred to as the *peak height velocity*, is reached about one year after breast budding, about one and one-half years before menarche, and about two years earlier than in normal males. There is very limited growth after menarche. Thus, girls who experience early menarche tend to be shorter in stature than those who first menstruate at a later age.

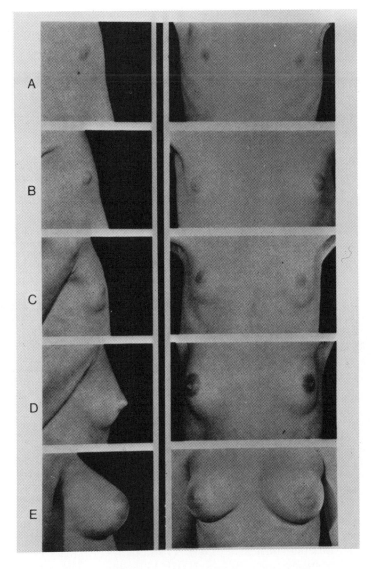

Figure 46–1 Stages of breast development: *A,* Stage 1: prepubertal breast. *B,* Stage 2: breast bud stage. *C,* Stage 3: further breast and areolar enlargement. *D,* Stage 4: areola and papilla form a secondary mound. *E,* Stage 5: mature stage. Only papilla projects, areola recessed to general contour of breast. (Reproduced with permission from Styne DM, Grumbach MM: Puberty in the male and female: Its physiology and disorders. In Yen SCC, Jaffe RB (eds): Reproductive Endocrinology. Philadelphia, W B Saunders Co, 1978, p 191.)

Body Composition

Prior to puberty, males and females have approximately the same lean body mass, skeletal mass, and body fat composition. These relationships change as males acquire an increasing proportion of lean body mass and skeletal mass, and females an increased proportion of fat.

HORMONAL CHANGES AT PUBERTY

Gonadotropins

After the first or second year of life, the gonadotropins, follicle-stimulating hormone (FSH) and luteinizing hormone (LH), remain low until puberty. In the peripubertal period, there is first an enhanced release of LH, which initially occurs only during sleep. FSH and LH are secreted in episodic bursts of increasing frequency and magnitude. These pulsatile bursts are believed to be secondary to the synthesis and episodic release of gonadotropin-releasing hormone (GnRH) from the maturing hypothalamus.

Sex Steroids

Estradiol, secreted by the ovary, is the major sex steroid in the female. Estradiol concentrations rise throughout the stages of puberty and reach adult levels as Graafian

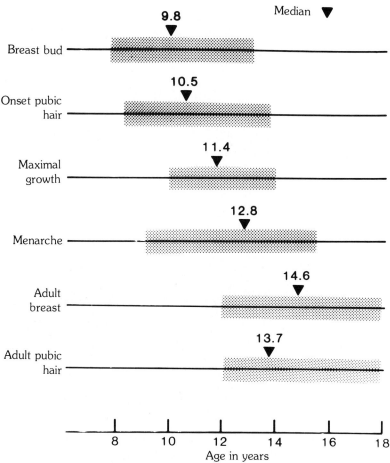

Figure 46–2 Chronological relationship of pubertal events. (Reproduced with permission from Speroff L, Glass RH, Kase NG: Clinical Gynecologic Endocrinology and Fertility. 3rd ed. Baltimore, Williams & Wilkins, 1983, p 371.)

follicles are recruited by FSH and LH and begin to mature. The adrenal androgens, dehydroepiandrosterone (DHEA) and dehydroepiandrosterone sulfate (DHEA-S), increase during early pubertal development. These increases, which precede changes in gonadotropins and estradiol, are associated with and may influence the development of pubic and axillary hair. The role of these adrenal androgens in the onset of puberty is not well understood.

CONTROL OF THE ONSET OF PUBERTY

Gonadostat Theory

The hypothalamic-pituitary-gonadal system is believed to be suppressed to very low levels during infancy and childhood. Before puberty, the hypothalamus and pituitary are apparently very sensitive to negative feedback by even the lowest levels of sex steroids. These low levels of sex steroids inhibit the secretion of FSH and LH. As puberty approaches there is a progressive decrease in the sensitivity of the hypothalamus and pituitary to sex steroids, resulting in increased release of GnRH and increased secretion of gonadotropins. Increased gonadotropin secretion then stimulates steroid output from the gonads, resulting in the development of secondary sexual characteristics.

The change in hypothalamic-pituitary sensitivity to the negative feedback of sex steroids takes place with or without a functioning gonad and must, therefore, be intrinsic to the central nervous system. This principle is clearly demonstrated in women with gonadal dysgenesis who have a biphasic pattern of FSH and LH secretion similar to that of

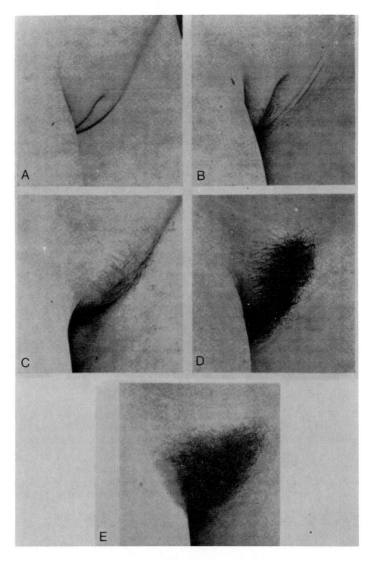

Figure 46–3 Stages of pubic hair development. *A,* Stage 1: no pubic hair. *B,* Stage 2: sparse hair on labia majora. *C,* Stage 3: darker, coarser hair extending to mons pubis. *D,* Stage 4: adult hair without spread to medial thighs. *E,* Stage 5: adult hair with spread to medial thighs. (Reproduced with permission from Styne DM, Grumbach MM: Puberty in the male and female: Its physiology and disorders. In Yen SCC, Jaffe RB (eds): Reproductive Endocrinology. Philadelphia, W B Saunders Co, 1978, p 192.)

normal women, even though the gonads are nonfunctional. The secretion of gonadotropins during the midchildhood years in patients with gonadal dysgenesis is similar to that of normal individuals, and the rise in pituitary output of gonadotropins in response to the absence of ovarian estrogen does not occur until the peripubertal years. During childhood, the low levels of gonadotropins that are secreted can be further suppressed by the administration of small amounts of exogenous sex steroids.

Factors that trigger the transition in hypothalamic-pituitary negative feedback sensitivity are not known. With the progression of puberty, the negative feedback mechanism becomes less sensitive to the suppressive effects of sex steroids. With further maturation of this system, the second, or positive, feedback mechanism becomes activated, establishing the fully mature ovulatory mechanism. This positive feedback mechanism is operative at midcycle and leads to the midcycle LH surge.

Body Composition Theory

Based on cross-sectional data, a relationship between critical body weight, amount of body fat, and the timing of the onset of puberty has been proposed. The onset of menarche is earlier in moderately obese girls, and later in those with chronic diseases and malnutrition. An "invariant mean weight" of 48 kg has been suggested as necessary for menarche in healthy girls. However, it has yet to be proven by direct prospective measurements that there is a metabolic signal leading to the onset of puberty.

PRECOCIOUS PUBERTY

Precocious puberty is a rare condition in which secondary sexual characteristics and accelerated growth appear at an early age. Because sexual development in normal girls usually begins at a mean age of 11, precocious puberty in females is defined as sexual development before the age of 8, which is two and a half standard deviations below the mean. Precocious puberty occurs in approximately 1 child out of 10,000 in North America. It is more common in females than in males.

Precocious puberty can be classified several ways. *True precocious puberty* is associated with increased secretion of sex steroids that are dependent on premature activation of the hypothalamic-pituitary-gonadal axis. The clinical manifestations of true precocious puberty are shown in Table 46–1. *Pseudoprecocious puberty* is associated with an excessive secretion of sex steroids unrelated to increased gonadotropin secretion. *Isosexual precocious puberty* implies that the changes are appropriate to the phenotype—that is, feminization occurs in girls and virilization in boys. *Heterosexual precocious puberty* implies that the changes are inappropriate to the phenotype—that is, feminization occurs in boys due to excessive estrogen production, or virilization occurs in girls due to excessive androgen production.

Complete sexual precocity implies development of the full panoply of secondary sexual characteristics, while *incomplete sexual* *precocity* implies development of only isolated secondary sexual characteristics.

True Precocious Puberty

True precocious puberty, which is always complete, isosexual precocity, is more common in girls than boys. In girls, 80 percent of cases are *constitutional or idiopathic* and manifest as progressive breast and pubic hair development and progressive enlargement of the external genitalia. If untreated, sexual maturation follows the normal sequence but at an obviously younger age. These girls respond to the diagnostic administration of exogenous gonadotropin-releasing hormone (*GnRH stimulation test*), with a rise in gonadotropins similar to that seen in normal pubertal girls.

Central nervous system disorders can cause complete isosexual precocity, but this occurs much more commonly in boys than in girls. Tumors of the hypothalamus, pineal, or cerebral cortex, such as gliomas, ependymomas, and hamartomas, may be responsible. They are believed to alter the neural pathways that would normally inhibit the release of gonadotropin-releasing hormone before puberty. Infections, such as meningitis, encephalitis, or brain abscess, may cause sexual precocity, as may a number of miscellaneous conditions, such as head trauma, suprasellar cysts, and cerebral sarcoidosis.

The *McCune-Albright syndrome,* or polyostotic fibrous dysplasia, is a condition in which precocious development is seen in association with fibrous dysplasia, cysts of the skull and long bones, and irregularly edged *café au lait* skin spots. This syndrome is more common in females. The reason for the pre-

TABLE 46–1   CLINICAL FINDINGS IN TRUE PRECOCIOUS PUBERTY

FINDINGS	IDIOPATHIC	CNS TUMOR	McCUNE-ALBRIGHT	HYPOTHYROID
Breast enlargement	Yes	Yes	Yes	Yes
Pubic hair	Yes	Yes	Yes	Unusual
Vaginal bleeding	Yes	Yes	Yes	Yes
Virilizing signs	No	No	No	No
Bone age	Advanced	Advanced	Advanced	Normal or Retarded
Neurologic deficit	No	Yes	Yes	No
Abdominopelvic mass	No	No	No	No

Modified with permission from Ross GT, Vande Wiele RL: The ovaries. In Williams RH (ed): Textbook of Endocrinology. 6th ed. Philadelphia, W B Saunders Co, 1981, p 379.

cocious development is not known but is thought to be central in origin. In some patients, hyperplasia of both the adrenal and thyroid glands has been documented, suggesting a form of multiple endocrine adenomatosis.

Chronic severe juvenile hypothyroidism may be associated with premature sexual precocity and galactorrhea. Although the mechanism is unknown, gonadotropins are elevated in this condition, possibly secondary to thyroid-releasing hormone (TRH) stimulation of follicle-stimulating hormone (FSH).

Pseudoprecocious Puberty

Sexual maturation in patients with pseudoprecocious puberty occurs in the absence of pubertal levels of hypothalamic-pituitary hormones. Therefore, the production of sex steroids in these patients is independent of the secretion of FSH and LH by the pituitary. The clinical manifestations of pseudoprecocious puberty are shown in Table 46–2.

Autonomously functioning *follicular cysts*, which secrete estrogens, may cause pseudoprecocious puberty in young girls, as may estrogen-secreting *granulosa-theca cell tumors* of the ovary. The latter are generally palpable on physical examination. They are associated with elevated plasma estradiol levels that can be used to document total removal of the tumor and to screen for recurrence.

Exogenous *administration of estrogen* can produce sexual precocity. Children may ingest or absorb estrogen from lotions, creams, tonics, or oral contraceptives. Inquiry concerning access to and use of such materials should be a part of the history.

Tumors secreting human chorionic gonadotropin (hCG) have been associated with isosexual precocity in males. These tumors are generally *hepatomas* or *hepatoblastomas,* and they produce their effects by means of hCG stimulation of testosterone production by the testicular Leydig cells. Ovarian neoplasms secreting hCG in girls are not associated with signs of puberty, unless the neoplasm is also secreting estrogen because hCG does not induce estrogen production by the ovary.

Incomplete Sexual Precocity

Incomplete pubertal development can be seen in young girls as a consequence of premature thelarche and premature adrenarche. *Premature thelarche* is premature breast development, either unilateral or bilateral, with no other signs of sexual maturation. This usually occurs before the age of four years. It is normally a self-limiting disorder and is associated with normal and appropriate sexual development at a later age. The condition is probably secondary to intermittent secretion of ovarian estrogen. Breast enlargement rarely persists beyond a few months.

Premature adrenarche is the appearance of pubic and/or axillary hair without other signs of puberty. This condition, more common in girls than in boys, usually appears after the age of six. It is also associated with the normal sequence of secondary sexual maturation at the appropriate age. Plasma concentrations of DHEA-S are elevated. This con-

TABLE 46–2 CLINICAL FINDINGS IN PREMATURE THELARCHE, PREMATURE ADRENARCHE, AND PSEUDOPRECOCIOUS PUBERTY

| | | | PSEUDOPRECOCIOUS PUBERTY | | | | |
| | | | Isosexual | | | Heterosexual | |
FINDINGS	PREMATURE THELARCHE	PREMATURE ADRENARCHE	Ovarian Tumor	Adrenal Tumor	Exogenous Estrogens	Ovarian Tumor	Adrenal Tumor
Breast enlargement	Yes	No	Yes	Yes	Yes	Yes	Yes
Pubic hair	No	Yes	Yes	Yes	Yes	Yes	Yes
Vaginal bleeding	No	No	Yes	Yes	Yes	Yes	Yes
Virilizing signs	No	No	No	Yes	No	Yes	Yes
Bone age	Normal	Normal to Minimally Advanced	Advanced	Advanced	Advanced	Advanced	Advanced
Neurologic deficit	No	No	No	No	No	No	No
Abdominopelvic mass	No	No	Usually	No	No	Occasional	No

Modified with permission from Ross GT, Vande Wiele RL: The ovaries. In Williams RH (ed): Textbook of Endocrinology. 6th ed. Philadelphia, W B Saunders Co, 1981, p 379.

dition is probably related to premature activation of the adrenal gland.

Heterosexual Precocity

Virilization in girls is most commonly seen at birth in association with *congenital adrenal hyperplasia*. The high excess androgen levels lead to the development of ambiguous genitalia *in utero*. If left untreated, this condition leads to progressive virilization during infancy and childhood (see Chapters 27 and 48). *Androgen-producing tumors* are rare in children.

EVALUATION OF PRECOCIOUS PUBERTY

Clinical History

The chronologic order of the sexual development should be detailed, and inquiry should be made about any central nervous system symptoms, such as headaches or seizures. The growth record should be noted, and a history of possible exposure to exogenous steroids should be sought. Past history should include inquiry regarding any chronic illness, CNS infection, head trauma, or bony fracture. The family history is also important.

Physical Examination

Physical examination must include measurement of height and weight and a thorough description of the secondary sexual development. The skin must be examined for abnormal pigmentation and neurofibromas. Neurologic examination should seek subtle lateralizing signs. An abdominal and pelvic examination must also be performed (under general anesthesia, if necessary).

Investigations

Radiologic examination should include determination of bone age and views of the sella turcica and skull. A CT scan of the brain, with particular emphasis on the hypothalamic and sellar regions, is the most sensitive radiologic means of identifying a central nervous system tumor associated with sexual precocity. A pneumoencephalogram, electroencephalogram, and visual field testing are frequently valuable when a CNS tumor or other lesion is suspected. Radiographs of the long bones should be obtained if there is any suspicion of the McCune-Albright syndrome. Ultrasound can identify ovarian tumors.

Laboratory evaluation should include measurement of serum LH, FSH, estradiol, DHEA-S, TSH, and possibly T3 resin uptake and T4 by radioimmunoassay. Differentiation between true precocious puberty and pseudoprecocious puberty is sometimes aided by the LH response to GnRH. Heterosexual precocity in girls suggests congenital adrenal hyperplasia, which can be diagnosed by measurement of serum 17-OH progesterone and 11-desoxycortisol. Elevations of these hormones indicate 21-hydroxylase or 11-hydroxylase deficiencies, respectively.

Treatment

Most patients with sexual precocity fall into the *idiopathic or constitutional* category and have no underlying organic disease. However, there are important reasons for treating these girls to retard the precocity. The psychologic impact of advanced sexual development can be significant. Psychologic development is consistent with chronologic age, not sexual development—a relationship easily forgotten by teachers and peers. Although the true precocious puberty patient is often tall for her age, she will usually achieve a short adult stature because of premature epiphyseal fusion. Fifty percent of girls with untreated idiopathic precocious puberty reach an adult height of less than five feet. Therefore, medical therapy is indicated to arrest secondary sexual development and premature epiphyseal fusion.

Medical treatment includes use of agents that inhibit pituitary gonadotropin secretion by negative feedback on the hypothalamus and/or pituitary. *Medroxyprogesterone acetate* (Provera) has long been the standard therapy. Although it suppresses breast development and menses, it does not consistently arrest the early growth spurt or prevent early fusion of the long bones. *Cyproterone acetate* is similarly effective, but has no advantage over medroxyprogesterone acetate and is not available in the United States. *Danazol*, an antigonadotropin and weak androgen, is also effective, but no more so than medroxyprogesterone acetate, and it may cause virilization.

Synthetic *gonadotropin-releasing hormone (GnRH) analogues* have recently shown great promise in arresting the changes associated with true precocious puberty. Agonist-analogues of GnRH suppress gonadotropins by down regulation of the pituitary, with resulting decreased gonadal steroid production. Preliminary experience with these agents in patients with true precocious puberty shows that they can arrest secondary sexual development and delay epiphyseal fusion.

If a specific treatable entity is diagnosed, treatment is directed against this cause. CNS tumors must be approached surgically, although many of the histologically benign tumors (e.g., hamartomas) are only biopsied to allow diagnosis because their locations preclude surgical removal. Such patients are then treated medically. Hypothyroidism causing sexual precocity is treated with thyroxine. Congenital adrenal hyperplasia is treated with glucocorticoid and mineralocorticoid replacement therapy. Hepatic and ovarian tumors are excised.

SUGGESTED READING

Comite F, Cutler GB Jr, Rivier J, et al: Short-term treatment of idiopathic precocious puberty with a long-acting analogue of luteinizing hormone-releasing hormone. N Engl J Med 305:1546, 1981.

Marshall WA, Tanner JM: Variations in pattern of pubertal changes in girls. Arch Dis Child 44:291, 1969.

Speroff L, Glass RH, Kase NG: Abnormal puberty and growth problems. In Clinical Gynecologic Endocrinology and Infertility. Baltimore, Williams & Wilkins, 1983, p 363.

Styne DM, Grumbach MM: Puberty in the male and female: Its physiology and disorders. In Yen SSC and Jaffe RB (eds): Reproductive Endocrinology. Philadelphia, W B Saunders Co, 1978, p 189.

Zacharias L, Rand WM, Wurtman RJ: A prospective study of sexual development and growth in American girls: The statistics of menarche. Obstet Gynecol Surv 31:325, 1976.

Chapter Forty-Seven

AMENORRHEA AND ABNORMAL UTERINE BLEEDING

JOHN MARSHALL

AMENORRHEA

Amenorrhea is defined as the absence of menses for at least six months. It is a symptom, not a diagnosis. *Physiologic amenorrhea* occurs before menarche, during pregnancy, during the puerperium and lactation, and following menopause. Nonphysiologic, but easily understood, amenorrhea occurs following hysterectomy.

Pathologic amenorrhea may be primary or secondary. *Primary amenorrhea* is the failure of menstruation to occur within two years of full development of secondary sexual characteristics or by age 18. *Secondary amenorrhea* is the cessation of menstruation after it has been established. Unfortunately, this simple classification is of limited clinical value.

Clinical and Laboratory Evaluation

Evaluation should be initiated if (1) secondary sexual characteristics have not begun to appear by age 14; (2) menses have not occurred by age 16 in the presence of normal secondary sexual characteristics; and (3) secondary amenorrhea persists for longer than six months. In certain obvious special situations (e.g., Turner's syndrome), evaluation should not be delayed if the patient presents earlier than the appointed age.

The use of algorithms and categorization according to physiologic principles permits a logical and systematic approach to the diagnosis and management of amenorrhea. The algorithms presented in this chapter depict the logic of the diagnostic evaluation.

The initial evaluation divides patients into three categories based upon data gathered at physical examination (Fig. 47–1). This is helpful in the subsequent evaluation because it separates patients according to the underlying pathophysiology. Patients with ambiguous external genitalia have all had exposure to excessive androgens *in utero*. Patients with no secondary sexual characteristics have had no prior exposure to estrogen. Patients with normal secondary sexual characteristics who have not had prior exogenous estrogen administration have had, at one time, ovaries with responsive oocytes, production of both follicle-stimulating hormone (FSH) and luteinizing hormone (LH) by the pituitary, and production of gonadotropin-releasing hormone (GnRH) by the hypothalamus.

Ambiguous External Genitalia. Evaluation of patients with ambiguous external genitalia is indicated in Figure 47–2. These patients are usually identified by the pediatrician, not the gynecologist. The first step in the workup is the identification of the most common problem, congenital adrenal hyperplasia, which is accomplished by measurement of serum dehydroepiandrosterone sulfate (DHEA-S) and 17α-hydroxyprogesterone (see Chapter 48). A karyotype or buccal smear differentiates genotypic sex. History

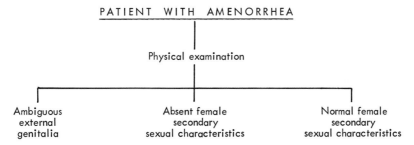

PATIENT WITH AMENORRHEA

Physical examination

| Ambiguous external genitalia | Absent female secondary sexual characteristics | Normal female secondary sexual characteristics |

Figure 47–1 Subdivision of patients with primary amenorrhea based upon findings on physical examination.

identifies individuals with familial male pseudohermaphroditism or maternal androgen exposure. For the remainder, laparotomy with bilateral gonadal biopsy provides the definitive diagnosis. Possibilities range from bilateral testis through true hermaphroditism to bilateral ovaries.

Absent Female Secondary Sexual Characteristics. The evaluation of patients with absent female secondary sexual characteristics is indicated in Figure 47–3. These patients will all present with a history of primary amenorrhea. They either have a central (hypothalamic or pituitary) abnormality resulting in inadequate secretion of gonadotropins, or ovarian unresponsiveness to gonadotropin stimulation.

The first step in the evaluation is measurement of FSH, which separates patients with a central cause (low or normal levels) from those with ovarian failure or dysfunction (el-

evated levels). The karyotype identifies patients with a Y chromosome. All phenotypic females with a Y chromosome should have their gonads removed to prevent the occurrence of a gonadal neoplasm, which can occur in up to 25 percent of such patients. The uterus and tubes should *not* be removed.

Normal Secondary Sexual Characteristics. Evaluation of patients with normal secondary sexual characteristics and no history of prior estrogen therapy is indicated in Figure 47–4. Although these patients may have a variety of diagnoses, the work-up need not be complicated. It usually involves, at most, a history and physical examination, a progestin withdrawal test, and measurement of FSH, LH, thyroid-stimulating hormone (TSH), and prolactin. Some patients may require a coned down x-ray or CT scan of the sella turcica.

The evaluation is divided into four main steps. Step I identifies any *congenital abnor-*

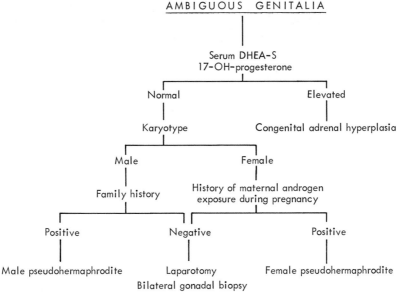

AMBIGUOUS GENITALIA

Serum DHEA-S
17-OH-progesterone

Normal — Elevated

Karyotype — Congenital adrenal hyperplasia

Male — Female

Family history — History of maternal androgen exposure during pregnancy

Positive — Negative — Positive

Male pseudohermaphrodite — Laparotomy Bilateral gonadal biopsy — Female pseudohermaphrodite

Figure 47–2 Evaluation of patients with amenorrhea and ambiguous external genitalia.

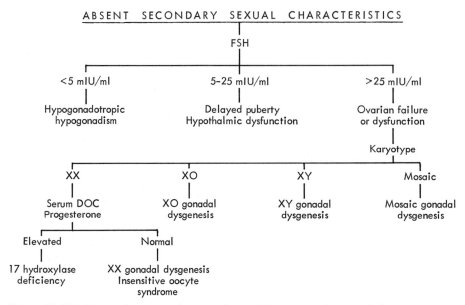

ABSENT SECONDARY SEXUAL CHARACTERISTICS

Figure 47–3 Evaluation of patients with amenorrhea and absent secondary sexual characteristics.

malities of the uterus, cervix, or vagina. Step II identifies any *abnormality of the endometrium*. Step III identifies any *abnormality of pituitary function* using gonadotropin measurements and correlated historic and physical examination data. Step IV identifies any *abnormalities associated with pituitary and/or hypothalamic dysfunction,* particularly focusing on causes of hyperprolactinemia.

The possibility of a *congenital abnormality* of the uterus, cervix, or vagina preventing menstruation is suggested by a history of primary amenorrhea in the presence of normal secondary sexual characteristics. Obviously, a congenital obstruction of the genital tract cannot be the cause of secondary amenorrhea, but this is the only point in the evaluation where the differentiation between primary and secondary amenorrhea is of diagnostic help.

After pregnancy has been appropriately ruled out, patients lacking congenital abnormalities are evaluated for *endometrial abnormalities* by the progestin and estrogen-progestin withdrawal tests. Progestin withdrawal is accomplished by administering either 100 mg of progesterone in oil intramuscularly or 10 mg of medroxyprogesterone acetate (Provera) orally for five days and then awaiting withdrawal bleeding. Any bleeding is considered positive, and is indicative of both a responsive endometrium and sufficient levels of circulating estrogens to cause appropriate endometrial proliferation. The progestin in-

duces a secretory endometrium that bleeds following the progestin withdrawal. The greater the bleeding, up to a normal period, the more normal the underlying endometrium and the circulating estrogen levels.

Because there are two unknowns in the progestin withdrawal test, namely endometrial responsiveness and estrogen concentration, the absence of bleeding may indicate either an insufficiency of estrogen or an inadequacy of the endometrium. Administration of sufficient estrogen (conjugated equine estrogens—Premarin—1.25 mg per day for 10 days) followed by progestin withdrawal (as above) should result in bleeding if the endometrium is normally responsive. The most common cause of failure to bleed following estrogen-progestin withdrawal is *Asherman's syndrome.*

Patients who respond with bleeding are evaluated in Step III for *pituitary-hypothalamic dysfunction.* Serum FSH and LH concentrations are determined, since high levels indicate ovarian failure (i.e., either absent or unresponsive oocytes). Women with ovarian failure who are less than 30 years of age should have a karyotype to identify a Y chromosome for the reason indicated previously. Patients with anorexia nervosa, exercise or weight loss amenorrhea, or polycystic ovarian syndrome are identified by history and physical examination.

The remaining patients proceed to *evaluation of the pituitary and hypothalamus* by

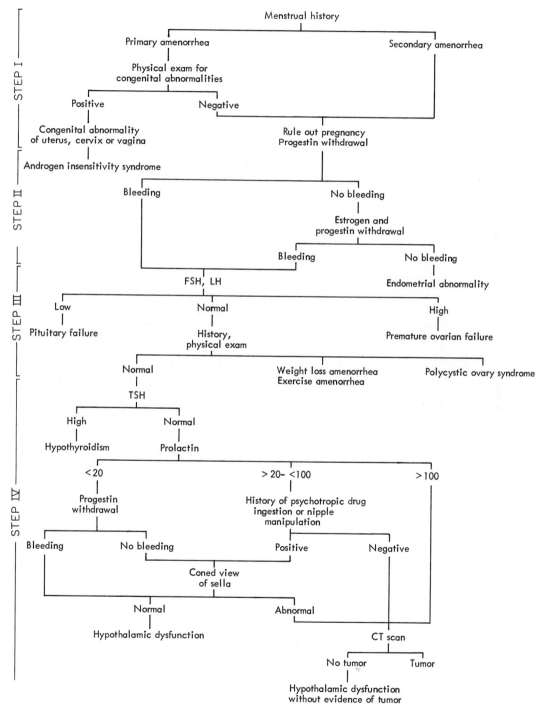

Figure 47–4 Evaluation of patients with amenorrhea and normal female secondary sexual characteristics.

means of *TSH* and *prolactin* measurements and radiologic evaluation of the *sella turcica*. Clinically inapparent hypothyroidism can be a cause of anovulation and amenorrhea and is identified by means of an elevated TSH. Routine thyroid function tests are inadequate to rule out hypothyroidism because they may be normal secondary to a compensatory increase in TSH secretion that is also often associated with hyperprolactinemia.

Euthyroid patients are next evaluated by measurement of serum prolactin. Patients with a normal prolactin who have bled in response to progestin withdrawal are presumed to have a form of hypothalamic dysfunction. The absence of bleeding suggests inadequate estrogen levels. These patients need a coned down x-ray of the sella turcica. Patients with a moderately elevated prolactin should be questioned concerning use of psychotropic drugs or nipple stimulation, both of which can elevate prolactin. Patients with a positive history require a coned view of the sella turcica, while patients with a negative history should have a CT scan of the sella turcica. The coned view needs careful interpretation. A double floor of the sella turcica is often seen in the absence of enlargement or demineralization and should be interpreted as a normal variant rather than indicative of tumor. A normal coned view suggests hypothalamic dysfunction. An abnormal coned view should be further evaluated by CT scan. Patients with persistently elevated prolactin levels without evidence of tumor and those with tumor who are being followed without surgery should have CT scans repeated yearly.

SPECIFIC ABNORMALITIES

Ambiguous External Genitalia

Congenital Adrenal Hyperplasia. Occasionally, patients with mild adult onset congenital adrenal hyperplasia will first present with amenorrhea (see Chapter 48). External genitalia may be ambiguous, and there is usually some evidence of additional androgen excess which becomes evident as hirsutism at puberty. The most common form is a 21-hydroxylase enzyme deficiency, which results in increased production of DHEA-S and 17α-hydroxyprogesterone. The karyotype is 46 XX.

Treatment with adrenocorticoid replacement results in suppression of the excess androgens and restoration of menses. Occasionally, the clitoromegaly may require surgical correction.

Male Pseudohermaphroditism. Male pseudohermaphroditism can be due to either deficient testosterone synthesis secondary to an enzyme deficiency or androgen resistance. All patients have XY karyotypes and testicles (see Chapter 27).

Therapy is dependent upon the degree of masculinization of the external genitalia. If the genitalia are only mildly feminized, glucocorticoid and androgen therapy can be utilized and the patient raised as a male. If the penis is deficient, it is usually preferable to remove the penis and testicles, feminize with estrogens, create a surgical neovagina, and have the patient function as a female. Obviously, this is best accomplished at an early age to avoid unnecessary psychologic difficulty.

Female Pseudohermaphroditism. Female pseudohermaphrodites are females having a 46 XX karyotype and normal ovaries who were exposed to androgens *in utero* (see Chapter 27). These patients undergo spontaneous thelarche and menarche, and demonstrate normal ovulation, menses, and fertility. Thus, they present with ambiguous external genitalia, not with amenorrhea, and are included here only for completeness.

Absent Secondary Sexual Characteristics

Failure of the pituitary to secrete sufficient gonadotropin results in failure of ovarian follicular maturation and sex steroid hormone production and the absence of secondary sexual characteristics and menses. Failure may result from inadequate stimulation by the hypothalamus or from primary pituitary disease.

Central Nervous System Disorders. *Kallmann's syndrome* is a familial syndrome of sexual immaturity and anosmia or hyposmia associated with midline cranial defects. The primary abnormality is probably hypothalamic dysfunction. Estrogen replacement induces sexual maturation and menses. Ovulation can be induced with gonadotropins.

Disorders of hypothalamic control of pituitary gonadotropins are associated with third ventricle tumors, parapituitary tumors, or suprasellar neoplasms. Neuroendocrinologic evaluation identifies the specific diagnosis.

Delayed Puberty. Constitutional delayed puberty, although more common in boys than girls, does occur. It tends to occur repeatedly in families, so obtaining a thorough family history is helpful. Menarche with normal fertility has been reported as late as 20 years. Despite its late appearance, the eventual pubertal sequence and fertility are normal. Therapy, consisting of estrogen and progestin replacement, is given for psychologic rather than physiologic reasons.

Ovarian Failure. This term describes a failure of end organ response manifest by elevated serum gonadotropin levels secondary to either a lack of oocytes or oocytes that fail to respond to gonadotropin stimulation. The term gonadal dysgenesis describes a number of specific entities, all of which share gonads consisting of bilateral streaks of fibrous stroma without germ cells. This is the most common error in fetal gonadal differentiation, and it occurs in about 1 per 2500 newborn phenotypic females. Sometimes gonadal differentiation proceeds differently on the two sides giving rise to unusual combinations of male and female gonads. The specific etiology is determined by karyotype. About 50 percent of patients with gonadal dysgenesis will have a 45 XO complement. About 25 percent have sex chromosomal mosaicism without X rearrangements, usually 45 X/46 XX; the remainder have X or Y rearrangements or no detectable chromosomal abnormality.

Turner's Syndrome (45 XO). Patients with this karyotype have streak gonads containing dense fibrous stroma without oocytes. The external genitalia usually differentiate as expected for females, but remain infantile because of inadequate estrogen. The uterus, cervix, and fallopian tubes are structurally normal but also infantile. Secondary sexual characteristics fail to develop. The patients are usually short, and 97 percent are less than 5 feet tall. Intelligence is usually normal. Somatic abnormalities are frequently present. More common ones include short broad neck (about 75 percent), low nuchal hair line (70 percent), hypoplasia or malformation of the nails (65 percent), pigmented nevi (60 percent), cubitus valgus (50 percent), shield chest (50 percent), short fourth metacarpals (50 percent), pterygium-coli (45 percent), renal abnormalities (40 percent), high arched palate (35 percent), and coarctation of the aorta or ventricular septal defect (15 percent).

The pathophysiology of the streak ovaries is interesting. The number and migration of the primordial germ cells into the ovaries is normal, but oocytes degenerate shortly after formation of the primordial follicle, apparently because the follicular layer is incomplete.

Therapy consists of estrogen-progestin replacement to induce growth, secondary sexual characteristics, and menstruation. Unfortunately, most patients never grow to normal stature, and breast development is frequently regarded as less than optimal. Menstruation occurs, and sexual function is normal. Virtually all patients are sterile. If a Y chromosome is not present, there is no increased likelihood of gonadal tumor formation, so gonadal extirpation is not indicated.

XY Gonadal Dysgenesis (Swyer's Syndrome). Patients with a 46 XY karyotype and streak gonads are uncommon. Only about 100 cases have been reported. About 10 percent have a familial history. Patients are of normal height but eunuchoid, and have an infantile vagina, uterus, and fallopian tubes. Somatic abnormalities are uncommon, although ambiguous external genitalia can occur.

Therapy consists of estrogen-progestin replacement to induce secondary sexual characteristics and menstruation. The gonads must be extirpated because approximately 25 percent of cases will develop dysgerminomas or gonadoblastomas. The uterus and tubes should not be removed.

Mosaic Gonadal Dysgenesis. Gonadal dysgenesis can be associated with various mosaic chromosomal patterns. Somatic abnormalities are dependent upon the specific mosaic chromosomal complement, but are usually less than those seen with 45 XO gonadal dysgenesis. Therapy consists of hormonal replacement and gonadal extirpation if a Y chromosome is present.

46 XX Gonadal Dysgenesis ("Pure Gonadal Dysgenesis"). These patients are also uncommon. About 10 percent have a familial history. The external genitalia and streak gonads are indistinguishable from those of a patient who has 46 XO gonadal dysgenesis. However, these patients are of normal height and eunuchoidal. Somatic abnormalities are uncommon. Therapy consists of hormonal replacement.

17α-Hydroxylase Deficiency. Deficiency of

the enzyme 17α-hydroxylase results in diminished synthesis of cortisol, androgens, and estrogens, and increased production of desoxycorticosterone and corticosterone. Patients manifest hypertension, hypokalemic alkalosis, infantile female external genitalia, absence of pubescence, and primary amenorrhea with elevated gonadotropins. Most of these patients will be identified at birth and will rarely present with primary amenorrhea.

Estrogen-progestin replacement therapy results in sexual maturation and menstruation but does not restore fertility.

Insensitive Ovary Syndrome. This term describes patients with amenorrhea and elevated gonadotropins despite the presence of ovarian follicles. The pathophysiologic basis for this failure to respond to gonadotropin stimulation is unknown, but it could be due to a lack of gonadotropic receptors in the follicles or to an inability of the follicular cells to synthesize estrogen. Because these patients do not respond to high doses of exogenous gonadotropins, it is probably not due to an abnormality of the endogenous gonadotropin molecules. Therapy consists of estrogen-progestin replacement.

Normal Secondary Sexual Characteristics

Congenital abnormalities of the uterus, cervix, or vagina are discussed in Chapter 27.

Androgen Insensitivity Syndrome (Testicular Feminization). Patients with androgen insensitivity syndrome are genetic males with 46 XY karyotypes and bilateral testicles. Because of an inability to respond to testosterone, wolffian duct structures do not develop and external genitalia do not masculinize. However, because of müllerian regression or inhibition factor secreted by testicular tubular cells, müllerian ductal structures do not develop. Thus, these patients manifest female phenotypes with normal female external genitalia, a short vagina, and absent cervix, uterus, and fallopian tubes. Diminished pubic and axillary hair and larger than average breasts are also usually present. Testicles may be located in the labia majora, inguinal canal, or abdominal cavity.

Therapy consists of psychologic support, extirpation of the testicles, and female hormonal replacement. It is usually best not to tell these patients that they are males.

Endometrial Abnormality (Asherman's Syndrome). Although an endometrial abnormality may be either primary or secondary to curettage, in reality only the latter condition is seen. The characteristic history is that of a pregnancy followed by retained products of conception, endometritis, and uterine curettage. This results in removal of the endometrium, scarring, subsequent obliteration of the endometrial cavity, and amenorrhea. Multiple synechiae can be seen on hysterogram and confirmed by hysteroscopy.

Treatment consists of dilatation and curettage and/or direct lysis of adhesions via the hysteroscope. Following these procedures, either an intrauterine device (IUD) or a pediatric Foley catheter should be placed in the endometrial cavity. The patient should be treated with high doses of estrogen.

Pituitary Failure. Patients demonstrating low pituitary gonadotropins in the presence of normal secondary sexual characteristics by definition must have secondary pituitary failure. This is an uncommon cause of amenorrhea and must be due to some destruction of the pituitary gland. The most common causes are a *pituitary tumor* or postpartum pituitary necrosis *(Sheehan's syndrome)*. A history of postpartum hemorrhage and hypotension is usually present in patients with Sheehan's syndrome. In both situations, the onset of hypopituitarism is generally insidious. Gonadotropin failure commonly appears first, followed by a deficiency of TSH and, finally, a deficiency of ACTH. Therapy consists of hormonal replacement.

Premature Ovarian Failure. Premature ovarian failure describes a condition of unknown etiology wherein the complement of oocytes is depleted sooner than usual (i.e., before age 35). It could occur secondary to a decreased number of primordial follicles or an increased rate of disappearance. The latter is probably more likely. Specific causes include 46 XX gonadal dysgenesis, mosaic gonadal dysgenesis, or various autoimmune disorders sometimes associated with detectable ovarian antibodies. A karyotype should be performed if the patient is less than 30 years of age. If a Y chromosome is present, the gonads should be excised to avoid the possibility of malignant transformation. Although for most patients premature ovarian failure is permanent, some patients have been reported who have subsequently resumed ovulation and become pregnant. The pathophysiology of this phenomenon is not understood.

Therapy consists of estrogen and progestin replacement. The estrogen sometimes enhances follicular responsiveness to gonadotropins and can be associated with ovulation.

Anorexia Nervosa. Anorexia nervosa is primarily a psychologic disorder manifested by hypothalamic dysfunction. It is associated with amenorrhea and weight loss greater than 25 percent of ideal body weight. It is most common in white, middle to upper class, success- and achievement-oriented females. Patients generally deny they are underweight and may manifest lanugo, bradycardia, hyperactivity, constipation, hypotension, or hypercarotenemia. Because death can occur in severe cases, recognition and effective management are important.

Therapy consists of explanation, general counseling, and, most importantly, a sufficient caloric intake. In some patients, hormonal replacement and psychiatric care may be required.

Exercise and Weight Loss Amenorrhea. Women engaged in vigorous or stressful physical exercise frequently manifest amenorrhea. Both the level of exercise and the level of stress appear to be determinants. Women who weigh less than 50 kg and lose more than 5 kg while exercising most often demonstrate menstrual abnormality. At least part of the explanation may be related to suppressed GnRH pulsations secondary to the increased level of endorphins associated with exercise.

Weight gain reverses the process, but these women are frequently unwilling to forego the exercise and diet that leads to the weight loss and the problem. In such patients, hormonal replacement is necessary to prevent osteoporosis.

Polycystic Ovarian Syndrome. Amenorrhea is present in about 55 percent of patients with polycystic ovarian syndrome. Irregular bleeding is present in 25 percent, and some degree of hirsutism in 70 percent (see Chapter 48). Therapy is dependent upon the patient's wishes, but menstruation usually occurs with periodic progestin withdrawal.

Hypothyroidism. Hypothyroidism is a rare cause of amenorrhea. Routine thyroid function tests will not identify all hypothyroid patients because the increased TSH secretion may result in a compensatory elevation of thyroxine levels. The definitive test is measurement of serum TSH. Treatment consists of thyroid hormone replacement.

Anovulatory Hypothalamic Dysfunction. More patients with amenorrhea and normal secondary sexual characteristics will probably fall into this diagnostic category than any other. These patients do not ovulate, but have no discernible cause for their abnormality. The basic disturbance probably resides within the hypothalamus, although the mechanism is not known. Therapy consists of cyclic administration of progestin and/or estrogen-progestin.

Hypothalamic Dysfunction with Idiopathic Hyperprolactinemia. These patients are similar to those with anovulatory hypothalamic dysfunction, except that they also manifest a mild degree of hyperprolactinemia without evidence of a pituitary tumor. The etiology of the hyperprolactinemia is unknown. Therapy should consist of observation or treatment with bromocriptine.

Drug or Nipple Manipulation-Induced Hyperprolactinemia and Anovulation. Selected psychotropic drugs or chronic manipulation of the nipple can result in hyperprolactinemia with resultant anovulation/amenorrhea. Therapy consists of removal of the cause.

Pituitary Tumors. Pituitary tumors have recently been recognized as a cause of amenorrhea with increasing frequency, probably because of the availability of serum prolactin determinations and an effective means of examination of the sella turcica. Most patients are asymptomatic, except for amenorrhea and, perhaps, galactorrhea. Galactorrhea, with or without amenorrhea, indicates an increased probability of a pituitary tumor but does not materially change the diagnostic evaluation.

Tumors are classified as *microadenomas* if less than 1 cm in diameter and as *macroadenomas* if greater than 1 cm. Most tumors are microadenomas contained within the sella turcica. Patients with these small tumors do not manifest visual field defects or other evidence of extrasellar enlargement, as found in patients with macroadenomas.

An elevated serum prolactin is present in about 10 percent of amenorrheic women, many of whom ultimately demonstrate a prolactin-producing pituitary adenoma. Computerized tomography is the definitive diagnostic technique, and most patients with hyperprolactinemia should have a CT scan of the sella turcica. Complicated endocrine stimulation and suppression tests have not proven useful. The choice of therapy is compounded by the fact that up to 25 percent of autopsy examinations of pituitary glands reveal adenomas. Most adenomas enlarge very slowly.

Therapy may consist of observation, surgical removal, radiation, or therapy with bromocriptine. *Transphenoidal resection* usually achieves complete remission with resumption of menses in about 40 percent of patients with macroadenomas and 80 to 90 percent of patients with microadenomas. Most complications are relatively mild. *Radiation therapy* is not generally satisfactory because it is slow to effect change and is associated with an unacceptably high incidence of panhypopituitarism. *Bromocriptine* is a dopamine agonist that binds to dopamine receptors and thereby inhibits pituitary prolactin secretion. Most adenomas regress with bromocriptine therapy, although neither the prolactin suppression nor the tumor regression persist after discontinuation of bromocriptine.

Current recommended therapy for macroadenomas is bromocriptine followed by surgery. Therapy for microadenomas is more complicated. If fertility or relief of breast discomfort is desired, the patient should receive bromocriptine. Trans-sphenoidal resection, however, is also appropriate. Patients who have no symptoms other than amenorrhea and who demonstrate withdrawal bleeding following progestins are probably best treated by progestin replacement therapy. Estrogen replacement in hypoestrogenic patients with adenomas is controversial because of the risk of stimulating growth of the tumor.

Patients with pituitary microadenomas who become pregnant while taking bromocriptine can carry the pregnancy and breast feed safely, although they should be observed carefully for signs and/or symptoms of pituitary enlargement. If possible, the drug should be discontinued after pregnancy is diagnosed. However, if it is required to control enlargement of a pituitary tumor, bromocriptine appears to be without hazard to the fetus.

"Postpill" Amenorrhea. Amenorrhea occurring following discontinuation of oral contraceptives should not be presumed to be due to a continuing suppressive effect of the contraceptives. The etiologies of amenorrhea occurring in patients who have previously taken oral contraceptives are not different from those in other patients. Therefore, these patients should be worked-up in the manner described for patients having normal secondary sexual characteristics.

Therapy

Psychologic Support. For most women, the bearing of a child is the ultimate indication of femininity. Menstruation is the penultimate indicator of fertility, followed, in turn, by the development of secondary sexual characteristics. Consequently, either the failure to initiate menstruation or the cessation of menstruation has profound psychologic import. It is necessary that the physician recognize the psychologic importance of amenorrhea and specifically address it therapeutically. The physician must help the patient maintain a positive image of herself as a competent woman who can function effectively sexually and who will continue to be desired as a companion and sexual partner.

Amenorrheic women see physicians because of fear of an unknown disease, lack of fertility, or concern because of loss of femininity. Unless the physician identifies specifically which of these concerns is present, management may be unsuccessful.

Hormonal Therapy. Hormonal therapy in the amenorrheic patient has two functions. First, if estrogen is present in quantities sufficient to cause endometrial proliferation, progestin is given to cause periodic endometrial shedding to prevent the development of endometrial hyperplasia and/or carcinoma. Second, if insufficient estrogen is available, estrogen is given to provide sufficient estrogen to effect secondary sexual characteristics and menstruation in pubertal females and to prevent osteoporosis. Patients who receive estrogen will usually also need progestin withdrawal.

The progestin medroxyprogesterone acetate (Provera), 10 mg per day, is given for the first 13 days of each calender month. This converts an estrogen-primed proliferative endometrium to a secretory endometrium. Withdrawal results in complete endometrial shedding.

Amenorrheic patients who do not bleed following progestin withdrawal or who have absent secondary sexual characteristics should receive replacement estrogen and progestin. A simple, easily remembered technique is as follows: *medroxyprogesterone acetate*, 10 mg per day, is given for the first 13 days of each calendar month; *conjugated equine estrogens* (Premarin), 1.25 mg per day, is given daily. Menstruation usually occurs approximately three days following cessation of the medroxyprogesterone acetate. This regimen provides 12 cycles per year and is simpler and easier than most other techniques. In general, oral contraceptives should not be used for induction of menses in amenorrheic women unless contraception is desired because oral contraceptives do not provide normal hormonal replacement.

Induction of Ovulation. In many patients, amenorrhea is accompanied by anovulation. If such patients desire fertility, induction of ovulation will be required (see Chapter 50).

ABNORMAL UTERINE BLEEDING

Classification

Abnormal uterine bleeding may be classified as follows:

1. **Hypermenorrhea or menorrhagia**: Cyclic menstrual bleeding that is excessive in amount or duration. Hypermenorrhea is most often due to anatomic abnormalities of the uterus, such as uterine myomas, but can be due to endometrial hyperplasia secondary to anovulation.

2. **Hypomenorrhea**: Diminished menstrual flow. This is also sometimes called spotting. This may occur premenopausally or during oral contraceptive usage.

3. **Polymenorrhea**: Episodes of bleeding occurring at less than 21-day intervals. This is frequently due to anovulation.

4. **Oligomenorrhea**: Episodic bleeding occurring at greater than 35-day intervals. This is also frequently due to anovulation.

5. **Metrorrhagia**: Uterine bleeding between periods. This is most likely due to organic pathology, such as endometrial or cervical polyps or carcinomas, but can be due to anovulation or estrogen withdrawal.

6. **Menometrorrhagia**: Uterine bleeding that is irregular in frequency and excessive in amount. This can be due to either organic pathology, an endocrine abnormality, or a complication of early pregnancy.

7. **Postmenopausal bleeding**: Any bleeding occurring more than one year following the menopause must be assumed to be due to malignancy and must be evaluated by histologic examination of the endometrium.

Dysfunctional Uterine Bleeding

When abnormal uterine bleeding occurs from nonsecretory endometrium secondary to anovulation and the consequent absence of progesterone, it is called dysfunctional uterine bleeding. Anovulation is usually due to a dysfunction of the hypothalamus that fails to initiate appropriate cyclic release of pituitary gonadotropins. Dysfunctional uterine bleeding can vary from spotting to menometrorrhagia and can be severe enough to require hospitalization and blood replacement.

In the absence of progesterone, endometrial proliferation continues and results in an endometrium that finally outgrows its estrogen-stimulated blood supply, then bleeds irregularly and sheds incompletely. This is the cause of the dysfunctional uterine bleeding. Dysfunctional uterine bleeding occurs most commonly in postmenarchial girls and premenopausal women because anovulation occurs more commonly at these ages.

Treatment of Dysfunctional Uterine Bleeding

Therapy can be conveniently divided into three phases: (1) endometrial stabilization and control of bleeding; (2) induction of controlled menstruation; and (3) long-term therapy. *Stabilization and control of bleeding* are accomplished by administration of high-dose estrogen-progestin oral contraceptives. The particular combination is relatively immaterial, but should be given as one pill four times a day for five to seven days. Bleeding usually stops within 12 to 14 hours. The second phase, *induction of controlled menstruation*, occurs when the oral contraceptives are withdrawn. This usually results in five to seven days of heavy bleeding that cleanly and thoroughly removes the hyperplastic endometrium.

Because anovulation is a recurrent problem, therapy cannot stop with the control of bleeding and induction of menses. It must be continued for several months until either regular ovulation occurs in young women or true menopause has taken place in older women.

If contraception is not desired, *long-term therapy* in the younger patient consists of cyclic medroxyprogesterone acetate, 10 mg per day, for the first 13 days of each month. Both contraception and endometrial control can be obtained through a low-dose estrogen-progestin combination oral contraceptive. After approximately six months, therapy should be stopped to see whether or not spontaneous cyclic ovulatory menstruation occurs.

In the premenopausal patient, long-term treatment also consists of medroxyprogesterone, 10 mg per day, for the first 13 days of each month. This therapy should be continued as long as withdrawal bleeding occurs. Not all patients will respond favorably with progestin-only control. Nonresponders may have inadequate production of estrogen and may require sequential administration of estrogen and progestin. Oral contraceptives should not be given to women over 40 years of age.

SUGGESTED READING

Chang RJ: Hyperprolactinemia and menstrual dysfunction. Clin Obstet Gynecol 26:736, 1983.

Chang RJ, Keye WR Jr, Young JR, et al: Detection, evaluation, and treatment of pituitary microadenomas in patients with galactorrhea and amenorrhea. Am J Obstet Gynecol 128:356, 1977.

Ross GT: Diagnosis and treatment of primary amenorrhea, secondary amenorrhea, and dysfunctional uterine bleeding. In DeGroot LH, Cahill GF, Odell WD, et al (eds): Endocrinology. New York, Grune & Stratton Inc, 1979, p 1419.

Simpson JL: Disorders of Sexual Differentiation. New York, Academic Press, 1976.

Speroff L, Glass RH, Kase NG: Amenorrhea. In Clinical Gynecologic Endocrinology and Infertility. 3rd ed. Baltimore, Williams & Wilkins, 1983, p 141.

Wallach EE, Kempers RD: Modern Trends in Infertility and Conception Control, Vol 2. Birmingham, American Fertility Society, 1982.

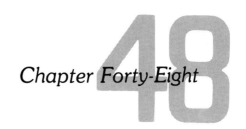
VIRILISM AND HIRSUTISM

R. JEFFREY CHANG

Virilism and hirsutism are clinical manifestations of increased androgen effect. Androgens are produced by the ovaries and adrenal glands in women. The effects of these hormones are related to their production rates, their transportation in the circulation, and the target organ response. The most common abnormality is an increased production rate, which may arise from a functional or neoplastic process. Thus, the evaluation of virilism and hirsutism is directed toward exclusion of an androgen-secreting tumor and identification of the site of hormone production.

NORMAL ANDROGEN METABOLISM

Androgens represent a class of steroid hormones that are structurally related to estrogens and progestins. The formation of androgens results from the metabolism of cholesterol via the Δ^5 or Δ^4 pathway (Fig. 48–1). Glucocorticoids (cortisol), mineralocorticoids (aldosterone), estrogens, and progestins are also derived from the metabolic breakdown of cholesterol. The most commonly studied androgens are testoster-

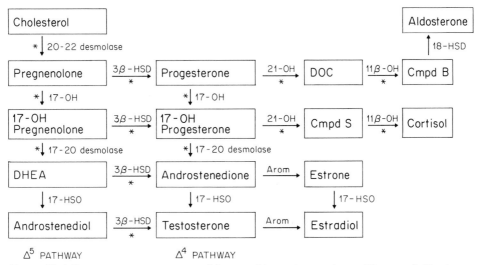

Figure 48–1 Diagrammatic representation of the steroid biosynthetic pathways. The asterisk (*) refers to specific enzyme defects that result in congenital adrenal hyperplasia. OH = hydroxylase; HSD = hydroxysteroid dehydrogenase; HSO = hydroxysteroid oxidoreductase; Arom = Aromatase.

429

one, androstenedione, dehydroepiandrosterone (DHEA), and dehydroepiandrosterone sulfate (DHEA-S). Other androgens exist that may possess greater or lesser biologic potency. The stimulus for ovarian androgen production is pituitary luteinizing hormone (LH), that for the adrenal gland is pituitary adrenocorticotropin (ACTH).

Approximately one-half of serum testosterone and androstenedione originates from the ovary, while the other half arises from the adrenal gland. DHEA and DHEA-S are chiefly products of adrenal androgen production and, as such, serve as markers for this tissue. The circulating levels, rates of production, and metabolic clearance rates of the common androgens are shown in Table 48–1. After secretion by the ovaries or adrenals, most androgens are bound to specific protein hormones in the circulation. In the bound form, androgens are biologically inactive. For example, in normal women, approximately 99 percent of serum testosterone is protein-bound and, thus, inactive. The active non-protein-bound or free fraction represents only about 1 percent of the total circulating testosterone.

When androgens reach the target tissue, they are further metabolized, which may result in more potent intracellular hormones. Testosterone is converted within the cell to dihydrotestosterone, which possesses greater biologic potency than its precursor. The skin is capable of this conversion. The pilosebaceous unit in the skin consists of the sebaceous gland and hair follicle, both of which are sensitive to androgens. The development, growth, and activity of these units appear to be regulated by hormonal as well as genetic factors. The sebaceous component is more sensitive to androgen stimulation than is the hair follicle.

ABNORMAL ANDROGEN METABOLISM

Hirsutism and virilism are the principal clinical signs of excess androgen production. *Hirsutism*, defined as excessive body hair, is most commonly manifested by excessive facial hair on the sideburns, chin, and upper lip. Increased body hair occurs as an extension of pubic hair toward the umbilicus, on the chest, or in the periareolar area of the breast. Frequently, hirsutism is accompanied by oily skin and acne. If the hyperandrogenism is severe, *virilizing signs* may be present. These include temporal balding, deepening of the voice, a male body habitus, or clitoromegaly.

Functional Adrenal Disorders

Functional disorders of the adrenal gland resulting in hirsutism or virilism are comprised of two major conditions: congenital adrenal hyperplasia and Cushing's syndrome.

Congenital Adrenal Hyperplasia. This is a general term used to describe an assortment of clinical entities that arise from inborn errors of steroid synthesis. Symptomatology associated with each entity is due to steroid overproduction, or underproduction, or both, secondary to an enzyme deficiency. Although there have been six enzyme deficiency states associated with congenital adrenal hyperplasia, only three lead to androgen overproduction and hirsutism or virilism.

The most common condition is *21-hydroxylase deficiency*. In 20 percent of cases, the defect is complete, whereas in 80 percent it is incomplete or partial. The most severe form of the disease usually occurs in the neonate and is manifest by ambiguous geni-

TABLE 48–1   MEAN VALUES FOR THE PLASMA CONCENTRATION, PRODUCTION RATE, AND METABOLIC CLEARANCE RATE (MCR) OF VARIOUS ANDROGENS IN NORMAL PREMENOPAUSAL WOMEN*

ANDROGEN	PLASMA CONCENTRATION (ng/ml)	PRODUCTION RATE (mg/day)	MCR (liters/day)
Testosterone	0.31	0.27	830
Androstenedione	1.90	3.44	1900
DHEA	4.20	6.34	1500
DHEA-S	1700.00	28.90	17

*Modified with permission from Abraham GE: Adrenal androgens in hirsutism. In Genazzani AR, Thijssen JHH, Siiteri PK (eds): Adrenal Androgens. New York, Raven Press, 1980, p 268.

talia in female newborns and life-threatening salt-wasting. Fortunately, in the majority of cases, the enzyme deficiency is only partial, which accounts for lack of salt-wasting in 50 percent of patients.

Recently, this disorder has been recognized in young women soon after puberty (*late onset 21-hydroxylase deficiency*). In these patients, the diagnosis is discovered after an evaluation of hirsutism or virilization. The diagnosis is suggested by an adolescent onset of severe hirsutism or virilism, particularly in the presence of regular menstrual function.

Since 21-hydroxylase is responsible for the conversion of 17-hydroxyprogesterone to desoxycortisol (compound S), a deficiency of this enzyme results in an accumulation of the precursor hormone, which is detectable in the circulation (Fig. 48–1). As a result, this specific enzyme disorder is marked by an elevated serum 17-hydroxyprogesterone level, as well as increases in its Δ4 metabolites androstenedione and testosterone. This disease is inherited as an autosomal recessive trait, and there is also a familial tendency of occurrence. Thus far, only 21-hydroxylase deficiency has been found to exhibit this familial tendency.

The second most common condition is *11-β hydroxylase deficiency,* which is associated with hirsutism or virilism and hypertension due to excessive production of androgens and mineralocorticoids. In contrast to 21-hydroxylase deficiency, salt-retention may exist due to an accumulation of desoxycorticosterone (DOC). Testosterone and androstenedione are usually elevated, whereas DHEA-S is uncommonly increased.

A rare cause of congenital adrenal hyperplasia resulting in androgen excess is *3-β hydroxysteroid dehydrogenase deficiency.* This condition is marked by a decrease of testosterone, mineralocorticoid, and glucocorticoid. However, DHEA-S is elevated. Affected genetic males fail to develop normal external genitalia secondary to a lack of testosterone, while females are slightly masculinized by the overproduction of DHEA-S.

Cushing's Syndrome. The second major adrenal disease leading to excess androgen production is Cushing's syndrome in which a constellation of clinical features occur as a result of hypercortisolism. Characteristic manifestations include truncal obesity, moon-like facies, hypertension, impaired glucose tolerance, muscle wasting, osteoporosis, ab-dominal striae, and easy bruisability. Other symptoms include hirsutism, acne, and irregular menstrual function. Emotional lability is common in Cushing's syndrome. This disorder may arise from a cortisol-producing tumor or from excessive ACTH production, which serves to overstimulate the adrenal glands.

Adrenal Neoplasms

Adrenal tumors resulting in androgenization without symptoms and signs of glucocorticoid excess are rare. Glucocorticoid-producing adenomas are usually associated with minimal, if any, elevation of androgens. Adenomas, which produce androgens only, generally secrete large amounts of DHEA-S. Adrenal carcinomas may produce large amounts of both glucocorticoids and androgens.

Functional Ovarian Disorders

Polycystic Ovarian Syndrome. In general, 1 to 4 percent of reproductive age women suffer from polycystic ovarian syndrome (PCO) (Fig. 48–2). The hallmark features of this disorder are: (1) androgen excess, (2) chronic anovulation, and (3) anabolic effect. Clinically, the most common symptoms are hirsutism (90 percent), menstrual irregularity (90 percent), and infertility (75 percent). Obesity is found in approximately one-half of cases, and 15 percent of patients are virilized. In most patients, the ovaries contain multiple follicle cysts that are inactive and arrested in the midantral stage of development. The ovarian stroma consists of luteinized thecal cells that produce androgens.

In PCO, hyperandrogenism commonly results from an overproduction of androgen by both the ovary and adrenal gland. These hormonal abnormalities may represent a vicious cycle of events that perpetuate the syndrome. Pituitary LH levels are increased and stimulate excess ovarian androgen production leading to hirsutism and acne. The excessive amounts of androgen are peripherally converted to estrogen. Since patients with PCO fail to ovulate, their estrogen secretion is acyclic and unopposed by progesterone. The unopposed estrogens may cause adenomatous hyperplasia of the endometrium or even endometrial carcinoma. Other important effects of the increased estrogen

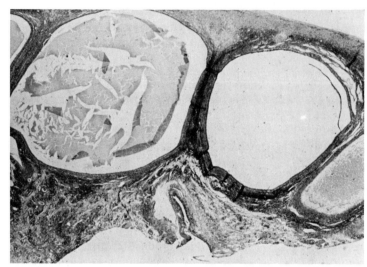

Figure 48–2. Low-power magnification of a polycystic ovary showing multiple cystic follicles with dense overlying cortical stroma.

secretion are the stimulation of pituitary LH release and the inhibition of FSH release. Increased LH results in the continued androgen production, while decreased FSH is largely responsible for the chronic anovulation.

PCO is unique in that excessive androgen production originates from both the adrenal glands and ovaries. The mechanism of excess adrenal androgen production is unknown. Basal ACTH concentrations in PCO are similar to those of normal ovulating women. The secretion pattern of ACTH over 24 hours in this disease has not been reported, although normal circadian rhythms of cortisol have been observed, which suggest that corresponding ACTH release is normal. These findings imply that in PCO, either factors other than ACTH stimulate adrenal androgen production or adrenal androgen responsiveness to ACTH is altered, or both.

A pituitary factor other than ACTH may contribute to stimulation of adrenal steroidogenesis, in particular adrenal androgens. This putative adrenal androgen-stimulating factor (CASH) has not been identified as yet. Moreover, the precise relationship of CASH to ACTH is not clear.

Hyperthecosis and Hilus Cell Hyperplasia. Hyperthecosis and hilus cell hyperplasia are also examples of chronic stimulation of the ovarian stroma due to disruption of feedback signals to the hypothalamus and pituitary. In hyperthecosis, nests of luteinized stroma are seen. The appearance of the remainder of the ovary is similar to PCO. Hyperthecosis may be simply one part of the spectrum of the ovarian response to overstimulation.

Hilus cell hyperplasia is seen most often when estrogen feedback from ovarian follicles is minimal or absent due to gonadal dysgenesis, menopause, or, occasionally, gonadotropin-resistant ovary syndrome. The resulting elevation of gonadotropin leads to hilus cell hyperplasia, which is functionally significant in only a minority of patients with the above disturbances.

Ovarian Neoplasms

Androgen-producing ovarian tumors are extremely uncommon. An arrhenoblastoma or *Sertoli-Leydig cell tumor* usually gives rise to a palpable mass, a large overproduction of testosterone, and a lesser increase of androstenedione. *Hilus cell tumors* are often nonpalpable and similarly give rise mainly to an increase in testosterone. *Lipoid cell tumors*, probably stromal in origin, are also frequently nonpalpable and produce androstenedione and testosterone in large amounts. Finally, there are virilizing conditions associated with hyperplasia of the stroma surrounding neoplasms, which themselves generally do not produce androgens. These tumors include cystic teratomas, Brenner tumors, serous cystadenomas, and Krukenberg's tumors, all of which are frequently associated with increased androstenedione production.

Idiopathic Hirsutism

Occasionally, some patients exhibit mild to moderate hirsutism without an elevation in circulating levels of androgens. This condition has been referred to as "familial," "constitutional," or "idiopathic" hirsutism. Serum 3-α-androstanediol glucuronide levels are increased in these individuals, compared with those of normal women. Because 3-α-androstanediol glucuronide is derived from intracellular testosterone metabolism, the excess hair growth may occur as a result of increased tissue utilization of testosterone.

EVALUATION

Hirsutism and virilism are evaluated by history, physical examination, and laboratory assessment.

History

Functional disorders often first appear in the pubertal period and tend to progress slowly, with the signs of androgen excess developing over several years. In contrast, neoplastic disorders can occur at any time. However, they most often arise several years after puberty, and their manifestations appear abruptly. Progression is rapid, and these patients frequently present with frank virilism. There is some overlap with functional disorders, as 15 percent of PCO patients can also exhibit signs of virilization, particularly temporal balding or clitoromegaly.

Evaluation of a Tumor

Physical Examination. A bimanual pelvic examination may identify ovarian enlargement. Asymmetrical ovarian enlargement associated with the rapid onset of virilizing signs usually indicates an androgen-producing tumor. Adrenal neoplasms are usually nonpalpable, and laboratory techniques are required for their diagnosis.

Laboratory Evaluation. The laboratory evaluation of patients with virilism and/or hirsutism is aimed primarily at identification of a neoplastic disorder. The most appropriate screening tests are measurement of serum total testosterone and DHEA-S. DHEA-S serves as a marker of adrenal androgen production and is extremely useful in the detection of an adrenal neoplasm. Values of DHEA-S in excess of 8000 ng/ml should be viewed as highly suspicious for an adrenal tumor.

Marked elevations of testosterone may in-dicate the presence of an ovarian or adrenal androgen-producing tumor. About 80 percent of patients with an androgen-producing ovarian tumor have peripheral testosterone concentrations over 200 ng percent. Since only rare patients with functional disorders have levels above 200 ng percent, such a finding demands that a neoplasm be ruled out.

Almost 20 percent of patients with tumors have levels under 200 ng percent, and there is a broad overlap with functional disease. In this group of patients, clinical features, such as the sudden onset and rapid progression of signs, are important in raising sufficient suspicion to go on to more definitive evaluation. Virilism is present in 98 percent of tumors, regardless of the peripheral level of testosterone.

A *pelvic sonogram* should be done whenever any high-risk features are present and the ovaries cannot be adequately delineated clinically. Androgen-secreting tumors of the adrenal may occasionally be detected by *CT scan. Magnetic resonance imaging* of the adrenal glands may prove very helpful.

If any of the above factors suggests the presence of an androgen-secreting tumor and it cannot be located by pelvic examination, sonogram, or adrenal CT scan, selective *venous catheterization* should be carried out and androgens measured in the venous blood from each adrenal gland and ovary. Selective venous catheterization is well-suited to the localization of an ovarian neoplasm, particularly one measuring 5 cm or less in diameter.

Evaluation of a Functional Disorder

Once an androgen-producing tumor has been excluded, attention is focused on possible functional disorders. With respect to the ovary, the presence of hirsutism and oligomenorrhea indicates PCO in the vast majority of cases.

Physical Examination. Approximately half of the patients are obese and many exhibit evidence of acne. On physical examination, the ovaries are usually bilaterally cystic and enlarged, although in some women ovarian enlargement does not occur. The diagnosis is based primarily on the history and physical examination, with an assessment of circulating androgens to rule out a neoplasm.

Laboratory Tests. SERUM 17α-HYDROXY-

PROGESTERONE. In the presence of regular menstrual cycles, congenital adrenal hyperplasia due to 21-hydroxylase deficiency should be considered. The appropriate screening test for this condition is a serum 17α-hydroxyprogesterone obtained at 8:00 A.M. The time of day is important. Steroid levels are greatest in the early morning due to the normal diurnal adrenal secretion pattern. Concentrations above 3 ng/ml warrant an ACTH stimulation test as the definitive method of diagnosis. Since ACTH regulates steroid production by the adrenal gland, subtle enzyme deficiencies are exaggerated by its administration.

ACTH STIMULATION TEST. One milligram of dexamethasone is given at bedtime on the night prior to testing. This will suppress endogenous ACTH secretion, which may interfere with the steroid response. The following morning, after an overnight fast, ACTH (Cortrosyn), 0.25 mg, is injected intravenously. Blood samples are obtained before and one hour after injection. In normal individuals, baseline 17α-hydroxyprogesterone levels are less than 3 ng/ml and rise two- to threefold in response to ACTH. In most instances, maximal stimulation does not exceed 5 ng/ml. In patients with 21-hydroxylase deficiency, the 17α-hydroxyprogesterone response to ACTH is greater than that of normals and may achieve peak levels in excess of 100 ng/ml.

DEXAMETHASONE SUPPRESSION TEST. If Cushing's syndrome is suspected, an overnight dexamethasone suppression test should be done. Dexamethasone, 1 mg, is given orally at bedtime, and blood is drawn at 8:00 A.M. after an overnight fast. This dose of dexamethasone will suppress serum cortisol concentrations to less than 5 μg/100 ml in the normal person. Occasionally, false-positive (> 5 μg/100 ml) results are found, which can be due to obesity or a poor night of sleep. If cortisol levels are nonsuppressible, then a formal low-dose, high-dose dexamethasone suppression test should be done.

TREATMENT

Treatment of hirsutism or virilism is determined by the nature of the underlying disease, the clinical symptoms and signs, and the ultimate desires of the patient. If an ovarian or adrenal neoplasm exists, surgical removal of the tumor is indicated. In premenopausal women, unilateral salpingo-oophorectomy is usually sufficient for an ovarian tumor and preserves future childbearing potential. In postmenopausal women, the treatment of choice is a total abdominal hysterectomy and bilateral salpingo-oophorectomy.

PCO is by far the most common functional ovarian disorder causing hirsutism. If necessary, therapy for the hirsutism is ovarian suppression, which is best achieved by administration of an estrogen-progestin oral contraceptive. Estrogen-progestin treatment suppresses gonadotropins, which allows regression of the testosterone and androstenedione overproduction by the ovary. The estrogen component also stimulates sex hormone-binding globulin, which decreases free testosterone. Estrogen-progestin also causes regular cyclic bleeding and progestin opposition to the estrogenic stimulation of the endometrium. The use of an estrogen-progestin combination is not without risk, particularly in women who are smokers and over the age of 35.

Treatment of functional adrenal androgen excess is determined by the type of disorder. Congenital adrenal hyperplasia is treated by the administration of glucocorticoid, which replaces any deficient cortisol and provides sufficient negative pituitary feedback to restore normal ACTH secretion. Cushing's syndrome should be treated by surgical removal of the source of excess cortisol or ACTH.

Corticosteroid administration is not without risk. Significant long-term complications include osteoporosis and adrenal atrophy. Bothersome side effects, such as weight gain, fluid retention, and emotional disturbances, may also occur.

Antiandrogenic Agents

Antiandrogenic agents have recently been advocated for the treatment of hirsutism, particularly when ovarian or adrenal suppression has failed or is contraindicated. The most commonly used drug in the United States is *spironolactone*. This aldosterone antagonist competes for testosterone-binding sites, thereby exerting a direct antiandrogenic effect at the target organ. In addition, spironolactone interferes with steroid enzymes and decreases testosterone production. Since this medication opposes the action of aldosterone, serum potassium levels may rise and, therefore, should be monitored.

Cyproterone acetate, a potent antiandrogen that has received wide acceptance, particularly in Europe, has demonstrated a beneficial effect in the vast majority of patients treated. Clinical trials with this drug have recently been instituted in the United States. Another antiandrogen is *cimetidine*. However, its utility in the treatment of hirsutism has not been fully substantiated.

Cosmetic Treatment

Suppression of abnormal androgen production will generally halt hair growth, but will not immediately cause the hirsutism to disappear. Improvement of the hirsutism may not be observed for up to one year, at which time most old hairs have degenerated and fallen out. In order to obtain good cosmetic results, some local hair removal is usually required in addition to the biochemical manipulation. Local methods include shaving or plucking of individual hairs, waxing, depilatory creams, and electrolysis.

Treatment of Infertility

Since most women suffering from androgen excess also exhibit infrequent or absent menses, infertility is a common problem. In this group of women, it is often necessary to induce ovulation with clomiphene citrate or human menopausal gonadotropin, sometimes coupled with corticosteroid suppression (see Chapter 50). Overall, these methods have proven extremely successful, and pregnancy outcomes have been good.

SUGGESTED READING

Abraham GE: Adrenal androgens in hirsutism. In Genazzani AR, Thijssen JHH, Siiteri PK (eds): Adrenal Androgens. New York, Raven Press, 1980, p 267.

Abraham GE: Ovarian and adrenal contribution to peripheral androgens during the menstrual cycle. J Clin Endocrinol Metab 39:340, 1974.

Chang RJ, Mandel FP, Wolfsen AR, Judd HL: Circulating levels of plasma adrenocorticotropin in polycystic ovarian disease. J Clin Endocrinol Metab 54:1265, 1982.

Goldzieher JW: Polycystic ovarian disease. Fertil Steril 35:371, 1981.

Grumbach MM, Conte FA: Disorders of sex differentiation. In Williams RH (ed): Textbook of Endocrinology. 6th ed. Philadelphia, W B Saunders Co, 1981, p 423.

Liddle GW: The adrenals. In Williams RH (ed): Textbook of Endocrinology. 6th ed. Philadelphia, W B Saunders Co, 1981, p 249.

Meldrum DR, Abraham GE: Peripheral and ovarian venous concentrations of various steroid hormones in virilizing ovarian tumors. Obstet Gynecol 53:36, 1979.

Parker LN, Odell WD: Control of adrenal androgen secretion. Endocr Rev 1:392, 1980.

Yen SSC: The polycystic ovary syndrome. Clin Endocrinol 12:177, 1980.

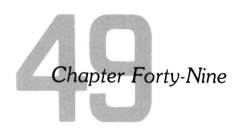

Chapter Forty-Nine

MENOPAUSE

HOWARD L. JUDD

According to the 1980 census, there are 116 million women in the United States, 32 million of whom are 50 years of age or older. The average woman goes through the menopause at 49 to 50 years of age. At this age, a woman can expect to live another 28 years. Thus, a large minority of women are without ovarian function, and these women live approximately one third of their total lifetime following ovarian failure. With the older portion of the population increasing, the care of women with climacteric symptoms becomes one of the very important issues in gynecology. This chapter reviews the relevant concerns about this issue.

TERMINOLOGY

There has been some inconsistency regarding the meaning of certain words related to this area; however, the following definitions are used in this chapter. The *climacteric* is that phase in the aging process during which a woman passes from the reproductive to the nonreproductive stage. The signals that this period of life has been reached are referred to as climacteric symptoms or, if more serious, as climacteric complaints (not as menopausal symptoms or complaints). The *menopause* is the final menstruation; it occurs during the climacteric. *Premenopause* refers to the part of the climacteric before the menopause during which the menstrual cycle is likely to be irregular and when other climacteric symptoms or complaints may occur. *Postmenopause* refers to the phase of life that comes after the menopause. It is uncertain whether this term should refer to the remainder of a woman's life or just to the period in which climacteric symptoms are present. Spontaneous cessation of menses before age 40 is called *premature menopause* or *premature ovarian failure*.

TYPES OF MENOPAUSE

There are two types of menopause: *physiologic* and *induced or artificial*. Physiologic menopause occurs in women because oocytes responsive to gonadotropins disappear from the ovary, and the few remaining ones do not respond. Isolated oocytes can be found in postmenopausal ovaries on very careful histologic inspection. Some of them show a limited degree of development, but most reveal no development in the presence of excess endogenous gonadotropins.

Cessation of menstruation and the development of climacteric symptoms and complaints can occur shortly after menarche. The reasons for premature ovarian failure are unknown. The menopause can be hastened by excess exposure to ionizing radiation, chemotherapeutic drugs (particularly alkylating agents), and surgical procedures that impair ovarian blood supply. Disease processes, especially severe infections or tumors, can also occasionally damage the ovaries so severely as to precipitate the menopause.

Induced or artificial menopause is the permanent cessation of ovarian function caused by surgical removal of the ovaries or destruction of the ovaries by radiation. Artificial menopause is employed as a treatment for endometriosis and estrogen-sensitive neoplasms of the breast and endometrium. More frequently, artificial menopause is a consequence of bilateral salpingo-oophorectomy for some ovarian problem such as infection or neoplasia.

HORMONAL CHANGES

The premenopause represents the transition from regular cycles to permanent amenorrhea and is characterized by marked menstrual irregularity. The duration of this transition varies greatly among women. The irregular vaginal bleeding represents irregular follicular maturation. These follicles secrete subnormal amounts of estradiol. Vaginal bleeding can occur after a rise and fall of estradiol without secretion of progesterone, such as occurs in anovulatory menses. Luteal phase defects can also occur, as demonstrated by either small and/or short elevations of progesterone. Although it is not known whether or not ovulation actually occurs during any of these cycles, the potential for conception during this time is minimal.

Androgen, estrogen, progesterone, and gonadotropin secretion all change with the menopause, mostly because of cessation of ovarian follicular activity. How soon after the last period these changes occur is not known, but they are definitely present within six months.

Androgens

During reproductive life, the principal ovarian androgen is *androstenedione*, which is the major secretory product of developing follicles. With the menopause, circulating androstenedione levels are reduced to approximately one-half of those found in young women, reflecting the absence of follicular activity.

The postmenopausal ovary continues to secrete *testosterone*, resulting in mean concentrations that are only minimally lower than in premenopausal women, but are distinctly higher than the levels observed in ovariectomized young women. The hilar cells and luteinized stromal cells (hyperthecosis) present in postmenopausal ovaries probably produce the testosterone. This continued secretion of testosterone by the ovary, coupled with a reduction of estrogen production, may partially explain the defeminization, hirsutism, and even virilism occasionally seen in older women.

Dehydroepiandrosterone and *dehydroepiandrosterone sulfate* levels begin to decline in the fourth decade and ultimately reach levels that are 60 and 80 percent lower, respectively. The primary source of these androgens is the adrenal glands, the ovaries contributing less than 25 percent. This marked decrease of adrenal androgen secretion has been called the *adrenopause*. The responsible mechanism is unknown, but is independent of ovarian function.

Estrogens

Estrogen production usually declines following the menopause. The greatest decrease is in *estradiol*. Postmenopausal levels are lower than those found during any phase of the menstrual cycle and similar to those seen in premenopausal women following ovariectomy. After the menopause, the circulating level of *estrone* is higher than estradiol, and there is overlap with estrone values seen during the early follicular phase in premenopausal women. The adrenal gland is the major source of both estradiol and estrone, but there is minimal direct secretion of either hormone from the adrenal gland or the ovary. Most estrone results from the peripheral aromatization of androstenedione, which occurs in fat, muscle, liver, bone marrow, brain, fibroblasts, and hair roots. Peripheral conversion of estrone, and to a lesser extent testosterone, account for most estradiol in postmenopausal women.

Progesterone

Postmenopausal progesterone levels are only 30 percent of follicular phase levels. The source of this progesterone is presumably the adrenal gland.

Gonadotropins

With the menopause, both *luteinizing hormone* (LH) and *follicle-stimulating hormone* (FSH) levels rise substantially due to the absence of the negative feedback of ovarian steroids and, possibly, inhibin on gonadotropin release. The circulating levels of both gonadotropins randomly oscillate because of pulsatile pituitary secretion that is triggered by the episodic release of hypothalamic gonadotropin-releasing hormone. The pulsatile bursts of gonadotropins occur every one to two hours. This frequency is similar to that seen during the follicular phase in premenopausal subjects, but the amplitude is much greater.

CLINICAL FINDINGS DURING THE CLIMACTERIC

Reproductive Tract

Alteration of menstrual function is usually the first clinical evidence of the climacteric, although a gradual reduction of fertility starts by age 35, and some premenopausal women complain of hot flashes. The most common pattern is a gradual decrease in both amount and duration of menstrual flow, tapering to spotting only and eventually to cessation. Cycle irregularity is common. A minority of patients have more frequent or heavier vaginal bleeding. Bleeding between periods may also occur. Abrupt cessation of menstruation is fairly rare because the decline of ovarian function usually proceeds slowly.

The diagnosis of permanent cessation of menses is, of necessity, retrospective. Amenorrhea lasting six months to one year is commonly accepted as establishing the diagnosis. Only rarely will vaginal bleeding reflecting ovarian follicular activity recur after one year of amenorrhea.

Because estrogen causes growth of the female reproductive tract, menopause is associated with regression of all the reproductive organs. Most postmenopausal women experience varying degrees of vaginal epithelial atrophy. The rugae progressively flatten. As the epithelium thins, the capillary bed shines through as a diffuse or patchy reddening. Minimal trauma with douching or coitus may result in slight vaginal bleeding. Bacterial invasion of the epithelium may occur and lead to vaginitis. Atrophy of both the endometrium and myometrium also occurs, and uterine myomas and foci of endometriosis shrink.

Urinary Tract

Marked estrogen deficiency can cause atrophic changes in the bladder and urethra. This may give rise to atrophic cystitis, characterized by urinary urgency, frequency, and incontinence. Loss of urethral tone, with pouting of the meatus and thinning of the epithelium, favors the formation of a *urethral caruncle* with resultant dysuria, meatal tenderness, and, occasionally, hematuria.

Breasts

Decrease in breast size during and after the menopause is psychologically distressing to some women. To those who have been bothered by cyclic symptoms of chronic cystic mastitis, the disappearance of these symptoms is a great relief.

Hot Flashes

About three fourths of women experience an episodic disturbance consisting of sudden flushing and perspiration, referred to as the *hot flash* or *flush*. Of those who experience flashes, approximately 80 percent have the disturbance for more than one year, and 25 to 80 percent are symptomatic for more than five years. About 15 to 20 percent of women in the United States seek medical attention for these symptoms.

A hot flash frequently begins with a sensation of pressure in the head, much like a headache, which increases in intensity until the flash is experienced. Palpitations may also be noted. The actual flush is characterized as a feeling of heat or burning in the affected areas. This is followed immediately by an outbreak of perspiration that affects the entire body but is particularly prominent over the head, neck, upper chest, and back. Patients frequently complain of "night sweats" and insomnia. There is a close temporal relationship between the occurrence of hot flashes and waking episodes. This is partially responsible for the measurable deterioration in memory and the increase in anxiety in these patients. Less commonly associated symptoms include weakness, fatigue, faintness, and vertigo. The average duration of a whole episode is four minutes, but this can vary from a few moments to as long as 10 minutes. The frequency varies from one or two an hour to one or two a week. In women with severe flashes, the mean frequency is approximately one every 60 minutes.

Physiologic changes associated with hot flashes include cutaneous vasodilation, perspiration, decrease in core temperature, and

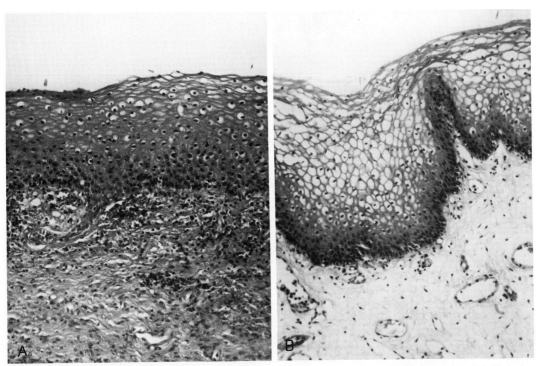

Figure 49–4 Vaginal epithelium in a postmenopausal woman *(A)* before estrogen, and *(B)* during estrogen. Note the marked increase in surface epithelial cells.

need for combined estrogen-progestin therapy has not been established for patients who do not have a uterus.

For patients with symptoms of vaginal atrophy who also have liver-related contraindications to estrogen therapy, low dosage local therapy may be useful. One gram of conjugated estrogen vaginal cream every other day will correct the vaginal symptoms in the average woman with no measurable effect on hepatic function. It should be remembered, however, that a portion of the local estrogen is absorbed into the blood stream, and application of large amounts can result in significant systemic effects.

Progestins alone also block hot flashes. Clonidine, an alpha-adrenergic antagonist, is more effective than placebo, but is associated with side effects. Vitamins E and K, mineral supplements, belladonna alkaloids in combination with mild sedatives, tranquilizers, sedatives, and antidepressants have all been used, but their efficacies have not been critically evaluated. Calcium supplements help to inhibit bone loss. A daily dosage of 1.5 gm of elemental calcium is recommended.

If the above principles are followed, the care of women during the climacteric years should provide relief of distressing symptoms with as high a degree of safety as possible.

SUGGESTED READING

Campbell S, Whitehead M: Estrogen therapy and the postmenopausal syndrome. Clin Obstet Gynecol 4:31, 1977.

Judd HL: Hormonal dynamics associated with the menopause. Clin Obstet Gynecol 19:775, 1976.

Judd HL: Menopause and postmenopause. In Benson RC (ed): Current Obstetric and Gynecologic Diagnosis and Treatment. 5th ed. Los Altos, CA, Lange Medical Publishers, 1984, p 570.

Judd HL, Cleary RE, Creasman WT, et al: Estrogen replacement therapy. Obstet Gynecol 58:267, 1981.

Judd HL, Meldrum DR, Deftos LJ, et al: Estrogen replacement therapy: Indications and complications. Ann Intern Med 98:195, 1983.

Lindsay R, Hart DM, Forrest C, et al: Prevention of spinal osteoporosis in oophorectomized women. Lancet 2:1151, 1980.

Stadel BV: Oral contraceptives and cardiovascular disease (Two Parts). N Engl J Med 305:612, 672, 1981.

Weiss NS, Ure CL, Ballard JH, et al: Decreased risk of fractures of the hip and lower forearm with postmenopausal use of oestrogen. N Engl J Med 303:1195, 1980.

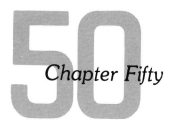

Chapter Fifty

INFERTILITY

DAVID R. MELDRUM

A couple is considered infertile after unsuccessfully attempting pregnancy for one year. Infertility is termed *primary* when it occurs without any prior pregnancy and *secondary* when it follows a previous conception. Some conditions, such as azospermia, endometriosis, and tubal occlusion, are more common in women with primary infertility, but virtually all conditions occur in both settings, making the distinction of little clinical benefit.

Conception requires the juxtaposition of the male and female gametes at the optimal stage of their maturation, followed by transportation of the conceptus to the uterine cavity at a time when the endometrium is supportive to its continued development and implantation. For these events to occur, the male and female reproductive systems must be both anatomically and physiologically intact, and coitus must occur with sufficient frequency for the semen to be deposited in close temporal relationship to the release of the oocyte from the follicle. Even when fertilization occurs, it is estimated that over 70 percent of resulting embryos are abnormal and fail to develop or become nonviable shortly after implantation. Therefore, it is not surprising that 10 to 15 percent of couples experience infertility. The physiology of conception is fully discussed in Chapter 3.

Considering the vast complexity of the reproductive process, it is remarkable that 80 percent of couples achieve conception within 1 year. More precisely, 25 percent conceive within the first month, 60 percent within 6 months, 75 percent by 9 months, and 90 percent by 18 months. The steadily decreasing rate of monthly conception demonstrated by these figures most likely reflects a spectrum of fertility extending from highly fertile couples through to those with relative infertility. After 18 months of exposure to pregnancy, the remaining couples have a very low monthly conception rate without treatment, and many may have absolute defects preventing fertility (sterility).

GENERAL PRINCIPLES OF EVALUATION

Conception requires adequate function of multiple physiologic systems in both partners. Infertility may result from either one major deficiency (e.g., tubal occlusion) or multiple minor deficiencies. Failure to realize this important dictum may lead the inexperienced practitioner to overlook additional factors that might be more amenable to treatment than the one that has been identified. About 40 percent of infertile couples have multiple causes. Therefore, with rare exceptions, a complete infertility evaluation should be performed on each couple.

Age substantially decreases the rate of conception because of decreased coital frequency and other poorly defined effects on fertility. From a large study of donor insemination, the strictly age-related reduction appears to be about one third in women aged 35 to 45. The tendency to embark on investigations and therapy at an earlier point in these older couples should be tempered by the expected delay and the consequence that unnecessary risks and expenses may be induced. A reasonable compromise is to telescope somewhat the testing and treatments during the second year of infertility in women over 35.

Basic Evaluations

Evaluation and therapy may be started at an earlier point when obvious defects are identified, or it may be delayed, for instance, when a correctable coital factor, such as infrequent intercourse, is identified. Generally, the first six to eight months of evaluation involve relatively simple and noninvasive tests and the performance of a radiologic evaluation of tubal patency (hysterosalpingogram), which can sometimes have a therapeutic effect. Operative evaluation by laparoscopy is thus reserved for the small proportion of couples (5 to 10 percent) who have not conceived by 18 to 24 months or who have specific abnormalities.

In order to keep the status of the evaluation in mind, it is helpful to arrange the work-up under a series of five categories that can be mentally reviewed at each visit. Table 50–1 shows the approximate incidence and the tests involved in the evaluation of each category. In 5 to 10 percent of couples, no explanation will be found (*idiopathic infertility*).

Effects of Social Trends

Modern social trends, such as delayed childbirth, use of the intrauterine device (IUD), and the "sexual revolution," with its accompanying epidemic of salpingitis, have made infertility more common. According to the National Center for Health Statistics, infertility increased 177 percent among married women aged 20 to 24 between 1965 and 1982. In addition, the legalization of abortion and the increased acceptance of single motherhood have largely removed the principal alternative of adoption. The infertile couple, therefore, has little choice but to go through a complex, expensive, and often lengthy series of evaluations and treatments.

Psychologic Effects

The infertility specialist must be aware of, and sensitive to, the psychologic stresses associated with infertility. The expectations of friends and family, the loss of self-esteem associated with the inability to fulfill this basic function, the associated stresses to the marital and sexual relationship, and the inability of the couple to plan their personal lives and careers, all contribute to the emotional impact of the condition. At the same time, the couple can be reassured that with the exception of effects on libido and occasional transient anovulation, there is no evidence of any significant effect of these psychologic stresses on fertility. A supportive relationship with the physician, frank discussion on the sometimes lengthy nature of various treatments, realistic expectations as to their prognosis, and participation in support groups such as *Resolve* all help these couples to adjust successfully to their condition.

Prognosis

Without therapy, spontaneous conception occurs at a decreased rate in infertile couples. Treatments are thus aimed at increasing the rate, as well as the likelihood, of conception. Unfortunately, most therapeutic regimens are based on collective clinical experience rather than controlled clinical trials. With a thorough evaluation and application of current treatments short of *in vitro* fertilization or ovum transfer, 50 to 60 percent of infertile couples will conceive. With the full development of the latter techniques, it is anticipated

TABLE 50–1   THE COMMON INFERTILITY FACTORS

FACTOR	INCIDENCE (%)	BASIC INVESTIGATIONS
Male-coital	40	Semen analysis, postcoital test
Ovulatory	15–20	Basal body temperature, serum progesterone, endometrial biopsy*
Cervical	5–10	Postcoital test
Uterine-tubal	30	Hysterosalpingogram, laparoscopy
Peritoneal	40	Laparoscopy

*Investigations when menses are regular (q 22 to 35 days); oligoamenorrhea requires additional testing (see Chapter 47).

that most couples who pursue all available treatment methods will eventually be successful.

ETIOLOGIC FACTORS

Male Coital Factor

History. The history from the male partner should cover any pregnancies previously sired; any past history of genital tract infections, such as prostatitis or mumps orchitis; surgery or trauma to the male genitals or inguinal region (e.g., hernia repair); and any exposure to lead, cadmium, radiation, or chemotherapeutic agents. Excessive consumption of alcohol or cigarettes or unusual exposure to environmental heat should be elicited.

Physical Examination. Lack of sexual hair or masculine build may indicate insufficient testosterone production. The normal location of the urethral meatus should be assured. Testicular size is estimated by comparison to a set of standard ovoids. The presence of a varicocele is elicited by asking the patient to perform Valsalva's maneuver in the standing position. Rectal massage of the prostate and seminal vesicles will bring forth sufficient secretions at the urethral meatus to allow microscopic examination for white blood cells.

Investigations. A *semen analysis* should be performed following a two- to three-day period of abstinence. The entire ejaculate should be collected in a clean glass container. Until relatively recently, the full range of normal variation has not been appreciated. Characteristics of a normal semen analysis are shown in Table 50–2.

An excessive number of leukocytes (over ten per high power field) may indicate infection, but special stains are required to differentiate polymorphonuclear leukocytes from immature germ cells. Semen quality varies markedly with repeated samples. A conclusion of normality should be based on at least two specimens, and an accurate appraisal of abnormal semen requires at least three analyses. Periodic reassessment is necessary. A few weeks should pass between each sample to reflect fluctuations in spermatogenesis. Although infertility does not occur until semen quality is below the above levels, fecundability continues to increase as the count,

TABLE 50–2 CHARACTERISTICS OF A NORMAL SEMEN ANALYSIS

CHARACTERISTIC	QUANTITY
Semen volume	2–5 ml
Sperm count	Greater than 20 million/ml
Sperm motility	Greater than 50 percent
Normal forms	Greater than 60 percent
White blood cells	Less than 10 per high power field

percentage, and quality of motility and percentage of morphologically normal sperm increase.

Endocrine evaluation of the male with subnormal semen quality may uncover a specific cause. Hypothyroidism can cause infertility, but there is no place for the empiric therapeutic use of thyroxine. Low levels of gonadotropins and testosterone may indicate hypothalamic-pituitary failure. An elevated prolactin concentration suggests the presence of a prolactin-producing pituitary tumor. An elevated level of follicle-stimulating hormone (FSH) generally indicates substantial parenchymal damage to the testes, since inhibin, produced by the Sertoli cells of the seminiferous tubules, provides the principal feedback control of FSH secretion. A response to any treatment is unlikely in the presence of an elevated level of FSH.

Treatment. The couple should be advised to have intercourse approximately every two days during the periovulatory period (e.g., days 10 through 18 and particularly days 12 through 16 of a 28-day cycle). Since infrequent coitus is a common contributing factor, firm advice in this regard can be very beneficial. However, this "scheduled intercourse" can be very disruptive and stressful, and insemination may relieve considerable pressure on a couple whose biologic drives do not match the physiologic necessity.

Lubricants and postcoital douching should be avoided, and the woman should be advised to lie on her back for at least 15 minutes following coitus with her knees bent and even a pillow under the buttocks to prevent rapid loss of semen from the vagina.

Smoking should be reduced or stopped, as should alcohol intake. Use of saunas, hot tubs, or tight underwear should be discouraged, as should exposure to other environments that raise scrotal temperature, as these factors may affect spermatogenesis.

Low semen volume may provide insufficient contact with the cervical mucus for adequate sperm migration to occur. This may be remedied by *artificial insemination* with the husband's semen (AIH). Following liquefaction (20 to 30 minutes), 0.1 ml of the semen is placed in the endocervical canal and the remainder in a cup over the cervix. When a high semen volume coexists with a low count, the sperm can be concentrated by collecting the specimen as a "split ejaculate." In most instances, the first small portion of the ejaculate contains most of the sperm and can be used for insemination.

If low sperm density (oligospermia) or low motility (asthenospermia) is due to *hypothalamic-pituitary failure,* injections of human menopausal gonadotropins (HMG) are effective. The suppressive effects of *hyperprolactinemia* on hypothalamic function can be reversed by the administration of bromocriptine, a dopamine agonist. When low semen quality coexists with a *varicocele* (dilation and incompetence of the spermatic veins), improved semen quality, particularly motility, may occur with ligation of this venous plexus. Various medications (clomiphene, human chorionic gonadotropin [hCG], testosterone, and HMG) have been tried where no etiology is apparent *(idiopathic oligoasthenospermia).* Although still inconclusive, the bulk of information does suggest a therapeutic role for clomiphene, but it is not yet approved for this purpose. Since approximately three months are required for spermatogenesis and transportation, frequent semen checks during treatment are unnecessary and only serve to discourage the patient.

If semen quality cannot be improved, intrauterine insemination with or without close timing of the insemination to the precise point of ovulation is effective. By washing and concentrating the sperm into a small volume by slow centrifugation, large numbers of sperm can be placed into the uterus. Without washing, intrauterine insemination must be limited to very small amounts of semen, due to marked cramping. Accurate timing may be accomplished either by measurement of daily luteinizing hormone (LH) concentrations or by controlled stimulation of the cycle with clomiphene or HMG, followed by administration of hCG when follicular diameter by ultrasound indicates maturity. Insemination may then be carried out within a few hours of ovulation, which occurs 36 to 44 hours following the LH surge or hCG injection.

In vitro fertilization is also used to treat the male factor, since a relatively small number of sperm is required to inseminate each oocyte. Finally, artificial insemination with donor sperm (AID) is very effective when the male factor is refractory to treatment.

Ovulatory Factor

History. Most women with regular cycles (every 22 to 35 days) are ovulating, particularly if they have premenstrual molimina (e.g., breast changes, bloating, and mood change).

Investigations. The simplest screening tests to confirm reasonably normal ovulation are the *basal body temperature* (BBT), which assesses the duration of luteal function, and the *midluteal level of serum progesterone,* which assesses the level of luteal function.

The BBT is the temperature on awakening before any activity. It rises about 0.4° F at ovulation due to the thermogenic effect of progesterone, and should remain elevated for at least 11 days (Fig. 50–1). The point of rise does not have a precise relationship to ovulation, and the BBT should not be used to predict the best time for the couple to attempt pregnancy. A progesterone level of greater than 5 ng/ml indicates ovulatory activity, but midluteal concentrations usually exceed 10 ng/ml in cycles capable of conception.

In spite of ovulation, an inadequate luteal phase may be responsible for infertility. If there are suggestions that a *luteal phase defect* may be present (abnormal BBT, history of spontaneous abortion or endometriosis, poor cervical mucus), an endometrial biopsy should be taken from the upper anterior aspect of the uterine fundus and the histologic development carefully dated. If the day of the biopsy, retrospectively determined by its relationship to the onset of the next menses, lags by more than two days in at least two cycles, a luteal phase defect is present.

Treatment. Correction of a *luteal phase defect* is generally possible by the use of vaginal progesterone suppositories, 25 mg twice daily, beginning on the second or third day of the temperature rise. Response should be documented in a subsequent cycle by repeat biopsy. Clomiphene citrate or HMG may be used if simple progesterone supplementation does not result in correction of the

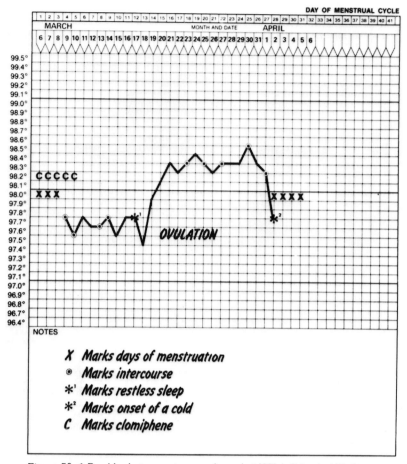

Figure 50–1 Basal body temperature graph used at UCLA School of Medicine.

defect or pregnancy. By resulting in higher levels of FSH, these latter treatments more directly treat the underlying pathophysiology (insufficient FSH stimulation of the follicle) and may correct accompanying defects of oocyte maturation or extrusion. However, they are accompanied by an increased risk of multiple pregnancy.

In women whose menses are less frequent than every 35 days (*oligoamenorrhea*), it is helpful to induce more frequent ovulation, thus increasing the opportunity for pregnancy and improving the ability to time coitus. Luteal activity associated with infrequent ovulation is often abnormal. Ovulation induction should always be preceded by a thorough work-up, as discussed in Chapter 47, because conditions causing anovulation may be worsened by pregnancy or may complicate it.

Choice of the most appropriate technique for ovulation induction is determined by the patient's specific diagnosis. With this approach, regular ovulation can be restored in over 90 percent of anovulatory women. Provided these patients persist with treatment for an adequate period of time and no other infertility factors are present, their fertility should approximate that of normal women.

Pituitary insufficiency requires the intramuscular administration of purified FSH and LH, which are extracted from menopausal urine and, therefore, are called human menopausal gonadotropins (HMG). *Hypothalamic amenorrhea* is due to infrequent or absent pulsatile release of gonadotropin-releasing hormone (GnRH). The latter is highly effective when administered in small pulses subcutaneously or intravenously in these patients every 90 to 120 minutes by a small portable infusion pump. *Hyperprolactinemia* and its suppressive effect on the hypothalamus is specifically treated by use of the dopamine agonist bromocriptine (Parlodel).

Most of the remaining patients with anovulation have some form of *polycystic ovarian syndrome* (PCO) and generally respond to clomiphene, an orally active antiestrogen. Anovulation occurs in patients with PCO because of chronic, mild suppression of FSH release and the antagonistic effect of androgens on the response of the follicle to FSH. These women often have both increased ovarian and increased adrenal androgen production. Clomiphene, by inhibiting the negative feedback effect of endogenous estrogen, causes a rise of FSH and stimulation of follicular maturation.

Two other treatments have been used to decrease the inhibitory effect of androgens. Surgical excision of androgen-producing ovarian stroma *(wedge resection)* induces ovulation, but it is not as effective as clomiphene treatment and may cause infertility by inducing periadnexal adhesions. *Dexamethasone* suppresses adrenal androgens. In those anovulatory women with levels of dehydroepiandrosterone sulfate above the mean for normal women, clomiphene treatment is more effective in inducing ovulation and pregnancy at lower dose levels when dexamethasone is given concomitantly. If ovulation does not occur at a maximal clomiphene dose, follicular development may be occurring, but the normal LH surge may fail to occur. This results in lack of follicular rupture. Assessment by serial pelvic ultrasounds and carefully timed hCG may lead to normal ovulation. If follicular maturation is not occurring, ovulation induction will require HMG/hCG with or without clomiphene pretreatment.

COMPLICATIONS OF OVULATION INDUCTION. The main complications are related to excessive stimulation of the ovaries. Substantial enlargement of the ovary with clomiphene citrate can generally be avoided by examining the adnexae before each treatment course and by using the lowest effective dose. *Cystic ovarian enlargement* is not an uncommon complication of HMG treatment. The *hyperstimulation syndrome* is a critical illness associated with marked ovarian enlargement and exudation of fluid and protein into the peritoneal and pleural cavities. The use of serum estradiol measurements with HMG treatment has virtually eliminated the hyperstimulation syndrome, provided hCG is withheld if the estradiol concentration is excessive. *Multiple pregnancy* occurs in 6 to 8 percent of clomiphene citrate conceptions, but more than twins is unusual (less than 1 percent). Multiple gestation occurs in 20 to 30 percent of HMG conceptions and 5 percent are more than twins. Ultrasound monitoring appears to reduce this risk if the hCG is withheld in the presence of an excessive number of mature follicles.

Cervical Factor

During the few days before ovulation, the cervix produces a profuse watery mucus that exudes out of the cervix to contact the seminal ejaculate. To assess its quality, the patient must be seen during the immediate preovulatory phase (day 12 to 14 of a 28-day cycle).

Investigations. The amount and clarity of the mucus are recorded. The *spinnbarkeit* may be tested by contacting the mucus with a piece of pH paper and lifting vertically. The mucus should thread out to at least 6 cm. The pH should be 6.5 or greater. A *postcoital (Sims'/Huhner) test* is done two to four hours after intercourse to assess the number and motility of spermatozoa that have entered the cervical canal. However, the number of sperm does not correlate well with semen quality, recovery of sperm from the cul-de-sac, or subsequent fertility. If the number of sperm is greater than 20 per high-power field, it is probable that the semen analysis is normal and that there is a better prognosis for fertility. When 0 to 20 sperm are seen, which is the case in most infertile couples, limited information is gained. For this reason, and because psychosexual stress can occur when coitus must occur at a prescribed time, it is important to emphasize to the couple that they should not be concerned if problems arise, since mucus quality can still be evaluated.

Treatment. Any cervical infection is treated by prescribing a 10-day course of doxycycline, 100 mg twice daily, for both partners. Persistent chronic cervicitis is treated with cryotherapy if antibiotic treatment fails. If the pH of the mucus is low, particularly if this is associated with a low number of active sperm, sperm migration and viability may be improved by advising a gentle douche with sodium bicarbonate (NaHCO$_3$) (1 tablespoon in a quart of water) 30 minutes before coitus. Poor mucus quality can be treated with a small dose of estrogen from day 7 until ovulation, but intrauterine insemination of washed sperm appears to be more effective.

Uterine-Tubal Factor

Abnormalities of the uterine cavity are seldom the cause of infertility. Large submucous myomata or endometrial polyps may rarely be associated with infertility but more often are associated with first trimester spontaneous abortions. The role of intramural myomata is not clear, although myomectomy has been associated with conception in 40 to 50 percent of couples in uncontrolled series.

Tubal occlusion may occur at three locations: the fimbrial end, the midsegment, or the isthmus-cornu. *Fimbrial occlusion* is by far the most common. Prior salpingitis and use of the intrauterine device are common etiologies, although about one half are unassociated with any such history. *Midsegment occlusion* is almost always secondary to tubal

sterilization. Such occlusion in the absence of this history suggests tuberculosis. *Isthmic-cornual occlusion* can be congenital, or due to endometriosis, tubal adenomyosis, or prior infection. In 90 percent of the cases, the occlusion is located in the isthmus near the cornu or may involve the superficial portion of the intramural tubal lumen.

Investigations. Tubal abnormalities may be diagnosed by *hysterosalpingography* or *laparoscopy.* To perform a *hysterosalpingogram* (HSG), an occlusive cannula is placed in the cervix, and the instillation of a radio-opaque dye is followed under fluoroscopy with image intensification. Selected radiographs are taken for permanent documentation (Fig. 50–2). Anesthesia is generally not required. A water-soluble dye is used initially to confirm tubal patency because of the adverse effects of sequestration of an oil-based dye within the lumen of an occluded tube. If patency is confirmed, an oil-based dye is then instilled

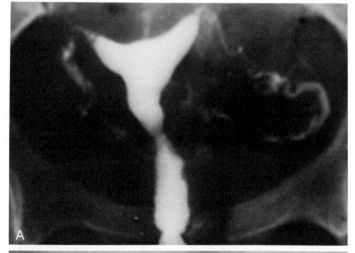

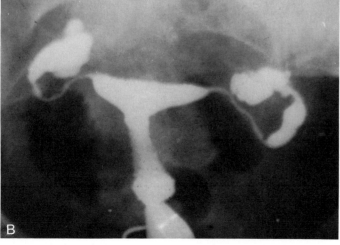

Figure 50–2 *A,* Normal hysterosalpingogram showing free spill of contrast; *B,* bilateral hydrosalpinges.

because of its prominent therapeutic effect in women with unexplained infertility. If only one tube fills with dye, the HSG should be considered normal, since this finding is usually, although not invariably, due to the dye following the path of least resistance.

Serious infections can result from HSG. A normal pelvic examination, normal erythrocyte sedimentation rate, and prophylactic doxycycline are precautions that should reduce this risk to essentially zero.

If no cause for the infertility is identified, *laparoscopy* should be delayed for six months to see if pregnancy occurs. The couple should be sure to have coitus at least once during each preovulatory period during the following six months in order to achieve the maximum probability of conception.

The *Rubin's test* is an older method for evaluating tubal patency. Carbon dioxide is insufflated through the cervix under controlled pressure, and patency is confirmed by shoulder pain. The test provides little information and little or no therapeutic effect, so should be considered obsolete.

Treatment. In most circumstances, *microsurgical tuboplasty* is more effective than conventional surgical techniques for reversal of tubal occlusion. About 60 to 80 percent of patients achieve pregnancy after reversal of sterilization using microsurgical techniques, with a decreasing prognosis for the following types of reanastomoses: isthmic-isthmic, isthmic-cornual, ampullary-isthmic, ampullary-ampullary, ampullary-cornual. *Neosalpingostomy,* which is required following fimbriectomy, is associated with a success rate of about 40 to 50 percent. For an isthmic-cornual occlusion due to disease, clearing of the obstruction with danazol has been reported when the occlusion coexists with peritoneal endometriosis. Microsurgical resection and reanastomosis is associated with a 50 to 60 percent pregnancy rate. If the intramural portion of the tube is occluded, a *reimplantation* is required, with a new opening being made into the endometrial cavity. A substantially lower rate of success is achieved in this circumstance.

At least 10 percent of conceptions following repair of diseased tubes will be ectopic in the tube. Reanastomosis of healthy tubes carries an ectopic risk of about 5 percent. This possibility must always be considered in the management of an early pregnancy following tuboplasty.

Peritoneal Factor

Laparoscopy will identify previously unsuspected pathology in 30 to 50 percent of women with unexplained infertility. Endometriosis is the most common finding. Periadnexal adhesions may be found that may hold the fimbriae away from the ovarian surface or entrap the released oocyte.

Endometriosis interferes with fertility in a number of ways. It may interfere with tubal motility, cause tubal obstruction, or cause adhesions that directly disturb the pick-up of the oocyte by the fimbriae. The inflammation caused by retrograde menstruation and the ectopic endometrium induces an increased number of peritoneal macrophages, each of which is more active in engulfing sperm, thus reducing the number of sperm available to penetrate the oocyte-cumulus complex. The presence of endometriosis is also associated with an increased incidence of *luteinized unruptured follicle (LUF) syndrome,* where, in spite of the presence of the usual indirect signs of ovulation, the oocyte is not released from the follicle. The presence of ectopic endometrium in the pelvic cavity also induces subtle alteration of luteal function with a delayed and shortened elevation of progesterone. Luteal phase defects are twice as common in women with endometriosis. If conception occurs with active endometriosis, the incidence of spontaneous abortion is 30 to 40 percent compared with the normal rate of 10 to 20 percent.

Treatment. Treatment of *endometriosis* depends on its extent and is fully discussed in Chapter 32. If substantial adhesions or endometriomas are present, surgery is preferable, since these will generally not respond to medical management. Intermediate amounts of disease may respond similarly to hormonal or surgical therapy (the latter being slightly more effective), with the choice depending largely on the prejudices of the patient against one or the other modality. Danazol or oral medroxyprogesterone acetate are highly effective, with continuous oral contraception therapy being generally inferior. If minimal disease with scattered implants is found, simple cautery at the time of laparoscopy should suffice, particularly since recent studies have suggested that minimal to mild degrees of endometriosis may not interfere with fertility.

Periadnexal adhesions may be lysed by

operative laparoscopy or may require laparotomy. Microsurgical techniques diminish adhesions. The single, most effective adjunct in preventing recurrent scarring is the placement of 32 percent dextran 70 in the pelvic cavity at the end of surgery. The dextran separates the raw surfaces during the early period of healing. An early postoperative laparoscopy may also be helpful, since the immature adhesions are filmy and avascular and can be released readily during the procedure. The advent of *in vitro* fertilization (IVF), which requires good ovarian accessibility, may make this procedure even more important in the future.

UNEXPLAINED INFERTILITY

No cause is found for infertility in 5 to 10 percent of cases. The problem appears to be primarily one of sperm transport, since intrauterine insemination with washed sperm appears to increase the rate of conception.

In other cases, a defect in the ability of the sperm to fertilize the egg may be present, since some infertile males have sperm that are unable to penetrate zona-free hamster eggs in spite of entirely normal semen parameters. Also, a lower rate of fertilization is noted in couples with unexplained infertility who undergo IVF, compared to those with a tubal cause for their infertility.

Treatment of idiopathic infertility should start with a hysterosalpingogram with oil-based dye if it has not been done previously. Intrauterine insemination, eventually with ovulation induction and hCG timing, is next employed. The final therapy is IVF.

IN VITRO FERTILIZATION

The last resort for infertile couples with any of the above factors and failure of lesser treatments is the procedure of *in vitro* fertilization and embryo transfer (IVF-ET). In some cases of tubal occlusion where the rate of success with tubal repair is low (less than 30 percent), IVF appears to be preferable to surgery because of the more rapid conception rate and the lower ectopic pregnancy rate.

Technique

Clomiphene and/or HMG is given to induce the maturation of multiple follicles, the growth of which is monitored by serum estradiol levels and pelvic sonography. An injection of hCG is given to induce the resumption of meiosis and to ready the oocytes for fertilization. Thirty-six hours after the hCG injection, multiple oocytes are aspirated under either laparoscopic or ultrasonic guidance. After a further 5 to 8 hours of *in vitro* maturation, washed sperm are added. Fertilization may be identified 14 to 18 hours after insemination by the visualization of two pronuclei. The conceptuses are then transferred to the uterine cavity two to three days after oocyte retrieval by means of a tiny catheter.

Outcome

In the best centers, the total pregnancy rate is 20 to 30 percent, the clinical pregnancy rate is 15 to 25 percent, the term pregnancy rate is 10 to 20 percent, and ectopic pregnancies occur rarely. The fetal abnormality rate to date has been lower than in spontaneous cycles.

OVUM TRANSFER

A very recent development has been the transfer of an early fertilized ovum from a volunteer donor. In this procedure, the cycles of the donor and infertile recipient are synchronized, the donor is artificially inseminated with the sperm of the male of the infertile couple, and five days later, the uterine cavity is flushed. If a conceptus is identified, it is transferred to the uterine cavity of the recipient as with IVF-ET.

This technique avoids the need for laparoscopy. It is applicable to women whose ovaries are not available for oocyte retrieval, to women whose ovaries have failed or have been removed, and to women with genetically transmittable disease. It has the disadvantage of using a donated egg.

HABITUAL ABORTION

The inability to carry pregnancy to viability is a form of infertility that is even more psychologically devastating than the inability to conceive. Since 20 to 25 percent of all pregnancies abort largely as a result of chromosomal defects unrelated to parental defects, the occurrence of two consecutive abortions is not uncommon. For this reason, and because of the complexity of the evaluation, habitual abortion is defined as the occurrence of three or more consecutive losses. Even after such a history, at least 50 percent will carry a subsequent pregnancy without therapy.

Repeated expulsion of the conceptus prior to viability may occur due to a genetic abnormality of one of the parents, lack of sufficient space for growth of the pregnancy, infection, hormonal deficiency leading to abnormal uterine contractility, or excessive similarity of histocompatibility antigens.

Genetic defects of one of the partners occur in 5 to 10 percent of couples. Gross chromosomal anomalies may be found, but more commonly a balanced translocation may be responsible, which may be detected only by staining ("banding") techniques that show more detailed structure within each chromosome. Although the testing is expensive, the finding of a chromosomal defect indicates the high likelihood of further abortions and the necessity for amniocentesis to allow determination of the fetal karyotype during any continuing pregnancy.

Abnormalities of the uterine cavity most often cause second trimester abortions. They are detected by either hysterography or hysteroscopy, or, in the case of an incompetent cervix, by a history of painless cervical dilatation. Uterine anomalies, particularly a septate uterus, uterine myomata, intrauterine synechiae (Asherman's syndrome), or a small T-shaped uterus resulting from *in utero* exposure to diethylstilbestrol (DES), are all associated with an increased rate of early fetal loss.

Correction of uterine anomalies, or myomectomy, reduces the rate of fetal loss to almost normal. Intrauterine synechiae are currently treated by hysteroscopic lysis of the adhesions, estrogen therapy to stimulate endometrial growth, and placement of an intrauterine device to prevent recurrence of adhesions during the healing phase. There is no available treatment of the DES uterus, but eventually the majority of such women are able to achieve a viable pregnancy.

Colonization with T-*Mycoplasma* (Ureaplasma urealyticum) is more common in women with habitual abortion. Appropriate cultures or empiric treatment of both partners with doxycycline is currently recommended, although absolute proof awaits the demonstration of a reduced abortion rate in a pro-spective double-blind study of this treatment. *Chronic nonspecific endometritis* can also be a cause of habitual abortion. This can be identified by the presence of a plasma cell infiltrate in the endometrial biopsy specimen.

Luteal phase defects can cause habitual abortion in addition to infertility, and have been reported in up to 30 percent of patients with habitual abortion. The abortion is postulated to occur because of insufficient relaxation of the myometrium secondary to the progesterone deficiency. Diagnosis and treatment are identical to that for associated infertility (see Ovulatory Factor section). Especially important is the continuation of progesterone replacement therapy until 10 to 12 weeks of gestation. The major source of progesterone secretion shifts from the corpus luteum to the placenta at six to seven weeks.

Some couples with habitual abortion have more sharing of *histocompatibility (HLA) antigens* than control couples. Basic animal investigations on the paradoxic immunotolerance of the fetal autografts also indicate that genetic dissimilarity somehow protects against rejection, perhaps by stimulating some sort of blocking antibodies. Immunotherapy by infusion of paternal lymphocytes is currently being investigated as a possible new treatment for habitual abortion in such couples.

OVERALL SUCCESS OF INFERTILITY THERAPY

Conventional therapies result in conception in 50 to 60 percent of infertile couples. The application of the new treatments described above should enable most couples who are willing to exhaust all measures to reach their goal.

SUGGESTED READING

Buttram VC, Malinak R, Cleary R, et al (Adhesion study group): Reduction of postoperative pelvic adhesions with intraperitoneal 32% dextran 70: A prospective, randomized clinical trial. Fertil Steril 40:612, 1983.

Daly DC: Endometrial biopsy during treatment of luteal phase defects is predictive of therapeutic outcome. Fertil Steril 40:305, 1983.

Daly DC, Walters CA, Soto-Albors CE, et al: A randomized study of dexamethasone in ovulation induction with clomiphene citrate. Fertil Steril 41:844, 1984.

Garcia CR, Mastroianni L Jr, Amelar RD, et al (eds):

Current Therapy of Infertility 1984–1985. Philadelphia, BC Decker, 1984.

Gomel V: An odyssey through the oviduct. Fertil Steril 39:144, 1983.

Guzick DS, Rock JA: A comparison of danazol and conservative surgery for the treatment of infertility due to mild or moderate endometriosis. Fertil Steril 40:580, 1983.

Hammond MG, Halme JK, Talbert LM: Factors affecting the pregnancy rate in clomiphene citrate induction of ovulation. Obstet Gynecol 62:196, 1983.

Hurley DM, Brian RJ, Burger HG: Ovulation induction with subcutaneous pulsatile gonadotropin-releasing hormone: Singleton pregnancies in patients with previous multiple pregnancies after gonadotropin therapy. Fertil Steril 40:575, 1983.

Lopata A: Concepts in human *in vitro* fertilization and embryo transfer. Fertil Steril 40:289, 1983.

Marshall JR: Infertility. In Benson RC (ed): Current Obstetric and Gynecologic Diagnosis and Treatment. Los Altos, California, Lange, 1982.

Schwabe MG, Shapiro SS, Haning RV: Hysterosalpingography with oil contrast medium enhances fertility in patients with infertility of unknown etiology. Fertil Steril 40:604, 1983.

Speroff L, Glass RH, Kase NG (eds): Clinical Gynecologic Endocrinology and Infertility. 2nd ed. Baltimore, Williams and Wilkins, 1983.

IV

GYNECOLOGIC ONCOLOGY

Jonathan S. Berek — SUBEDITOR

Chapter Fifty-One

PRINCIPLES OF CANCER THERAPY

NEVILLE F. HACKER

The standard modalities for the management of gynecologic cancer are surgery, chemotherapy, radiation therapy, and hormonal therapy. In this chapter, the principles of chemotherapy, radiation therapy, and hormonal manipulation are discussed. Immunotherapy and hyperthermia are currently experimental modalities and are not included.

CHEMOTHERAPY

One of the major advances in medicine since the 1950s has been the successful treatment of certain disseminated malignancies, including choriocarcinoma and some ovarian tumors, with chemotherapy. Prior to reviewing the agents used to treat gynecologic tumors, a brief review of the relevant cellular biology is presented.

Cellular Biology

The characteristic feature of malignant tumor growth is its uncontrolled cellular proliferation, which requires replication of deoxyribonucleic acid (DNA). There are two distinct phases in the life cycle of all cells: *mitosis* (M phase), during which cellular division occurs, and *interphase*, the interval between successive mitoses.

Interphase is subdivided into three separate phases (Fig. 51–1). Immediately following mitosis is the G_1 *phase*, which is of variable duration and is characterized by a diploid content of DNA. DNA synthesis is absent, but ribonucleic acid (RNA) and protein synthesis occur. During the shorter *S phase*, the entire DNA content is duplicated. This is followed by the G_2 *phase*, which is characterized by a tetraploid DNA content and by continuing RNA and protein synthesis in preparation for cell division. When mitosis occurs, a duplicate set of chromosomal DNA is inherited by each daughter cell, thus restoring the diploid DNA content. Following mitosis, some cells leave the cycle temporarily or permanently and enter the G_0 or resting phase.

The *growth fraction* of the tumor is the proportion of actively dividing cells. The higher the growth fraction, the fewer the number of cells in the G_0 phase and the faster the tumor doubling time. As tumors enlarge, their vascularity becomes compromised, and there is a progressive decrease in their growth fraction.

Chemotherapeutic agents and radiation kill cells by first-order kinetics, which means that a constant proportion of cells is killed for a given dosage, regardless of the number of cells present. Both modalities of therapy are most effective against actively dividing cells, since cells in the resting (G_0) phase are better able to repair sublethal damage. By surgically removing bulky, hypoxic tumor masses in patients with ovarian cancer, the growth fraction of the residual tumor is increased, thereby rendering it more susceptible to chemotherapy or radiation therapy. Unfortu-

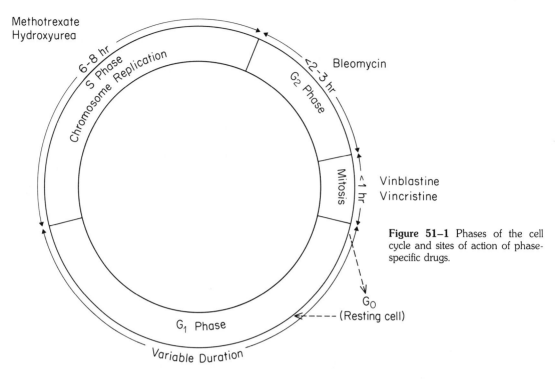

Figure 51–1 Phases of the cell cycle and sites of action of phase-specific drugs.

nately, both therapeutic modalities also suppress rapidly dividing normal cells, such as those in the gastrointestinal mucosa, bone marrow, and hair follicles.

Classification of Chemotherapeutic Agents

Chemotherapeutic agents act primarily by disrupting nuclear DNA, thus inhibiting cellular division. They may be subdivided into two categories according to their mode of action relative to the cell cycle:

1. *Cycle-specific agents,* such as alkylating agents and *cis*-platinum, which exert their damage at any phase of the cell cycle. They may damage resting as well as cycling cells, but the latter are much more sensitive.

2. *Phase-specific agents*, which exert their lethal effects exclusively or primarily during one phase of the cell cycle. Examples include hydroxyurea and methotrexate, which act primarily during the S phase; bleomycin, which acts in the G_2 phase; and the vinca alkaloids, which act in the M phase.

Principles of Chemotherapy

Chemotherapeutic agents are selected on the basis of previous experience with partic-

ular agents for any given tumor, although much current research is being undertaken to develop an effective assay for *in vitro* chemotherapy sensitivity testing. The drugs are usually given systemically so that the tumor can be treated regardless of its anatomic location. To increase the local concentration, certain drugs may occasionally be administered topically, by intra-arterial infusion, or by intrathecal or intracavitary instillation.

Chemotherapy is generally not administered if the white cell count is less than 3000 per cu mm or the platelet count less than 100,000 per cu mm. Nadir blood counts are obtained 7 to 14 days following treatment, and subsequent doses may need to be reduced, depending on the degree of myelosuppression. Dosage reduction may also be necessary because of toxicity to other organs, such as the gastrointestinal tract, liver, or kidneys.

Resistance to chemotherapeutic agents may be temporary or permanent. *Temporary resistance* is related mainly to the poor vascularity of bulky tumors, which results in poor tissue concentrations of the drugs and an increasing proportion of cells in the relatively resistant G_0 phase of the cell cycle. *Permanent resistance* is mainly due to spontaneous mutation to phenotypic resistance, and occurs most commonly in bulky tumors.

Permanent resistance may also be acquired by frequent exposure to chemotherapeutic agents. The smaller the tumor burden, the fewer the number of cycles required to eliminate the disease, thereby decreasing the likelihood of acquired chemotherapeutic resistance.

Chemotherapeutic Agents

The common agents used in the management of gynecologic malignancies may be classified as shown in Table 51–1. A summary of the main indications and side effects of these drugs is presented in Table 51–2.

Alkylating Agents. The cytotoxicity of alkylating agents is due to their ability to cause alkylation to deoxyribonucleic acid (DNA), resulting in cross-linkage between DNA strands and prevention of DNA replication. Although not phase-specific, these agents are most effective during the S phase when DNA is being replicated. Nonreplicating cells are able to enzymatically repair DNA damage. There is cross resistance among the various alkylating agents.

Antimetabolites. Antimetabolites are compounds that closely resemble normal intermediaries, for which they may substitute in biochemical reactions and thereby produce a metabolic block. Methotrexate competitively inhibits the enzyme *dihydrofolate reductase*, thus preventing the conversion of dihydrofolate to tetrahydrofolate. The latter is required for the methylation reaction necessary for the synthesis of purine and pyrimidine subunits of nucleic acid. 5-Fluorouracil (5-FU) is a fluoridated analogue of uracil, one of the two pyrimidine bases in ribonucleic acid. It may be converted to the nucleotide 5-fluorodeoxyuridine monophosphate (5-FdUMP), which inhibits *thymidylate synthetase*, an essential enzyme in DNA synthesis.

Antibiotics. The antibiotics are naturally occurring antitumor agents elaborated by certain species of *Streptomyces*. They have no single clearly defined mechanism of action, but many agents in this group intercalate between strands of the DNA double helix, thereby inhibiting both DNA and RNA synthesis and causing oxygen-dependent strand breaks.

Vinca Alkaloids. The vinca alkaloids are derived from the periwinkle plant. They are spindle toxins that interfere with cellular microtubules and cause metaphase arrest.

Other Drugs. *Cis-platinum*, one of the newer but more important drugs in gynecologic oncology, causes inhibition of DNA synthesis by forming interstrand and intrastrand linkages.

Hexamethylmelamine is an active agent against ovarian cancer, but its mechanism of action has not been elucidated. It does not display cross-resistance with the alkylating agents.

RADIATION THERAPY

Radiation may be defined as the propagation of energy through space or matter.

Types of Radiation

There are two main types of radiation: (1) electromagnetic and (2) particulate.

Electromagnetic Radiation. Examples of electromagnetic radiation include:

1. Visible light
2. Infrared light
3. Ultraviolet light
4. X-rays (photons)
5. Gamma rays (photons)

X-rays and gamma rays are identical electromagnetic radiations, differing only in their mode of production. X-rays are produced by bombardment of an anode by a high-speed electron beam; gamma rays result from the decay of radioactive isotopes, such as cobalt-60 (^{60}Co).

TABLE 51–1 CHEMOTHERAPEUTIC AGENTS COMMONLY USED IN GYNECOLOGIC ONCOLOGY

I. Alkylating Agents
   A. Melphalan (Alkeran)
   B. Chlorambucil (Leukeran)
   C. Cyclophosphamide (Cytoxan)

II. Antimetabolites
   A. Methotrexate (Methotrexate)
   B. 5-Fluorouracil (Fluorouracil)

III. Antibiotics
   A. Actinomycin-D (Cosmegen)
   B. Doxorubicin (Adriamycin)
   C. Bleomycin (Blenoxane)

IV. Vinca Alkaloids
   A. Vinblastine (Velban)
   B. Vincristine (Oncovin)

V. Other Drugs
   A. *Cis*-diamminedichloroplatinum (Platinol)
   B. Hexamethylmelamine (Hexamine)

TABLE 51–2 INDICATIONS, SIDE EFFECTS, AND PRECAUTIONS FOR COMMONLY USED CHEMOTHERAPEUTIC AGENTS

DRUG	MAIN INDICATIONS	SIDE EFFECTS	PRECAUTIONS
Chlorambucil	Ovarian carcinoma	Bone marrow depression	
Melphalan	Ovarian and tubal carcinoma	Bone marrow depression, leukemia	Avoid prolonged courses (>12 cycles) to avoid leukemia
Cyclophosphamide	Ovarian carcinoma, germ cell tumors, squamous carcinomas, sarcomas	Bone marrow depression, nausea and vomiting, alopecia, hemorrhagic cystitis, sterility	Maintain adequate fluid intake to avoid cystitis
Methotrexate	Gestational trophoblastic disease	Bone marrow depression, nausea and vomiting, stomatitis, alopecia, liver and renal failure, dermatitis	Ensure normal renal and liver function
5-Fluorouracil	Vaginal and vulvar intraepithelial neoplasia (topical application)	Pain and ulceration	
Actinomycin-D	Gestational trophoblastic disease	Bone marrow depression, nausea and vomiting, diarrhea, stomatitis, alopecia, dermatitis, local tissue necrosis	Administer through running IV infusion to avoid extravasation
Adriamycin	Ovarian carcinoma, recurrent endometrial carcinoma, sarcoma	Bone marrow depression, nausea and vomiting, cardiomyopathy, cardiac arrhythmias, alopecia, local tissue necrosis	Administer through running IV infusion; do not exceed total dose of 550 mg/m^2 to avoid cardiac toxicity; avoid if significant heart disease
Bleomycin	Germ cell tumors, squamous carcinomas	Pneumonitis and pulmonary fibrosis, alopecia, stomatitis, cutaneous reactions	Do not exceed total dose of 400 units; monitor pulmonary function with carbon monoxide diffusion capacity
Vinblastine	Germ cell tumors, sarcomas	Bone marrow depression, nausea and vomiting, stomatitis, diarrhea, local tissue necrosis	Administer through running IV infusion
Vincristine	Germ cell tumors, sarcomas	Neurotoxicity, constipation, alopecia, local tissue necrosis, bone marrow depression less marked	Administer through running IV infusion; prophylactic cathartics may be helpful
Cis-platinum	Ovarian carcinoma, germ cell tumors, squamous carcinomas	Renal toxicity, ototoxicity, neurotoxicity, severe nausea and vomiting, bone marrow depression less marked, hypokalemia, hypomagnesemia	Administer IV fluids to maintain urinary output of 100 cc/hr during infusion; discontinue if creatinine clearance <35 cc/hr
Hexamethylmelamine	Ovarian carcinoma	Bone marrow depression, nausea and vomiting, neurotoxicity, depression	

X-rays and gamma rays (photons) are differentiated from electromagnetic radiations of longer wavelength by their greater energy, which allows them to penetrate tissues and cause ionization.

Particulate Radiation. Particulate radiation consists of moving particles of matter. Their size varies over a wide range, and their energy consists of the kinetic energy of the moving particles.

$$Energy = 0.5 \ Mass \times Velocity^2$$

The particles vary greatly in size and include:

1. Neutrons (uncharged)
2. Protons (positive charge)
3. Electrons (negative charge)

The most commonly used particles are electrons. These may be derived from a linear accelerator, the beam of electrons being directed into the patient without first striking a metal target and producing x-rays. Alternatively, high-energy electrons (called *beta particles*) may be derived from the radiodecay of an unstable isotope, such as phosphorus-32 (^{32}P). Particulate radiation penetrates tissues less than photons but also produces ionization.

Units of Radiation Measurement

The *rad* is the most commonly used unit of absorbed dose. One rad is equivalent to an energy absorption of 100 ergs per gram of any material. Recently, the Gray has been defined and is equivalent to an absorbed dose of 1 joule/kg (1 Gray = 100 rad).

Inverse Square Law

The intensity of electromagnetic radiation is inversely proportional to the square of the distance from the source. Thus, the dose of radiation 2 cm from a point source will be 25 percent of the dose at 1 cm.

Biologic Considerations

Ionization of Molecules. Radiation damage is caused by the ionization of molecules in the cell, with the production of free radicals. Since approximately 80 percent of a mammalian cell is water, most of the cellular radiation damage is mediated by ionization of water and the production of the free radicals H^+ (hydrogen) and OH^- (hydroxyl). Free radicals may cause irreversible damage to DNA, making it impossible for the cell to continue replication. Minor or sublethal damage to DNA, which the cell is capable of repairing, may also occur. RNA, protein, and other molecules in the cell are also damaged, but these molecules can be more readily repaired or replaced.

Oxygen Effect. In the absence of oxygen, cells show a two- to threefold increase in their capacity to survive radiation exposure—that is, hypoxic cells are less radiosensitive than fully oxygenated cells. The enhancement of the lethal effects of radiation by oxygen is presumed to occur because the oxygen will combine with the free radicals split from cell targets by the radiation. This prevents the recombination of the free radicals with the targets, which would restore the integrity of the targets.

The effect of oxygen has important clinical implications. First, anemic patients should be transfused prior to radiation therapy. Second, bulky tumors are usually poorly vascularized and, therefore, are hypoxic, particularly in the center. Such areas are likely to be relatively resistant to radiation so that viable tumor cells may remain in spite of marked shrinkage of the tumor. This principle is used in recommending extrafascial hysterectomy following radiation therapy for bulky Stage Ib cervical cancer in order to decrease the incidence of central recurrence.

Pharmacologic Modification of the Effects of Radiation. A variety of chemical compounds are being developed to enhance the lethal effects of radiation, particularly in hypoxic tissues. The most common of these *radiosensitizing compounds* are the electron affinic agents, such as metronidazole (Flagyl). These substances act like oxygen in preventing repair of radiation damage, but because they are not metabolized like oxygen, they can penetrate and act in the hypoxic centers of tumors. Chemicals may also interact with radiation by preferentially killing cells more resistant to radiation. For example, cells are most resistant to radiation in the S phase of the cell cycle. Hydroxyurea is an S phase-specific drug, so it acts in conjunction with radiation to achieve maximum cell kill. *Radioprotective agents*, such as the sulfhydryl-containing compounds and other reducing substances, act in the reverse fashion and tend to make cells more resistant.

Time-Dose Fractionation of Radiation. Successful radiation therapy requires a delicate balance between dosage to the tumor and that to the surrounding normal tissues. A dose of radiation that is too high will sterilize the tumor but result in an unacceptably high complication rate because of the destruction of normal tissues.

Most normal tissues, such as gastrointestinal mucosa and bone marrow, have a remarkable capacity to recover from radiation damage by the division of stem cells, as well as by repair of sublethal radiation damage. Tumors, in general, have less ability to repair and repopulate. This difference can be exploited by administering the radiation in multiple fractions, thereby allowing some recovery, particularly of normal cells, between fractions.

If the interval between each fraction increases, the total dose must increase to produce the same biologic effect because of the amount of recovery that will occur in the interval. Cells that survive the acute effects of radiation usually repair sublethal damage within 24 hours; therefore, conventionally fractioned radiation is usually given in daily increments.

When treating the pelvis with external radiation, each fraction is usually 180 to 200 rad. In treating the whole abdomen, fractions are decreased to 100 to 120 rad, because the tolerance of normal tissues decreases as the volume irradiated increases. The exact reason for this phenomenon is unclear. The converse of this principle allows a small radiation field (e.g., one pelvic sidewall) to be boosted to a higher dose without significant risk to normal tissues. This may be important in treating a patient found to have fixed, positive lymph nodes on one side of the pelvis. The major factors influencing the outcome of radiation therapy are summarized in Table 51–3.

Modalities of Radiation Therapy

The modalities used to deliver radiation therapy are listed in Table 51–4. In general, there are two radiation techniques: teletherapy and brachytherapy. In *teletherapy*, a device quite removed from the patient is used, as with external beam techniques. In *brachytherapy*, the radiation source is placed either within or close to the target tissue, as with

TABLE 51–3 MAJOR FACTORS INFLUENCING THE OUTCOME OF RADIATION THERAPY

1. Normal tissue-tolerance
2. Malignant cell type
3. Total volume irradiated
4. Total dose delivered
5. Total duration of therapy
6. Number of fractions
7. Type of equipment used
8. Tissue oxygen concentration

intracavitary and interstitial techniques. In contrast to external beam therapy, intracavitary and interstitial techniques allow a high dose of radiation to be delivered to the tumor itself. Dosages to surrounding normal tissues are considerably lower and determined by the inverse square law.

External Beam Therapy. As the energy of the electromagnetic radiation increases, the penetration of the tissues increases, resulting in a relative sparing of the skin and an increased dosage to deeper tissues. At megavoltage energies (one million electron volts or greater), there is no differential absorption of energy by bone.

Orthovoltage machines are no longer used, except to treat skin cancers. Cobalt machines, developed in the early 1950s, have also been largely replaced by linear accelerators, which have a higher range of energies. The advantages of megavoltage therapy over the earlier orthovoltage machines (thousand electron volts) are demonstrated in Table 51–5.

External radiation allows a uniform dose to be delivered to a given field. The tolerance

TABLE 51–4 MODALITIES OF RADIATION THERAPY

1. *External Beams*
   a. Kilovoltage ("orthovoltage") (125–400 kV)
   b. Cobalt-60 machine (1.25 meV)
   c. Linear accelerator (4–35 meV)
   d. Betatrons (20–42 meV)
   e. Particle accelerators (e.g., electrons, protons, neutrons)

2. *Intracavitary* (radium or cesium)
   a. Rigid applicators (e.g., Ernst)
   b. After-loading applicators (e.g., Fletcher-Suit)
   c. Intraperitoneal (e.g., ^{32}P, ^{198}Au)

3. *Interstitial*
   a. Permanent
      1. Seeds (e.g., ^{198}Au, ^{125}I)
   b. Removable
      1. Ribbons (e.g., ^{192}Ir)
      2. Needles (e.g., ^{226}R, ^{137}C)

TABLE 51-5 ADVANTAGES OF MEGAVOLTAGE THERAPY

1. Skin sparing
2. Greater dose at deeper depth in tissues
3. Shorter treatment times
4. No differential bone absorption (therefore no bone necrosis)
5. Can treat larger fields easily (e.g., whole abdomen)

of the normal tissues (for example, bowel, bladder, liver, kidneys) limits the total dosage that can be delivered. External radiation is usually used to shrink a large tumor mass prior to brachytherapy. When used alone, it is generally useful only when there is small residual macroscopic or microscopic disease following surgery, such as when whole pelvic radiation is given following total abdominal hysterectomy and bilateral salpingo-oophorectomy for Stage I endometrial cancer or when whole abdominal radiation is given following surgical removal of gross disease in Stage III ovarian cancer. With highly radiosensitive tumors (e.g., dysgerminoma), external radiation alone may sterilize even bulky disease.

Intracavitary Radiation. Intracavitary therapy is used particularly in the treatment of cervical cancer, Stage II endometrial cancer, and vaginal cancer. All applicators now in use should be *"afterloaded,"* which means that they are placed in the patient and their

position checked by x-ray prior to the radioactive radium or cesium being loaded into the applicator. The correct placement of the applicator is critical if the tumor is to receive the maximum dose and the surrounding tissues the minimum dose. The ability to afterload these devices has improved the accuracy of their placement, and spared medical and paramedical personnel from excessive radiation exposure. The Fletcher-Suit afterloading device, used in the treatment of cervical and endometrial cancer, is shown in Figure 51-2.

Radioactive colloids, such as gold (^{198}Au) and chromic phosphate (^{32}P), may be instilled directly into the peritoneal or pleural cavities to treat malignant effusions or minimal residual disease, particularly in patients with ovarian cancer. To be effective, these agents must achieve a uniform distribution throughout the cavity. Prerequisites for uniform distribution include instillation in an adequate fluid volume, frequent positional change after instillation, and freedom from physical barriers such as adhesions. ^{32}P is a pure beta (electron) emitter, in contrast to ^{198}Au, which also emits the more penetrating gamma rays; therefore, radiation safety is enhanced with the use of ^{32}P.

Interstitial Radiation. Interstitial therapy (in which the radioactive source is placed directly in the tumor) may be delivered by removable implants or permanent implants. *Permanent implants* are used for inaccessible

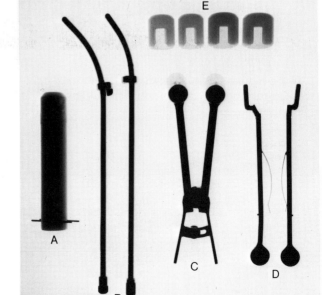

Figure 51-2 Devices for intracavitary radium or cesium: (1) vaginal cylinder, *A*; (2) components of the Fletcher-Suit afterloading device: uterine tandems, *B*; vaginal colpostats, *C*; afterloading devices for colpostats, *D*; vaginal spacers, *E*.

tumors. They utilize radioisotopes such as radon (^{222}Rn) or iodine (^{125}I) seeds and are usually placed in an unresectable tumor nodule at the time of laparotomy.

Removable implants are placed in tumors that are accessible (e.g., cervical or vaginal tumors). Interstitial therapy has the theoretical advantage of better dose distribution within the tumor, but the disadvantage that it is easier to overdose normal tissues, therefore increasing the complication rate. Interstitial therapy should be performed only by therapists who have had adequate experience with the technique. As with intracavitary devices, afterloading devices are now available for interstitial therapy. Figure 51–3 illustrates the Syed-Nesbit template used for treating pelvic malignancies. The radioisotope of choice for afterloading interstitial implants is iridium (^{192}Ir).

Complications Associated with Radiation

The success of radiation therapy depends on an exploitable gradient of susceptibility to injury in favor of normal tissue. Unfortunately, most malignant tumors are only marginally more sensitive to radiation than normal tissues, so the total dose that can be delivered, and therefore the radiocurability, is limited by the associated complications.

Acute Complications. Acute reactions to radiation include the following pathologic changes:

1. Rapid cessation of mitotic activity
2. Cellular swelling
3. Tissue edema
4. Tissue necrosis

In the management of gynecologic tumors, these acute reactions may produce the following effects:

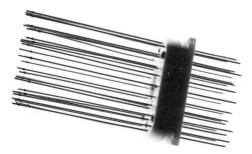

Figure 51–3 Syed-Nesbit template for interstitial radiation with iridium (^{192}I). Note that the needles have been loaded into the template.

1. *Acute cystitis*, manifested by hematuria, urgency, and frequency
2. *Proctosigmoiditis*, manifested by tenesmus, diarrhea, and passage of blood and mucus in the stool
3. *Enteritis*, manifested by nausea, vomiting, diarrhea, and colicky abdominal pain
4. *Bone marrow depression*, which is uncommon with pelvic radiation but common with pelvic and abdominal radiation, particularly if the patient has had previous cytotoxic chemotherapy

Chronic Complications. Chronic complications occur 6 to 24 months after completion of radiation and are characterized pathologically by the following changes:

1. Internal thickening and obliteration of small blood vessels (endarteritis)
2. Fibrosis
3. Permanent reduction in the epithelial and parenchymal cell populations

These changes may be slowly progressive over several years. The poor vascularization of irradiated tissues results in an increased susceptibility to injury and a reduced capacity for repair, both of which must be considered when operating on irradiated tissues.

Common chronic complications of radiation include:

1. *Radiation enteropathy.* Significant intestinal injuries occur in about 5 percent of patients receiving 5000 rad or more of pelvic radiation. Previous surgery, with resultant loops of adherent small bowel fixed in the pelvis, predispose the patient to radiation injury, particularly when intracavitary or interstitial radiation is used in addition to teletherapy.

   Large bowel injuries, which are best diagnosed by sigmoidoscopy or colonoscopy, may include:
   a. *Proctosigmoiditis*, manifested by pelvic pain, tenesmus, alteration in bowel habits, anorexia and weight loss
   b. *Ulceration*, manifested by rectal bleeding
   c. *Rectovaginal fistula*, manifested by passage of stool through the vagina
   d. *Rectal or sigmoid stenosis*, manifested by progressive large bowel obstruction.
   Small bowel injuries usually present with symptoms of an incomplete small bowel obstruction.
2. *Vaginal vault necrosis.* This is associated with severe pain and tenderness of the

vaginal vault, and hemorrhage may occur. The condition may mimic recurrent cancer, but biopsy other than by fine needle aspiration cytology should be delayed until the necrosis has cleared or a fistula may be produced.

3. *Urologic injuries.* These may include:
   a. *Hemorrhagic cystitis*, which may necessitate frequent blood transfusions and, occasionally, urinary diversion. Cystoscopy confirms the diagnosis.
   b. *Vesicovaginal fistula*, in which the patient complains of the constant leakage of urine. Methylene blue instilled into the bladder passes immediately into the vagina.
   c. *Ureterovaginal fistula*, also manifested by constant leakage of urine, and demonstrable with an intravenous pyelogram.
   d. *Ureteric stenosis*, manifested by progressive hydronephrosis.

HORMONAL THERAPY

The estrogen-receptor (ER) status of primary and metastatic breast cancer has been shown to be of therapeutic and prognostic significance. More recently, research has been directed to the measurement of estrogen and progesterone receptors (PR) in gynecologic cancers, and the potential significance of this information is being evaluated.

Mechanism of Action of Hormonal Receptors

Most steroid hormones influence their target tissues by the following series of steps:

1. Passive diffusion of the hormone through the cell membrane
2. Specific binding in the cytoplasm with the hormone receptor
3. Translocation of the receptor-hormone complex to the nucleus
4. Binding of the receptor-hormone complex to an "acceptor" site on the chromatin
5. Transcription of DNA in a manner characteristic of the specific hormone-target cell interaction, resulting eventually in either an increase or a decrease in specific protein synthesis

Of the naturally occurring estrogens, estradiol has the highest affinity for the estrogen receptor. The synthetic, nonsteroidal estrogen, diethylstilbestrol, also binds readily to estrogen receptors. Tamoxifen binds with the ER and is translocated to the nucleus, where it binds to chromatin. It does not influence gene transcription, so functionally, tamoxifen acts as an antiestrogen.

Estrogen exposure increases the production of both ER and PR, while progesterone inhibits production of both ER and PR. This suggests that patients whose tumors are ER-positive should also be PR-positive, which is usually true. It also suggests that tumors should not contain PR in the absence of ER. However, in practice, some such tumors will be found.

Clinical Applications

Since tumor growth in patients who are ER- and PR-positive is likely to be stimulated by estrogen exposure, tumor regression should occur if endogenous estrogen production is abolished or if the patient is exposed to a progestin or antiestrogen. In breast cancer, patients whose tumors are ER- and PR-positive have an 80 percent response rate to hormonal manipulation, while less than 10 percent of receptor-poor tumors respond. In addition, prognosis in primary, operable cases is better in receptor-rich tumors.

Objective response to progestin therapy occurs in about one third of patients with recurrent or metastatic endometrial carcinoma. It has been known for many years that progestin therapy is more effective among well-differentiated endometrial adenocarcinomas, and it has recently been demonstrated that these tumors are the ones that are most likely to contain ER and PR. The presence of steroid receptors is a more reliable guide to response to progestin therapy than histologic grade.

Recently, ER and PR have been demonstrated in some ovarian adenocarcinomas, but the therapeutic implications of these findings await further investigation.

SUGGESTED READING

DiSaia PJ, Creasman WT: Clinical Gynecologic Oncology. St. Louis, CV Mosby Co, 1981.

Ehrlich CE, Young PCM, Cleary RE: Cytoplasmic progesterone and estradiol receptors in normal, hyperplastic, and carcinomatous endometria: Therapeutic implications. Am J Obstet Gynecol 141:539, 1981.

Hoffman PG, Siiteri PK: Sex steroid receptors in gynecologic cancer. Obstet Gynecol 55:648, 1980.

Morrow CP, Townsend DE: Synopsis of Gynecologic Oncology. 2nd ed. New York, John Wiley and Sons, 1981.

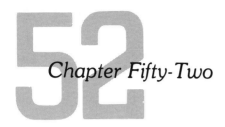

Chapter Fifty-Two

UTERINE CORPUS CANCER

RONALD S. LEUCHTER and MACLYN E. WADE

Cancer of the endometrium is the most common gynecologic malignancy, being twice as common as carcinoma of the cervix. It is the fourth most common malignancy found in American women after breast, colorectal, and lung cancer. There has been a recent increase in the incidence of endometrial cancer that may be related in part to the increased use of estrogen by postmenopausal women. The majority of tumors associated with this medication are of low stage and grade.

EPIDEMIOLOGY AND ETIOLOGY

The median age for endometrial cancer is about 60 years. The risk factors associated with the development of carcinoma of the endometrium are listed in Table 52–1. Some of these factors are associated with prolonged stimulation of the endometrium with unopposed estrogen. If the proliferative effects of estrogen are not counteracted by progester-

TABLE 52–1 RISK FACTORS IN ENDOMETRIAL CANCER

Obesity and tallness
Nulliparity
Late menopause
Diabetes mellitus
Hypertension
Gallbladder disease
Breast, colon, or ovarian cancer
Chronic unopposed estrogen stimulation

one, endometrial hyperplasia, which may be a precursor of endometrial cancer, can result (see Chapter 30).

Obesity results in an increased extraovarian aromatization of androstenedione to estrone. The androstenedione is secreted by the adrenal glands, while the increased peripheral conversion occurs predominantly in fat depots but also in the liver, kidneys, and skeletal muscles. *Granulosa–theca cell tumors* of the ovary produce estrogen, and up to 15 percent of patients with these tumors have an associated endometrial cancer.

Unopposed estrogen stimulation also occurs in premenopausal patients who are anovulatory, such as those who have *polycystic ovarian syndrome* (Stein-Leventhal syndrome), and postmenopausal women taking *estrogen replacement* without progesterone for menopausal symptoms. In the latter group, the risk of developing cancer appears to be both dose- and duration-dependent. This increased risk varies from two- to fourteenfold compared with nonusers. The addition of an oral progestogen during the last ten days of the month eliminates this risk. Fertile patients who use oral contraceptives have been shown to have a lower incidence of subsequent development of endometrial cancer.

SCREENING OF ASYMPTOMATIC WOMEN

Screening for endometrial cancer in asymptomatic women is less effective than screening for cervical cancer, since only about 40 percent of cases of endometrial cancer can be detected with a Papanicolaou (Pap) smear. Furthermore, routine endometrial sampling of all postmenopausal women has not been shown to be practical or cost-effective. Outpatient techniques for endometrial sampling include use of the Kevorkian curette, Vabra aspirator, or Gravlee jet washer. These techniques have a diagnostic accuracy of about 90 percent.

Premenopausal patients who have polycystic ovarian syndrome should have their endometrium sampled to exclude endometrial hyperplasia or carcinoma. Similarly, postmenopausal women using unopposed oral estrogen therapy should ideally have an endometrial biopsy annually. Other high-risk patients, such as those who are obese and nulliparous with hypertension or diabetes, should also undergo endometrial sampling.

SYMPTOMS

The most common symptom of endometrial cancer is abnormal vaginal bleeding. Postmenopausal bleeding is always abnormal and must be investigated. The most common conditions associated with postmenopausal bleeding are listed in Table 52–2. While a single episode of vaginal spotting is most likely due to a nonmalignant lesion, the physician must exclude malignancy. The older the patient, the more likely it is that she has cancer. In a premenopausal patient, menorrhagia or intermenstrual bleeding may be present.

SIGNS

General physical examination may reveal obesity, hypertension, and stigmata of diabetes mellitus. Evidence of metastatic disease is unusual at initial presentation, but the chest should be examined to exclude a pleural effusion and the abdomen carefully palpated and percussed to exclude ascites, hepatomegaly, or evidence of upper abdominal masses.

On pelvic examination, the external genitalia and vagina are usually normal. The cervix is also usually normal, but should be carefully inspected and palpated for evidence of involvement. A patulous cervical os or a firm, expanded cervix may indicate extension of disease from the corpus to the cervix. The

TABLE 52–2 ETIOLOGY OF POSTMENOPAUSAL BLEEDING

FACTOR	APPROXIMATE PERCENTAGE
Exogenous estrogens	30
Atrophic endometritis/vaginitis	30
Endometrial cancer	15
Endometrial or cervical polyps	10
Endometrial hyperplasia	5
Miscellaneous (e.g., cervical cancer, uterine sarcoma, urethral caruncle, trauma)	10

uterus may be of normal size or enlarged, depending on the extent of the disease and the presence or absence of other uterine conditions, such as adenomyosis. The fornices should be carefully palpated for evidence of extrauterine metastases or of an ovarian neoplasm. A granulosa cell tumor or an endometrioid ovarian carcinoma may occasionally coexist with an endometrial cancer.

DIAGNOSIS

Any woman who presents with postmenopausal bleeding should have a Pap smear, an endocervical curettage, and an endometrial biopsy performed as an outpatient. If the endometrial biopsy reveals endometrial cancer, definitive treatment can be arranged. If the endometrial biopsy is negative or reveals endometrial hyperplasia, a *fractional dilatation and curettage* should be performed under general anesthesia. Specimens from the endometrium and endocervix should be submitted separately for histologic evaluation to determine if the tumor has extended to the endocervix. Diagnosis of endometrial cancer in a premenopausal patient requires a high index of suspicion, but in a patient with high-risk factors and abnormal uterine bleeding, a similar work-up should be undertaken.

STAGING

The official International Federation of Gynecology and Obstetrics (FIGO) staging for endometrial cancer is a clinical staging; i.e., it is based on the physical examination and a limited number of nonoperative investigations (Table 52–3). These investigations

TABLE 52–3 FIGO* STAGING OF CARCINOMA OF THE CORPUS UTERI

Stage 0	Carcinoma in situ.
Stage I	The carcinoma is confined to the corpus.
Stage Ia	The length of the uterine cavity is 8 cm or less.
Stage Ib	The length of the uterine cavity is more than 8 cm.
It is desirable that the Stage I cases be subgrouped with regard to the histologic grade of the adenocarcinoma as follows:	
G1	Highly differentiated adenomatous carcinoma.
G2	Moderately differentiated adenomatous carcinoma with partly solid areas.
G3	Predominantly solid or entirely undifferentiated carcinoma.
Stage II	The carcinoma has involved the corpus and the cervix but has not extended outside the uterus.
Stage III	The carcinoma has extended outside the uterus but not outside the true pelvis.
Stage IV	The carcinoma has extended outside the true pelvis or has obviously involved the mucosa of the bladder or rectum. A bullous edema as such does not permit a case to be allotted to Stage IV.
Stage IVa	Spread of the growth to adjacent organs.
Stage IVb	Spread to distant organs.

*International Federation of Gynecology and Obstetrics

should include a chest x-ray and skeletal x-rays if bone pain is present.

PREOPERATIVE INVESTIGATIONS

In addition to the radiologic studies performed for staging purposes, a general medical evaluation should consist of a complete blood count, urinalysis, clotting studies, blood urea nitrogen or serum creatinine, blood sugar, liver function tests, and an electrocardiogram. An intravenous pyelogram should be obtained preoperatively, and in postmenopausal women, a barium enema is necessary to exclude a concurrent primary colonic neoplasm.

PATHOLOGY

Several histologic types of endometrial carcinoma exist. About 75 percent of the cases are pure *adenocarcinomas*. When benign squamous elements are present, the tumor is called an *adenoacanthoma*. Lesions that contain malignant squamous epithelium are called *adenosquamous carcinomas* and carry a poorer prognosis. Rarely, *clear cell* or *squamous carcinomas* occur in the endometrium.

Invasive adenocarcinoma of the endometrium demonstrates proliferative glandular formation with minimal or no intervening stroma. Tumor grade is determined by the degree of abnormality of the glandular architecture. A lesion that is well-differentiated (grade 1) forms a glandular pattern similar to normal endometrial glands (Fig. 52–1). A moderately well-differentiated lesion (grade 2) has glandular structures admixed with papillary, and occasionally solid, areas of tumor. In a poorly differentiated lesion (grade 3), the glandular structures have become predominantly solid with a relative paucity of identifiable endometrial glands (Fig. 52–2).

PATTERN OF SPREAD

Endometrial cancer spreads by (1) direct extension, (2) exfoliation of cells that are shed through the fallopian tubes, (3) lymphatic dissemination, and (4) hematogenous dissemination.

The most common route of spread is *direct extension* of the tumor to adjacent structures. The tumor may invade through the myometrium and eventually penetrate the serosa. It may also grow downward and involve the cervix. Although very uncommon, progressive direct extension may eventually involve the vagina or parametrium. *Exfoliated cells* that pass through the fallopian tubes may implant on the ovaries, the visceral or parietal peritoneum, or the omentum. *Lymphatic spread* occurs most commonly in patients with significant myometrial penetration. Spread occurs mainly to the pelvic lymph nodes and subsequently to the periaortic lymph nodes. The incidence of lymph node metastases is dependent upon the tumor grade and the depth of myometrial invasion. In Stage I endometrial cancer, the overall incidence of pelvic lymph node metastases is about 12 percent, and periaortic lymph node metas-

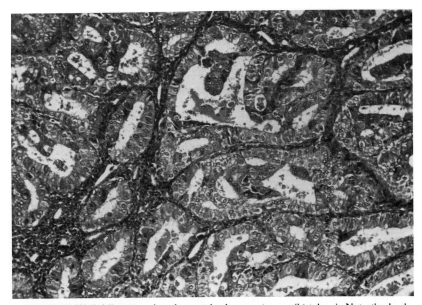

Figure 52–1 Well-differentiated endometrial adenocarcinoma (histology). Note the back-to-back glands with minimal intervening stroma and the gland-within-gland formation.

tases are present in about 8 percent of cases. However, in patients with deeply invasive, poorly differentiated Stage I adenocarcinomas, pelvic lymph node metastases occur in up to 40 percent of patients. Lymphatic spread is also responsible for vaginal vault recurrences. *Hematogenous dissemination* is less common, but it results in parenchymal metastases, particularly in the lungs and/or liver.

TREATMENT

Stage I

Surgery. The primary treatment of Stage I endometrial cancer is surgical. In the past, it was common practice to use preoperative intracavitary radiation in an attempt to ster-

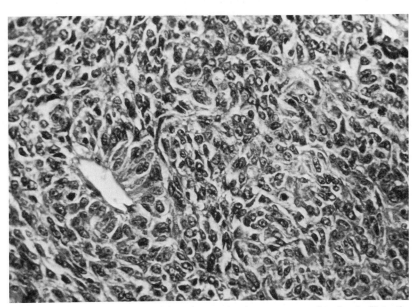

Figure 52–2 Poorly differentiated endometrial adenocarcinoma (histology). Note the predominantly solid nature of the tumor with minimal gland formation.

TABLE 52–4 HIGH-RISK FACTORS IN STAGE I ENDOMETRIAL CANCER

1. High tumor grade
2. Deep myometrial invasion
3. Pelvic and/or periaortic lymph node metastasis
4. Occult cervical involvement
5. Occult adnexal spread
6. Occult upper abdominal spread
7. Positive peritoneal cytology

ilize the disease prior to surgical intervention. Currently, it is generally considered preferable to operate primarily to allow proper identification of risk factors (Table 52–4). Adjuvant postoperative therapy can then be given more appropriately.

An exploratory laparotomy with total abdominal hysterectomy and bilateral salpingo-oophorectomy is performed on all patients, unless there are absolute medical contraindications (Fig. 52–3). To prevent potential spillage of cancer cells through the fallopian tubes, the fimbriated ends are tied off prior to performing the operation. On entering the peritoneal cavity, any free fluid is submitted for cytologic evaluation. If there is no free fluid and no macroscopic evidence of tumor dissemination, saline washings are taken from the pelvis, paracolic gutters, and subdiaphragmatic areas and sent separately for cytologic evaluation. Approximately 12 percent of patients with Stage I disease have positive peritoneal cytology. Retroperitoneal spaces should be opened and evaluated, and any enlarged pelvic or periaortic lymph nodes should be biopsied.

Radiation Therapy. An algorithm summarizing the treatment of Stage I endometrial cancer is presented in Figure 52–4. After exploratory laparotomy and an evaluation of the histopathology and peritoneal cytology, adjuvant radiation is given to selected patients. The depth of myometrial invasion cannot be determined preoperatively, so some patients with superficial invasion only may be spared pelvic radiation if the surgery is done initially.

Most patients who require additional treatment are candidates for *external beam pelvic radiation*, which is given in an attempt to prevent recurrent disease at the vaginal vault and pelvic side wall. Any patient with a poorly differentiated (grade 3) carcinoma or with invasion beyond the inner one third of the myometrium should receive whole pelvic irradiation postoperatively.

In patients with a superficially invasive, well-differentiated (grade 1) carcinoma, the incidence of recurrent disease is so low that no adjuvant therapy is indicated. If a superficially invasive grade 2 carcinoma is present, *intracavitary radiation to the vaginal vault*, which carries virtually no morbidity, may be given to prevent a vault recurrence.

In patients with periaortic lymph node involvement, *extended field radiation* to include

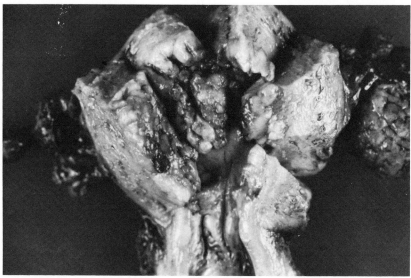

Figure 52–3 Specimen from a total abdominal hysterectomy and bilateral salpingo-oophorectomy. The uterus has been opened to reveal an exophytic carcinoma on the posterior wall of the corpus.

TREATMENT OF ENDOMETRIAL CANCER:

STAGES I + II OCCULT

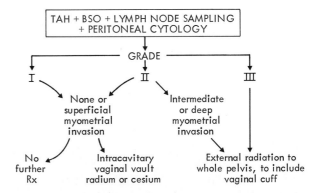

Figure 52–4 Algorithm of the treatment of Stage I and occult Stage II endometrial cancer.

the pelvis and periaortic area is indicated. The management of patients who have positive peritoneal cytology is controversial. *Whole abdominal radiation* or *intraperitoneal radioactive phosphorus* (^{32}P) has been advocated, although these treatments are associated with significant morbidity, and no randomized prospective study has been done to demonstrate proven benefit.

In patients medically unfit for surgery, radiation therapy without surgery may be employed. A combination of intracavitary plus external beam radiation is used. The overall five year survival is about 25 percent lower than for patients treated with hysterectomy.

Stage II

If the cervix is grossly normal and involvement is detected only on the histologic evaluation of the endocervical curettings (occult Stage II disease), treatment may be the same as for Stage I disease (i.e., total abdominal hysterectomy, bilateral salpingo-oophorectomy, surgical staging, and postoperative radiotherapy).

If the cervix is grossly enlarged, preoperative external beam and intracavitary radiation are indicated, followed by total abdominal hysterectomy and bilateral salpingo-oophorectomy six weeks later. An alternative approach is to use preoperative external radiation only, followed in six weeks by a modified radical hysterectomy and bilateral salpingo-oophorectomy. This avoids a second anesthetic for the placement of the intracavitary radium or cesium.

Advanced Stages

For advanced disease, treatment is individualized. The uterus, tubes, and ovaries are best removed, if possible, for palliation of bleeding and other pelvic symptoms. If gross disease is present in the upper abdomen, tumor metastases that are readily removable, such as an omental "cake," should be extirpated in an attempt to improve the patient's quality of life by temporarily decreasing abdominal discomfort and ascites. In addition to pre- or postoperative radiation, patients with advanced disease will also require hormonal therapy, with or without chemotherapy.

Recurrent Disease

Seventy-five percent of recurrences occur within two years after treatment, and a further 10 percent occur by the end of the third year. If recurrent disease is detected, the patient should undergo a complete physical examination and metastatic work-up. If the disease appears to be limited to the vaginal vault, surgery, radiation, or a combination of the two may be effective, particularly if radiation was not used as part of the primary therapy. Metastases in other sites, such as the upper abdomen, lungs, or liver are treated initially with high-dose progestins or antiestrogens. Medroxyprogesterone acetate (Provera), 50 mg three times daily; Depo-Provera, 400 mg intramuscularly weekly; or megestrol acetate (Megace), 80 mg twice daily, may be given. If disease progresses on progestins, chemotherapy may be offered. Doxorubicin (Adriamycin) appears to be the most active single agent, but the response rate is only about 35 percent, and most responses are partial and of short duration.

Hormone Receptors

Recently, it has been shown that about one third of recurrent endometrial carcinomas contain estrogen and progesterone receptors. The frequency of positive receptors is dependent upon the grade of the tumor, the more well-differentiated tumors being more likely to contain these receptors. As with breast cancer, the likelihood of a patient responding to progestin treatment is increased in patients whose tumors are receptor-positive. Approximately 80 percent of such patients respond to progestin therapy, compared with less than 10 percent of receptor-negative patients.

PROGNOSIS

Operative findings do not change the FIGO stage, but they may change the prognosis. Prognosis is dependent on several variables identifiable at laparotomy, including uterine size, stage of tumor, histologic type, grade of tumor, depth of myometrial penetration, status of lymph nodes, status of peritoneal cytology, and presence or absence of occult adnexal metastases. These factors are generally interrelated. The more poorly differentiated tumors (grade 3) have a greater propensity for deep myometrial invasion and, conse-

quently, an increased incidence of lymph node metastases. Positive peritoneal cytology also frequently coexists with other poor prognostic factors but may occur as an independent poor prognosticator. About one third of patients with positive washings develop recurrence in the peritoneal cavity. Of all the criteria used, the size of the uterine cavity is the least significant because the uterus can be enlarged by fibroids or adenomyosis, benign entities that do not alter the prognosis.

Five-year survivals for each stage of endometrial cancer are presented in Table 52–5. Stage for stage, prognosis is similar to that for cervical cancer.

UTERINE SARCOMAS

Uterine sarcomas are rare. They arise from the stromal components of the uterus, either the endometrial stroma or the mesenchymal and myometrial tissues. As a group, sarcomas tend to be more advanced at the time of diagnosis, are more likely to disseminate hematogenously, and have much lower two- and five-year survival rates.

Classification

A classification system for uterine sarcomas is presented in Table 52–6. Uterine sarcomas can be classified as either *pure,* in which the only malignant tissue is of mesenchymal origin, or *mixed,* in which malignant mesenchymal and malignant epithelial tissues are present. They may also be classified as *homologous,* implying that the tissue that is malignant is normally present in the uterus (e.g., endometrial stroma, smooth muscle);

TABLE 52–5 CARCINOMA OF THE CORPUS UTERI*

STAGE	PATIENTS TREATED		FIVE-YEAR SURVIVAL	
	No.	%	No.	%
I	8550	74.3	6340	74.2
II	1690	14.7	970	57.4
III	822	7.2	240	29.2
IV	314	2.7	30	9.6
No stage	125	1.1	76	60.8
Total	11,501	100.0	7656	66.6

*Distribution by stage and five-year survival rate in different stages

Reproduced with permission from the Editorial Office of the Annual Report on the Results of Treatment in Gynecological Cancer. Vol 18. Stockholm, Sweden, 1982, p 61.

TABLE 52–6 CLASSIFICATION OF UTERINE SARCOMAS

TYPE	HOMOLOGOUS	HETEROLOGOUS
Pure	Leiomyosarcoma Stromal sarcoma (i) endolymphatic stromal myosis (ii) endometrial stromal sarcoma	Rhabdomyosarcoma Chondrosarcoma Osteosarcoma Liposarcoma
Mixed	Carcinosarcoma	Mixed mesodermal sarcoma

or *heterologous,* implying that the tissue that is malignant is not normally present in the uterus (e.g., bone or cartilage). The majority of "pure" uterine sarcomas are leiomyosarcomas and endometrial stromal sarcomas.

Leiomyosarcoma

Leiomyosarcomas may be associated with a benign leiomyoma of the uterus, but the risk of malignant transformation in a benign fibroid is less than 1 percent. The most important histologic criterion for distinguishing leiomyosarcomas from leiomyomas is the mitotic index. If the tumor's most highly mitotic areas contain 10 or more mitoses per 10 high-power fields (hpf), the lesion is malignant. Lesions with fewer than 5 mitoses per 10 hpf are generally benign, while tumors with 5 to 9 mitoses per 10 hpf can behave in a malignant fashion if the cells are atypical cytologically.

Clinically, the mean age of patients with a leiomyosarcoma is about 55 years. Patients with this disease may present with either menometrorrhagia or postmenopausal bleeding. A vaginal discharge or a sensation of pressure or fullness in the pelvic area may also be noted.

Most cases are not diagnosed preoperatively, but are discovered at the time of exploratory surgery for probable uterine myomata. Endometrial curettings are usually negative. If on pelvic examination the uterus appears to be rapidly enlarging, the suspicion of a uterine malignancy exists.

Leiomyosarcomas tend to spread by local extension, as well as by hematogenous and lymphatic dissemination. Isolated pelvic recurrences are uncommon; most patients die with disease in distant organ parenchyma, particularly the lungs and liver.

The treatment of a uterine leiomyosarcoma is a total abdominal hysterectomy and bilateral salpingo-oophorectomy. In the absence of obvious tumor dissemination, peritoneal cytology and selective pelvic and periaortic lymph node biopsies should be obtained, as with endometrial adenocarcinoma. Following surgery, patients whose tumors are confined to the uterus and contain fewer than 5 mitoses per 10 hpf require no adjuvant therapy. Patients whose lesions have a high mitotic index should receive adjuvant postoperative radiation, either pelvic, extended field, or possibly whole abdominal, depending on the opera-tive findings. While pelvic radiation does appear to decrease local pelvic recurrence, it does not prolong survival, as most patients develop distant metastases.

Chemotherapy has not proven to be effective in this disease. The most commonly used drugs include doxorubicin, *cis*-platinum, cyclophosphamide, vincristine, and actinomycin-D. The most active of these agents appears to be doxorubicin, but objective response rates in patients with metastatic disease are only 25 to 30 percent. The use of adjuvant chemotherapy in patients with Stage I disease has not been shown to improve survival.

Endometrial Stromal Sarcoma

There are three types of stromal sarcomas: (1) endometrial stromal nodule, (2) endolymphatic stromal myosis, and (3) endometrial stromal sarcoma. The first of these, the *stromal nodule,* is a rare benign condition. The mitotic index is very low, typically 3 or fewer per 10 hpf. A hysterectomy is curative.

Endolymphatic stromal myosis is a low-grade sarcoma. Histologically, there is minimal to absent cellular atypism, with usually fewer than 5 mitoses per 10 hpf. There is always evidence of vascular channel invasion. These patients usually present with abnormal vaginal bleeding and, often, pelvic pain. This condition is diagnosed at the time of exploratory surgery for presumed benign leiomyomata. About 30 percent of the tumors have extrauterine extension discovered at laparotomy, which consists of multiple wormlike, rubbery growths in the pelvis.

Most patients are cured with a total abdominal hysterectomy and bilateral salpingo-oophorectomy. With local pelvic extension, a radical or modified radical hysterectomy and bilateral pelvic lymphadenectomy may be necessary to resect all of the disease. Incompletely resected lesions will often respond to pelvic radiation. Local recurrences may occur even 10 to 20 years later, and require re-exploration and resection of disease. Distant metastases also rarely occur. High-dose progesterone therapy has been shown to result in tumor regression in some patients with metastatic disease.

Endometrial stromal sarcoma generally causes menometrorrhagia or postmenopausal bleeding and, occasionally, pelvic pain. The diagnosis can often be made by endometrial biopsy or by cervical dilatation and curettage of the uterus.

Histologically, there are 10 or more mitoses per 10 hpf, and the lesion is composed of rather poorly differentiated stromal cells. Aggressive myometrial invasion occurs, and tumor is commonly seen in lymphatic spaces.

About half of the patients present with evidence of metastatic disease, usually to distant organs, particularly the liver or lungs. Recurrence in these sites is high in patients who had disease apparently confined to the uterus at the time of diagnosis.

The treatment of endometrial stromal sarcomas is the same as that for leiomyosarcoma. Postoperative pelvic radiation improves local control but does not improve survival. In patients with metastatic disease, progestogens or chemotherapy should be offered, but response rates are low.

Mixed Müllerian Sarcoma

Mixed müllerian sarcomas account for about 40 percent of uterine sarcomas. Most patients are postmenopausal and present with vaginal bleeding or discharge. About one third of patients have tumor growing through the cervix into the vagina as a polypoid mass. As opposed to a "fibroid" uterus, these lesions are usually soft to palpation. About 50 percent of patients with this lesion have evidence of metastatic disease at the time of diagnosis.

Histologically, either the carcinoma or the sarcoma may be the predominant component. As with endometrial stromal sarcomas, these tumors aggressively invade the myometrium and disseminate via the lymphatics and the blood stream.

The primary treatment of mixed müllerian sarcoma is the same as that for leiomyosarcoma.

Prognosis

The prognosis for uterine sarcomas is poor, the overall 5-year survival rate being about 35 percent. Patients with mixed müllerian sarcomas have a poorer overall survival than patients with a leiomyosarcoma or endometrial stromal sarcoma. However, when compared stage for stage, all three uterine sarcomas have the same prognosis. Patients with a Stage I uterine sarcoma have about a 50 percent five-year survival.

SUGGESTED READING

Aalders J, Abeler V, Kolstad P, Onsrud M: Postoperative external irradiation and prognostic parameters in Stage I endometrial carcinoma: Clinical and histopathologic study of 540 patients. Obstet Gynecol 56:419, 1980.

Berman ML, Ballon SC, Lagasse LD, Watring WG: Prognosis and treatment of endometrial cancer. Am J Obstet Gynecol 136:679, 1980.

Boronow RC, Morrow CP, Creasman WT, et al: Surgical staging in endometrial cancer: Clinical pathologic findings of a prospective study. Obstet Gynecol 63:825, 1984.

Cox JD, Komaki R, Wilson F, Greenberg M: Locally advanced adenocarcinoma of the endometrium: Results of irradiation with and without subsequent hysterectomy. Cancer 45:715, 1980.

Creasman WT, Boronow RC, Morrow CP, et al: Adenocarcinoma of the endometrium: Its metastatic lymph node potential: A preliminary report. Gynecol Oncol 4:239, 1976.

Jones HW Jr: Treatment of adenocarcinoma of the endometrium. Obstet Gynecol Surv 30:147, 1975.

Landgren RD, Fletcher GH, Gallager HS, Declos L, Wharton JT: Treatment failure sites according to irradiation technique and histology in patients with endometrial cancer. Cancer 40:131, 1977.

Malkasian GD: Carcinoma of the endometrium: Effect of stage and grade on survival. Cancer 41:966, 1978.

Salazar OM, Bontfiglio TA, Pattern SF, et al: Uterine sarcomas: Natural history, treatment, and prognosis. Cancer 42:1152, 1978.

Salazar OM, Feldstein ML, DePapp EW, et al: The management of clinical Stage I endometrial carcinoma. Cancer 41:1016, 1978.

Soper JT, Creasman WT, Clarke-Pearson DL, et al: Intraperitoneal chronic phosphate P^{32} suspension therapy of malignant peritoneal cytology in endometrial carcinoma. Am J Obstet Gynecol 153:191, 1985.

Zaloudek CJ, Norris HJ: Mesenchymal tumors of the uterus. Prog Surg Pathol 3:1, 1981.

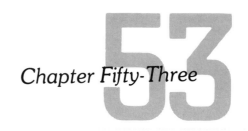

Chapter Fifty-Three

CERVICAL DYSPLASIA AND CANCER

EDWARD SAVAGE

In the United States, cervical cancer ranks sixth among cancers in women, with 16,000 new cases diagnosed annually. The incidence has decreased markedly since the 1930s. Part of the decline in cervical cancer is probably related to the advent of the Papanicolaou (Pap) smear, which permits detection of preinvasive disease. Therapy for preinvasive disease is usually curative and prevents the subsequent development of invasive cancer. The incidence of preinvasive disease of the cervix has been increasing over the past decade.

ETIOLOGY AND EPIDEMIOLOGY

Cervical cancer and its precursors have been associated with several epidemiologic variables (Table 53–1). Cervical carcinoma is

TABLE 53–1 RISK FACTORS FOR CERVICAL CANCER

Young age at first coitus (under 20 years)
Multiple sexual partners
Young age at marriage
Young age at first pregnancy
High parity
Divorce
Lower socioeconomic status
Smoking

relatively rare before the age of 20 years, the average age of this occurrence being 47 years. In the lower socioeconomic groups and in some geographic areas, the average age has been reported to be as low as 39 years.

The adolescent cervix is believed to be more susceptible to carcinogenic stimuli because of the active process of squamous metaplasia, which occurs within the transformation zone during that period of development. This squamous metaplasia is normally a physiologic process, but under the influence of a carcinogen, cellular alterations may occur that result in an *atypical transformation zone*. These atypical changes initiate a process called *cervical intraepithelial neoplasia* (CIN), which is the preinvasive phase of cervical cancer.

Cervical intraepithelial neoplasia represents a spectrum of disease beginning as a change called mild dysplasia (CIN I), which may gradually progress to moderate dysplasia (CIN II) and to severe dysplasia and carcinoma *in situ* (CIN III). This process is not always continuously progressive and may remain in an earlier phase or regress entirely. About 20 percent of patients with carcinoma *in situ* eventually develop invasion beyond the basement membrane, resulting initially in microinvasive carcinoma, then frankly invasive carcinoma.

It is estimated that approximately 10 to 15 percent of mild to moderate dysplasias progress to invasive cancer if not treated. The

475

length of time for this progression varies, and even a fairly advanced form of dysplasia may require 3 to 20 years to become invasive cancer.

Although herpes type II virus has been implicated as an etiologic agent in the past, more recent studies have documented a stronger link between cervical carcinoma and the human papilloma virus (HPV). The HPV virus can now be "typed" using DNA hybridization techniques. Types 6 and 11 have been frequently associated with cervical condylomata, whereas types 16 and 18 have been associated with noninvasive and invasive cervical neoplasia. Some investigators have related cervical carcinogenesis to contact with human sperm, but these data are controversial.

SCREENING OF ASYMPTOMATIC WOMEN

The current recommendation of the American College of Obstetricians and Gynecologists is that all women, once they have become sexually active, should undergo an annual physical examination, including a Pap smear. There has been some controversy regarding this recommendation because women who do not have the high-risk features outlined above have a significantly lower rate of cervical cancer. Less rigorous screening, such as every two to five years following two or three normal Pap smears, has been proposed by some as being more "cost-effective" for this low-risk group. Both the endocervical canal and the ectocervix should be sampled when taking the Pap smear.

Although cervical cytology generally correlates with the histologic diagnosis, a biopsy is absolutely necessary for the definitive diagnosis prior to therapy. With the Pap smear, the false-positive rate is less than 1 percent, whereas the false-negative rate is between 10 and 20 percent. With simultaneous use of Pap smears and colposcopically directed biopsies, almost all squamous cervical lesions can be detected on initial evaluation. However, false-negative Pap smears have been reported in as many as 40 to 45 percent of patients ultimately diagnosed as having cervical adenocarcinomas. The latter usually arise in the endocervical canal.

CERVICAL TOPOGRAPHY

In order to understand the concepts of colposcopy, it is important to understand cervical topography. During early embryonic development, the cervix and upper vagina are covered with columnar epithelium. Progressively, during intrauterine development, the columnar epithelium of the vagina is replaced by squamous epithelium. At birth, the vagina is usually covered with squamous epithelium, and the columnar epithelium is limited to the endocervix and the central portion of the ectocervix. In about 4 percent of normal female infants and about 30 percent of those exposed to diethylstilbestrol *in utero*, the columnar epithelium extends onto the vaginal fornices. Macroscopically, the columnar epithelium has a red appearance because it is only a single cell layer thick, allowing blood vessels in the underlying stroma to show through it.

The squamous and columnar epithelia of infants are designated the *original* or *native* squamous and columnar epithelia, respectively. The junction between them is called the *original squamocolumnar junction*. Throughout life, but particularly during adolescence and the first pregnancy, metaplastic squamous epithelium covers the columnar epithelium so that a new squamocolumnar junction is formed more proximally. This junction moves progressively closer to the external os, then up the endocervical canal. The *transformation zone* is the area of metaplastic squamous epithelium located between the original squamocolumnar junction and the new squamocolumnar junction (Fig. 53–1).

EVALUATION OF A PATIENT WITH AN ABNORMAL PAP SMEAR

Although there is no uniformly accepted system for the classification of Pap smears, the one shown in Table 53–2 is a reasonable approximation of most that have been devised. Any patient with a grossly abnormal cervix should have a punch biopsy performed. The following discussion refers to patients who have an *abnormal* Pap smear and a *grossly normal* appearing cervix.

An algorithm for the evaluation of patients with abnormal Pap smears is presented in

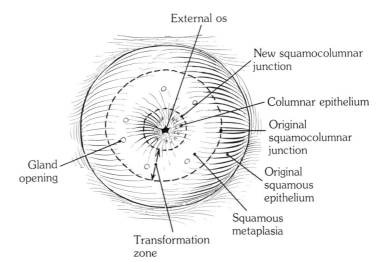

Figure 53–1 Schematic representation of the transformation zone.

Figure 53–2. Patients with a Class II Pap smear require evaluation for, and management of, inflammatory conditions (see Chapter 33). Patients with a persistent Class II smear and all those with a Class III or worse smear require colposcopic evaluation of the cervix.

Colposcopy

The colposcope is a stereoscopic binocular microscope of low magnification, usually 10 to 40× (Fig. 53–3). Illumination is centered, and the focal length is between 12 and 15 cm.

To perform colposcopy, an appropriately sized speculum is inserted to expose the cervix, which is cleansed with a cotton pledget soaked in 3 percent acetic acid to remove adherent mucus and cellular debris. It may be necessary to reapply the acetic acid at intervals during a prolonged examination. With direct illumination from the white light, surface features of the cervix can usually be identified. A green filter can be employed to accentuate the vascular changes that fre-

quently accompany pathologic alterations of the cervix. Cameras are available for attachment to colposcopes, and photographs may sometimes be useful to facilitate follow-up when conservative treatment is used.

Colposcopic Findings. Colposcopically, the original or native squamous epithelium appears gray and homogeneous. The columnar epithelium is red and grape-like in appearance. The transformation zone can be identified by the presence of gland openings that are not covered by the squamous metaplasia and by the paler color of the metaplastic epithelium compared to the original squamous epithelium. Nabothian follicles may also be seen in the transformation zone. Normal blood vessels are branching like a tree.

The colposcopic hallmark of *cervical dysplasia* is an area of sharply delineated acetowhite epithelium—that is, epithelium that appears white after the application of acetic acid. It is thought that the acetic acid dehydrates the cells, and there is increased light reflex from areas of increased nuclear density (that is, areas of CIN). Within the acetowhite areas, there may or may not be abnormal vascular patterns.

There are two basic changes in the vascular architecture in patients with CIN: (1) punctation and (2) mosaicism. Punctation is caused by single looped capillaries lying within the subepithelial papillae, seen endon as a "dot" as they course toward the surface of the epithelium. Mosaicism is due to a fine network of capillaries disposed parallel to the surface in a mosaic pattern. Punc-

TABLE 53–2 CLASSIFICATION OF ABNORMAL SQUAMOUS CELL CYTOLOGY

Class I	Normal
Class II	Inflammatory atypia
Class III	Dysplasia
Class IV	Carcinoma *in situ*
Class V	Invasive carcinoma

EVALUATION OF THE ABNORMAL PAPANICOLAOU SMEAR

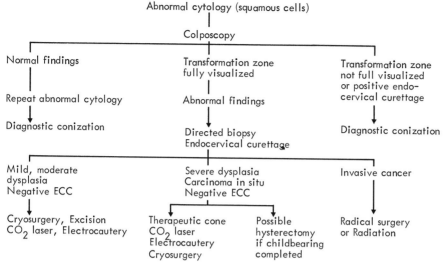

Figure 53–2 Algorithm for evaluation of patients with an abnormal Papanicolaou smear and a grossly normal appearing cervix.

tate and mosaic patterns may be seen together within the same area of the cervix.

The more dilated and irregular the punctate and mosaic capillaries and the greater the intercapillary distance, the more atypical is the tissue on histologic examination. Similarly, the whiter the lesion, the more severe the dysplasia. True branching vessels have not been observed in dysplasia or carcinoma *in situ*.

With *microinvasive carcinoma*, extremely irregular punctate and mosaic patterns are found, as well as small atypical vessels. The irregularity in size, shape, and arrangement of the terminal vessels becomes even more striking in frankly invasive carcinoma, with exaggerated distortions of the vascular architecture producing comma-shaped, corkscrew-shaped, and dilated, blind-ended vessels.

Directed Biopsy and Endocervical Curettage

If the colposcopic examination is *satisfactory*, which implies that the entire transformation zone has been visualized, a punch biopsy is taken from the worst area(s), together with an endocervical curettage (ECC). The endocervical curettage is not performed in patients who are pregnant.

If the colposcopic examination is *unsatisfactory*, the endocervical curettings are positive, there is significant discrepancy between the biopsy and Pap smear, or microinvasion is present on the biopsy, conization should be performed (see Chapter 43).

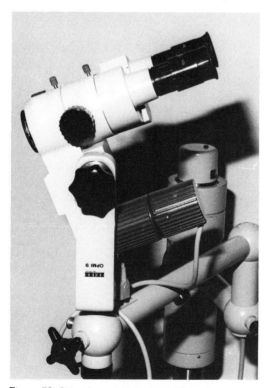

Figure 53–3 A colposcope, used to evaluate patients with an abnormal Papanicolaou smear and a grossly normal cervix.

Schiller's Test

The superficial cells of the normal mature squamous epithelium of the vagina and cervix contain glycogen. Therefore, when a dilute aqueous solution of Lugol's iodine is applied, the epithelium stains brown almost immediately. When no glycogen is present, as is usually the case with carcinoma *in situ* and cervical dysplasia, the involved area fails to stain. The nonstaining areas are designated Schiller-positive, or iodine-negative. Many benign conditions of the cervix, including ectropions, atrophic epithelium, nonmalignant ulcers, and columnar epithelium, are also Schiller-positive. The test is, therefore, not specific for malignant lesions. In addition, Schiller-negative areas have been described in patients with intraepithelial neoplastic disease. Schiller staining may serve as a complementary technique to colposcopic examination but should never replace it.

SYMPTOMS

Preinvasive disease (dysplasia and carcinoma *in situ*) does not produce symptoms. The discharge frequently seen in preinvasive disease is most often due to accompanying infection. Clinical symptoms of *microinvasive carcinoma* are also either nonexistent or nonspecific and, therefore, are of no assistance in making the diagnosis.

The most common symptoms of *invasive cervical carcinoma* are abnormal bleeding and vaginal discharge. Approximately 80 to 90 percent of patients experience some abnormal bleeding. The bleeding may be postcoital, abnormal menstrual bleeding, or intermenstrual spotting. Some patients may present with postmenopausal bleeding. The only symptom in some patients may be a vaginal discharge. The character of the discharge may be serous, purulent, or mucoid. It is not necessarily malodorous, except with fairly advanced disease. Other symptoms, such as pelvic pain, leg swelling, and urinary frequency, are usually only seen with advanced disease. A minority of patients are completely asymptomatic.

PHYSICAL FINDINGS

Patients with cervical cancer usually have a normal general physical examination. Weight loss occurs late in the disease. With advanced disease, there may be enlarged

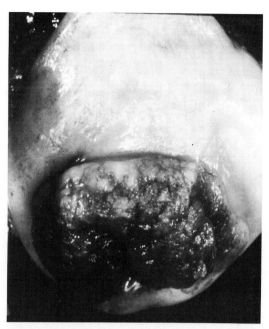

Figure 53–4 Squamous cell carcinoma of the cervix. A granular, nodular lesion that bleeds easily on contact is seen replacing the ectocervix.

inguinal or supraclavicular lymph nodes, edema of the legs, ascites, pleural effusion, or hepatomegaly, but these are not commonly seen.

The pelvic examination in early disease may reveal a cervix that appears normal, especially if the lesion is endocervical. Visible disease may take several forms: ulcerative, exophytic, granular, or necrotic. It may be friable and bleed on palpation. There is often an associated serous, purulent, or bloody discharge. The lesion may involve the upper portion of the vagina and extend toward the introitus. The cervix may be distorted or completely replaced by tumor (Fig. 53–4).

The rectovaginal examination is essential to determine the extent of involvement. The degree of cervical expansion and any spread to the parametria is much more easily detected with the rectal finger in this examination, as is extension into the vaginal fornices or uterosacral ligaments. Occasionally, a palpable mass on the pelvic wall representing an enlarged node can be felt.

PATHOLOGY

Most uterine cervical cancers are squamous in origin. Adenocarcinomas and adenosquamous carcinomas, which appear to be increasing in incidence, account for about 15 percent of cases. Melanomas and sarcomas occur rarely.

Cervical Intraepithelial Neoplasia

The cellular changes associated with atypia are related to the loss of the normal maturation of the epithelium. There is a tendency for the basal and parabasal cells to proliferate abnormally, with distortion of the normal architecture and lack of the usual differentiation. The severity of the lesion may be judged by the percentage of epithelium involved. Thus, involvement of the inner one third of the epithelium represents mild dysplasia (CIN I), involvement of the inner one half to two thirds represents moderate dysplasia (CIN II), and full thickness involvement represents severe dysplasia or carcinoma *in situ* (CIN III). In carcinoma *in situ*, the cells are indistinguishable from those of frankly invasive cancer, except that the basement membrane remains intact (Fig. 53–5).

Microinvasive Carcinoma

With progression to microinvasive carcinoma, there is a breakthrough of the basement membrane with malignant cells invading into the cervical stroma. There is no official International Federation of Gynecology and Obstetrics (FIGO) definition of microinvasive (Stage Ia) cervical cancer. Most gynecologists accept penetration into the stroma up to 3 mm from the basement membrane, provided there is no lymphatic or vascular space invasion. Some use the criterion of confluency of the invading plugs or attempt to define the lesion in terms of volume of invading tumor. The diagnosis of microinvasive carcinoma can only be made on the basis of a cone biopsy of the cervix, which allows multiple step-sections to be taken at 2-mm intervals. With a punch biopsy, the sampling of the cervix is too limited, and a more frankly invasive focus may be missed. The concept of microinvasive carcinoma should be applied only to squamous cell carcinomas. All invasive adenocarcinomas should be regarded as frankly invasive.

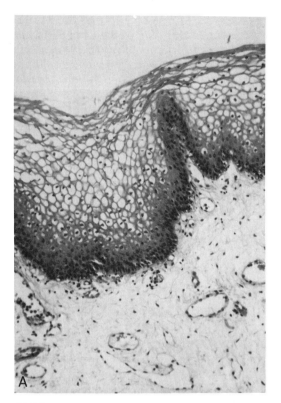

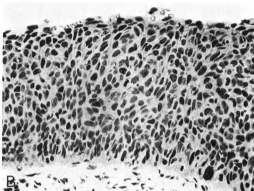

Figure 53–5 Histology of *(A)* normal cervical squamous epithelium and *(B)* carcinoma *in situ* of the cervix. In the normal epithelium, note the orderly maturation from the basal layer to the parabasal cells, glycogenated intermediate cells, and flattened superficial cells. In the carcinoma *in situ*, the entire thickness of the epithelium is replaced by immature cells that are variable in size and shape and have irregular nuclei. Mitotic figures are seen in the lower two thirds of the epithelium.

Invasive Carcinoma

Squamous carcinomas, which account for 80 to 85 percent of all invasive lesions, can be divided into the small-cell carcinoma, which is a poorly differentiated lesion, and the better differentiated large-cell carcinoma.

Large-cell carcinomas may be nonkeratinizing or keratinizing. Some pathologists use simpler terminology: poorly differentiated, moderately differentiated, and well differentiated.

About 10 to 20 percent of invasive cervical cancers are adenocarcinomas or mixed adenosquamous carcinomas. The most poorly differentiated adenosquamous carcinoma is the "glassy cell" carcinoma. Rare cervical lesions, such as melanomas, sarcomas, and lymphomas, together account for less than 1 percent of cases.

PREOPERATIVE INVESTIGATIONS FOR INVASIVE CERVICAL CANCER

Clinical Staging

The official FIGO staging for cervical cancer is a clinical staging method based on physical examination and noninvasive testing (Table 53–3).

The studies used for the FIGO staging of cervical cancer include biopsies, cystoscopy, sigmoidoscopy, chest and skeletal x-rays, intravenous pyelography, and liver function tests. Cystoscopy and sigmoidoscopy seldom reveal mucosal invasion, unless the central disease is advanced. Lung metastases are seen in about 5 percent of patients with advanced disease and almost never in early disease.

Other tests that may be useful, especially in advanced or recurrent disease, include a bipedal lymphangiogram, liver-spleen scan, barium enema, and computerized tomography of the abdomen and pelvis. Results of these latter tests are not used for FIGO staging, but may be helpful in establishing the extent of the disease and in guiding management.

Laboratory studies may reveal abnormalities with advanced disease, the most common being anemia from bleeding, elevated blood urea nitrogen and creatinine if the ureters are obstructed, and abnormal liver function tests if there are liver metastases. Ureteral obstruction occurs in about 30 percent of patients with Stage III disease and 50 percent of patients with Stage IV disease. Hypercalcemia may denote advanced disease, sometimes without bone involvement.

Surgical Staging

Less than two decades ago, several investigators began to use surgical staging prior to

TABLE 53–3 FIGO* STAGING OF CERVICAL CARCINOMA

PREINVASIVE CARCINOMA

Stage 0	Carcinoma *in situ,* intraepithelial carcinoma
	Cases of Stage 0 should not be included in any therapeutic statistics for invasive carcinoma

INVASIVE CARCINOMA

Stage I	Carcinoma strictly confined to the cervix (extension to the corpus should be disregarded)
Stage Ia	Microinvasive carcinoma (early stromal invasion)
Stage Ib	All other cases of Stage I; occult cancer should be marked "occ"
Stage II	The carcinoma extends beyond the cervix, but has not extended onto the pelvic wall. The carcinoma involves the vagina, but not the lower third.
Stage IIa	No obvious parametrial involvement
Stage IIb	Obvious parametrial involvement
Stage III	The carcinoma has extended to the pelvic wall. On rectal examination there is no cancer-free space between the tumor and the pelvic wall. The tumor involves the lower third of the vagina. All cases with a hydronephrosis or nonfunctioning kidney should be included, unless they are known to be due to another cause.
Stage IIIa	No extension onto the pelvic wall
Stage IIIb	Extension onto the pelvic wall and/or hydronephrosis or nonfunctioning kidney
Stage IV	The carcinoma has extended beyond the true pelvis or has clinically involved the mucosa of the bladder or rectum. Bullous edema of the bladder alone does not permit a case to be allotted to Stage IV
Stage IVa	Spread of the growth to adjacent organs
Stage IVb	Spread to distant organs

*International Federation of Gynecology and Obstetrics.

radiation therapy to better determine the extent of disease. The stimulus was the occasional finding of periaortic lymph node metastases at the time of radical hysterectomy for early stage disease. Many centers now use surgical staging to define the extent of the disease and to plan optimal radiation therapy. The incidence of periaortic lymph node metastases is approximately 20 percent in Stage II disease and 30 percent in Stage III. Approximately 10 percent of patients with Stage II lesions or greater have unsuspected peritoneal, adnexal, or liver metastases diagnosed at surgery. Occasionally, patients may be down-staged because of surgical findings that do not represent carcinoma, such as endometriosis. In some series, the incidence of complications following radiation, particularly bowel injuries, has been higher after surgical staging. If a retroperitoneal approach is used rather than a transperitoneal approach, there is no significantly increased incidence of post-radiation complications. Periaortic irradiation appears to improve survival in patients whose periaortic metastases are microscopic.

TREATMENT

Intraepithelial Neoplasia

The ability to locate and precisely define the size and distribution of the intraepithelial lesion by colposcopy in most patients has allowed a more conservative approach to the disease. Superficial ablative techniques, such as local excision, cryosurgery, CO_2 laser, or electrocoagulation, may be appropriate. For these more conservative forms of management, the entire transformation zone must be visible and accessible to the method to be employed. The more conservative methods are particularly preferred in patients who desire to maintain their childbearing capacity and may be repeated should failure occur, as long as invasive disease has been excluded.

Cryosurgery. Cryosurgery is probably most widely used for the treatment of CIN in this country. The advantages of this method are: (1) it is relatively painless, (2) there is minimal or no blood loss, (3) it is inexpensive, (4) it is an outpatient procedure, and (5) it has no appreciable effect on childbearing capacity. The major side effect is a rather copious vaginal discharge that persists for several weeks. Another disadvantage is that the squamocolumnar junction frequently recedes into the endocervical canal, making colposcopic evaluation less valuable in the follow-up of these patients. The failure rate is approximately 20 percent but may be higher with gland involvement or with more advanced or larger lesions.

Laser. The CO_2 laser (*l*ight *a*mplification by *s*timulated *e*mission of *r*adiation) is a more recent technique for the treatment of CIN. The technique has the advantages of precision, rapid tissue destruction, and minimal scarring. Treatment without anesthesia may be painful, and cervical bleeding may sometimes occur. The entire transformation zone should be destroyed. Post-treatment surveillance by colposcopy is more likely to be satisfactory, because the squamocolumnar junction is not moved into the endocervical canal by treatment. When properly used, failure rates are approximately 10 to 15 percent. This technique is more expensive than cryotherapy.

Electrocoagulation. Success rates of up to 97 percent have been reported for electrocoagulation. However, it causes more discomfort than the other techniques and, therefore, requires general anesthesia. Cervical stenosis may occasionally occur.

Cervical Conization. Once widely used for diagnosis, this technique is also sometimes used for treatment. Therapeutic indications for cone biopsy are extension of the lesion into the endocervix or the presence of extensive carcinoma *in situ*. Provided the margins of resection are clear, cure rates are as high as with hysterectomy. Compared with simpler techniques, the advantage is that an optimal portion of tissue is submitted for pathologic evaluation.

Hysterectomy. Since this method has a high cure rate, it is acceptable to employ it to treat CIN III in patients who have completed childbearing. Hysterectomy is particularly applicable in the following circumstances: (1) when there is a positive margin on the cervical cone, (2) when the lesion is anaplastic, and (3) when there is deep endocervical glandular involvement. It is the preferred technique when sterilization is desired for other reasons or when there is concomitant uterine or adnexal disease.

Persistence or recurrence rates combined are approximately 2 to 3 percent after hysterectomy. This number should be significantly reduced by using colposcopy and

Schiller's staining preoperatively, since it is likely that most of the disease is persistent because of an inadequate surgical resection of the vaginal cuff.

Stage Ia (Microinvasive Carcinoma)

Because microinvasive carcinoma has not been well-defined, the management remains controversial. The crux of the problem is finding the point in the evolution of this disease from intraepithelial to invasive carcinoma at which the lesion changes its biologic behavior and becomes capable of lymphatic metastasis.

For Stage Ia disease, surgery is almost always employed, except when medically contraindicated. Intracavitary radium or cesium may be used under such exceptional circumstances. When the depth of invasion on cone biopsy is less than 3 mm, and there is no lymphatic or vascular space involvement, an extrafascial abdominal hysterectomy is appropriate treatment. Cervical conization alone may be used in special circumstances in which the patient desires to maintain her childbearing capacity and the cervical cone margins are clear of disease.

Stage Ib

Stage Ib disease may be treated by either radical hysterectomy and bilateral pelvic lymphadenectomy or radiation therapy. The advantage of surgery is that the ovaries may be spared in premenopausal women. There may also be less interference with coital function. Complications involving the rectum, ureters, or bladder are less common following radical hysterectomy than following radiation therapy, and repair is more likely to be successful if injury does occur.

The results of treatment by either method are similar when both the surgeon and the radiotherapist are knowledgeable and skilled. However, radiation is usually chosen when the lesion is expanded beyond 4 cm because a more extensive surgical resection is required, which increases the likelihood of postoperative bladder dysfunction. Some patients may require self-catheterization for the rest of their lives after an extensive radical hysterectomy.

A Stage Ib *barrel-shaped* carcinoma of the cervix is one in which the entire length of the cervix is markedly expanded so that the junction between the lower uterine segment and the large cervical lesion cannot be appreciated. Even when these lesions are treated with radiation, it is common practice to perform an extrafascial hysterectomy six weeks following completion of radiation in order to reduce the incidence of central pelvic recurrence.

Radical Hysterectomy. Radical hysterectomy is an operation for the removal of the uterus with adjacent portions of the vagina, cardinal ligaments, uterosacral ligaments, and bladder pillars (see Fig. 43–5). Surgery is easier to do in thin patients and should be preferred in those with colonic diverticular disease or chronic pelvic inflammatory disease, where radiation may induce pelvic abscesses. It may also be chosen for patients who have a fear of radiation therapy or in whom rapid treatment is desirable (that is, psychologically compromised patients).

The most serious complication of radical hysterectomy is ureteric fistula or stricture. These are less common than they once were. In recent years the incidence of ureteric complications has declined from 10 to 15 percent to 1 to 2 percent. This has occurred because surgeons avoid extensive stripping of the ureter from the parietal peritoneum, as was once the case. There is also general use of suction drainage of the retroperitoneal spaces, which helps minimize infection.

The most common complication of radical hysterectomy is bladder dysfunction. This occurs as a result of interruption of the portion of the autonomic nerve supply traversing the cardinal and uterosacral ligaments. Although normal bladder function is usually restored within one to three months after surgery, dysfunction can be prolonged and is occasionally permanent. A suprapubic catheter is generally placed at the time of radical hysterectomy and removed when satisfactory voiding occurs.

A less common, but life-threatening, complication of radical hysterectomy is deep venous thrombosis with pulmonary embolism. The incidence of pulmonary embolism can probably be reduced with the use of early ambulation, together with prophylactic low-dose subcutaneous heparin or external pneumatic calf compression at the time of surgery and prior to adequate postoperative mobilization.

Radiation Therapy. For patients with Stage Ib disease, radiation may be the only modality of therapy, in which case both external and intracavitary therapy are required. Radiation may be given preoperatively in an attempt to shrink bulky cervical lesions and make them amenable to more limited surgical procedures. Postoperative pelvic radiation may also be used for patients with lymph node metastases or inadequate surgical margins. Radiation therapy is well-tolerated by most patients with medical contraindications to surgery.

If radiation alone is to be used, the treatment plan is based primarily on the extent and distribution of the disease. Treatment is directed at the upper vagina, cervix, paracervical tissues, and the lymph nodes on the pelvic wall. Therapy usually begins with external radiation in an attempt to shrink the central lesion and improve the dosimetry of the subsequent intracavitary therapy. The relative proportion of external radiation versus intracavitary radium or cesium is determined by the size of the primary tumor, its response to the external therapy, and the capacity of the vagina for the intracavitary applicators. Most patients will require a minimum of 4500 to 5000 rad external radiation to the pelvis.

Stage IIa

In patients with minimal involvement of the vaginal fornix, radical surgery or radiation therapy may be employed the same as for patients with Stage Ib lesions. With more extensive upper vaginal involvement, radiation therapy alone is the treatment of choice.

Stage IIb

Most patients with Stage IIb lesions are treated with a combination of external beam and intracavitary radiation therapy. Some patients with bulkier lesions may be selected for an adjunctive extrafascial hysterectomy following radiation therapy in an effort to reduce the risk of persistent central disease. If positive periaortic or high common iliac lymph nodes are detected by surgical staging or CT scan-directed fine needle aspiration cytology, extended field radiation may be employed to treat all of the periaortic lymph nodes up to the diaphragm.

Stages IIIa and IIIb

These patients are treated almost exclusively with radiation therapy, usually external therapy followed by intracavitary radium or cesium. There are study protocols using combinations of chemotherapy and radiation in an effort to improve the cure rates, since many of these patients have occult distant metastases.

In patients with locally advanced disease, distortion of the cervix and vagina may make intracavitary radiation therapy difficult to apply. Therefore, a higher dose of external therapy, up to 6000 to 7000 rad, may be necessary. Alternatively, interstitial radiation may be given to get a better dose distribution than would be possible with intracavitary therapy (see Chapter 51).

Stage IVa

Pelvic radiation therapy is used in most of these patients. If radiation therapy results in only partial tumor regression, a "salvage" pelvic exenteration may be performed. Primary pelvic exenteration is performed only rarely, usually when the patient presents with a rectovaginal or vesicovaginal fistula.

Stage IVb

These patients may receive some pelvic radiation therapy to palliate bleeding from the vagina, bladder, or rectum. However, because distant metastases are present, chemotherapy is often employed, but is only palliative.

Recurrent or Metastatic Disease

Chemotherapy. The effectiveness of chemotherapy is limited in the treatment of cervical cancer because most cervical carcinomas are relatively resistant. In addition, many patients have had previous radiation, which decreases the vascularity of the tissues so that optimal tissue levels of the drug are not reached. Some tumors may be bulky, with fairly large necrotic centers that act as pharmacologic sanctuaries. Other factors that may limit the use of chemotherapy are: (1) diminished marrow reserve secondary to radiation; (2) ureteral obstruction, which affects excretion of the drug; and (3) sepsis and fistulae, which may occur following administration of the chemotherapy.

Several drugs have been tested and found to be active in up to 35 percent of cases. Most responses are partial, and the patients soon relapse and die of their disease. The most active agents are *cis*-platinum, bleomycin, mitomycin C, methotrexate, and cyclophosphamide.

Pelvic Exenteration. Pelvic exenteration is generally reserved for those patients who have a *central recurrence* following pelvic radiation. The operation involves removal of the pelvic viscera, including the uterus, tubes, vagina, ovaries, bladder, and rectum (Fig. 53–6). Depending on the site and extent of the recurrence, the operation may be limited to an *anterior exenteration*, which spares the rectum, or a *posterior exenteration*, which spares the bladder.

Following the extirpative surgery, *pelvic reconstruction* is necessary. If the bladder is removed, the ureters must be implanted into a portion of the small or large bowel that has been isolated from the remainder of the gastrointestinal tract to form a conduit. When the disease is confined to the upper vagina and rectovaginal septum, the lower rectum and anal canal may be preserved and reanastomosed to the sigmoid colon. A temporary colostomy is required to protect the reanastomosis because of the prior radiation. Vaginal reconstruction can be performed simultaneously using a split-thickness skin graft or bilateral gracilis myocutaneous grafts. This helps to reconstruct the pelvic floor, thereby significantly decreasing the risk of a perineal hernia or an enteroperineal fistula.

Relatively few patients with recurrent cancer of the cervix are suitable for pelvic exenteration, because of metastases outside the pelvis or fixation of the tumor to structures that cannot be removed, such as the pelvic

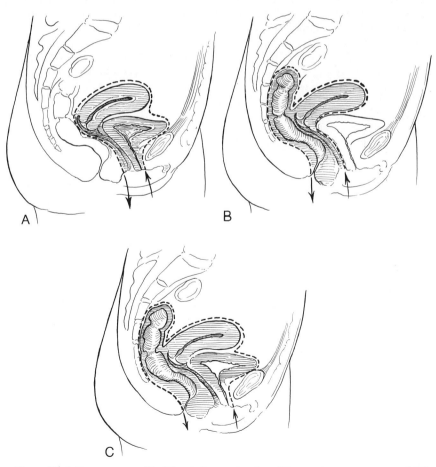

Figure 53–6 Organs removed in *(A)* anterior exenteration, *(B)* posterior exenteration, and *(C)* total pelvic exenteration.

side wall. If an extensive metastatic work-up is negative, patients undergo exploratory laparotomy with a view to pelvic exenteration. If the tumor is discovered to have spread to pelvic or periaortic lymph nodes or to intra-abdominal viscera, the procedure is abandoned because of the low likelihood of cure in such circumstances. Palliative exenteration is not advisable.

In selecting patients who may be suitable for pelvic exenteration, the triad of unilateral leg edema, sciatic pain, and ureteral obstruction is ominous and suggests unresectable disease in the pelvis. Obesity, advanced age (over 65 years), and systemic disease are relative contraindications, considering the serious morbidity associated with this operation. Some patients may be unsuitable for psychologic reasons. A few patients regard the surgery as too mutilating and would prefer to die of disease rather than undergo the procedure.

CERVICAL CARCINOMA IN PREGNANCY

Carcinoma of the cervix associated with pregnancy usually implies diagnosis during pregnancy or within 12 months postpartum. It is relatively uncommon, invasive carcinoma occurring in approximately 1 out of 2200 pregnancies. The proportion of patients with invasive cancer who are pregnant is about 1 in 34 cases, and the average age is about 34 years.

Symptoms

The symptoms are similar to those in nonpregnant patients, painless vaginal bleeding being the most common. During pregnancy, this symptom can readily be attributed to conditions such as threatened abortion or placenta previa, so there is often unnecessary delay in diagnosis even though the patients are under regular medical surveillance.

Diagnosis

Methods of diagnosis are generally the same as in nonpregnant patients. Screening cervical cytology leads to the diagnosis in most cases. The pregnant cervix lends itself to colposcopic evaluation because the columnar eversion that occurs during pregnancy facilitates adequate visualization of the transformation zone. Pregnancy tends to exaggerate the colposcopic features of cervical intraepithelial neoplasia, so overdiagnosis is more likely than the reverse. Endocervical curettage should not be performed during pregnancy because of the risk of rupturing the membranes. Cone biopsy, if required, is best performed during the second trimester to avoid the possibility of induced abortion in the first trimester and severe hemorrhage and premature labor in the third trimester. Unfortunately, about half of the patients are not diagnosed until the postpartum period. The later the diagnosis is made, the more likely is the cancer to be in an advanced stage.

Management

Carcinoma *in situ* diagnosed during pregnancy should be managed conservatively, with the pregnancy allowed to proceed to term, vaginal delivery anticipated, and appropriate therapy carried out six to eight weeks postpartum. Microinvasive carcinoma of the cervix diagnosed by conization of the cervix during pregnancy may also be managed conservatively, the pregnancy being allowed to continue to term with colposcopic surveillance of the cervix every six weeks. At term, either cesarean hysterectomy or vaginal delivery followed by postpartum extrafascial hysterectomy is appropriate.

Frankly invasive cancer requires relatively urgent treatment. After 22 to 26 weeks, it is reasonable to continue the pregnancy until fetal viability, if the patient desires. The general principles of treatment are essentially the same as in the nonpregnant patient. For early lesions, radical hysterectomy may be performed. Before 20 weeks' gestation, this is done with the fetus *in situ*. After that time, hysterotomy through a high incision in the uterine fundus is performed to remove the fetus, followed by radical hysterectomy and bilateral pelvic lymphadenectomy.

For many patients with early disease and for all patients with advanced disease, the alternative to radical surgery is radiation therapy. For patients with disease diagnosed in the first trimester, external irradiation is started in order to shrink the tumor. Abortion usually occurs spontaneously during the course of external therapy; if it does not, uterine curettage should be performed prior to intracavitary radium or cesium insertion. After the first trimester, it is preferable to perform a hysterotomy through a high incision in the corpus before instituting radiotherapy.

If a decision is made to await fetal viability, it is important to be certain by ultrasonography that the baby is apparently healthy, and to obtain a mature lecithin:sphingomyelin ratio to ensure fetal lung maturity before delivery. Because of the increased risk of hemorrhage and infection likely to be associated with delivery through a cervix containing gross cancer, classic cesarean section is the preferred method of delivery. However, for patients in whom inadvertent vaginal delivery has occurred, there is no evidence to suggest that prognosis is altered.

Prognosis for Cervical Cancer

Prognosis is related directly to clinical stage (Table 53–4) and the frequency of pelvic and periaortic lymph node metastasis. With higher stage disease, the frequency of nodal metastasis escalates and the five-year survival diminishes.

Adenocarcinomas and adenosquamous carcinomas have a somewhat lower five-year survival than squamous carcinomas, stage for stage. This may be because these lesions are more likely to occur in older women and are usually endophytic (the growth initiates from the endocervical canal), so they may not be detected as readily as squamous carcinomas.

Patients with a central recurrence treated by pelvic exenteration have a five-year survival rate of about 40 to 50 percent. For cervical cancer in pregnancy, the overall prognosis for all stages of disease is similar to that in nonpregnant women. This is because of the higher proportion of patients with Stage I disease during pregnancy. For more advanced disease, pregnancy has an unfavorable effect on prognosis. The reason for this is not clear but may be related to problems associated with radiation dosimetry in pregnancy or interruptions to the radiation therapy necessitated by genital tract sepsis.

TABLE 53–4 FIVE-YEAR SURVIVAL OF CERVICAL CANCER BY CLINICAL STAGE

| | FIVE-YEAR SURVIVAL | | |
STAGE	Patients Treated	Patients Alive	Percent
I	10,933	8680	79.4
II	12,561	7306	58.2
III	9,139	2873	31.4
IV	1,461	122	8.4
Total	34,094	18,981	55.7

Adapted from The Editorial Office of the Annual Report on the Results of Treatment in Gynecological Cancer. Vol 18. Stockholm, Sweden, 1982, p 47.

SUGGESTED READING

Berek JS, Castaldo TW, Hacker NF, et al: Adenocarcinoma of the uterine cervix. Cancer 48:2734, 1981.

Charles EH, Savage EW: Cryosurgical treatment of cervical intraepithelial neoplasia. Obstet Gynecol Surv 35:539, 1980.

Coppleson LW, Brown B: Observations on a model of the biology of carcinoma of the cervix: A poor fit between observation and theory. Am J Obstet Gynecol 122:127, 1975.

Crum CP, Ikenberg H, Richart RM, et al: Human papillomavirus type 16 and early cervical neoplasia. N Engl J Med 310:880, 1984.

DiSaia PJ, Creasman WT (eds): Invasive cervical cancer. In Clinical Gynecologic Oncology. 2nd ed. St. Louis, CV Mosby Co, 1984, p 61.

Hacker NF, Berek JS, Lagasse LD, et al: Carcinoma of the cervix associated with pregnancy. Obstet Gynecol 59:735, 1982.

Kolstad P, Stafl A: Atlas of Colposcopy. 2nd ed. Baltimore, University Park Press, 1982.

Nelson JH, Boyce J, Macasaet M, et al: Incidence, significance, and follow-up of para-aortic lymph node metastases in late invasive carcinoma of the cervix. Am J Obstet Gynecol 128:336, 1977.

Novak ER, Woodruff JD (eds): Novak's Gynecologic and Obstetric Pathology with Clinical and Endocrine Relations. 8th ed. Philadelphia, W B Saunders Co, 1979.

Odell LD, Savage EW: Colposcopy. In Wynn RM (ed): Obstetrics and Gynecology Annual. New York, Appleton-Century-Crofts, 1974, p 473.

Savage EW: Microinvasive carcinoma of the cervix. Am J Obstet Gynecol 113:708, 1972.

Van Nagell JR Jr, Greenwell N, Powell DF, et al: Microinvasive carcinoma of the cervix. Am J Obstet Gynecol 145:981, 1983.

Chapter Fifty-Four

OVARIAN CANCER

JONATHAN S. BEREK

Ovarian cancer is the fifth most common cancer among females in the United States, accounting for one fourth of all gynecologic malignancies. It is the leading cause of death from gynecologic cancer because it is difficult to detect prior to its dissemination. In 1984, there were over 18,000 new cases and about 12,000 deaths from this disease. Most women who develop ovarian cancer are in their fifth or sixth decade of life.

ETIOLOGY AND EPIDEMIOLOGY

The cause of ovarian cancer is unknown. The patient characteristics found to be associated with an increased risk for epithelial ovarian cancer include Caucasian race, late age of menopause, family history of cancer of the ovary or endometrium, and prolonged intervals of ovulation uninterrupted by pregnancy. Pedigrees of several ovarian cancer families have revealed multiple adenocarcinomas in siblings and offspring, suggesting some genetic predisposition. There is an increased prevalence of ovarian cancer in unmarried women, nuns, and nulliparous married women.

The use of oral contraceptives has been found to protect against ovarian cancer, possibly beause of suppression of ovulation. It has been postulated that incessant ovulation may predispose to malignant transformation in the ovary. Postmenopausal estrogen use has not been shown to cause ovarian cancer.

It has also been postulated that an etiologic agent could enter the peritoneal cavity through the lower genital tract. For example, the perineal use of asbestos-contaminated talc has been linked to the development of epithelial ovarian cancer. However, this possibility remains controversial. The role of the mumps virus is also controversial, although more recent epidemiologic data suggest that a prior history of infection with this agent probably does predispose the patient to the subsequent development of epithelial ovarian malignancies.

The incidence of ovarian cancer varies in different geographic locations. Western countries, including the United States, have rates three to seven times greater than Japan. Second generation Japanese immigrants to the United States have an incidence of ovarian cancer similar to that of American women. White Americans develop ovarian cancer about one and one-half times more frequently than do black Americans.

CLINICAL FEATURES

Symptoms

Unfortunately, most patients who develop ovarian cancer are relatively asymptomatic prior to disease dissemination. In early stage disease, the patient may complain of nonspecific symptoms or irregular menses if she is premenopausal. Symptoms of a mass compressing the bladder or rectum, such as urinary frequency or constipation, may bring the patient to a physician. Sometimes the patient will complain of a lower abdominal or pelvic "fullness" or of dyspareunia. Only rarely does a patient present with acute symptoms, such as pain secondary to torsion, rupture, or intracystic hemorrhage.

In advanced stage disease, patients most often present with abdominal pain or swelling. The latter may be from the tumor itself or from associated ascites. On careful questioning, there has usually been a history of vague abdominal symptoms, such as bloating, constipation, nausea, dyspepsia, anorexia, or early satiety. Premenopausal patients may complain of irregular menses or heavy vaginal bleeding. Postmenopausal bleeding occasionally is a symptom of ovarian neoplasms, particularly functional stromal tumors.

Signs

Pelvic examination is critical to the diagnosis of ovarian cancer. The disease is frequently misdiagnosed for several months because patients with nonspecific abdominal symptoms do not receive a vaginal and rectal examination. A solid, irregular, fixed pelvic mass is very suggestive of ovarian cancer, and if combined with upper abdominal masses and/or ascites, the diagnosis is almost certain. In a woman two or more years postmenopausal, any palpable ovarian mass is suspicious, since the ovaries should then be atrophic and not clinically palpable. This circumstance has been referred to as the "*postmenopausal palpable ovary syndrome.*"

Preoperative Evaluation

The diagnosis and management of any ovarian neoplasm requires laparotomy. Routine preoperative hemotologic and biochemical studies should be obtained, as should a *chest x-ray* and *intravenous pyelogram*. However, extensive preoperative evaluation of the patient with pelvic and abdominal CT scan, liver-spleen scan, and bone scan is not indicated.

A *Pap smear* should be obtained to evaluate the cervix, but this test is of limited value in detecting ovarian cancer. An endometrial biopsy and endocervical curettage are necessary in patients with abnormal vaginal bleeding, as concurrent primary tumors occasionally occur in the ovary and endometrium. In the presence of a pelvic mass, it is preferable not to perform abdominal paracentesis for cytologic evaluation of ascitic fluid because seeding of the abdominal wall may occur.

An *abdominal x-ray* may be useful in a younger patient to locate calcifications associated with a benign cystic teratoma (dermoid cyst), which is the most common neoplasm in patients under 25 years of age. In patients over 45 years of age, a *barium enema* should be obtained to rule out a primary colon cancer with ovarian metastasis. Similarly, an upper gastrointestinal barium study is important if there are significant gastric symptoms. Breast cancer may also metastasize to the ovaries, so bilateral mammograms should be obtained if there are any suspicious breast masses.

Pelvic ultrasonography may be useful for smaller (less than 8 cm) masses in premenopausal women. Masses that are predominantly solid or multilocular have a higher probability of being neoplastic, whereas unilocular cystic masses are generally functional cysts.

Several tumor markers have been investigated, but none has been consistently reliable. If elevated, carcinoembryonic antigen (CEA) may be useful in following patients, but this test is not sufficiently sensitive or specific for screening patients. The tumor-associated antigen, CA-125, which can be detected by a murine monoclonal antibody serum assay (OC-125), is present in many women who have documented ovarian cancer. This assay is currently being studied for evaluation of its utility in detecting early ovarian cancer or for following the clinical course of patients with documented disease.

Differential Diagnosis

Ovarian malignancies must be differentiated from benign neoplasms and functional cysts of the ovaries. In addition, a variety of gynecologic conditions can simulate a neoplastic process, including tubo-ovarian abscess, endometriosis, and pedunculated uterine leiomyoma. Nongynecologic causes for a pelvic tumor must also be excluded, such as inflammatory or neoplastic disease of the colon or a pelvic or "horseshoe" kidney.

Mode of Spread

Ovarian cancer typically spreads by exfoliating cells that disseminate and implant throughout the peritoneal cavity. The distribution of intraperitoneal metastases tends to follow the circulatory path of peritoneal fluid, so metastases are commonly seen on the posterior cul-de-sac, paracolic gutters, right hemidiaphragm, liver capsule, and omentum. Implants are also common on the bowel serosa and its mesenteries. Generally, they grow around the intestines, encasing them with tumor, without invading the bowel lumen. Widespread bowel metastases can lead to a functional obstruction known as *carcinomatous ileus*.

Lymphatic dissemination to the pelvic and periaortic nodes is common, particularly with advanced disease. Extensive blockage of the diaphragmatic lymphatics is at least partially responsible for the development of ascites. Hematogenous metastases are not common, and parenchymal metastases to the liver and lungs are seen in only about 2 to 3 percent of patients at initial presentation.

Death from ovarian cancer usually results from progressive encasement of abdominal organs leading to anorexia, vomiting, and inanition. The bowel obstruction caused by tumor growth is often incomplete and intermittent and may last for several months prior to the patient's demise.

STAGING

The standard staging system for ovarian cancer is presented in Table 54–1. It is based on *surgical* exploration of the patient in addition to the clinical examination. Ovarian cancer is the only gynecologic cancer in which surgery is formally incorporated into the In-

TABLE 54–2 REQUIREMENTS FOR A "STAGING" OR "SECOND-LOOK" OPERATION*

I. Multiple Cytologic Assays
   A. Free ascitic fluid, if present
   B. Peritoneal "washings" (50 cc normal saline)
      1. Pelvic cul-de-sac
      2. Both paracolic gutters
      3. Both hemidiaphragms

II. Multiple Intraperitoneal Biopsies
   A. Pelvis
      1. Cul-de-sac peritoneum
      2. Bladder peritoneum
      3. Pedicles of infundibulopelvic ligaments
      4. Any adhesions
   B. Abdomen
      1. Both paracolic gutters
      2. Bowel serosa and mesenteries
      3. Omentum
      4. Any adhesions

III. Extraperitoneal Biopsies
   A. Pelvic and periaortic lymph nodes

*Procedures performed in patients with no visible evidence of metastatic disease.

TABLE 54–1 FIGO* STAGING OF OVARIAN TUMORS

STAGE	CHARACTERISTICS
Stage I	Growth limited to the ovaries
Stage Ia	Growth limited to one ovary; no ascites
	i. No tumor on the external surface; capsule intact
	ii. Tumor present on the external surface, capsule ruptured, or both
Stage Ib	Growth limited to both ovaries; no ascites
	i. No tumor on the external surface; capsules intact
	ii. Tumor present on the external surface, capsules ruptured, or both
Stage Ic	Tumor either Stage Ia or Ib, but with ascites† present or with positive peritoneal washings
Stage II	Growth involving one or both ovaries with pelvic extension
Stage IIa	Extension and/or metastases to the uterus and/or tubes
Stage IIb	Extension to other pelvic tissues
Stage IIc	Tumor either Stage IIa or Stage IIb, but with ascites† present or positive peritoneal washings
Stage III	Growth involving one or both ovaries with intraperitoneal metastases outside the pelvis, or positive retroperitoneal nodal involvement, or both
	Tumor limited to the true pelvis with histologically proven malignant extension to small bowel or omentum
Stage IV	Growth involving one or both ovaries with distant metastases. If pleural effusion is present, there must be positive cytology to allot a case to Stage IV. Parenchymal liver metastases equal Stage IV
Special category	Unexplored cases that are thought to be ovarian carcinoma

*International Federation of Gynecology and Obstetrics.
†Ascites is peritoneal effusion, which, in the opinion of the surgeon, is pathologic or clearly exceeds normal amounts.

ternational Federation of Gynecology and Obstetrics (FIGO) staging system.

Even though all microscopic disease may appear to be confined to the ovaries at the time of laparotomy, microscopic spread may have already occurred; thus patients must undergo a thorough "surgical staging." Procedures necessary to stage ovarian cancer are shown in Table 54–2.

CLASSIFICATION

The histogenetic classification of ovarian neoplasms is listed in Table 54–3. These lesions fall into four categories according to their tissue of origin. Most ovarian neoplasms (80 to 85 percent) are derived from coelomic

epithelium and are called epithelial carcinomas. Less common tumors are derived from primitive germ cells, specialized gonadal stroma, or nonspecific mesenchyme. In addition, the ovary can be the site of metastatic carcinomas, most often from the gastrointestinal tract or the breast.

EPITHELIAL OVARIAN CARCINOMAS

Pathology

The main histologic subtypes of epithelial tumors are serous, mucinous, endometrioid, clear-cell (mesonephroid), Brenner, and undifferentiated. The relative percentages of

TABLE 54–3 HISTOGENETIC CLASSIFICATION OF PRIMARY OVARIAN NEOPLASMS

DERIVATION OF NEOPLASM	TYPE OF TUMOR
Coelomic epithelial origin (80–85%)	A. "Common" epithelial tumors; benign, borderline, malignant 1. Serous tumor 2. Mucinous tumor 3. Endometrioid tumor 4. Clear-cell (mesonephroid) tumor 5. Brenner tumor B. Undifferentiated carcinoma C. Carcinosarcoma and mixed mesodermal tumors

Germ-cell origin (10–15%)	A. Teratoma
	 1. Mature teratoma
	  a. Solid adult teratoma
	  b. Dermoid cyst
	  c. Struma ovarii
	  d. Malignant neoplasms secondarily arising from teratomatous tissues (squamous carcinoma, carcinoid tumor, sarcoma, etc.)
	 2. Immature teratoma
	B. Dysgerminoma
	C. Endodermal sinus tumor
	D. Embryonal carcinoma
	E. Choriocarcinoma
	F. Gonadoblastoma*
	G. Mixed germ-cell tumors

Specialized gonadal stromal origin (3–5%)	A. Granulosa-theca tumors 1. Granulosa-cell tumor 2. Thecoma B. Sertoli-Leydig tumors 1. Arrhenoblastoma 2. Sertoli tumor C. Gynandroblastoma D. Lipid-cell tumors
Nonspecific mesenchymal origin (less than 1%)	A. Fibroma, hemangioma, leiomyoma, lipoma B. Lymphoma C. Sarcoma

*Combined germ-cell and specialized gonadal stromal elements.

Adapted with permission from Hart WR, Morrow CP: The ovaries. In Romney SL, Gray MJ, Little AO, et al (eds): Gynecology and Obstetrics: The Health Care of Women. 2nd ed. New York, McGraw-Hill, 1981.

TABLE 54–4 PERCENTAGE OF EPITHELIAL OVARIAN MALIGNANCIES BY HISTOLOGIC TYPE

TYPE	PERCENT
Serous	35–40
Endometrioid	15–25
Mucinous	6–10
Clear cell	5
Brenner	<1
Undifferentiated	15–30

Derived from Scully RE: Tumors of the ovary and maldeveloped gonads. Atlas of Tumor Pathology. Armed Forces Institute of Pathology, 2nd series, fasc. 16, 1979.

these subtypes are listed in Table 54–4. About 70 percent of serous, 85 percent of mucinous, and over 95 percent of Brenner tumors are benign, while almost all endometrioid and clear-cell tumors are malignant.

Serous tumors resemble fallopian tube epithelium histologically (Fig. 54–1). About 30 percent of patients with Stages I and IIa disease have bilateral involvement, while if all stages are included, about two thirds of patients have bilateral disease. On gross examination, serous carcinomas have an irregular and multilocular appearance (Fig. 54–2).

Mucinous tumors histologically resemble endocervical epithelium and are often quite large, measuring 20 cm or greater in diameter. They are bilateral in 10 to 20 percent of patients. *Pseudomyxoma peritonei* is occasionally associated with a mucinous carcinoma. In this condition, extensive tumor deposits are present throughout the peritoneal cavity, producing a thick mucinous ascites that ultimately leads to bowel obstruction. A mucocele or carcinoma of the appendix or gallbladder may occasionally be seen in conjunction with these tumors.

Endometrioid tumors closely resemble carcinomas of the endometrium and arise in association with a primary endometrial cancer in about 20 percent of cases. In early stage disease, they are bilateral in about 10 percent of cases. Approximately 10 percent of endometrioid ovarian carcinomas are associated with endometriosis, although malignant transformation of endometriosis occurs in less than 1 percent of patients.

Clear-cell carcinomas of the ovary are uncommon. They have been called mesonephroid carcinomas because their histologic features resemble tumors of mesonephric origin. They are only rarely bilateral, but in about 25 percent of cases they occur in association with endometriosis.

The *Brenner* tumor represents only 2 to 3 percent of all ovarian neoplasms, and less than 2 percent of these are malignant. About

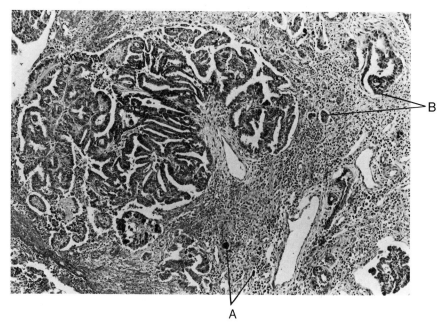

Figure 54–1 Histology of a grade 1 serous adenocarcinoma of the ovary. Note the papillary nature of the tumor and the well-formed glands. Psammoma bodies (calcifications) (*A*) and stromal invasion (*B*) are evident (× 60).

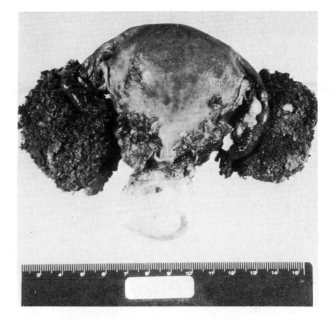

Figure 54–2 Bilateral serous cystadenocarcinomas. Note the papillary projections from the surface of both ovaries and the implants on the serosal surfaces of the uterus and fallopian tubes.

10 percent of Brenner tumors occur in conjunction with a mucinous cystadenoma or dermoid cyst in the same or the opposite ovary.

Tumors of *low malignant potential* or *borderline* histology exist for each histologic type. Approximately 5 to 10 percent of malignant serous tumors are borderline (Fig. 54–3), whereas 20 percent of malignant mucinous tumors fall into this category. The endometrioid, clear-cell, or Brenner tumors are only rarely borderline.

Management of Epithelial Ovarian Cancer

The initial approach to all patients with ovarian cancer is surgical exploration of the abdomen and pelvis.

Early Stage Disease. In patients with no gross evidence of disease beyond the ovary, the standard operation is total abdominal hysterectomy, bilateral salpingo-oophorectomy, infracolic omentectomy, and thorough surgical staging, as shown in Table 54–2.

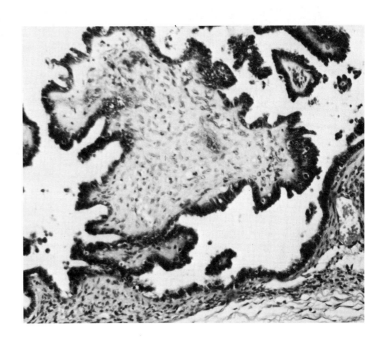

Figure 54–3 Histology of a "borderline" serous cystadenoma of the ovary. Note the multiple, papillary projections lined by pseudostratified columnar epithelium. There is no stromal invasion, as demonstrated by the clear delineation of the epithelium from the underlying stroma ($\times$ 60).

Patients who wish to preserve fertility may have a unilateral salpingo-oophorectomy, unless the tumor is poorly differentiated on frozen section. In patients with grade 1 or 2 tumors confined to one or both ovaries after surgical staging, no further treatment is necessary. Patients with poorly differentiated (grade 3) tumors are subsequently treated with systemic chemotherapy.

Advanced Stage Disease. In patients with advanced disease, cytoreductive surgery ("debulking") is required. The objectives are to remove the primary tumor and all of the metastases, if possible. If all macroscopic disease cannot be removed, an attempt should be made to reduce individual tumor nodules to 1.5 cm or less in diameter. Patients in whom this goal is achieved are said to have had "optimal" cytoreduction, which can be achieved in about 80 percent of patients. In addition to a total or subtotal abdominal hysterectomy, bilateral salpingo-oophorectomy, omentectomy, and resection of peritoneal metastases, optimal cytoreduction may necessitate bowel resection; therefore, all patients having surgery for suspected ovarian cancer should have a bowel preparation preoperatively. In retrospective studies, patients whose individual residual tumor nodules are 1.5 cm or less in diameter prior to the commencement of chemotherapy have been shown to have longer median survivals and more complete responses to therapy.

Following primary cytoreductive surgery, combination chemotherapy is given. Various combinations of drugs may be given, including *cis*-platinum, doxorubicin (Adriamycin), and cyclophosphamide (PAC); cyclophosphamide, hexamethylmelamine, Adriamycin, and *cis*-platinum (CHAP); or hexamethylmelamine, cyclophosphamide, methotrexate, and 5-fluorouracil (Hexa-CAF). These combination chemotherapy regimens, particularly those containing *cis*-platinum, have resulted in a greater number of responses and longer median survivals than were previously achieved with single alkylating agent therapy. Single agent therapy, typically melphalan (L-phenylalanine mustard, L-PAM), is still commonly used for frail or elderly patients. It is unclear whether or not patients with "metastatic" borderline tumors benefit from chemotherapy.

Whole abdominal radiation therapy has been used as primary therapy instead of chemotherapy, but it appears to have its major role in patients who have no gross residual disease following initial surgery. A comparison of combination chemotherapy with whole abdominal radiation as primary treatment in such patients has not been reported.

Second-Look Laparotomy. In patients who are clinically free of disease after completing a prescribed course of chemotherapy (usually 6 to 12 cycles), a "second-look" laparotomy should be performed to determine whether or not the patient has had a complete response to chemotherapy. Prolonged alkylating agent chemotherapy is associated with a significant risk for the subsequent development of acute nonlymphocytic leukemia. Therefore, it is desirable to use briefer, more intensive chemotherapeutic programs whenever feasible and to discontinue therapy when a complete surgical response has been documented. If there is no macroscopic or microscopic evidence of disease at second-look laparotomy, essentially the same procedures as are carried out for surgical staging should be performed (Table 54–2). If gross disease is present, an attempt should be made to resect persistent disease to facilitate a response to subsequent therapy.

Second-Line Therapies. Secondary systemic chemotherapy has been disappointing in patients with ovarian cancer who have failed primary combination therapy. Experimental approaches are currently being tried, including whole abdominal radiation, intraperitoneal chemotherapy, and intraperitoneal immunotherapy.

Prognosis

Patients with Stage I disease have five-year survivals of 50 to 99 percent, depending on the histology and grade. Almost all patients with carefully staged Stage Ia(i) grade 1 ovarian cancer are cured surgically, while the five-year survival of patients with poorly differentiated bilateral lesions is as low as 50 percent. The five-year survival for patients with Stage II disease is about 40 percent. In spite of aggressive primary surgery and combination chemotherapy, five-year survival for patients with advanced stage disease is generally no better than 20 percent. Patients with advanced stage disease who have a negative second-look laparotomy have a five-year survival of about 60 to 70 percent.

Patients who have borderline ovarian tumors can be expected to have a prolonged survival. If the disease is confined to the ovary, the vast majority of tumors never recur. Five- and 10-year survivals are 95 to 100 percent, but late recurrences may present and 20-year survivals are approximately 85 to 90 percent. Patients who initially present with metastatic disease are most likely to develop subsequent clinical evidence of disease, although the rate of progression is slow; most will live at least 5 years.

GERM-CELL TUMORS

Germ-cell tumors of the ovary account for only about 2 to 3 percent of all ovarian malignancies. They occur predominantly in young patients and frequently produce either human chorionic gonadotropin (hCG) or alpha-fetoprotein (AFP), which serve as tumor markers.

The most common germ-cell tumors are the dysgerminoma and immature teratoma. Endodermal sinus tumors, embryonal tumors, and nongestational choriocarcinomas are less common. Mixed germ-cell tumors are not uncommon.

Dysgerminomas

Dysgerminomas occur predominantly in children and young women. About 10 percent are bilateral. These tumors are occasionally seen in patients with gonadal dysgenesis or the testicular feminization syndrome. In such patients, the dysgerminoma may arise in a gonadoblastoma. In about two thirds of cases, the disease is confined to the ovaries at the time of diagnosis. About 10 percent of dysgerminomas are associated with other germ-cell malignancies. Pure dysgerminomas do not produce the tumor markers hCG or AFP.

Treatment. In patients who have a unilateral tumor that is less than 10 cm in diameter, the contralateral ovary and uterus can be preserved. Surgical staging, as outlined earlier in this chapter, is important. Particular attention should be paid to the pelvic and periaortic lymph nodes because of the propensity of these tumors for lymphatic dissemination. If disease extends beyond one ovary, the treatment of choice is total abdominal hysterectomy, bilateral salpingo-oophorectomy, and postoperative radiation to the pelvis and abdomen, since dysgerminomas are uniquely radiosensitive. If there are metastases to the periaortic lymph nodes, the radiation field may include the mediastinal and supraclavicular lymph nodes. Recurrence after conservative surgery is also treated with radiation.

Chemotherapy is utilized primarily for treatment failures following radiation or for mixed germ-cell tumors. Regimens employed for these patients are usually vincristine, actinomycin-D, and cyclophosphamide (VAC); or vinblastine, bleomycin, and *cis*-platinum (VBP).

Prognosis. The overall five-year survival for patients with a pure dysgerminoma is approximately 90 percent for Stage I, 65 percent for Stage II, and 50 percent for Stage III. The five-year survival for patients with Stage Ia pure dysgerminoma treated with a unilateral oophorectomy is about 95 percent. Because of the radiosensitivity of dysgerminomas, recurrences following conservative surgery have about a 50 percent five-year survival.

Immature Teratomas

Immature teratomas are the second most common malignant ovarian germ-cell tumor. About 75 percent of malignant teratomas are encountered during the first two decades of life. Bilaterality is rare, although the other ovary may contain a benign dermoid cyst in about 5 percent of cases. Like other germ-cell tumors, immature teratomas grow fairly rapidly, cause pain early, and are found confined to the ovary in about two thirds of cases at the time of diagnosis. Pure immature teratomas do not produce hCG or AFP.

Histologically, the tumors can be graded from 1 to 3 according to the degree of differentiation, grade 3 tumors being the least differentiated. Neural elements are most frequently seen, but cartilage and epithelial tissues are also common.

Treatment. The primary tumor should be removed. However, in young patients, the uterus and contralateral ovary should be preserved to maintain fertility. All patients with other than Stage Ia, grade 1 immature teratomas should receive postoperative chemotherapy using either vincristine, actinomycin-D, and cyclophosphamide (VAC), or vinblastine, bleomycin, and *cis*-platinum (VBP). Therapy should be given for four to six cycles, and a second-look laparotomy is required to document a complete response prior to discontinuing treatment.

Prognosis. Survival correlates with grade and stage of disease. The 5-year survival for patients with grade 1 immature teratomas is about 80 percent, compared with 60 percent for grade 2 and 30 percent for grade 3.

Other Germ-Cell Tumors

The *endodermal sinus tumor* is a rare malignancy. It is also referred to as a "yolk sac" tumor. Endodermal sinus tumors produce alpha-fetoprotein, which can serve as a useful serum marker for this neoplasm. *Embryonal carcinomas* produce both hCG and AFP, while *choriocarcinomas* produce hCG. All occur in children and young women, and all grow rapidly. Most are confined to one ovary at the time of diagnosis. Bilaterality is rare.

Therapy for these lesions includes surgical resection of the primary tumor followed by systemic combination chemotherapy with VAC or VBP. Prior to the advent of effective chemotherapy, these tumors were usually fatal. The overall five-year survival is now about 60 percent.

SPECIALZED GONADAL-STROMAL TUMORS

This group of relatively uncommon tumors is derived from the specialized ovarian stroma. As such, they are often endocrinologically functional, many of them being capable of synthesizing gonadal or adrenal steroid hormones.

Since the ovarian stroma is sexually bipotential, hormones that are secreted can be either female or male. Estrogen and progesterone are typically associated with granulosa-theca tumors, while testosterone and other androgens may be secreted by many Sertoli-Leydig cell tumors. Rarely, lipid cell tumors, which are usually virilizing, produce adrenal corticoids and a clinical "cushingoid" syndrome.

Pathology

Granulosa-cell tumors are the most common stromal carcinomas. The granulosa tumors have a distinct histologic pattern; small groups of cells called Call-Exner bodies are the hallmark. They may secrete large amounts of estrogen and can be associated with endometrial cancer in adults or sexual pseudoprecosity in children.

Thecomas, which are only one third as common as granulosa-cell tumors, are rarely malignant. Mixtures of the two types of tumor exist.

Sertoli-Leydig cell tumors (arrhenoblastomas) contain both Sertoli and Leydig-type stromal cells and are classically associated with masculinization. Only 3 to 5 percent of these tumors are malignant.

Lipid-cell tumors are often referred to as hilar-cell tumors because they are located in the ovarian hilus. Only a rare lipid tumor, usually larger than 8 cm in diameter, behaves in a malignant fashion.

Treatment

Most stromal tumors occur in postmenopausal women, and a total abdominal hysterectomy and bilateral salpingo-oophorectomy is indicated in such cases. Conservation of the uterus and contralateral ovary is appropriate for carefully staged young patients with Stage I disease, provided the possibility of an associated adenocarcinoma of the endometrium has been excluded by dilatation and curettage. Postoperative radiation therapy to the pelvis is occasionally used in early stage disease. Effective chemotherapy is not available at this time.

Prognosis

Granulosa-cell tumors, which tend to be slow-growing tumors, are usually confined to one ovary at the time of diagnosis. The five-year survival is approximately 90 percent for Stage I cases. Recurrences are usually detected late and may result in death 15 to 20 years following removal of the primary lesion.

METASTATIC CANCERS

About 4 to 8 percent of ovarian malignancies are metastatic, most commonly from either the gastrointestinal tract or breast. The Krukenberg tumor is a specific type of metastatic tumor in which "signet-ring" cells are seen in the ovarian stroma histologically. Most Krukenberg tumors are bilateral and metastatic from the stomach. Rarely, it has not been possible to locate a primary focus, and removal of the ovarian disease has produced apparent cures.

FALLOPIAN TUBE CARCINOMA

Primary carcinoma of the fallopian tube accounts for only 0.1 to 0.5 percent of gynecologic cancers. Most carcinomas of the fallopian tube are adenocarcinomas, but sarcomas and mixed tumors can also occur. There is no official staging system for fallopian tube carcinoma, but generally it is staged like ovarian cancer because its mode of dissemination is similar. Bilateral carcinomas are seen in 10 to 20 percent of patients.

Clinical Features

Clinically, patients can present with a vaginal discharge that is typically serous in nature, vaginal bleeding, and/or pelvic pain. In postmenopausal patients, the vaginal discharge may be yellow, watery, and similar to the symptoms of a urinary fistula. Physical examination may reveal an adnexal mass. A fallopian tube cancer should be suspected in a postmenopausal patient whose bleeding or abnormal cytology is not explained by an endometrial or endocervical curettage. In most patients, the diagnosis is not made preoperatively.

Treatment

The treatment for fallopian tube carcinoma is total abdominal hysterectomy, bilateral salpingo-oophorectomy, and omentectomy. Surgical staging should be performed in patients whose disease appears to be confined to the pelvis, and cytoreductive surgery is appropriate in patients with metastatic disease. Postoperatively, combination chemo-therapy, including *cis*-platinum, Adriamycin, and cyclophosphamide, is usually used for patients with metastatic disease. Pelvic radiation or whole abdominal radiation may be given for patients with completely resected disease confined to the pelvis.

Prognosis

Prognosis for fallopian tube carcinoma is similar to that for ovarian cancer.

SUGGESTED READING

Barber HRK, Graber EA: The PMPO syndrome (post-menopausal palpable ovary syndrome). Obstet Gynecol 38:921, 1971.

Bast RC Jr, Klug TC, St John E, et al: A radioimmunoassay using a monoclonal antibody to monitor the course of epithelial ovarian cancer. N Engl J Med 309:883, 1983.

Berek JS, Hacker NF, Lagasse LD, et al: Second-look laparotomy in Stage III epithelial ovarian cancer: Clinical variables associated with disease status. Obstet Gynecol 64:207, 1984.

Berek JS, Hacker NF, Lagasse LD, et al: Survival following secondary cytoreductive surgery in ovarian cancer. Obstet Gynecol 61:189, 1983.

Curry SL, Smith JP, Gallagher HS: Malignant teratoma of the ovary: Prognostic factors and treatment. Am J Obstet Gynecol 131:845, 1978.

Dembo AJ, Bush RS, Beole FA, et al: The Princess Margaret Hospital Study of ovarian cancer: Stages I, II, and asymptomatic III presentations. Cancer Treat Rep 63:249, 1979.

Gordon A, Lipton D, Woodruff JD: Dysgerminoma: A review of 158 cases from the Emil Novak Ovarian Tumor Registry. Obstet Gynecol 58:497, 1981.

Hacker NF, Berek JS, Lagasse LD, et al: Primary cytoreductive surgery for epithelial ovarian cancer. Obstet Gynecol 61:413, 1983.

Hart WR: Ovarian epithelial tumors of borderline malignancy (carcinomas of low malignant potential). Hum Pathol 8:541, 1977.

Kurman RJ, Norris HJ: Malignant germ-cell tumors of the ovary. Hum Pathol 8:551, 1977.

Scully RE: Tumors of the ovary and maldeveloped gonads. Atlas of Tumor Pathology, Armed Forces Institute of Pathology. 2nd series, fasc. 16, 1979.

Webb MJ, Decker DG, Mussey E, et al: Factors influencing survival in Stage I ovarian cancer. Am J Obstet Gynecol 116:222, 1973.

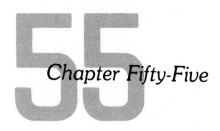

Chapter Fifty-Five

VULVAR AND VAGINAL CANCER

NEVILLE F. HACKER

VULVAR NEOPLASMS

Malignant tumors of the vulva are uncommon, representing about 3 to 4 percent of malignancies of the female genital tract. Most tumors are squamous cell carcinomas, with melanomas, adenocarcinomas, basal cell carcinomas, and sarcomas occurring much less frequently.

Squamous cell carcinoma of the vulva occurs mainly in postmenopausal women, and the mean age at diagnosis is 65 years. A history of chronic vulvar itching is common. Vulvar cancer tends to be found more frequently in patients who are obese and in those who have hypertension, diabetes mellitus, or arteriosclerosis. Other primary malignancies have been reported in up to 22 percent of cases, the most common primary site being the cervix.

Epidemiology

No specific etiologic agent has been identified for vulvar cancer. Because of the common association among squamous cancers of the lower genital tract, it has been postulated that a common pathogen may be involved. Herpes virus type II has been regarded as a possible carcinogen, as has the human papilloma virus. Approximately 5 percent of vulvar cancers develop within preexisting genital condylomas, and about 5 percent of patients have a positive serologic test for syphilis. In the latter group of patients, vulvar cancer occurs at an earlier age and carries a graver

prognosis. Although rarely seen in the United States, vulvar cancer also occurs in association with lymphogranuloma venereum and granuloma inguinale.

Vulvar dystrophies that show cellular atypia on biopsy carry a small risk of malignant transformation, particularly if untreated. With adequate treatment, however, a vulvar dystrophy should not significantly predispose the patient to the development of vulvar cancer. The malignant potential of carcinoma *in situ* of the vulva is also uncertain but appears to be low, except in elderly patients and those who are immunosuppressed.

INTRAEPITHELIAL NEOPLASIA

The International Society for the Study of Vulvar Disease recognizes two varieties of intraepithelial neoplasia, namely, squamous cell carcinoma *in situ* (Bowen's disease) and Paget's disease.

Squamous Cell Carcinoma *In Situ*

During the past two decades, the incidence of carcinoma *in situ* of the vulva has increased. Younger patients are being affected, and the mean age is approximately 45 years.

Clinical Features. Itching is the most common symptom, although some patients present with palpable or visible abnormalities of

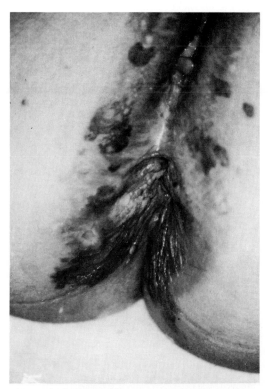

Figure 55–1 Carcinoma *in situ* of the vulva. Note the pigmented and multicentric nature of the lesions and the extensive perianal involvement in this patient.

the vulva. Approximately half of the patients are asymptomatic. There is no absolutely diagnostic appearance. Most lesions are elevated, but the color may be white, red, pink, gray, or brown (Fig. 55–1). Approximately 20 percent of the lesions have a "warty" appearance, and the lesions are multicentric in about two thirds of cases.

Diagnosis. Careful inspection of the vulva in a bright light, with the aid of a magnifying glass, if necessary, is the most useful technique for detecting abnormal areas. In a patient with pruritus vulvae and no gross abnormality, colposcopic examination of the entire vulva after the application of 2 percent acetic acid is helpful. The toluidine blue dye test (*Collin's test*) may also help direct biopsies. Because the dye fixes to cell nuclei, *false-negative* results may be seen in the presence of hyperkeratosis, and *false-positive* results may be seen in the presence of excoriations. A liberal number of directed biopsies must be taken to establish the diagnosis and rule out invasive carcinoma.

Management. A number of methods of treatment are used for carcinoma *in situ* of the vulva. In the past, total vulvectomy was usually performed. It is now clear, however, that the incidence of recurrence following total vulvectomy (about 30 percent) is not less than that following local excision of the individual lesions. Because of the distressing psychologic consequences of vulvectomy, *local excision* is now considered the mainstay of treatment.

The microscopic disease seldom extends beyond the macroscopic lesion, so that margins of about 5 mm are usually adequate. For extensive lesions involving most of the vulva, a *skinning vulvectomy*, in which the vulvar skin is removed and replaced by a split-thickness skin graft, may be used. Because the subcutaneous tissues are not excised, the cosmetic result is superior to vulvectomy. *Topical 5-fluorouracil cream* is effective in about 50 percent of cases, but patient tolerance is low because of the painful ulceration that results. *Laser therapy* is also effective, particularly for multiple small lesions. When large areas of the vulva are treated with laser therapy, postoperative pain is severe and patient tolerance for this procedure is low. Topical chemotherapy and laser therapy offer the optimal cosmetic outcome, but because no specimen is available for histology, a liberal number of biopsies must be taken prior to treatment to exclude invasive disease.

Bowenoid Papulosis of the Vulva

Bowenoid papulosis is a new entity that affects younger individuals. It is characterized clinically by multiple reddish-brown or violaceous papules on the vulva or penis. Histologically, it is indistinguishable from carcinoma *in situ*. A viral etiology has been postulated but not proven. Treatment should be by local excision or laser therapy.

Paget's Disease

Paget's disease of the vulva predominantly affects postmenopausal Caucasian women.

Clinical Features. Itching and tenderness are common and may be longstanding. The affected area is usually well-demarcated and eczematoid in appearance, with the presence of white plaque-like lesions. As growth progresses, extension beyond the vulva to the mons pubis, thighs, and buttocks may occur; rarely, it may extend to involve the mucosa of the rectum, vagina, or urinary tract. In about 20 percent of cases, Paget's disease is associated with an underlying adenocarcinoma.

Histology. The disease is characterized by large, pale, pathognomonic Paget's cells, which are seen within the epidermis and skin adnexa. They are rich in mucopolysaccharide, a diastase-resistant PAS-positive substance. The intracytoplasmic mucin may also be demonstrated by Mayer's mucicarmine stain. The histogenesis of this lesion has been controversial, but it is currently believed to be a type of adenocarcinoma *in situ*. The Paget's cells are typically located adjacent to the basal layer, both in the epidermis and in the adnexal structures.

Management. Unlike Bowen's disease, the histologic extent of Paget's disease is frequently far beyond the visible lesion. Hence, very wide local excision is required to clear the lesion, and frozen sections should be obtained on the margins of resection. Recurrences still occur in approximately 30 percent of cases and may be treated by further excision or laser therapy. If an underlying invasive carcinoma is present, the treatment should be the same as for other invasive vulvar cancers, requiring at least a radical vulvectomy and bilateral inguinofemoral lymphadenectomy.

INVASIVE VULVAR CANCER

Squamous Cell Carcinoma

Squamous cell carcinoma accounts for about 90 percent of vulvar cancers.

Clinical Features. Patients generally present with a vulvar lump, although longstanding pruritus is common and may be associated with an underlying vulvar dystrophy. Other common presenting symptoms include vulvar pain, bleeding, discharge, or dysuria. The lesions may be raised, ulcerated, pigmented, or warty in appearance (Fig. 55–2), and definitive diagnosis requires biopsy under local anesthesia. Most lesions occur on the labia majora; the labia minora are the next most common sites. Less commonly, the clitoris or the perineum is involved. Approximately 5 percent of cases are multifocal.

Methods of Spread. Vulvar cancer spreads by *direct extension* to adjacent structures, such as the vagina, urethra, and anus, by

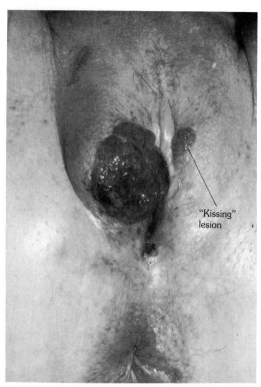

"Kissing" lesion

Figure 55–2 Squamous cell carcinoma of the right labium majus. Note the small "kissing" lesion on the left labium majus.

lymphatic embolization to regional lymph nodes and by *hematogenous spread* to distant sites, including the lungs, liver, and bone. In most cases, the initial lymphatic metastases are to the superficial inguinal lymph nodes, located between Camper's fascia and the fascia lata. From these superficial nodes, spread occurs to the femoral nodes located along the femoral vessels. Cloquet's node, which is situated beneath the inguinal ligament, is the most cephalad of the femoral node group. From the inguinofemoral nodes, spread occurs to the pelvic nodes, particularly the external iliac group (Fig. 55–3). Metastasis to the femoral nodes without involvement of the superficial inguinal nodes has occasionally been reported, but metastasis to pelvic nodes without initial involvement of the groin nodes is rare.

The incidence of lymph node metastases in vulvar cancer is approximately 30 percent. It is related to lesion size (Table 55–1) and also to the stage of the disease (Table 55–2). Approximately 5 percent of patients have metastases to pelvic lymph nodes. Such patients usually have three or more positive unilateral inguinofemoral lymph nodes.

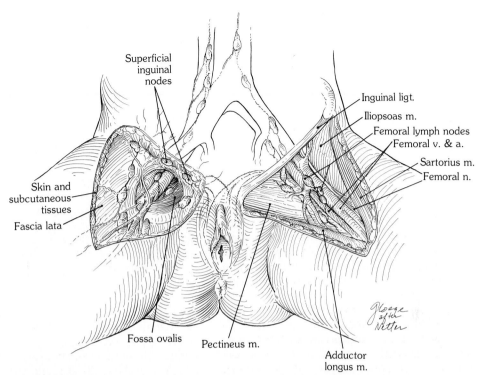

Figure 55–3 Lymphatic drainage of the vulva. Inguinal nodes displayed in the right groin and femoral nodes in the left groin.

Hematogenous spread usually occurs late in the disease and rarely occurs in the absence of lymphatic metastases.

Staging. Staging of vulvar cancer, which is shown in Table 55–3, is clinical, and is based on an evaluation of the primary tumor and regional lymph nodes and a limited search for distant metastases. Evaluation of the primary tumor may include cystoscopy and/or proctoscopy, with bladder or rectal biopsies as indicated. The metastatic work-up should include chest x-ray and, if indicated because of bone pain, skeletal x-rays. Although the clinical assessment of inguinal lymph nodes is helpful, false-positive and false-negative rates of 25 to 30 percent may be expected.

Management. During the past 40 years, *en bloc* radical vulvectomy and bilateral inguinofemoral lymphadenectomy, with or without pelvic lymphadenectomy, has been considered the standard treatment for invasive vulvar cancer. This operation involves removal of the lymph nodes and fatty tissue in the femoral triangle and overlying the inguinal ligament, together with the entire vulva between the labiocrural folds, from the perineal body to the upper margin of the mons pubis. The vulvar dissection is carried down to the level of the fascia overlying the symphysis pubis, which is coplanar with the inferior fascia of the urogenital diaphragm and the fascia lata. If necessary to obtain adequate surgical margins, the distal portions of the urethra and vaginal wall are included in the *en bloc* dissection.

Pelvic lymphadenectomy is not performed routinely, but should be undertaken in patients with three or more positive unilateral

TABLE 55–1 INCIDENCE OF LYMPH NODE METASTASES IN RELATION TO LESION SIZE IN VULVAR CANCER

LESION SIZE (cm)	NUMBER	POSITIVE NODES	PERCENT
1	40	2	5
1–2	81	13	16
2–4	33	11	33.3
>4	15	8	53.3

Source: Hacker NF, et al: Vulvar cancer. In Haskell CM (ed): Cancer Treatment. 2nd ed. Philadelphia, W B Saunders Co, 1985.

TABLE 55–2 INCIDENCE OF LYMPH NODE METASTASES
IN RELATION TO STAGE OF DISEASE IN VULVAR CANCER

STAGE	NUMBER OF CASES	POSITIVE NODES	PERCENT
I	140	15	10.7
II	145	38	26.2
III	137	88	64.2
IV	18	16	88.9

Combined data from Green TH Jr (Obstet Gynecol 52:462, 1978); Iverson T, et al (Gynecol Oncol 9:271, 1980); and Hacker NF, et al (Obstet Gynecol 61:408, 1983).

groin nodes. Pelvic radiation is a comparable alternative to pelvic lymphadenectomy for these patients. Although direct lymphatic channels to the pelvic lymph nodes have been demonstrated from the clitoris and Bartholin's gland, the involvement of pelvic lymph nodes with these tumors is very uncommon in the absence of inguinofemoral lymph node metastases; therefore, tumors in these sites should be managed in the standard way.

With an *en bloc* approach, prolonged hospitalization is common because of postoperative wound breakdown. Chronic leg edema also occurs in about 50 percent of patients. In order to decrease this postoperative morbidity, *separate incisions* may be utilized for the groin dissections. This allows the wounds to be closed without tension and significantly improves the incidence of wound breakdown. The technique leaves a skin bridge between the primary tumor and the draining lymph nodes. Metastases in this skin bridge are rare unless the patient has clinically suspicious (N 2) groin nodes, which are a contraindication to the separate incision technique.

Complications. Utilizing the separate incision technique, major wound breakdown in the groins may be reduced from about 45 to about 15 percent. Anterior thigh anesthesia from injury to the cutaneous branches of the femoral nerve is common in the immediate postoperative period, but usually progressively resolves with time. Less common acute complications include groin seromas, cellulitis, thrombophlebitis, and pulmonary embolus. Chronic complications include leg edema, genital prolapse, urinary stress incontinence. Rarely, introital stenosis, pubic osteomyelitis, femoral hernia, or rectoperineal fistula may occur.

Early Vulvar Cancer

During the past decade, a significant weight of evidence has suggested that it is possible to modify the standard radical approach to vulvar cancer for selected patients with Stage I disease, in an attempt to decrease both physical and psychologic morbidity. Modifications may involve either the lymphadenectomy or the primary tumor.

With respect to the lymphadenectomy, early reports suggested that patients with less than 5 mm of stromal invasion, usually measured from the basement membrane, were at very small risk for lymph node metastases. However, it has become apparent that patients with stromal invasion up to 5 mm have approximately a 10 percent risk of lymph node metastases, so the omission of lymphadenectomy for this group will compromise survival. It now seems clear that the only patients without significant risk of lymph node metastases are those in whom the depth of penetration is less than 1 mm from the overlying basement membrane. In this group of patients, groin dissection may be eliminated. For patients with midline lesions, bilateral groin dissection is necessary. If the lesion is situated laterally on the labia, unilateral inguinofemoral lymphadenectomy is an acceptable approach, although there is about a 1 percent risk of positive contralateral nodes.

With respect to the primary tumor, preliminary evidence suggests that a wide and deep local excision (*radical local excision*) may be as effective as radical vulvectomy in preventing local recurrence, provided the remainder of the vulva is normal. For patients with Stage I vulvar cancer, there is a 6 to 10 percent risk of local recurrence, even with radical vulvectomy, and this incidence appears to be no higher with radical local excision.

Advanced Vulvar Cancer

The standard management for patients with advanced vulvar cancer involving the proximal urethra, anus, or rectovaginal septum has been pelvic exenteration performed in conjunction with radical vulvectomy and bilateral inguinofemoral lymphadenectomy. Although the 5-year survival rate for such patients approximates 50 percent, the operative mortality is about 10 percent, and the cure rate is very low if there are any positive lymph nodes. More recently, some centers have been using preoperative radiation to shrink the primary tumor, followed by more conservative surgical excision. Survival does not seem to be compromised by this approach, and most patients can be spared pelvic exenteration.

Prognosis. The overall survival for vulvar carcinoma is about 70 percent. This reflects the trend toward earlier diagnosis. Survival correlates with the International Federation of Obstetrics and Gynecology (FIGO) stag-

TABLE 55–3 STAGING OF VULVAR CARCINOMA

TNM CLASSIFICATION OF CARCINOMA OF THE VULVA

T Primary Tumor

Tis	Preinvasive carcinoma (carcinoma *in situ*).
T 1	Tumor confined to the vulva—2 cm or less in largest diameter.
T 2	Tumor confined to the vulva—more than 2 cm in diameter.
T 3	Tumor of any size with adjacent spread to the urethra and/or vagina and/or perineum and/or anus.
T 4	Tumor of any size infiltrating the bladder mucosa and/or rectal mucosa, including the upper part of the urethral mucosa and/or fixed to the bone.

N Regional Lymph Nodes

N 0	No nodes palpable.
N 1	Nodes palpable in either groin, not enlarged, mobile (not clinically suspicious of neoplasm).
N 2	Nodes palpable in either one or both groins, enlarged, firm, and mobile (clinically suspicious of neoplasm).
N 3	Fixed or ulcerated nodes.

M Distant Metastases

M 0	No clinical metastases.
M 1a	Palpable deep pelvic lymph nodes.
M 1b	Other distant metastases.

FIGO* STAGING OF CARCINOMA OF THE VULVA

Stage 0

Tis	Carcinoma *in situ,* intraepithelial carcinoma.

Stage I

T1 N0 M0	Tumor confined to the vulva with a maximum diameter of 2 cm or less and no suspicious groin
T1 N1 M0	nodes.

Stage II

T2 N0 M0	Tumor confined to the vulva with a diameter greater than 2 cm and no suspicious groin nodes.
T2 N1 M0	

Stage III

T3 N0 M0	Tumor of any size with:
T3 N1 M0	(1) adjacent spread to the lower urethra, vagina, perineum, or anus, and/or
T3 N2 M0	(2) clinically suspicious lymph nodes in either groin.
T1 N2 M0	
T2 N2 M0	

Stage IV

T4 N0 M0	Tumor of any size with:
T4 N1 M0	(1) infiltration of the mucosa of the bladder, rectum, or proximal urethra, and/or
T4 N2 M0	(2) fixation to bone, and/or
All conditions	(3) fixed or ulcerated nodes in either groin, and/or
containing	(4) distant metastases.
N3 or M1a or	
M1b	

*International Federation of Gynecology and Obstetrics.

TABLE 55–4 SURVIVAL OF PATIENTS WITH VULVAR CANCER TREATED WITH CURATIVE INTENT VERSUS STAGE OF DISEASE

STAGE	NUMBER	DEAD OF DISEASE	CORRECTED 5-YEAR SURVIVAL RATES (PERCENT)
I	306	25	91.8
II	259	51	80.3
III	215	100	53.5
IV	101	86	14.6
Total	881	262	70.3

Source: Hacker NF, et al: Vulvar cancer. In Haskell CM (ed): Cancer Treatment. 2nd ed. Philadelphia, W B Saunders Co, 1985.

ing, 5-year survival ranging from approximately 90 percent for patients with Stage I disease to 15 percent for Stage IV (Table 55–4). Survival also correlates significantly with lymph node status, since patients with positive nodes have a 5-year survival of about 50 percent, while those with negative nodes have a 5-year survival of about 90 percent. Patients with one positive node have a good prognosis, regardless of stage, while those with three or more positive nodes do poorly, regardless of stage.

Malignant Melanoma

Malignant melanoma is the second most common type of vulvar cancer. Melanomas may arise *de novo* or from a pre-existing junctional or compound nevi. They occur predominantly in postmenopausal Caucasian women and most commonly involve the labia minora or clitoris (Fig. 55–4).

Diagnosis and Staging. Any pigmented lesion on the vulva requires excisional biopsy for histologic diagnosis. The staging of vulvar cancer as used for squamous cell carcinomas does not apply well to melanomas, which are usually smaller lesions and tend to metastasize earlier. The prognosis correlates more closely with the depth of penetration into the dermis, and those lesions that penetrate to a depth of 1 mm or less from the granular layer of the epidermis rarely metastasize. Clark's levels are not readily applicable to vulvar melanomas.

Management. For the superficial lesions referred to above, radical local excision is adequate therapy. For more invasive tumors, *en bloc* radical vulvectomy and bilateral inguinofemoral lymphadenectomy should be performed. Adjuvant therapy with nonspecific immunostimulants or chemotherapeutic agents has been disappointing. However, estrogen receptors have recently been demonstrated in melanomas, and responses to tamoxifen (Nolvadex) have been reported.

Prognosis. The overall 5-year survival for vulvar melanomas is approximately 30 per-

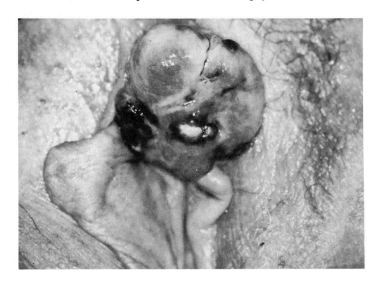

Figure 55–4 Malignant melanoma arising from the clitoris.

cent, which is comparable to that for cutaneous melanomas of nongenital origin.

Verrucous Carcinoma

Verrucous carcinoma is a variant of squamous cell carcinoma and was originally described in the oral cavity. The lesions, which are "cauliflower-like" in nature, may occur in the cervix, vulva, or vagina. Invasion occurs with a broad "pushing" front, and unless the base of the lesion is submitted for histologic examination, these tumors may be difficult to differentiate from a condyloma acuminatum or squamous papilloma. Metastasis to regional lymph nodes is rare, but the tumors are locally aggressive and prone to local recurrence, unless wide surgical margins are obtained. Radiation therapy may induce anaplastic transformation and is contraindicated.

Bartholin's Gland Carcinoma

Adenocarcinomas, squamous cell carcinomas, and, rarely, transitional cell carcinomas may arise from Bartholin's gland. A history of preceding inflammation of Bartholin's gland is present in about 10 percent of patients, and malignancies may be mistaken for benign cysts or abscesses. Treatment consists of radical vulvectomy and bilateral inguinofemoral lymphadenectomy, with pelvic lymphadenectomy reserved for patients with positive groin nodes. Stage for stage, the prognosis is similar to that for squamous cell carcinoma, although diagnosis is often delayed because of the deep location of the gland.

Basal Cell Carcinoma

Basal cell carcinomas of the vulva are rare. They commonly present as a rolled edge "rodent" ulcer, although nodules and macules may occur. They are locally aggressive but nonmetastasizing, so wide local excision is adequate treatment.

Vulvar Sarcoma

Vulvar sarcomas represent 1 to 2 percent of vulvar malignancies. Many histologic types have been reported, including leiomyosarcomas, fibrosarcomas, neurofibrosarcomas, liposarcomas, rhabdomyosarcomas, angiosarcomas, and epithelioid sarcomas. Leiomyosarcomas are the most common, and prognosis correlates with lesion size, mitotic activity, and growth patterns. Recurrence is most likely with lesions larger than 5 cm, with infiltrating margins, and with 5 or more mitotic figures per 10 high power fields.

VAGINAL NEOPLASMS

Intraepithelial Neoplasia

Carcinoma *in situ* of the vagina is much less common than its counterpart in the cervix or vulva. Most lesions occur in the upper third of the vagina, and the patients are usually asymptomatic.

Etiology. The etiology is unknown, but patients with a past history of *in situ* or invasive carcinoma of the cervix or vulva are at increased risk, suggesting that the squamous epithelium of the lower genital tract may respond to the same carcinogenic factors. Some lesions may occur after irradiation for cervical cancer.

Diagnosis. The diagnosis is usually entertained because of an abnormal Pap smear in a woman who has either had a hysterectomy or has no demonstrable cervical abnormality. Definitive diagnosis requires vaginal biopsy, which should be directed by colposcopy or Lugol's iodine staining. Colposcopic findings are similar to those seen with cervical lesions, although thorough colposcopy of all vaginal walls is technically more difficult. In postmenopausal patients, a four-week course of topical estrogen prior to colposcopy is indicated to enhance the colposcopic features and eliminate those patients with Pap smear abnormalities due to inflammatory atypia.

Management. Surgical excision is the mainstay of therapy, and this usually requires excision of the vaginal apex. At times, extensive disease requires total vaginectomy and creation of a neovagina using a split-thickness skin graft. More recently, laser therapy has increased in popularity. Topical 5-fluorouracil is another alternative to surgical excision.

Squamous Cell Carcinoma of the Vagina

Squamous cell carcinoma of the vagina is very uncommon, and the etiology is unknown. The mean age of patients is about 60 years. Symptoms consist of abnormal vaginal bleeding, vaginal discharge, and urinary symptoms. On physical examination, ulcerative, exophytic, and infiltrative growth patterns may be seen. About half of the lesions are in the upper third of the vagina, particularly on the posterior wall. Punch biopsy is required to confirm the diagnosis.

Patterns of Spread. Vaginal cancer spreads by direct invasion, as well as by lymphatic and hematogenous dissemination. Direct tumor spread may result in involvement of the bladder, urethra, or rectum, or progressive lateral extension to the pelvic sidewall. The lymphatic drainage from the upper vagina is to the obturator, hypogastric, and external iliac nodes, while the lower vagina drains primarily to the inguinofemoral nodes. Hematogenous spread is uncommon until the disease is advanced.

Staging. FIGO staging for vaginal cancer is clinical, as shown in Table 55–5. All patients should have at least a chest x-ray, intravenous pyelogram, cystoscopy, and sigmoidoscopy. A pelvic and abdominal CT scan may be useful to detect lymph node metastases, which can be confirmed by fine needle aspiration, but a finding of positive nodes does not alter the FIGO stage.

Management. Radiotherapy is the main method of treatment for primary vaginal cancer. Initial treatment usually consists of 4500–5000 rad external irradiation to the pelvis to shrink the primary tumor and treat the pelvic lymph nodes and paravaginal tissues. Small tumors may then be treated with intracavitary vaginal applicators, but, in general,

interstitial therapy is preferable because of the higher dosages that can be delivered to deeper tissues. When the lower third of the vagina is involved, the groin nodes should be either included in the treatment field or surgically removed.

Radical surgery has a limited role in the management of vaginal cancer. Radical hysterectomy, partial vaginectomy, and pelvic lymphadenectomy may be performed for early lesions in the posterior fornix. Surgery should otherwise be reserved for medically fit patients who develop a central recurrence following radiation. Pelvic exenteration with creation of a neovagina may be appropriate in such patients, provided there are no lymph node metastases at the time of exploratory laparotomy and adequate surgical margins can be attained.

Prognosis. The overall 5-year survival for vaginal cancer is about 50 percent. When corrected for death from intercurrent disease, 5-year survival should be approximately 85 to 90 percent for Stage I lesions, 55 to 65 percent for Stage II, 30 to 35 percent for Stage III, and 5 to 10 percent for Stage IV.

Rare Vaginal Cancers

Adenocarcinoma. Most adenocarcinomas of the vagina are metastatic, usually from the cervix, endometrium, or ovary, but occasionally from more distant sites, such as the kidney, breast, or colon. Most primary vaginal adenocarcinomas are clear-cell carcinomas in female offspring of women who ingested diethylstilbestrol (DES) during pregnancy (see later in this chapter). Non-DES-related primary adenocarcinomas of the vagina are rare but may arise in residual glands of müllerian (paramesonephric) origin, Gartner's duct (a remnant of the embryonic wolffian or mesonephric duct), or foci of endometriosis.

Malignant Melanoma. Vaginal melanomas account for less than 2 percent of vaginal malignancies. The mean age at diagnosis is 55. The carcinoma usually occurs on the distal anterior wall. Radiation therapy is not effective treatment, so radical surgery is required to achieve the best results. This may require radical hysterectomy and vaginectomy or some type of pelvic exenteration, depending on the location and extent of disease. The prognosis is poor, with an overall 5-year survival of 5 to 10 percent.

TABLE 55–5 FIGO STAGING OF VAGINAL CANCER*

STAGE	DESCRIPTION
Stage I	Carcinoma limited to the vaginal wall
Stage II	Carcinoma has involved the subvaginal tissue but has not extended onto the pelvic sidewall
Stage III	Carcinoma has extended to the pelvic sidewall
Stage IV	Carcinoma has extended beyond the true pelvis or has involved the mucosa of the bladder or rectum
IVa	Spread to bladder or rectum
IVb	Spread to distant organs

*International Federation of Gynecology and Obstetrics.

Sarcoma. Vaginal sarcomas are rare. In adults, leiomyosarcomas are most common, while in infants and children, *sarcoma botryoides* predominates. The latter term comes from the Greek *botrys*, a bunch of grapes, which these lesions usually grossly resemble. The mean age at diagnosis of sarcoma botryoides is 2 to 3 years, with a range of 6 months to 16 years. They are usually multicentric, and histologically the tumor is an embryonal rhabdomyosarcoma. Treatment consists of surgical resection of gross disease followed by adjuvant chemotherapy, with or without radiation.

DIETHYLSTILBESTROL EXPOSURE *IN UTERO*

In 1971, an association between *in utero* exposure to diethylstilbestrol (DES) and the later development of clear-cell adenocarcinoma of the vagina was reported. Since that time, numerous non-neoplastic uterine and vaginal anomalies have been reported in young women exposed *in utero* to DES. *Vaginal adenosis* (vaginal columnar epithelium) is the most common anomaly and is present in about 30 percent of exposed females. This tissue behaves similarly to the columnar epithelium of the cervix and is replaced initially by immature metaplastic squamous epithelium. Colposcopically, the latter resembles dysplasia, mainly because of the frequent occurrence of mosaic pattern and punctation. With progressive squamous maturation, complete resolution of this anomaly usually occurs.

Structural changes of the cervix and vagina occur in about 25 percent of exposed females. Possible changes include a transverse vaginal septum, cervical collar (Fig. 55–5), cockscomb (a raised ridge, usually on the anterior cervix), or cervical hypoplasia. Most of these changes tend to disappear as the individual matures. Pregnancy hastens their maturation. The occurrence of these anomalies is related to the dosage of medication given and the time of first exposure. The risk is insignificant if administration was begun after the twenty-second week.

In addition to these changes in the lower genital tract, upper genital tract anomalies also occur in at least half of the patients and may be associated with exposure later in pregnancy. The most common abnormalities are a T-shaped uterus and a small uterine cavity (less than 2.5 cm in length). Exposed individuals have an increased risk of miscarriage, premature delivery, or ectopic pregnancy, but most are able to deliver a viable infant successfully.

Clear-Cell Adenocarcinoma

Since 1971, over 400 cases of clear-cell adenocarcinoma of the cervix or vagina have been reported to the Registry for Research on Hormonal Transplacental Carcinogenesis in Chicago. The risk for developing clear-cell adenocarcinoma following DES exposure *in utero* is somewhat less than 1 in 1000. The

Figure 55–5 A cervical collar in a patient exposed to diethylstilbestrol *in utero*. (Courtesy of Dr. William Growdon, Department of Obstetrics and Gynecology, UCLA School of Medicine.)

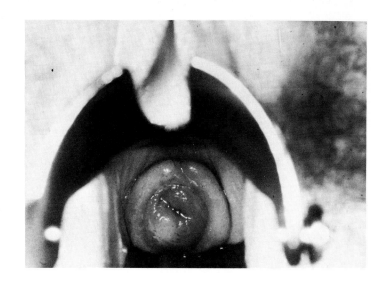

tumors are rare before age 14, and the mean age of patients is about 19 years. Very few cases have been reported after 30 years of age. Diagnosis is best made by thorough inspection and palpation of the entire vagina and cervix, with biopsies taken of any abnormal areas. Pap smears should be obtained from the cervix and vagina, but colposcopy is necessary only for the evaluation of an abnormal Pap smear. A young woman exposed to DES *in utero* should be examined at menarche, or at about 14 years of age if menstruation has not occurred. Any vaginal bleeding or discharge in a prepubertal child should be investigated by examination under anesthesia. For early tumors, radical hysterectomy and vaginectomy (with creation of a neovagina) or radiation therapy are effective. Overall, the 5-year survival is about 80 percent, which is considerably better than that for squamous cell cancer of the cervix or vagina.

SUGGESTED READING

Benedet JL, Murphy KJ, Fairey RN, et al: Primary invasive carcinoma of the vagina. Obstet Gynecol 62:715, 1983.

Boronow RC: Combined therapy as an alternative to exenteration for locally advanced vulvo-vaginal cancer: Rationale and results. Cancer 49:1085, 1982.

Buscema J, Woodruff JD, Parmley TH, et al: Carcinoma in situ of the vulva. Obstet Gynecol 55:225, 1980.

Chung AF, Woodruff JM, Lewis JL Jr: Malignant melanoma of the vulva. Obstet Gynecol 45:639, 1975.

Creasman WT, Gallager HS, Rutledge F: Paget's disease of the vulva. Gynecol Oncol 3:133, 1975.

Crum CP, Braun LA, Shah KV: Vulvar intraepithelial neoplasia: Correlation of nuclear DNA content and the presence of a human papilloma virus (HPV) structural antigen. Cancer 49:468, 1982.

Hacker NF, Berek JS, Lagasse LD, et al: The management of regional lymph nodes in vulvar cancer and their influence on prognosis. Obstet Gynecol 61:408, 1983.

Hacker NF, Berek JS, Lagasse LD, et al: Individualization of treatment for Stage I squamous cell vulvar carcinoma. Obstet Gynecol 63:155, 1984.

Herbst AL, Cole P, Norusis MJ, et al: Epidemiologic aspects and factors related to survival in 384 Registry cases of clear cell adenocarcinoma of the vagina and cervix. Obstet Gynecol 135:876, 1979.

Leuchter RS, Hacker NF, Voet RL, et al: Primary carcinoma of the Bartholin gland: A report of 14 cases and review of the literature. Obstet Gynecol 60:361, 1982.

Morley GW: Infiltrative carcinoma of the vulva: Results of surgical treatment. Am J Obstet Gynecol 124:874, 1976.

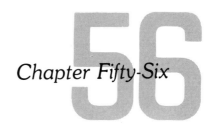

Chapter Fifty-Six

GESTATIONAL TROPHOBLASTIC NEOPLASIA

JONATHAN S. BEREK

Gestational trophoblastic neoplasia (GTN) represents a unique spectrum of diseases that includes benign *hydatidiform mole*; *invasive mole* (chorioadenoma destruens), which can metastasize; and the frankly malignant variety, *choriocarcinoma*. About 3000 hydatidiform moles are diagnosed annually in the United States. The majority of patients (80 to 90 percent) with GTN follow a benign course, with their disease spontaneously remitting. Most patients with metastatic disease can be effectively cured with chemotherapy. This diverse group of diseases has a sensitive tumor marker, the beta subunit of human chorionic gonadotropin (β-hCG), which is secreted by all of these tumors and allows accurate follow-up and assessment of the disease.

EPIDEMIOLOGY AND ETIOLOGY

The incidence of molar pregnancy is about 1 in every 1500 to 2000 pregnancies among Caucasians in the United States. There is a much higher incidence among Oriental women in the United States (1 in 800) and an even higher incidence among Oriental women in the Far East, for example, Taiwan (1 in every 125 to 200 pregnancies). The risk of developing a second molar pregnancy is 1 to 3 percent or as much as 40 times greater than that of the first.

While the cause of GTN is unknown, it is known to occur more frequently in women under 20 years and in those older than 40 years. It appears that GTN may result from defective fertilization, a process that is more common in both younger and older individuals. Diet may play an etiologic role. The incidence of molar pregnancy has been noted to be higher in geographic areas where people consume less beta-carotene (a retinoid) and folic acid.

Cytogenetics

The cytogenetic analysis of tissue obtained from molar pregnancies offers some clue to the genesis of these lesions. Figure 56–1 illustrates the genetic compositon of molar pregnancies. The majority of hydatidiform moles are "complete" moles and have a 46 XX karyotype. Specialized studies indicate that both of the X chromosomes are paternally derived. This androgenic origin probably results from fertilization of an "empty egg" (that is, an egg without chromosomes) by a haploid sperm (23 X), which then duplicates to restore the diploid chromosomal complement (46 XX). Only a few percent of lesions are 46 XY. Complete molar pregnancy is only rarely associated with a fetus, and this may represent a form of twinning.

In the "incomplete" or partial mole, the karyotype is usually a triploid, often 69 XXY (80 percent). The majority of the remaining lesions are 69 XXX or 69 XYY. Occasionally, mosaic patterns occur. These lesions, unlike

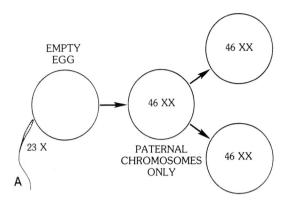

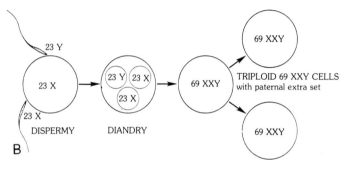

Figure 56–1 Cytogenetic makeup of hydatidiform mole: *A,* Chromosomal origin of a complete mole. A single sperm fertilizes an "empty egg." Reduplication of its 23 X set gives a completely homozygous diploid genome of 46 XX. A similar result follows fertilization of an empty egg by two sperms with two independently drawn sets of 23 X or 23 Y; note that both karyotypes, 46 XX and 46 XY, can ensue. *B,* Chromosomal origin of the triploid, partial mole. A normal egg with a 23 X haploid set is fertilized by two sperms that can carry either sex chromosome to give a total of 69 chromosomes with a sex chromosome configuration of XXY, XXX, or XYY. A similar result can be obtained by fertilization with a sperm carrying the unreduced paternal genome 46 XY (resulting sex complement, XXY only). (Reproduced with permission from Szulman AE: Syndromes of hydatidiform moles: Partial vs complete. J Reprod Med 29:789–790, 1984.)

complete moles, often present with a coexistent fetus. The fetus is usually triploid and defective.

Genetic analysis of choriocarcinomas usually reveals aneuploidy or polyploidy, typical for anaplastic carcinomas.

CLASSIFICATION

The term gestational trophoblastic neoplasia (GTN) is of clinical value because often the diagnosis is made and therapy instituted without definitive knowledge of the precise histologic pattern. GTN may be benign or malignant and nonmetastatic or metastatic (Table 56–1).

The benign form of GTN is called *hydatidiform mole.* While this entity is usually confined to the uterine cavity, trophoblastic tissue can occasionally embolize to the lungs. The malignant forms of GTN are invasive mole and choriocarcinoma. *Invasive mole* (chorioadenoma destruens) is usually a locally invasive lesion, although it can be associated with metastases. This lesion accounts for the majority of patients who have persistent hCG titers following molar evacuation. *Choriocarcinoma* is the frankly malignant form of GTN.

Metastatic GTN can be subdivided into "good prognosis" and "poor prognosis" groups, depending on the sites of metastases and/or other clinical variables (Table 56–2).

PATHOLOGY

Grossly, a *hydatidiform mole* appears as multiple vesicles that have been classically described as a "bunch of grapes" (Fig. 56–2).

TABLE 56–1 CLASSIFICATION OF GESTATIONAL TROPHOBLASTIC NEOPLASIA (GTN)

1) Benign
   Hydatidiform mole
   a) Complete mole
   b) Incomplete ("partial") mole

2) Malignant
   a) Invasive mole ("chorioadenoma destruens")
   b) Choriocarcinoma

   Malignant GTN may be:
   a) Nonmetastatic
   b) Metastatic
      i) Good prognosis
      ii) Poor prognosis

TABLE 56–2 CLINICAL FEATURES OF POOR PROGNOSIS METASTATIC GTN

1. Urinary hCG titer greater than 100,000 IU/24 hours or serum hCG titer greater than 40,000 IU.

2. Disease present more than four months from the antecedent pregnancy.

3. Metastasis to the brain or liver (regardless of hCG titer or duration of disease).

4. Failure to respond to prior single agent chemotherapy.

5. Choriocarcinoma after a full-term delivery.

The characteristic histopathologic findings associated with a complete molar pregnancy are (1) hydropic villi, (2) absence of fetal blood vessels, and (3) hyperplasia of trophoblastic tissue (Fig. 56–3). Invasive mole differs from hydatidiform mole only in its propensity to invade locally and to metastasize.

A *partial mole* has some hydropic villi, while other villi are essentially normal. Fetal vessels are seen in a partial mole, and the trophoblastic tissue exhibits less striking hyperplasia.

Choriocarcinoma in the uterus appears grossly as a vascular-appearing, irregular, and "beefy" tumor, often growing through the uterine wall. Metastatic lesions appear hemorrhagic and have a consistency of "currant jelly." Histologically, choriocarcinoma consists of sheets of malignant cytotrophoblast and syncytiotrophoblast with no identifiable villi.

HYDATIDIFORM MOLE

Symptoms

Most patients with hydatidiform mole present with irregular or heavy vaginal bleeding during the first or early second trimester of pregnancy (Table 56–3). The bleeding is usually painless, although it can be associated with uterine contractions. In addition, the patient may expel molar "vesicles" from the vagina and occasionally may develop excessive nausea, even "hyperemesis gravidarum." Irritability, dizziness, and photophobia may occur, since some patients develop pre-eclampsia. Patients may occasionally exhibit symptoms relating to hyperthyroidism, such as nervousness, anorexia, and tremors.

Signs

The patient's vital signs may reveal tachycardia, tachypnea, and hypertension, reflecting the presence of pre-eclampsia or clinical hyperthyroidism. Funduscopic examination may show arteriolar spasm. In the rare case of trophoblastic emboli to the pulmonary system, wheezing and rhonchi may be noted on chest examination. Abdominal examination may reveal an enlarged uterus. Auscultation of the uterus will typically be remarkable for the absence of fetal heart sounds.

On pelvic examination, the grape-like vesicles of the mole may be detected in the vagina. Blood clots may be present. About one half of patients with molar pregnancy present with a uterine size that is greater than

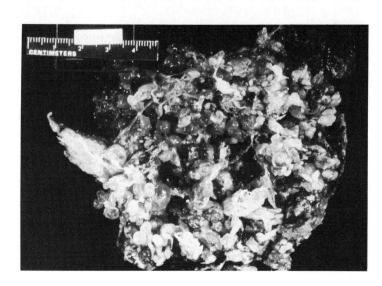

Figure 56–2 Complete hydatidiform mole. Multiple hydropic villi (vesicles), resembling a "bunch of grapes," are admixed with areas of necrosis (white areas) and hemorrhage. Note the absence of a fetus.

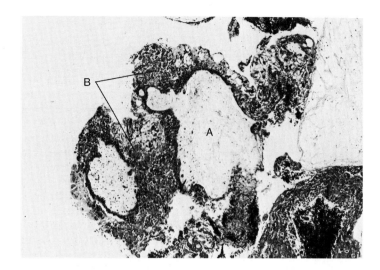

Figure 56–3 Histology of a complete hydatidiform mole. Note the *(A)* hydropic, avascular villi and *(B)* increased trophoblastic proliferation. In the bottom right corner is an area of hemorrhage and necrosis (× 60).

expected based on their last menstrual period, while about one fourth each have a size compatible with or smaller than gestational age. Ovarian enlargement by *theca-lutein cysts* occurs in about one third of women with molar pregnancies. This may be difficult to detect until the uterus has been evacuated.

Diagnosis

Beta-hCG titers can be very high for early pregnancy. This should alert the physician that the patient might have GTN or multiple gestation. The condition must also be distinguished from a threatened spontaneous abortion or an ectopic pregnancy.

TABLE 56–3 DIAGNOSIS OF HYDATIDIFORM MOLE

1) *Clinical data*
   a) Bleeding in the first half of pregnancy
   b) Lower abdominal pain
   c) Toxemia before 24 weeks' gestation
   d) Hyperemesis gravidarum
   e) Uterus large for dates (only 50 percent of cases)
   f) Absent fetal heart tones and fetal parts
   g) Expulsion of vesicles

2) *Diagnostic Studies*
   a) Chest x-ray
   b) Urinary hCG greater than 500,000 IU/24 hours
   c) Ultrasound
   d) Amniocentesis and amniography (rarely required)

Adapted from Morrow CP, Townsend DE (eds): Gestational trophoblastic neoplasia. In Synopsis of Gynecologic Oncology. 2nd ed. New York, John Wiley and Sons, 1981, p 329.

Definitive diagnosis of hydatidiform mole can usually be made by *ultrasonography* (Fig. 56–4). The ultrasound test is noninvasive and produces a "snow storm" pattern that is diagnostic. Another test that can be employed is *amniography*, a procedure in which water soluble radio-opaque dye is introduced into the uterus. It produces an irregular, "moth-eaten" appearance in the absence of a fetus. This test is only used when the diagnosis is in question.

Investigations

Patients who have the presumptive or definitive diagnosis of hydatidiform mole should undergo a complete blood count in order to exclude anemia, which might require a transfusion. They require an assessment of the platelet count, prothrombin time (PT), partial thromboplastin time (PTT), and a fibrinogen level, since an occasional patient may develop disseminated intravascular coagulation. Liver and renal function tests should be obtained. Blood should be typed and cross-matched in the event that excessive bleeding is encountered at the time of evacuation of the mole. A chest x-ray should be obtained and an EKG performed if tachycardia is present or if the patient is over 40 years of age.

Treatment

Evacuation. The standard treatment of hydatidiform mole is suction evacuation followed by sharp curettage of the uterus, re-

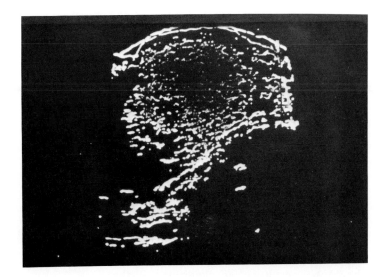

Figure 56–4 An ultrasound of a hydatidiform mole. Note the "snow storm" pattern without evidence of a fetus.

gardless of the duration of pregnancy. This should be performed in the operating room with general or regional anesthesia. Intravenous oxytocin is given simultaneously to help stimulate uterine contractions and reduce blood loss. This technique is associated with a low incidence of uterine perforation and trophoblastic embolization.

Most patients have an uncomplicated course in the immediate postoperative period. However, some require transfusion because of excessive blood loss. Abnormal clotting parameters should be treated with fresh frozen plasma and platelet transfusions, as indicated. Rarely, a patient can develop acute respiratory distress from *trophoblastic embolization* or fluid overload. Such patients may require respiratory support via a ventilator and careful cardiopulmonary monitoring.

Monitoring β-hCG Titers. Following the evacuation of a hydatidiform mole, the patient must be monitored with weekly serum assays of β-hCG. Because the titers drop to a very low level, a nonspecific pregnancy test cannot be utilized because of cross-reactivity with luteinizing hormone (LH). The radioimmunoassay, sensitive to levels of 1 to 5 mIU/ml, should be utilized. Following the evacuation, the β-hCG titers should steadily decline to undetectable levels, usually within 12 to 16 weeks. A normal regression curve for β-hCG titers following evacuation of a molar pregnancy is shown in Figure 56–5.

Chemotherapy. Of patients with a molar pregnancy, 80 to 90 percent have spontaneous remissions, so prophylactic chemotherapy is not indicated. If the β-hCG titers

plateau or rise at any time, chemotherapy should be initiated. This is discussed later in this chapter.

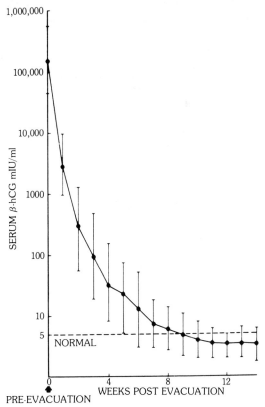

Figure 56–5 Normal regression curve of β-hCG following molar evacuation. (Reprinted with permission from Morrow CP, et al: Clinical and laboratory correlates of molar pregnancy and trophoblastic disease. Am J Obstet Gynecol 128:428, 1977.)

PARTIAL MOLE

The incomplete or partial mole is usually associated with a developing fetus. Patients with a partial mole display most of the pathologic and clinical features of a complete mole, although usually in a less severe form. Partial moles are usually diagnosed later than complete moles and generally present as a spontaneous or missed abortion.

It is unusual for a partial mole to be detected prior to the spontaneous termination of a pregnancy. An ultrasound performed for other indications may indicate possible "molar degeneration" of the placenta associated with the developing fetus. Under these circumstances, an amniocentesis should be performed to determine if the karyotype of the coexisting fetus is normal.

Uterine enlargement is much less common; most patients with partial moles are actually small for dates. When pre-eclampsia occurs with a partial mole, it may be severe, but the condition usually occurs between 17 and 22 weeks, about one month later than with a complete mole. The most striking difference between partial and complete moles is related to the malignant potential of the two lesions. Partial moles have not been reported to metastasize, and only rarely will there be need for chemotherapy because of plateaued or rising β-hCG titers.

INVASIVE MOLE

Invasive mole is usually a locally invasive tumor. It constitutes about 5 to 10 percent of all molar pregnancies, representing the majority of those with persistent β-hCG titers following molar evacuation. The lesion may penetrate the entire myometrium, rupture through the uterus, and result in hemorrhage into the broad ligament or peritoneal cavity. Rarely, invasive mole is associated with metastases, particularly to the vagina or lungs, although brain metastases have been documented.

Histologic confirmation of invasive mole is almost always made at the time of hysterectomy. The latter is usually performed in patients with persistent β-hCG titers following evacuation of a molar pregnancy, or in those with persistent titers despite chemotherapy, who have no evidence of metastatic disease. The hysterectomy is usually curative.

CHORIOCARCINOMA

The frankly malignant form of gestational trophoblastic neoplasia is choriocarcinoma. About one half of patients with gestational choriocarcinoma have had a preceding molar pregnancy. In the remaining patients, the disease is preceded by either a spontaneous or induced abortion, ectopic pregnancy, or normal pregnancy. Trophoblastic disease following a normal pregnancy is always choriocarcinoma. The tumor has a tendency to disseminate hematogenously, particularly to the lungs, vagina, brain, liver, kidneys, and gastrointestinal tract.

Symptoms

Most patients with choriocarcinoma present with symptoms of metastatic disease. Vaginal bleeding is a common symptom of uterine choriocarcinoma or vaginal metastasis. Because of the gonadotropin excretion, amenorrhea may develop, simulating early pregnancy. Hemoptysis, cough, or dyspnea may occur as a result of lung metastasis. In the presence of central nervous system metastases, the patient may complain of headaches, dizzy spells, "blacking out," or other symptoms referable to a space-occupying lesion in the brain. Rectal bleeding or "dark stools" could represent disease that has metastasized to the gastrointestinal tract.

Signs

The signs, like the symptoms, are common to many pathologic entities. Uterine enlargement may be present, with blood coming through the os, as seen on speculum examination. A tumor metastatic to the vagina may present with a firm, discolored mass. Occasionally, the patient will present with an acute abdomen because of rupture of the uterus, liver, or theca-lutein cyst. Neurologic signs, such as partial weakness or paralysis, dysphasia, aphasia, or unreactive pupils, indicate probable central nervous system involvement.

Diagnosis

Choriocarcinoma is a great imitator of other diseases, so unless it follows a molar pregnancy, diagnosis may not be suspected.

In females of reproductive age, a β-hCG titer to screen for choriocarcinoma should be performed when any unusual symptoms or signs develop.

Investigations

If the β-hCG titer is positive, the work-up of a patient with choriocarcinoma is the same as that for patients with hydatidiform mole, but should also include a CT scan of the abdomen, pelvis, and head. In addition, a lumbar puncture should be performed if the brain CT scan is negative, because simultaneous evaluation of the β-hCG titer in the cerebrospinal fluid (CSF) and serum may allow detection of very early cerebral metastases. Since the beta subunit does not readily cross the blood-brain barrier, a ratio of serum to CSF β-hCG levels of less than 40 to 1 suggests central nervous system involvement, with secretion of the β-hCG directly into the cerebrospinal fluid.

TREATMENT OF GESTATIONAL TROPHOBLASTIC NEOPLASIA (GTN)

If the β-hCG titers plateau or rise, chemotherapy is required. Because of the sensitivity of this tumor marker, chemotherapy is usually initiated without histologic confirmation of disease. Prior to initiating chemotherapy, a full metastatic work-up must be done to determine whether or not there is metastatic disease present and, if so, whether or not the liver and/or brain are involved.

Nonmetastatic and Good Prognosis Metastatic GTN

The chemotherapy most often employed is either methotrexate or actinomycin-D (Table 56–4). Methotrexate is usually given as a daily dose for five consecutive days or every other day for eight days, alternating with folinic acid (leukovorin). This folinic acid "rescue" regimen is associated with significantly less bone marrow, gastrointestinal, and liver toxicity. Actinomycin-D is given for five consecutive days intravenously or every other week as a single dose.

In appropriately selected patients, hysterectomy may be the primary therapy for hy-

TABLE 56–4 CHEMOTHERAPY FOR MOLAR PREGNANCY

Standard Chemotherapy Regimens
Actinomycin-D
   10–12 μg/kg/day IV for 5 days
              OR
Methotrexate
   0.4 mg/kg/day IM or IV for 5 days

Repeat cycle after minimum gap of 7 days if: granulocytes greater than 1500/mm³; platelets greater than 100,000/mm³; stomatitis and gastrointestinal toxicity recovered; SGOT, SGPT, BUN, and bilirubin levels normal.
Continue chemotherapy cycles
  (a) one or two courses past normal β-hCG titer (less than 1.0 mIU/ml), or
  (b) until β-hCG titers plateau or begin rising.
Obtain weekly β-hCG values and peripheral blood counts.
Before each treatment cycle, obtain SGOT, SGPT, BUN, bilirubin, CBC, and platelet count.
Obtain monthly β-hCG titers for 12 months, then every 2 months for 12 months.
Continue contraception for one year after remisssion induction.

Alternative Chemotherapy Regimens
Actinomycin-D
   1.25 mg/M² IV q 2 weeks
              OR
Methotrexate
   1.0 mg/kg/day IM or IV on days 1,3,5,7 followed 24 hours later by 0.1 mg/kg/day of folinic acid "rescue" on days 2,4,6,8

Adapted from Morrow CP, Townsend DE (eds): Gestational trophoblastic neoplasia. In Synopsis of Gynecologic Oncology. 2nd ed. New York, John Wiley and Sons, 1981, p 348.

datidiform mole. Women over 40 years of age have an increased incidence of choriocarcinoma developing after molar pregnancy. These patients may decrease their risk of malignant sequelae by undergoing hysterectomy.

Poor Prognosis Metastatic GTN

For patients with poor prognosis disease, combination chemotherapy is always utilized. Regimens that have been successfully employed include methotrexate, actinomycin-D, and cyclophosphamide (MAC), or the so-called "Bagshawe" regimen, which is an eight-drug, nine-day program of chemotherapy. The drugs used include hydroxyurea, actinomycin-D, vincristine, cyclophosphmide, methotrexate, melphalan, doxorubic and folinic acid. For patients who fail these agents, combinations of *cis*-platinum and etoposide (VP-16) have been used. Preliminary results with vinblastine, bleomycin, and *cis*-platinum (VBP) have also been encouraging.

In patients with disease metastatic to the brain or liver, radiation is often employed to these areas in conjunction with chemotherapy. The whole brain tolerates an initial dose of 2000 to 3000 rad, with fractions of approximately 200 rad per day. Together with systemic chemotherapy, a 50 percent cure rate can be expected. Liver metastases are usually treated with about 2000 rad.

Follow-Up Studies

Following three negative β-hCG titers, good prognosis patients should be followed with monthly titers for one year. Poor prognosis patients should have monthly titers for two or more years. Thereafter, titers should be checked every three months until five years have elapsed.

Patients should be advised not to become pregnant again within the first 12 months after molar evacuation and should be given a reliable contraceptive.

If a patient's titers become "negative" and later are found to be rising, a second metastatic work-up must be undertaken prior to the initiation of secondary therapy.

Prognosis

About 95 to 100 percent of patients with good prognosis GTN will be cured of their disease. Patients with poor prognostic features can be expected to be cured in only 50 to 70 percent of cases. The majority of the patients who die develop brain or liver metastasis.

SUGGESTED READING

Bagshawe KD: Risk and prognostic factors in trophoblastic neoplasia. Cancer 38:1373, 1976.

Berkowitz RS, Goldstein DP, Bernstein MR: Methotrexate with citrovorum factor rescue as primary therapy for gestational trophoblastic disease. Cancer 50:2024, 1982.

Curry SL, Hammond CB, Tyrey L, et al: Hydatidiform mole: Diagnosis, management and long-term follow-up of 347 patients. Obstet Gynecol 45:1, 1975.

Goldstein DP, Berkowitz RS: Gestational Trophoblastic Neoplasms. Philadelphia, W B Saunders Co, 1982.

Lurain JR, Brewer JI, Torok EE, et al: Natural history of hydatidiform mole after primary evacuation. Am J Obstet Gynecol 145:591, 1983.

McDonald TW, Ruffolo EH: Modern management of gestational trophoblastic disease. Obstet Gynecol Surv 38:67, 1983.

Morrow CP, Kletzky OA, DiSaia PJ, et al: Clinical and laboratory correlates of molar pregnancy and trophoblastic disease. Am J Obstet Gynecol 128:424, 1977.

Surti U, Szulman AE, O'Brien S: Dispermic origin and clinical outcome of three complete hydatidiform moles with 46 XX karyotype. Am J Obstet Gynecol 144:84, 1982.

Surwit EA, Hammond CB: Treatment of metastatic trophoblastic disease with poor prognosis. Obstet Gynecol 55:565, 1980.

INDEX

Your
MBA Game Plan

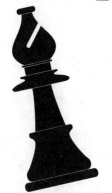

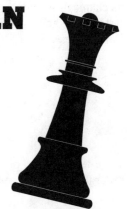

Proven Strategies for Getting Into the Top
Business Schools

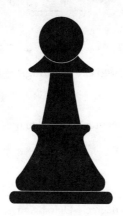

By
Omari Bouknight & Scott Shrum

CAREER
PRESS

The Career Press, Inc.
Franklin Lakes, NJ

YOUR MBA GAME PLAN
EDITED AND TYPESET BY NICOLE DEFELICE
Cover design by Lu Rossman/Digi Dog Design
Printed in the U.S.A. by Book-mart Press

To order this title, please call toll-free 1-800-CAREER-1 (NJ and Canada: 201-848-0310) to order using VISA or MasterCard, or for further information on books from Career Press.

The Career Press, Inc., 3 Tice Road, PO Box 687,
Franklin Lakes, NJ 07417
www.careerpress.com

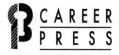

Library of Congress Cataloging-in-Publication Data

Bouknight, Omari, 1977-
    Your MBA game plan : proven strategies for getting into the top business schools / by Omari Bouknight and Scott Shrum.
        p. cm.
    Includes index.
    ISBN 1-56414-683-9 (pbk.)
    1. Master of business administration degree—United States. 2. Business education—United States—Planning. I. Title: MBA game plan. II. Shrum, Scott, 1975- III. Title.

HF1131.B68 2003
650'.071'1—dc21

2003051510

DEDICATION

Scott—Dedicated to the memory of James Bartlett, the most brilliant, principled, and steadfast friend anyone could ever hope to have.

Omari—For my parents, who showed me truth in God, power in education, and the burden of legacy.

ACKNOWLEDGMENTS

It's safe to say that we hardly knew what we were getting into when we first decided to write a book about getting into business school. Fortunately, the people below made the whole process much more bearable, and the final product a lot more valuable. We are truly thankful for their assistance along the way.

John Abbamondi; Kirsten Beucler; Alex Brown; Justin Crandall; Jon Crawford; Nicole DeFelice; Brian Dukes; Buckethead Section, Kellogg Class of 2004; Stacey Farkas; Brigid Ganley; Kavita Gunda; Shaan Kandawalla; Michael Lewis; Mark Lueking; Carolina Menezes; Campbell Murray; Matt Niksch; Tom Pusic; Sarah Richardson; Section A, HBS Class of 2004; Brian Schmidt; Brendan Sheehan; Misha Simmonds; Doug Stein; Anita Thekdi; Chad Troutwine; and Mike Worosz.

Also, this book probably wouldn't have happened if not for the supportive community of fellow b-school applicants on the *BusinessWeek* online forums. We'd like to thank everyone out there for putting up with our surveys and giving us great feedback as this book took shape.

Finally, a few people have been particularly helpful, patient, and supportive in this process. Scott would like to especially thank his wife, Anita, and his parents. Omari would like to especially thank his entire family and Kavita for their continual support. These people believed in us and stuck with us the whole way through.

CONTENTS

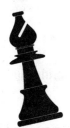
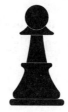
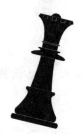

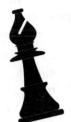
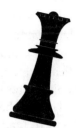

FOREWORD

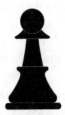

What are your stats? This is the most harmful phrase in the English language, as far as any business school applicant is concerned. In this case, "stats" refers to an applicant's basic quantifiable characteristics, such as "700 GMAT, 3.5 GPA at a top-25 undergrad, four years W/E in P/E." W/E in P/E???

Something is terribly wrong. That stream of numbers and letters tells us nothing about who the applicant really is. What does she like to do for fun? What kind of leadership roles has she taken on? Where does she want to be 10 years from now? We have no idea. Yet we've gotten to the point where many business school applicants immediately ask each other this question whenever they meet. It's a senseless secret handshake.

Make no mistake, the numbers do matter. You need to demonstrate a minimum level of intellectual ability in order to get into any business school. But even though the Stanfords and Whartons of the world boast GMAT averages in the low 700s, don't fool yourself into thinking that a 770 GMAT score means that you're definitely in. Even more importantly, don't think that a sub-700 score means that you're definitely out. The same goes for your undergraduate GPA. And your work experience. And anything else that you can slap a number on.

Unfortunately, the majority of applicants fall into this trap. They focus on one or two statistics and let the rest of their applications suffer. Even worse, they focus on the *wrong* things, and assume that ultra-high GMAT scores or impressive jobs (such as "four years W/E in P/E," which means that an applicant has four years of work experience in private equity) will carry them into business school. Or they think that a 620 GMAT score equals certain rejection from any "top 10" school, which couldn't be further from the truth.

We spoke with hundreds of fellow applicants while working on our own business school applications. Many of them were amazingly bright and were great at what they did, but sometimes they didn't seem to "get it." They would say things such as, "I took the GMAT three times, and I went from a 670 to a 690 to a 700. I'm thinking of enrolling in another GMAT prep class and taking the test a fourth time. What do you think? Don't worry; I'll get around to the essays eventually." To the admissions committee, applicants with great GMAT scores but so-so essays and recommendations are a dime a dozen, and "dime a dozen" won't get you into a top business school.

After seeing too many qualified business school candidates get rejected because of critical strategic mistakes in their applications, we decided to see if we could help. We examined the advice available on the market and realized that while there were some good books that target the business school application process, many of the applicants who were reading them were still asking the wrong questions. So we took a step back and tried to get to the root of the problem. We realized that many applicants are of top-business-school caliber, but don't understand what admissions committees are really looking for in an application.

We decided to build a new application framework. We took a close look at each part of the application process and asked, "What are admissions committees really looking for here, and how can applicants make sure that they're delivering it?" The result is a strategic approach to the business school application process. By applying this approach through your MBA game plan, you can greatly improve your chances of receiving admittance into the top programs.

We haven't made a living from providing college candidates with application advice, but we have managed to get into the top MBA programs during a very competitive year by using strategic analysis and targeted approaches. We've been in your shoes, and hope to share with you what we've learned over the course of the application process. We also hope we can save you from some of the most common mistakes that applicants make. If you can make it easy for admissions officers to see that you have a distinctive profile and would fit well with their schools' cultures, then you'll quickly get ahead of other candidates. And getting ahead of other candidates is probably what you were shooting for when you picked up this book in the first place.

Best of luck to you!

—Scott and Omari

1
NEW GAME,
NEW RULES

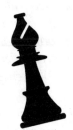
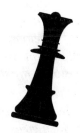
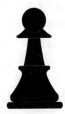

To my relief, the cab slowed down and the driver waved me over. I had been on the verge of running for the last 30 minutes, trying to reach my interview with Harvard Business School (HBS) on time. Sliding into the back seat of the taxi, I heavily exhaled directions to the admissions office, rejuvenated with confidence knowing that I would not arrive to the interview late. Now all I had to do was differentiate myself from the other 10,000 applicants and prove to the admissions committee that I embody HBS's culture and mission. Suddenly, it hit me. This would be no small task.

In many ways, the on-campus interview is a wake-up call. For many applicants, it is the first time that they interact directly with the competition and with their target schools. Stepping into the admissions office, my alarm went off as I began to discuss experiences, backgrounds, and objectives with other applicants who were waiting to interview. The conversations were enlightening, as gossip and advice on the application process were freely swapped. More so, however, these conversations were humbling. I spoke with a military pilot who had escorted the President around the country, a scientist in biotechnology who was working on a cancer-fighting antibody, and a dot-com entrepreneur who had executed a multi-million dollar initial public offering. What did I have to offer?

I no longer believed my family's frequent promises that I would be admitted. They obviously didn't understand what I was up against.

"Your interviewer is ready to see you now," the receptionist called out to me. Moments later, I was sitting across from an admissions officer. A 30-minute conversation ensued in which we discussed all aspects of my application, except for my GMAT score and GPA. Indeed, the interview was very similar to the several others in which I took part. Because most applicants to top business schools have the ability to succeed in the curricula, GPA and test scores are often ruled out as differentiating factors. So what remained to separate me from the thousands of other applicants?

The admissions officer asked questions about my story. What were my career goals and how would attending business school play a role in meeting those goals? How would my professional and personal experiences enhance the classroom dynamic? In what ways had I acted as a leader to my peers?

Fortunately, I was ready. My responses were well crafted and were supported with details that augmented the assertions. These responses were all part of a strategic approach that I developed to target the schools to which I applied. The interview transformed into a platform on which I established my case. The admissions officer became my audience, measuring my storyline against other applicants' stories and against the school's sense of "fit."

By the end of the interview, I felt satisfied. I had covered each of my points and made a convincing case for why I belonged at HBS. Exiting the interview, I didn't concern myself with finding a taxi. I wanted to savor my victory. Thanks to my preparation, I was one step closer to being admitted.

The Increasing Popularity of Business School

Business is a natural extension of all professions. Whether the occupation we pursue is in fashion, banking, technology, or healthcare, business permeates the fabric of the workplace. Perhaps this was never more evident than during the Internet craze of the late 1990s, when having an innovative business plan in the Silicon Valley became as cliché as having a ground-breaking movie script in Hollywood. While the subsequent economic downturn sent the majority of business plans to the trash, our entrepreneurial spirit and industrial mentality has remained undiminished. Indeed, the number of applications that were sent to top business schools during the 2002–2003 season reached an approximate 100,000 applications, an increase of more than 30 percent over the number of applications submitted a few years prior.

Over the last several years, the rules to the business school application game have changed drastically. As a result of the increase in applications, the competition among applicants has intensified. The average GMAT score and undergraduate GPA of admitted students to top business schools have risen to almost 690 and 3.45, respectively. The level of competition has heightened to the point that the acceptance rates for some schools have fallen to near single-digits. This has pushed schools to closely examine all aspects of the application beyond the basic statistics.

Many applicants, however, are responding to this increased competition by merely focusing on improving their GMAT scores. Any popular periodical's business school rankings prominently feature a school's average GMAT score next to its name, so it is only natural that applicants focus on this obvious component of the application. But while the GMAT may be the first challenge in the application process that must be navigated, high scores alone certainly won't win the business school application game.

MBA Application Strategy

Traditional strategic analysis examines the approach of a decision-maker given his environment and the tactics of other decision-makers who are in pursuit of similar objectives. As an applicant, you must succeed in an environment that demands differentiation against the competition and proper fit with the programs to which you apply. The ultimate questions that you as an applicant must answer are:

- ❏ How do I measure against the competition?
- ❏ How do I measure against my targeted business schools?

In our admittedly subjective estimation, the probability of gaining acceptance to top business school programs looks something like the following:

	Don't Fit Program	Fit Program
Differentiate From Competition	10%–20%	50%–70%
Don't Differentiate From Competition	0%–5%	10%–20%

The rest of this book focuses on developing answers to those two questions and getting you to the upper right-hand cell. It will do so in a functional and comprehensive manner, highlighting all aspects of the application process. You will learn how to position yourself based on your experiences and your target schools, how to write effective essays, and how to execute your application strategy.

Understanding the competition

When Omari first started the business school application process, one of the first pieces of insight he was given dealt with the number of candidates applying with his professional profile: *If you want to gain admittance to a top program, you must first find a way to differentiate yourself from the thousands of other consultants who are applying.* This is good advice for any applicant, regardless of the profile. Therefore, it is helpful to get into the minds of admissions officers and of other business school candidates with the knowledge that these candidates will have applications that cross the officers' desks before and after your own application. In general, there are two aspects of your application that admissions officers will compare with other candidates' applications: Your profile and your career goals.

Your profile

The first aspect of differentiation that you must understand as a business school candidate is that all applicants have an Achilles' heel. We all have a weakness in our profile that will be reflected in our application unless it is appropriately addressed. Whether the issue is number of years of work experience, lack of community service activities, low GPA, poor writing ability, low GMAT, unconvincing interview skills, or overconfidence, all candidates have an aspect of their profiles that, unaddressed, could lead to the dreaded "ding," as rejections are commonly called.

Your profile consists of your academic background, professional experiences, and personal interests and activities. As much as possible, the components in your profile should be multifaceted and consistent with an overall theme.

Multifaceted

Admissions officers are looking for candidates who demonstrate multiple dimensions through various interests. A common question that is asked during business school interviews is: "Outside of your professional activities, what are your personal interests and endeavors?" Top business schools want to ensure that they do not merely admit workaholic drones, but rather candidates who lead interesting and inspiring lives.

Consistent

Not too long ago, we spoke with Carrie, an applicant who was declined admittance to the Kellogg School of Management at Northwestern University. During her feedback session with an admissions officer, one of the messages that Carrie received was that she lacked community service experience. Actually, Carrie did have community service experience, but it was not consistent with the overall message that she conveyed in her application. The community service activities in which Carrie took part appeared to be events in which she participated purely so that they could be posted on her resume. Admission committee members are savvy enough to detect when an applicant's attempts to enhance her profile are contrived, so you therefore need to weave the components of your profile into your story in a logical and consistent manner.

The second and third chapters will assist you in differentiating your application story from the competition. Chapter 2 will outline the characteristics that are valued by admissions officers and show you how to demonstrate these characteristics in your own application. In highlighting those characteristics, you will ensure that your profile is multifaceted and consistent with a targeted story. This approach impresses top business schools, as they are searching for candidates who will add something unique to the classroom dynamic. Chapter 2 will also show you how to overcome certain weaknesses that your application may contain. Specific profiles will be covered in Chapter 3, detailing their typical strengths and weaknesses, and providing guidance on how to overcome the stereotypes and tendencies that are associated with them.

Your career goals

Where you are going is just as important as where you are coming from. Admissions officers often cite candidates' inability to articulate their post-graduation goals—and how the business school's curriculum will support those goals—as a contributing factor in a candidate's rejection.

As you communicate your career goals, you should convey an overall story that makes it easy for the admissions committee to see why an MBA makes sense for you. Typically, the career goal aspect of your story will either describe your motivation to make a career change or your intent to bolster your current career direction. Whichever career path you intend to pursue, the messages you communicate in the application should reflect innovation and an entrepreneurial spirit. That doesn't mean that all applicants should strive to start their own businesses, but rather that business schools are looking for candidates who want to contribute a fresh perspective and new insight to their chosen professions.

Use the application as a forum in which to display ambition and ingenuity as you discuss future objectives. Additionally, you should discuss the ways in which the targeted school's specific curriculum would aid you in achieving those objectives.

Chapter 4 will provide you with details on each component of the application process. Your story should be reflected in each of these components.

Understanding Your Business School Targets

Most business schools look for similar qualities in their applicants. They look for students who demonstrate academic aptitude, leadership, an ability to work well with peers and subordinates, integrity, and ambition, just to name a few.

So does this mean that the applications to your target schools should be the same? Of course not. Each school tends to emphasize certain traits over others and looks for examples to support these traits. A quick look at the essay questions from a few business school applications tells you that each school asks about these qualities in different ways. Here's the irony: Each school claims to look for a unique type of candidate, yet it seems that every year there are some applicants who manage to get into all of the top programs. Do these candidates really have *every* trait that all of these schools are looking for?

Probably not. More likely, they understand the emphasis that each school places on specific traits, and they know how to highlight those traits in their application. Successful applicants know that MIT Sloan values analytical ability, and they therefore stress their methodical approach to business problems. They know that Fuqua really does pride itself on its teamwork-oriented culture, and they highlight the success they've had while working in teams.

These are obvious examples, but this is an area where many applicants stumble. They either don't give enough thought to highlighting the traits that each school looks for, or they "tack on" one trite example in a half-hearted attempt to meet the requirement. The result is almost always a rejection because the applicants failed to demonstrate proper fit with their target schools.

What is "fit"?

In short, "fitting" with a school means demonstrating that you have the ability to succeed there, you are someone the school would be glad to have as part of its community, and you will serve as an ambassador for the school after you graduate.

In order to convey proper fit with a school, you should demonstrate that:

❒ You understand what the school stands for and why it is important. When you say, "Darden preaches leadership," you are able to give examples of what leadership means to you and explain why you want to further strengthen your own leadership abilities in business school.

❑ You embody the traits that the school most wants to see in its students. You don't need to have climbed Mount Everest to have demonstrated accomplishment or aced the GMAT to demonstrate quantitative excellence. You do need to be able to illustrate how your everyday life is peppered with examples of the traits for which the school looks.

❑ You will become very involved in your business school, from contributing to class discussions to running student organizations to being an active alum 20 years from now. One great way to communicate this is by pointing to similar experiences with your undergraduate school.

❑ You are the kind of person whom your classmates would want to work with on a team project at 3 a.m. Exhibiting a penchant for working in teams and a sociable personality will establish the basis for this.

One other extremely important question that an admissions officer asks about every applicant is, "Would he actually attend this school if he were accepted?" Admissions officers know that you're applying to multiple schools, and they know that their school may not be your first choice. But you need to convey enough knowledge and enthusiasm about the school to convince admissions officers that you would strongly consider attending their school if you were accepted. The history of business school applications is littered with stories of people with stellar credentials who were rejected by "safety" schools. If you don't sound sincere about wanting to attend a given school, you can expect that school to return the favor by not wanting you.

Demonstrating "fit" in your application

Your entire application should spell out how well you fit with your target school. Practically speaking, though, the parts of the application that will do this the most are your essays, recommendations, and interview. Think of these as your opportunities to talk about how your background and future direction correspond with what the school has to offer, and to discuss them in a way that lets your personality come through. Yes, you will answer specific questions for each school, but admissions officers inevitably want to know what's most important to you and why.

In essays, admissions officers most want to hear about actions that you have taken to solve a real problem or reach an actual goal, not what you would do in a hypothetical situation. They also want to hear what you learned from your experiences. Be as specific as possible in describing what you have accomplished and what you have learned in the process.

The same goes for recommendations. Everyone finds someone to write a positive recommendation for them, but a truly great recommendation will support your positioning by providing specific examples of how you demonstrated leadership, succeeded as part of a team, etc. We can't emphasize this enough: Be as specific as possible!

Before you put together your applications, you should know exactly what you want them to communicate. Chapter 6 will help you build your game plan, which will bring out the messages that you want to convey to each of your target schools.

Selecting your schools

As important as it is to establish proper fit in your applications, you must first select the schools to which you will apply. The game is reversed, as you must decide which schools fit you rather than having the schools decide that you fit them.

Selecting schools should be an introspective process. You should be warned, however that people who don't even know your name will have an opinion on where you should apply. Also remember that school rankings are just one piece of information to consider. Certainly rankings can be helpful tools in getting familiar with the schools' perceived strengths and weaknesses. Still, it's important that you do your own research. After all, no magazine or newspaper knows what really matters most to you.

Do not be enticed by prestige alone. While it certainly may be a factor in making your selections, there are plenty of other criteria that should be considered. Some of the selection criteria that you may want to use in evaluating schools include:

- ❏ Curriculum emphases.
- ❏ Typical career paths of graduates.
- ❏ Teaching style.
- ❏ Student culture.
- ❏ Compensation upon graduation.
- ❏ Financial aid opportunities.
- ❏ International perspective and access.
- ❏ Geographical location.
- ❏ Facilities.
- ❏ Diversity.
- ❏ Cost of tuition and living.
- ❏ Class size.
- ❏ Use of technology.

Fortunately, there is an abundance of resources available to help you evaluate these criteria. Some of the steps you should undertake are:

- ❏ Visit business school Websites.
- ❏ Review curriculum information.
- ❏ Speak with current students and alumni.
- ❏ Speak with faculty.
- ❏ Attend business school forums.
- ❏ Visit the schools.

We will discuss some of these resources and criteria in more detail later. We will also assist you in your evaluation of programs. Chapter 5 takes a look at the business school selection process and provides an overview of 30 top business schools, with perspectives on how to gain admittance to them. Finally, we've compiled a list of frequently asked questions (FAQs), which you will find at the end of most chapters. These are questions that we've heard a number of applicants ask. The FAQs have been placed in different chapters depending on their topics.

The B-school Decision

The decision to apply to business school is likely to be one of the most important decisions you'll make in your career. For full-time students, the investment is likely to be in excess of $100,000 before you even take opportunity costs (the salary you would have earned during those two years) into consideration. And with more than 70 percent of MBAs taking out loans to pay for at least a portion of their education, it's clear that you shouldn't just wake up one morning and decide that you want to go to business school.

Interestingly, that seems to be exactly the way some business school applicants arrived at their decision. Others (read: investment bankers and consultants) scheduled "apply to business school" in their Outlook calendars four years ago as if it's just another item to check off. Regardless of how you arrived at this decision, you should really spend some time thinking about what you want to get out of the business school experience.

The bottom line is that you absolutely have to be passionate about attending business school before making the decision to apply. Sure, the thought of going $100,000 into debt is intimidating, but there are plenty of ways in which you can balance the costs of b-school, including a large salary at the end of the rainbow. Perhaps the more daunting factor is the admissions process itself. Indeed, you must be passionate about b-school, because the application process will deter anyone who isn't dedicated to getting in. Certainly this book will help you with every step in that process, but unfortunately we can't do much to instill the dedication that it takes to get in. That part is up to you.

Thankfully, business school programs come in all sorts of shapes, sizes, and colors, so you should be able to select a program that fits your needs. Here are some of your options:

- ❏ **Full-time:** As the title would suggest, full-time programs are the most involved option. U.S. b-school programs are generally two years in duration, although there are some one-year programs, and require students to leave their professional positions. Students like this option, because it gives them full exposure to the b-school experience. Certainly the opportunity costs are higher than the other options, but the experience is richer, because of the amount of time spent with classmates, faculty, and speakers. Generally, full-time is seen as a good option for people who are considering some type of career transition, be it a new industry, function, or position. One of the benefits of full-time programs that allows this transition to occur is the summer internship. There is heated debate over whether there is actually any financial benefit to attending a full-time program. Although there is no clear answer, our personal experiences have shown that in addition to making a career transition, there are great intangible benefits to being surrounded by intelligent, motivated people for two years. Our focus, in terms of providing application strategy advice, will be on full-time programs. The application processes for part-time and distance learning programs, however, are very similar. You can still benefit from the advice in this book should you decide not to apply to a full-time program.

❏ **Part-time:** If you are satisfied with your current career path and can't fathom the thought of breaking away from the workforce for one or two years, a part-time program might be what you're looking for. Part-time students generally follow the same curriculum as their full-time counterparts, but take all of their classes during the evenings and on weekends. Most part-time students take three to five years to finish their degrees. Many part-timers report that the class load combined with their normal work load can be intense at times, but they are happy not to have to take on the extra debt load.

❏ **Distance-learning:** These programs are quickly rising in popularity as people become more comfortable with taking classes online. Typically, students will download course material and assignments from the b-school Website and have access, via the Internet, to faculty. On weekends, students will then meet in the classroom to discuss that week's material. Distance-learning programs are normally two or three years in length and feature curricula similar to that of full-time programs. The benefits are that you can continue your career in a location that isn't within close proximity of the program in which you're enrolled. B-schools are scrambling to see how they can capitalize on this trend and often refer to them as "eMBA" programs. Be aware that a large tradeoff you make in choosing a distance-learning program is that you will miss out on the opportunity to be surrounded by exceptional peers from all walks of life. If you are comfortable with this tradeoff and are mostly interested in the hard skills that an MBA can deliver (especially if you want to move ahead in your current job, rather than find a new job), then a distance-learning option may be right for you.

❏ **Executive MBA:** Executive MBA (EMBA) programs are similar to distance-learning programs in that they appeal to professionals who are further along in their careers than typical full-time applicants. Also like distance-learning programs, EMBA programs allow students to remain employed full-time. The main difference between the two program types is that EMBA students don't access course content online. Rather, students take all of their courses in the classroom on weekends. The majority of students in EMBA programs are sponsored by their companies. EMBA programs generally follow similar curricula as full-time programs and can take anywhere from two to five years to complete.

❏ **Executive programs:** For those who are further along in their careers and have specific aspects of business they would like to learn more about, executive education programs might be the way to go. Executive education programs generally run for one or two weeks and provide established executives with the opportunity to improve their competency in one of a variety of business topics from mergers and acquisitions to leading change in an organization to supply chain management. Their short length allows executives to rapidly get educated in an area without infringing upon their work schedule. These programs are also a nice way to get up to speed on a business topic without enduring lectures on topics with which you are already familiar. Executive programs are, however, notoriously expensive. You can expect one these programs to set you or your company back any-where from $2,000 to $20,000. Additionally, you won't receive any type of degree for your participation. At best, you can hope to receive some type of certification. Still, you will enjoy a fairly simple application process. Most applications request information on your professional background (no GMAT, no essays, no interview, no recommendations, etc.) and can be accessed directly from business schools' Websites. Overall, executive education programs are much more interested in your ability to pay than your qualifications. So if you're reading this book in order to develop a strategy to get into an executive education program, you can stop right now.

❒ **Ph.D.:** If you are enamored with thought of teaching business concepts, then you should consider going the Ph.D. route. Business schools are al-ways looking for fresh talent, knowing that faculty strength is a major dif-ferentiating factor in the eyes of applicants. Ph.D. programs generally take four to five years to complete and in many cases require you to take some MBA coursework before specializing. Although you will be in school much longer than with a full-time MBA program, you will receive considerably more financial assistance. You should know, however, that Ph.D. programs can be extremely difficult to gain admittance to, even more so than their MBA counterparts. Many Ph.D. programs at top schools only take a hand-ful of students per specialty each year. Additionally, landing your dream faculty position can be much more challenging than landing your dream business job because faculty spots at top schools are always limited.

In addition to these basic options, you should also consider whether you want to apply for a dual degree program or a specialty program. Dual degree programs provide you with the ability to earn an MBA degree and another advanced degree in less time than it would take to complete both degrees separately. Unfortunately, there's no two-for-one deal on the price of pursuing a dual degree. Some of the most popular degrees to combine with an MBA include:

❒ Law.
❒ Public policy.
❒ Education.
❒ International studies.
❒ Engineering.
❒ Medicine.
❒ Health administration.

If you decide to pursue a dual degree, you should make sure that you understand how the extra degree will be beneficial. You should be wary of pursuing it for the prestige of getting additional letters after your name. In fact, some companies might be slow to consider you during recruiting, because of the fear that they'd have to compensate you more for both degrees. Also, know that a dual degree may actually provide you with less flexibility. If, for instance, you get a dual degree in business and medicine, then firms outside of healthcare will immediately ask why you're interested in them, given your background. With that said, if you have a firm understanding of how the additional degree fits in with your career goals, are willing to pay the extra tuition, and don't mind spending the additional time, then a dual degree is probably worth pursuing.

Apart from dual degree programs, several schools offer specialization programs within their core business school curricula. These programs generally require you to take a few required MBA courses before following the specialization component of the curriculum. Examples of specialization programs include:

- ❏ Financial engineering.
- ❏ Computer engineering.
- ❏ Accounting.
- ❏ Healthcare.
- ❏ Manufacturing management.

Specialization programs are nice from the standpoint that they signal your dedication to a particular field. Recruiters from those areas tend to like that level of dedication, so if you're comfortable aligning yourself with a particular industry or function, you should consider specializing. Naturally, the flip side is that you are narrowing your business focus rather than broadening it. Also, specialization programs can sometimes be more difficult to gain acceptance to than their general management counterparts. Nonetheless, participants in these programs who have a clear career direction consistently speak highly about their experiences.

So there you have it; a whole world of opportunity from which you can select. It is of course a big decision to make. But once you make the decision to apply, we'll be there the rest of the way.

FAQs

How specific should I be in discussing my career goals?

Simply espousing generalities with regard to your career goals will not win you the gold. While you don't have to state that you want to be CEO of a specific company within five years, it is important that you convey a career direction in your application. Establishing a direction shows that you know what you want to get out of business school and aren't simply trying to boost your salary. As a general rule, you should be as specific as you feel comfortable discussing. In other words, don't discuss a career path in your application that you can't speak intelligently about. Overall, your career goals should make sense in the context of your application story and should be compelling, answering the question of why you want an MBA to pursue that career path. You should also be able to discuss how your career goals will have an impact on an industry, individuals, or society in general.

What if I'm not sure what my career goals are?

Use the application preparation process to gain a better understanding of your talents and ambitions. Talk to your friends and family about what they see you doing and match that with your background. Refine your ideas as you study business school curricula until you have your application story. Odds are that by the end of the business school application process you will have a much clearer picture of what your career goals are. After you get admitted to the school of your dreams, you can change your aspirations as many times as you please, but you don't want the admissions committee to view you as an aimless vagabond. This is particularly true if you come from a less business-oriented background, in which case having a concrete story for why an MBA makes sense for you is even more critical than for a typical applicant.

2
THE FOUR DIMENSIONS OF A PERFECT APPLICANT

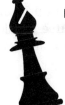
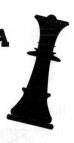
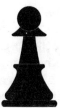

Becoming the perfect business school candidate is as much an exercise in understanding and cultivating your relative strengths as it is in identifying and addressing your relative weaknesses. We all have strengths. The main challenge is to reveal your strengths in your applications and convince admissions officers that those strengths aren't outweighed by your weaknesses.

For every Superman there is a kryptonite. For every applicant there is a weakness. That's okay! This is the first reality that must be understood as you develop your position and become the "perfect applicant." Remember, a 780 on the GMAT does not blind admissions officers to generic career goals any more than a great stereo system makes up for a car that looks like a rust bucket. To avoid this type of imbalance, you must express all four dimensions that every business school is in search of.

Leadership	Innovation
Teamwork	Maturity

Leadership

Probably more than anything else, business schools want to be known as institutions that produce leaders in their fields. Admissions committees are therefore in search of applicants who display leadership ability in all facets of their lives. This doesn't mean that you need to have started three new nonprofit organizations or replanted a forest. Candidates who successfully demonstrate leadership in their applications exhibit how they have provided others with direction, shown initiative, and managed difficult situations in their professional, personal, and academic careers.

It is not enough to merely state that you are a leader, but rather you must provide examples of demonstrated leadership. Ultimately, the admissions committee should identify you as a high potential leader because of supporting details rather than overt statements. A good rule of thumb is "Show, don't tell."

Innovation

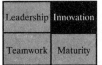

Innovation is a combination of traditional intellectual ability and creativity. Naturally, the former is reflected in the first line statistics (GMAT and GPA), but admissions committee members are also in search of the latter. Applicants who are visionaries are generally successful in establishing the trait of innovation. Innovation in this case can be as simple as finding a new solution to an everyday business problem. Candidates should strive to deliver application stories that speak to adding something new to their selected career paths, rather than merely becoming middle managers in mindless business conglomerates.

Teamwork

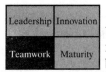

The success that Kellogg has had with integrating teamwork throughout its curriculum has spread over time to the other top business schools. Kellogg's success with a team-oriented curriculum has been supported by the way in which most companies now operate. Because companies utilize teams for virtually all of their functions, business schools are in search of applicants with strong team skills. A team-oriented attitude is now a baseline expectation of every applicant. This includes basic social skills and a willingness to share successes and take accountability for failures. While top business schools are certainly known for being competitive environments, operating in teams has become an integral part of conducting business, and as such is a key aspect of the business school experience.

Maturity

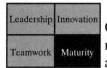

Work experience has become a vital part of candidates' applications. On average, admitted applicants to the top business schools have almost five years of full-time work experience. Although there are some applicants who are admitted directly from undergraduate programs, this remains the exception and not the rule. More important than the length of one's work experience, however, is the quality and depth of that experience.

Top business schools are in search of candidates who present multilayered experiences inside and outside of the workplace. An important aspect of the business school experience is that students teach one another based on their backgrounds. It is often said that everyone at business school, including faculty, are both teachers and students. Admissions committees therefore try to identify "mature" candidates who display professional maturity and integrity throughout their application.

As an applicant, your goal should be to weave each of these dimensions throughout all of the application components. In general, application components consist of: data sheets, essays, recommendations, resume, transcript, and interview. In Chapter 4, we will step through each of these components in detail and show ways in which successful applicants have expressed the four dimensions.

In order to help you gauge how well your profile supports these dimensions, you should take an inventory of your activities and achievements. This will allow you to identify your strengths and weaknesses and address them accordingly.

Activities and achievements that typically support the four dimensions include:

Community Service

Over time, community service has slowly transitioned from a "nice-to-have" to a "must-have" on the application. During feedback sessions with rejected applicants, admissions committee members have been known to bring it up as a reason for their decision. It should be stressed, however, that this is a quality (not quantity) activity. You shouldn't merely write down every humanitarian act that you've ever performed. Nor should you try to join half a dozen community service organizations to desperately demonstrate that you have a heart. Rather, it is important to show that you have aspirations of helping society as a whole and not just your personal bank account. Your goal should be to demonstrate deep impact through a few activities, not broad impact across several. Community service is a great way to express all of the four dimensions, but it can especially be powerful in communicating maturity and leadership abilities.

GMAT Score

While your GMAT score alone will never get you into a business school, it certainly can keep you out. As a general rule, if your score falls below a school's middle 80 percent range of scores, you will have to fight an uphill battle in order to be considered a contender. On the flip side, a GMAT score close to a school's mean indicates that you have the intellectual horsepower to excel in the business school classroom. Naturally, achieving a strong score on the GMAT gives you points in the innovation department. To avoid having to overcome a low score, you should review our section on the GMAT in Chapter 4.

Hobbies and Extracurricular Activities

Any hobby that can support one of the dimensions or give the admissions committee insight into your personality is worth mentioning. At the end of the day, business schools are looking to admit people, not numbers, and discussing hobbies is a great way to differentiate yourself from the competition. These activities can also display your strengths in areas such as teamwork and innovation. As such, it isn't really important what the hobby is, but rather what the hobby says about you as an applicant. Do you like fly fishing? Great. Now tell the admissions committee why.

International and Cultural Exposure

As the trend of globalization continues and the world gets smaller, business schools are in search of applicants who will have world impact. Use the application process as a platform to reveal your foreign language skills, multi-national experiences, and cultural awareness. Examples of this can be as grandiose as leading a business unit through a global merger across three continents, or as simple as working with a group of individuals with diverse professional and educational backgrounds. In general, including international or cultural experiences displays a willingness to explore beyond your comfort zone. In effect, it will help you to support the maturity and teamwork dimensions.

Professional Experience

For most applicants, professional experience will be the primary driver of the application. It will permeate the essays, recommendations, interviews, and resume. Because it has such wide-ranging usage, it should be utilized to support all four dimensions.

Undergraduate and Graduate Transcripts

Although your undergraduate and graduate transcripts can't be altered, you can emphasize different aspects of them to support your position. Perhaps you took myriad courses outside of your major during undergrad. You could use that multi-discipline approach to support your desire to attend a business school that focuses on general management. Naturally, a high Grade Point Average (GPA) helps to support the innovation dimension and indicates your ability to succeed in a rigorous academic environment.

Analyzing Your Strengths and Weaknesses

Odds are, you have some notable strengths that will make you a solid student and worthy contributor in business school, but you also have some weaknesses that might keep you out of your ideal school if they go unaddressed. That puts you in a pool that includes probably 99 percent of all business school applicants. This section will show you how to systematically identify and capitalize on your strengths while rooting out and neutralizing your weaknesses.

The grid

Surprisingly, many applicants don't spend any time analyzing or even just writing down their strengths and weaknesses. This might seem like a trivial task—especially because you know yourself better than anyone—but remember that your goal is to sell yourself to someone whose only contact with you is through your application and possibly a 30-minute interview. Therefore, you need to organize your thoughts and make sure that you know exactly what traits you will emphasize for the admissions committee.

It helps to start by drawing out the four dimensions and activity/achievement categories in a grid, like the one on the following page.

Start with an empty grid

Activities/Achievements	Characteristics			
	Leadership	Innovation	Teamwork	Maturity
Community Service				
GMAT Score				
Hobbies and Extracurricular Activities				
International/Cultural Exposure				
Professional Experience				
Transcript(s)				

Next, list your activities and achievements, according to the categories, that bring out one or more of the dimensions. This process shouldn't happen in one 10-minute session. Rather, it will likely take a few minutes here and there as other activities and achievements come to mind. The process might stretch over days or even weeks. Some things to think about when you are looking into your past are:

❐ What extracurricular activities did you participate in while in college? What did you volunteer for? What positions were you elected to?

❐ How have you gotten involved in your community since graduating from college? What have you enjoyed about these experiences? What have you learned that you didn't learn in school or on the job?

❐ What do you like to do in your spare time? What do you enjoy about each of these things? How have they helped you gain a new perspective or exercise your creative side?

❐ Where have you traveled? What languages do you know? What have you learned from your friends of different backgrounds?

❐ What have you done on the job that might exhibit one or more of the four desired dimensions? Did you lead a team, identify a problem and find a creative solution, deal with a problematic coworker, and achieve a goal that no one thought was possible?

❐ What about your undergraduate academic experience might stand out? Did you study abroad or develop your own independent study? Did you dedicate yourself to one academic field, or did you pursue multiple interests? What awards did you receive?

Start by being fairly generous with yourself. Put everything that comes to mind in the grid. You can pare down the overlaps and the weaker examples later on. Also, you may have participated in some activities that don't fit neatly into any of the above categories. As long as they help bring out one of the four main dimensions that you want to demonstrate, include them. You can create a catch-all "other" category if needed.

When you are done, your grid may look like an expanded version of this:

Activities/Achievements	Characteristics			
	Leadership	Innovation	Teamwork	Maturity
Community Service				
Volunteer at a local soup kitchen				X
Founded a student group that assists the eldery	X	X		X
GMAT Score				
High quantitative score		X		
Hobbies and Extracurricular Activities				
Writing		X		X
Photography		X		X
Play keyboard for a small jazz band	X	X	X	X
International/Cultural Exposure				
Conversant in Spanish				X
Participant on a global project team			X	X
Professional Experience				
Developed a strategic plan to enter a new market	X	X		
Led a team in implementing a new technology	X		X	
Led internal training for new hires	X			X
Transcript(s)				
Difficult course load in quantitative areas		X		
Graduated with honors		X		

Note that you will likely have more Xs in some categories than in others. That's perfectly fine. The idea is not to have a completely full grid, but rather to use the grid as a tool for visualizing what your strengths and weaknesses are. Hopefully, your activities and achievements will complement each other and help fill in each column of the table to some degree, but don't worry if this doesn't happen when you first fill it out.

Also note that some activities may only demonstrate one dimension while others may demonstrate three or four of them. That doesn't mean that the former is less valuable than the latter. Keep in mind that the most important thing is to adequately demonstrate all four desired dimensions. An activity that provides your only strong example of leadership may end up being the most important piece of your application story, rather than one of many activities that show that you demonstrated all four dimensions moderately well.

After you are confident that you have covered everything in your background that is relevant to your application, start to trim the list if needed. If you have 10 examples that demonstrate teamwork, try to evaluate them through an admissions officer's eyes and rank them from most important to least important. The question you should ask yourself in order to rank them should be, "How effectively does this achievement or activity demonstrate what I am trying to show?" It's tempting to include "glamorous" examples over more common ones, but being one small part of a CEO's task force on cost-cutting may do less to show off your traits than having led a lower-profile team within your own department.

Also look for activities and achievements that overlap. If you have done four things that all demonstrate leadership and maturity, you won't need to mention all four of them in your application. Just one or two will do.

What to Do About Your Weaknesses

In the event that you look at one row or column of your grid and see a lot of white space, don't panic! Most applicants will encounter this challenge. Remember that the table isn't the end, but rather it is the means for identifying what you might need to work on while you build your application.

Following are some areas where applicants typically have some holes in their grids, and some ideas for bolstering your position in each.

Community service

Not everyone has done a lot of community service, and it can be tempting to want to volunteer for five nonprofit organizations in the weeks leading up to your application deadline. Admissions committees can see right through this, however, so don't waste your time in a last-ditch attempt to look "involved."

If you simply do not have any community service activities to point to, look for other activities in your background that will demonstrate similar characteristics. Starting a volleyball club at the local gym won't solve world hunger, but it still shows that you like to get involved and can motivate others to do the same. If you find that your application is still lacking the altruistic angle that a community service activity might demonstrate, then make sure to bring out your human side in other ways, such as more subtle examples of how you helped a family member or someone on the job solve a problem. The bottom line is that you want to show that you like to get involved in the community around you, and that you are more than a GMAT score and fancy resume.

If you still have time before you begin the application process, be on the lookout for community service opportunities. Mentoring programs such as Big Brothers Big Sisters are great ways to show your willingness to give back to the community.

GMAT score

The good news about the GMAT is that it is one of the few achievements that you can work on and improve in a short amount of time (compared to community service or an undergraduate transcript from five years ago). The bad news is that some applicants can spend months studying for it and still fall short of their goal. If your GMAT score makes you look weak in the quantitative or verbal departments, be sure to bring out other examples in your application that will counterbalance these weaknesses.

If your quantitative score is low, highlight any tough analytical courses that you took as an undergrad. Or show how you use your quantitative skills to unravel tough problems on the job, or even as part of a volunteer opportunity in which you participated. Remember that demonstrating an analytical skill set doesn't have to mean showing that you know calculus. There are practical, everyday activities that can help you demonstrate your comfort with using numbers to make decisions. The bottom line is that you just need to show that you won't be helpless two weeks into your first-year finance course.

If your verbal score is low, then you will need to work extra hard to highlight your communication skills. You can do this through your essays and your interviews.

You can also enlist support from your recommenders, to address weaknesses in both the quantitative and/or verbal section. If your undergraduate transcript and your job don't help, consider enrolling in a statistics, finance, public speaking, or accounting course in a local community college. This shows a dedication to education and will impress the admissions committees. Many business schools are happy to suggest what kinds of courses they would consider as useful preparation for their programs.

Hobbies and extracurricular activities

This is usually the part of the application that gives applicants the least amount of trouble, as most of us have enough interests to keep us busy outside of school or work. Look at how your hobbies relate to your other activities, and they hopefully will provide a well-rounded picture of you as a person. If you already have the four desired dimensions covered reasonably well by your other activities and achievements, then use your hobbies as a way to provide a little extra depth and color to your application. If your hobbies don't add anything new, then de-emphasize them and let the other parts of your application stand on their own.

International and cultural exposure

For many people, this is a clear-cut have-or-don't-have issue. If you haven't worked, studied, or traveled abroad, don't despair. Business schools like to see experience in this area, but realize that not everyone has had a chance to see the world. If this is the case for you, be sure to emphasize the success that you have had in working with people of various backgrounds or even different points of view from your own. Even two people from the same school who work for the same company have a lot of differences between them. Show how you have overcome these differences to build success, and, even more importantly, demonstrate that you value these opportunities to grow and push yourself outside of your normal comfort zone.

Professional experience

People who worry about their professional experience are usually concerned with either the quality or quantity of the work that they have done. If you are worried about the amount of work experience that you have, take comfort in the fact that many business schools are reversing a decade-old trend and are actually pursuing younger applicants. They will still be interested in you as long as you have demonstrated success on the job, increased responsibility in your assignments, and a true understanding of what an MBA can do for you. If you are still an undergrad and are looking to go right into business school, your best chances of demonstrating leadership and maturity will be in your extracurricular activities and anything else where you took charge and made something happen outside of the classroom.

Quality issues around work experience can be tough, but can also be overcome. Have you stagnated in your job? Think about why this has happened and how an MBA will help you address the issue. Maybe you have hit a plateau in your career because you lack important managerial skills that an MBA will give you. The important thing in this case is to demonstrate that your lack of upward mobility does not correspond to a lack of ambition or aptitude for success.

Does your work not seem interesting or exciting enough? Don't worry too much about this issue, as business schools love people from a variety of backgrounds. Being a foreman at a corrugated box factory may seem dull to you, but if you can highlight what you have learned about business on the job—and what you still have to learn—then you can make a strong case for yourself.

Some applicants have holes in their work records, as they took sabbaticals to travel, to care for a sick loved one, or to simply try new things. As long as you can convince the admissions committee that you are indeed ambitious and committed to studying business, they will appreciate the unique perspectives that these experiences will give you.

Undergraduate and graduate transcripts

If your transcript shows weakness, don't worry. Not all "weak" transcripts are equally bad, and there are some things you can do to help yourself.

A Stanford admissions officer once said about transcripts, "We're forgiving of slow starts, but not as forgiving of slow finishes." Most business schools have the same attitude. If you got off to a rough start your freshman year but showed steady improvement while in college, then you are probably in good shape. Admissions officers like to see that you got more serious about your work and were able to turn the academic tide.

If you were consistently poor or did worse as time went on, however, your challenge will be to convince the admissions committee that you're serious about academics and have the brainpower to succeed in school. The former can be accomplished in your essays, where you will discuss what it is that you expect to get out of a business school curriculum. The latter can be made up for by the GMAT or, if that is also weak, by earning As in part-time courses at a local school.

Your transcript(s) may also be weak because you were simply too involved in extra-curricular activities as an undergrad. Use this opportunity to turn a weakness into a strength by demonstrating your commitment and initiative at your undergraduate school, and making the case for why you will be equally involved in business school. You must balance that out, however, with a demonstrated understanding of the importance of academics in business school. In other words, you should try and convince the admissions counselors that you will get the school/activities mix right this time around.

Final Word on Strengths and Weaknesses

In general, your strategy should be to counteract your perceived weaknesses with examples that show your strengths in those same (or similar) areas. The more that each part of your application can naturally complement and support the other pieces, the better off you will be. Some applicants will use the extra essay—which many schools provide as an option in their applications—to directly address a weakness such as a low GMAT score or undergraduate GPA. This is fine, but think of it as a last resort. One risk of devoting an entire essay to a weakness is that it highlights the very issue that you're trying to neutralize. There are times when the extra essay does help, however, and we will discuss these types of situations more in Chapter 4.

Conversation With Alex Brown

Alex Brown, Senior Associate Director of MBA Admissions at The Wharton School, has become one of the best-known personalities among business school applicants over the last several years. He has developed a reputation for being quick to respond to applicants' questions with candid advice through BusinessWeek's online b-school forums and through Wharton's own applicant-focused message board, known as student-2-student. We checked in with Alex to get his opinion on some of the best and worst things that business school applicants typically do.

What are some of the major mistakes that you see applicants make year after year?

Good applicants not presenting good applications. While that is a very general answer, it gets to the core of the issue. Specifically, I think one major error is not researching the school and understanding what the particular school offers, and how it fits the goals of the candidate. It's fine for us to learn that you are a strong candidate in general, but we are also looking for those who show good fit and who can make the most of our resources and learning culture. Those that have not done their homework on the school are sending a negative signal. This does not imply that there is only one right school for each candidate. There should be a "choice set" that is relevant to the candidate's goals, learning style, etc.

What do you look for in trying to distinguish between applicants with very similar professional backgrounds?

A deep understanding of how the MBA is relevant and the potential outcomes of the MBA, aside from the notion that it needs to be done to get ahead in that particular industry. We also look for how the candidate's overall profile, which includes interests outside of work, will add to the learning community of the school. Oftentimes, it is these interests and passions, and how they manifest themselves, that will be the key differentiator of someone with strong academics, a strong career, and a solid plan going forward.

What is your take on the GMAT exam, its importance and use by an admissions committee? What do applicants need to do to get in with a relatively low GMAT score?

It's all relative. Like all aspects of the application, it is important. (By the way, the weakest element of any application will be the most critical for each applicant, and for some that will be the GMAT.) The recent increases in GMAT scores at schools should not lead candidates to believe we focus more on the GMAT than we used to do. The reasons for the increases are simply that there are more resources available for people to prepare for the test, and the fact that the test is more flexible in terms of when it can be taken (this is not universal, which we understand). Given the increased ability to be fully prepared when taking the test, candidates are doing so. I would say that what we are seeing is candidates maximizing their potential GMAT score, and I do not think that was always the case.

The GMAT scores we publish are averages, so clearly we admit people with scores below that number. The score itself will be reviewed within the context of an applicant's academic work, and our goal is to admit people who will thrive in our academic curriculum. That will then allow students to be more involved in the overall program. In order for us to "look past" low GMAT scores, the scores must be due to demonstrated poor standardized test-taking, supported by strong academics, not due to lack of preparation for the test, which is a clear demonstration of lack of commitment to the application process and respect for the applicant pool.

We hear admissions committee members talk about looking for fit when evaluating applicants. What exactly does that mean? What helps you determine if someone will fit in at Wharton?

Fit can follow a couple of themes: fit for the learning culture and fit for the school's resources. Each school will have a certain learning culture that determines the spirit, attitude, and future direction of the school. We need to make sure we admit people that will fit into the culture that Wharton has developed. If we admit people who would not excel in that culture, the culture itself would change over time.

Fit also refers to how the student fits into the resources of the school (academic and extracurricular) and the goals of the student. Clearly, if the goals of the student going into the program are unrealistic given the school's resources, there is a disconnection.

Some candidates seem to place more importance on one aspect of the application over another. Is there one part of the application that you consistently see applicants falling short on?

I think this may vary based on the culture of the applicant. Some international cultures are less assertive in terms of expressing their qualities, passions, and interests, and simply approach the process as they would approach writing their resume. While we understand this, a candidate knows if he is applying to a U.S.–based school, so the candidate should learn how to approach U.S. schools more appropriately perhaps. Rather than simply listing accomplishments and experiences in essays, an applicant should discuss the outcomes and the learning opportunities, plus how these experiences have helped shape value systems, leadership perspectives, and team skills, for example.

What makes a really good essay? What makes a really bad one?

I want to get a sense that I really know the person after reading the essays. Don't just write what you think we want to hear, but tell it the way it is, centered on knowing some of the core themes we are looking for and of course answering the questions. A recent discussion on student-2-student referred to a candidate getting naked through the essays. While this may sound extreme, the attitude and approach makes sense. We are about transparency in our process and communications. We want our candidates to be similarly transparent.

How important is an applicant's enthusiasm for the program? Can you tell when an applicant is simply applying to Wharton along with every other top school, without really getting to know Wharton's program?

We know candidates apply to multiple schools, and there is nothing wrong with that. Our attitude is less, "Are we your first choice?" and more, "Are we a good choice?" Make that case and we are happy. How does Wharton fit your goals, given our resources, our culture, etc.? We hope that our marketing resources can help you understand exactly what our culture and resources are, and that you can make an effective case. Help us picture you sitting in a classroom at Wharton, or running a club here.

Any other pearls of wisdom?

I am passionate about what an MBA at Wharton can do for many different types of people. Don't be intimated by the process of applying. Use it as a chance to really find what is right for you. While our stats may be intimidating to some, they are only stats. We look at much, much more.

FAQs

How important is the strength of your undergraduate/graduate school's brand to the admissions committee?

Overall, what you did in college and what you've done since then are more important than what school you went to. Still, business schools do take your college's brand name into consideration, especially when considering your grades. Some schools are known to pay more attention to this than others. However, this should not be a major consideration when you apply. For every Princeton and Yale grad prowling the halls of these schools, there is also a student from a lesser-known school. All schools love to brag about the number of undergraduate institutions that are represented by their classes (the numbers generally range from 80 to 200). You definitely shouldn't spend all of your time trying to sell your school if it is not a well-known one. You should, however, be able to explain why you decided to attend the schools listed on your transcripts and discuss their merits. Outside of that, try to keep the focus on you. At the same time, if you did go to a college with a great reputation, don't rest on your laurels and expect to gain admission based on reputation alone. It's an asset, but one that will quickly fall by the wayside if your other application components are mediocre.

What if I have been laid off from my job?

First of all, don't panic! Getting laid off does not squash your chances of getting into a top business school. There are several things that you need to do. Most importantly, you need to convince the admissions committee that you're not simply applying to business school because you're out of work and have no better option. If admissions officers sense that this is the case, then you will indeed have squashed your chances. You can combat this perception by highlighting your career goals, and how business school fits into the picture. Also, while you absolutely should not dwell on the fact that you were laid off, acknowledge that it happened and be prepared to explain why (hopefully it's something out of your control), and move on. Admissions officers understand that even good employees sometimes lose their jobs.

Also, you will need to work extra hard to weave professional success stories throughout your application, to make it clear that you are a "winner" who just happened to get caught up in bad circumstances. Recommendations are especially important here, particularly if they come from your ex-boss who regrettably had to let you go. Showing that you were a positive contributor and that you left on good terms will help a great deal. Finally, show that you've been productive in your time off. A Tuck admissions officer once commented that she couldn't believe how some laid-off applicants were content to do nothing for a year. Even things outside of your career such as pro-bono work or volunteering can show that you're not someone who's content to sit back and take it when life deals you a bad hand.

3

APPLICANT

PROFILES

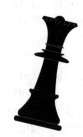

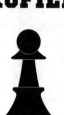

What you communicate in your application will be largely dictated by who you are and where you want to go in your career. However, where you've been speaks volumes about you, particularly in the eyes of business school admissions officers. If you are an investment banker, for example, they will assume that you have more in common with other banking applicants than with military or nonprofit applicants. This means that absent information that you tell admissions committees about yourself, they may assume that you have many of the traits (both positive and negative) that a typical banker has. It is your responsibility to be aware of these commonly held stereotypes and be ready to take advantage of them or overcome them, whatever the case may be.

While business schools rarely say so explicitly, it makes sense that your stiffest competition will come from those who are most like you. Schools don't necessarily operate off of hard quotas when admitting applicants with various professional backgrounds, but they can only take so many consultants, or so many accountants, marketers, educators, etc., before their classes start to become homogenous. So, you will be compared to other applicants with similar backgrounds, and your job will be to stand apart from these other applicants. This is a core part of any winning application game plan.

This chapter will help you achieve this goal. We will examine 11 of the most common applicant profiles (by profiles we mean professional backgrounds), name some perceived strengths and weaknesses for each, and discuss ways that an applicant with a given profile can set himself apart from others with the same background. Naturally, much of the advice that applies to one applicant profile may apply to another. Also, there's a good chance that you don't fit explicitly into one of these profiles. For example, many engineers go into consulting or investment banking. Still, getting a sense of how admissions counselors think about various profiles will help you in creating your differentiated position. We recommend using this chapter in conjunction with your strengths/weaknesses analysis from Chapter 2 to develop your application strategy. Above all else, your application needs to reflect who you are. Beyond that, use the material presented here to separate yourself from the pack.

Consulting

In many ways, consultants are made for business school. As a consultant, you most likely have a strong academic background, have had multiple experiences with myriad companies, and have finely tuned analytical and interpersonal skills. Additionally, you have direct access to a cadre of b-school graduates through your firm, who serve as great advisors.

Unfortunately, more applicants fall into the consultant category than probably any other profile type. As a result, it is also probably more difficult to differentiate yourself as a consultant. Consulting firms often have standardized analyst programs that "feed" business schools with applicants after they've had two or three years of experience. Over time, many b-schools have become somewhat wary of these programs, because of their tendency to produce applicants who are simply looking to "get their ticket punched."

You can avoid the perception that you're just trying to get your ticket punched by being explicit about how you intend to utilize an MBA to reach your career goals. That's not to say that you shouldn't express an interest in returning to consulting. But if you do go down that path, you need to make sure to discuss how you see yourself having an impact on the organization. Do you see an opportunity to increase your clients' revenues through Customer Relationship Management? Then discuss how you want to capitalize on this opportunity by studying the intersection of marketing and technology. The bottom line is that you have to provide tangible reasons for wanting to attend b-school. In many ways, if you intend to return to consulting, this is even more important than if you're planning on switching careers.

Along the lines of being explicit in your writing, try your best not to introduce consultant jargon into your essays and interviews. Consultants have a tendency to write essays that are high-level and ambiguous. Admissions counselors comment that consultants often fail to adequately explain their specific actions on projects and the results of those actions. To the extent that you can quantify both, you will stand out from the pack. Take a close look at Chapter 4 for additional guidance on how to write and interview effectively.

The average number of years of work experience at top business schools approaches five. Consultants, however, tend to apply to schools after only two to four years of experience. If you fall into this group, then you should expect to be questioned about it and should find ways to emphasize your maturity. One way to do that is by discussing activities in which you are involved outside of consulting. Because of the long hours associated with their profession, many applicants from consulting are unable to talk about anything that is unrelated to work. To the extent that you are able to weave activities outside of the consulting world into your story, you will be able to differentiate yourself.

Creative

If this header describes you, then you are what business schools and their students like to call a "poet." Whether you were previously a teacher, psychologist, musician, writer, chef, artist, or anything else that falls into this category, you bring something to the applicant pool that few others do. The trick will be to appear different enough to be interesting, but not so different that admissions officers will suspect that you can't hack it or fit in with your more business-minded peers.

First of all, don't let anyone tell you that you have no business applying. The fact that you want an MBA makes you qualified to apply. Whether or not you get in is up to the admissions counselors, but what they decide will be greatly influenced by how well you craft your application. Your past is history, but how you present it is entirely up to you.

When you describe your past experiences, don't simply write or talk about what you did. Go a level deeper and talk about why you have done these things. For instance, a sculptor got into a top business school by describing the satisfaction he got from turning his ideas into something of substance. He then effectively tied it back to business, describing how he wanted to acquire the tools to do the same thing for business ideas. You don't need to be this explicit in tying your background to business (especially if it will end up sounding forced), but try to think in this way as you develop your application game plan. Admissions officers will value you for the unique perspective that you can bring to the classroom, but it's up to you to show that you can connect the dots and apply your non-business experiences to business problems.

Most schools look for leadership skills more than anything else, and odds are that you've had a chance to display these skills at some point in your life. The more recent, the better, but don't be afraid to bring up examples of how you uniquely made a difference in a situation when you were younger. Even if the story has nothing to do with business, leadership examples are universal, and your application will be much stronger for it. Your recommendations can be helpful here, especially if you can get people with business backgrounds to vouch for your leadership skills and business potential.

Of course, business schools also look for a minimum level of quantitative skills, and this is one place where you won't get the benefit of the doubt. You absolutely must produce a GMAT score within range of your target schools' averages. Your best bet is to practice early and practice often, and give yourself enough time to take the exam more than once if needed. And plan on taking some pre-MBA courses in accounting and statistics before you apply. Doing so will demonstrate a sincere interest in earning an MBA, and answer questions in admissions officers' minds about you possibly applying to school as a dilettante who has nothing better to do. Taking these courses early will allow you to sell them in your application.

Entrepreneurship

Few applicants can say that they've built their own business, giving entrepreneurs a leg up in the business school admissions process. If you are an entrepreneur, the key will be to drive home the strengths that admissions officers typically associate with people like you, while addressing the questions of why you want a degree now and how well you will fit into the business school culture. Here we use the term "entrepreneur" broadly. As such, our advice can apply to people who have set out to build organizations in a variety of fields, from technology to hospitality to nonprofit.

By definition, entrepreneurs are people who like to strike out on their own and make things happen. It doesn't take much imagination to see how you can spin a story rich in leadership, creativity, and ambition, no matter what your venture was. Whether you built a whole organization or simply started up a new department within an existing company, you should have a lot of material to draw upon. When you discuss these experiences, be sure to not only talk about your accomplishments, but also about how you achieved them. Saying that you led your fledgling team to launch its first prototype on time is impressive, but it's more interesting to hear about how it happened. Stories about how you found the right people to build your team, how you motivated them, and how you helped them overcome obstacles will all paint a great portrait of you as a leader.

The most obvious challenge you will face is that you already set out to build a business, and only now are you applying to business school. Admissions officers will undoubtedly ask, "If you thought you could make it on your own two years ago, how come you now feel like you need to sit in a classroom and learn again?" Your reasons will obviously depend on your own situation, but a stronger answer will emphasize your desire to learn and move toward new goals, while a weaker one will focus on your desire to get away from the start-up scene.

The flipside of your perceived strengths is that an admissions committee may wonder if you have too much hubris for your own good. The key is for you to communicate your appreciation for rigorous business training and to spell out exactly what skills you want to attain and why. Admissions officers don't like to see someone who's too much of a maverick. You will need to demonstrate your penchant for teamwork, ideally through some of your past actions.

So far we have skirted the issue of whether or not your past ventures have been successful. Of course, it will be much easier to sell yourself if you have a long track record of success to point to, but you can also use failures to your advantage. The challenge will be to make sure that your business school application doesn't look like a "last resort" now that your entrepreneurial efforts haven't panned out. By emphasizing that you understand what went wrong and that you are now actively seeking learning opportunities in order to shore up your skills before you make another go at it, you can pull together a nice application story.

Engineering and Science

Engineers (here we will use "engineers" to refer to anyone coming from a science or engineering background) typically have strong quantitative skills, and that is one reason why you will find a good number of engineers at any top business school. Coming from engineering, however, you will find that you need to sell your interpersonal skills, and prove that you understand the "big picture" when it comes to business.

Few engineers ever fail to make the cut in business school admissions because of their quantitative abilities. Even if you don't have a superlative GMAT score, you should be able to point to your undergraduate degree and recent work experience as evidence of these skills. Even better, you will hopefully be able to demonstrate strong problem-solving skills by virtue of the work you've done. Even if your past experiences seem ho-hum to you, an admissions officer will be interested to hear how you solved an important problem, and why you went about it in the way that you did. A good example can be as mundane as improving the flow rate through a valve by 2 percent, or contributing to a small enhancement in the efficacy of a new drug. Being explicit about the significance of the problem—and which of your skills helped you arrive at the solution—will go a long way toward selling these abilities.

Many business-minded engineers also enjoy the advantage of having a good overall story for why they want to earn an MBA. Whereas a consultant or an investment banker may have to spend a lot of time proving that she isn't just getting her ticket punched for a higher salary, you can craft a strong story about how you've mastered one discipline, and now you want to move on to achieve a broader view of how a business is run. Admissions officers will appreciate any evidence that you can provide that shows you understand the importance of the functions in a company outside of its R&D department.

The stereotype that you will most likely have to overcome is in regard to your inter-personal skills. An admissions committee will look critically for evidence that you can reach goals that require you to work with others. Any teamwork examples that you can provide will help you a great deal here; particularly stories that demonstrate your ability to understand others' motivations and to deal with them constructively. These "empathy" examples will go a long way toward showing your ability to grow into the role of a leader.

You can also set yourself apart through extracurricular activities that demonstrate your interests outside of the workplace. They can show your desire to actively seek out opportunities to make the world around you better, rather than simply waiting for an engineering problem to be handed to you. Examples of community service, volunteering at your church, or simply pursuing a creative or athletic passion outside of the office will help you distinguish yourself from the other engineers in the crowd.

Government

One of the better known business school graduates of the last decade—Peter Robinson, author of *Snapshots from Hell: The Making of an MBA*—was a White House speech writer before entering Stanford. In his book, Robinson describes being told that he and his non-business-background classmates were the ones who were added to the class to add some variety. It's to your advantage that you bring this variety to the table, and it can help you a great deal if you are able to overcome what the top schools expect your weaknesses to be.

Whether you frequently dined on Air Force One or served as your town's dog-catcher, you can build your application story knowing that most other applicants will have far less unique stories to tell. You can start by emphasizing your strong principles and passion for making a difference. Business schools love people who are committed to making an impact wherever they go, and they know that people who have worked in government tend to exhibit this trait. No matter what specific field you worked in, or at what level, make sure that this passion and dedication are a central part of your application story.

You may also have excellent examples that demonstrate your interpersonal skills and communication abilities. To some degree, both will come through on their own in your essays and your interview, but be sure to explicitly sell these abilities at some point. Any examples of past successes where you put these skills to use will only help in winning over admissions officers.

One of the most common weaknesses of applicants coming from the public sector is a lack of quantitative skills. Government-types have a reputation for being great with words but less so with numbers, and you will need to overcome this stereotype with supporting evidence. If your past jobs included any kind of work with numbers, such as fundraisers, budgeting, or research, then be sure to mention it. You should also show a minimum level of comfort with quantitative problem-solving through the other common tools (GMAT, undergraduate coursework, and/or pre-MBA courses). Similarly, you will need to answer questions about your business experience, or lack thereof. Admissions officers are often willing to accept a lack of business experience as long as you can communicate an understanding of the value of business training and how it will help you. By communicating both messages, you will be able to help set yourself apart from other government employees. Additionally, you should convey a clear vision for how an MBA will help you and why.

Also, emphasize your desire to innovate and make things happen. Many government applicants will have impressive stories to share about their past experiences, but the most successful ones will present a convincing argument for how an MBA will help them shake up the status quo.

International

Clearly the international applicant (that is, international from the perspective of the 27 U.S. schools covered in this book) profile will overlap with at least one other profile. Still, it is invaluable for international applicants to understand how they are viewed by admissions counselors, based on their geographical status alone.

It should be stated up front that business schools are eager to maintain, or, in some cases, increase the percentage of their international students. B-schools and students find that having a large international presence is the best way to expand students' perspectives beyond ethnocentrism. It's an amazing experience to sit in a classroom and hear voices from around the world weigh in on a variety of issues. This alone ensures that business schools will continue to enthusiastically pursue international applicants for the foreseeable future. Still, there remains a gap in access to information on the business school application process in terms of domestic versus international applicants. At a holistic level, our hope is that this book contributes to minimizing that gap. At a more tactical level, however, it is important for international applicants to understand the stereotypical strengths and weaknesses with which they are automatically associated.

On the strengths side of the equation, a guaranteed plus is your cultural awareness. Interestingly, this tends to be a latent strength for international applicants on which they don't capitalize enough. As an international applicant, you're used to living in a truly global world and being exposed to various cultures, languages, and belief systems, so you accept this as a norm and don't emphasize these types of experiences as much as you should. Realize that the ability to speak several languages or dialects and expound on the social impacts of introducing economic liberalization policies is something most American applicants do not bring to the table. As such, demonstrate to the admissions committee your experiences in multicultural environments in order to show them how adding your voice to the classroom dialogue will appreciably improve the learning model.

Additionally, consider integrating your global perspective into your career goals. Your past cross-cultural experiences will lend career goals that extend beyond U.S. boundaries, a level of credibility that most American applicants will not be able to achieve. In terms of the ability to have a global impact, most international applicants have a natural advantage.

The lack of access to information on the application process reveals itself in a majority of applications from international candidates. In general, international applicants tend to produce applications that read more like records of accomplishments than stories. This hurts these applicants' chances of getting into b-school. The best way to put together an application that positively resonates with admissions officers is by reviewing application components produced by successful applicants and by understanding the admissions criteria of your target schools. To avoid the trap of obsessing over baseline GMAT, Test of English as a Foreign Language (TOEFL), and GPA statistics, you should live and breathe Chapters 4 and 5. These chapters go through each of the application components in great detail and outline strategies for gaining acceptance to top business schools. Make sure that you review each of the examples in order to gain an understanding of how admissions counselors will evaluate your application. Having a good understanding of how to assemble an application that tells a story, rather than an application that rattles off your achievements, is a great way to separate yourself from other international applicants.

One of the questions that admissions counselors will ask themselves when reviewing applications from international candidates is whether they will take the initiative to share their perspectives with their classmates. There is a common understanding that as an international applicant you have a unique perspective, but in the admissions committee's eyes that perspective is worthless if it isn't shared. The best way to address this question is to provide examples of instances in which you've provided your perspective in a multicultural environment. Better yet, emphasize your desire to express your viewpoints during your time in business school. In addition to getting this point across in your essays, it is crucial that you emphasize it during your interviews. This may be your one point of direct contact with the admissions committee, so you definitely want them to be comfortable with having you in the classroom.

Investment Banking and Finance

Business schools love bankers for their business training and analytical skills, and bankers love the schools because they often have no choice but to apply after a few years on the job. Your challenge will be to stand out from a sea of similar-looking applicants. You can do this by defeating the stereotypes that are most often associated with bankers and others coming from finance-related fields, including private equity and venture capital.

Let's start with the good news. As an investment banker, you will probably have to do very little selling of your business abilities. Schools will assume that you come with at least enough analytical skills to hack it in an MBA program. They will also expect that you are comfortable with big-picture business concepts and have enough polish to make yourself presentable to potential employers. While you should at least provide some evidence of these skills, know that b-schools will generally anticipate that you have these characteristics.

Of course, the hard part will be distinguishing yourself from the other gazillion bankers who also apply. You should therefore focus your story. Discuss not only what makes you a great banker, but on what makes you a *different* banker. To this end, any experiences where you demonstrated leadership and truly made a difference in the outcome of a project will help a great deal. Admissions officers will look hard for examples where you didn't simply follow your job description, but rather went a step further and did something that few others would have done in order to succeed. This can sometimes be difficult in this industry, but that's exactly why business schools value these kinds of experiences so much.

Extracurricular activities can be even more powerful in setting you apart from the pack. Any way in which you can show a desire to get involved and make things happen will distinguish you. Again, schools are looking for examples where you didn't merely do what was asked of you, but rather stepped outside of your comfort zone and made a difference.

One stereotype that you will need to overcome is the one that paints most investment bankers as overly competitive sharks. You most likely have had experiences where you worked with others to execute a deal; don't overlook the importance of these experiences when describing your professional history. As much as an admissions committee looks for a track record of success, it will pay even more attention to how you accomplished those tasks. An applicant who knifed and clawed his way to the top isn't someone whom most schools will welcome with open arms.

Finally, you know—and every school knows—that many bankers apply to business school because they have little choice. That won't be held against you. But you will really need to think about what you plan on doing with an MBA. Whether or not you plan on going back to banking, admissions officers will demand evidence that shows you really understand the value of an MBA, and that you're not simply out to get your ticket punched. Be prepared to discuss your strengths and weaknesses, and how an MBA will help you round out your personal traits and professional skills. To that end, explaining how an MBA will help you make a true difference is a great way to differentiate yourself from other bankers whose career objectives often come across as conventional.

Marketing

Marketing professionals usually have loads of relevant business experience to high-light in their applications. As a marketing professional, between previous schoolwork and your work experience, you should have ample evidence that shows you know how to get things done in a business setting. The challenge is to bring out the breadth of your business experience, especially when it comes to quantitative and leadership skills.

As a marketer, you will likely have little problem pointing to instances of innova-tion in your career. Most applicants with marketing backgrounds will have examples of creativity that they can draw upon, but you should think broadly and refer to ex-amples of how you innovated in a variety of business scenarios, whether it was devel-oping a creative new advertising campaign or finding a new solution to an old business problem. Choose broad examples over times when you simply developed a creative brochure or updated the look of your company's Website. Admissions officers will as-sume that, as a marketer, you have a good deal of creativity. It is up to you to demon-strate creativity in the broader, business-minded sense of the word.

Depending on what you did as a marketer, one challenge you might face is in pre-senting convincing evidence of your quantitative and analytical skills. Of course, many marketing jobs are quite quantitative, but admissions officers will look hard for proof of these skills. Naturally, the GMAT can go a long way toward making your case. If your GMAT score isn't as high as you would like, make a point of emphasizing the quantitative work that you've done on your job, whether it's analyzing market research data or budgeting for a project. No matter how mundane these experiences may seem, mentioning them can help a great deal. Also, if you didn't do much undergrad work in quantitative subjects, be prepared to take some courses in accounting or statistics be-fore you attend school (or, ideally, before you apply).

Leadership will really help to set you apart from the pack. As someone coming from marketing, you will likely find that you have more teamwork examples to share in your application than many other applicants. Be sure to emphasize your teamwork dimension in discussing these stories. However, in relating your examples, make sure to be clear about what *you* did, rather than only on what the team accomplished. Don't make admissions officers search all day to figure out what you specifically did on a project in order to make it a success. You should get comfortable with the idea of using the word "I" instead of "we" a little more than you're used to.

Also, the fact that you are already in business can actually present a challenge in terms of how you answer the "Why an MBA?" question. You won't necessarily have the obvious answer of wanting to change careers, and not every marketer ends up go-ing to business school (unlike consulting or banking, where leaving for business school is much more common). A skeptical admissions officer or interviewer may probe you on this. Valid reasons for pursuing an MBA can include the fact that you want to gain new, hard skills outside of what you already know, or that you want to bolster your leadership abilities. Whatever your reasons, be prepared to answer this question and be specific about the skills that you want to gain from an MBA.

Military

Applicants coming from the military are blessed with some of the best stories that anyone could possibly tell in a business school application. Tales of clearing a third-world playground of landmines and of whipping a motley platoon of new recruits into a well-oiled machine are the stuff of admissions officers' dreams. Unfortunately, nearly every military applicant has similarly impressive experiences to draw upon, and not many of these stories explicitly spell out your potential for success at business school.

One of your best strengths as a military applicant will likely be your leadership experience. Any stories that you can relate about directing a group of men and women to achieve a tangible goal will speak volumes about your ability to lead, and most business schools value this trait above all else. You are also likely to have great examples of teamwork, which will further help an admissions committee picture you fitting into a classroom at its school. Don't be shy about sharing these stories, even if you think they've been told a thousand times before. Focus on these accomplishments in your essays and interview, and—more importantly—spell out what you learned as a result, and how it will help you in your next career.

The most obvious challenge you could face is in cases when your great experiences have little to do with business. As a military applicant, you need to show the admissions committee that your skills are directly transferable to the business world. More to the point, you need to show that you see how these skills will translate, and that you know what your own strengths and weaknesses are. You may not know accounting or marketing, but you understand why it is important that you have knowledge of them. Moreover, you can demonstrate your desire to bolster your knowledge in these areas by taking a pre-MBA course. If you have taken any business-oriented courses that won't show up on your transcripts—or have simply embarked on a mission to read one good business book per month—be sure to let the admissions committee know about it. The committee will understand that you're relatively new to the business world, but will look critically for evidence that you have the ability and motivation to learn business principles.

The other challenge you will face is in setting yourself apart from the rest of the military crowd. Most of your fellow military applicants will also have great stories about leadership, teamwork, and problem solving, among others. You can stand out from the pack by demonstrating how you've gotten involved and contributed in situations outside of your military career. Just as a consultant needs to show how he has a life outside of his job, you will need to do the same. Also, many military applicants' leadership stories will be about "direct" leadership, in which there was a clear leader-subordinate hierarchy. Because the business world is often much murkier than this, providing examples of how you succeeded in a less-defined leadership role will further set you apart.

Nonprofit

Some of the most unique members of every business school class tend to come from a nonprofit background. Admissions committees love to round out their incoming student bodies with students who have taken the road less traveled, and as a nonprofit applicant, you can potentially fit this bill quite nicely. First, however, you will need to address the weaknesses that are most commonly associated with applicants coming from the nonprofit sector.

The good news is that you don't need to be shy about your nonprofit background. Just the contrary—even if you didn't gain a bit of "real" business experience during your career, your previous work will likely have given you a unique world perspective that few others can offer. You were willing to take risks with your career in order to make someone else's situation better. Admissions officers love to see passion and strong principles like these. Odds are, you gained some very relevant experience, even if it was as dull as maintaining volunteers' schedules or procuring supplies. The trap that some applicants fall into is in simply stating what they have done, without going two more steps and spelling out what they learned, and how it will help them in their future career. This will be critical because admissions committees will expect a "non-traditional" applicant like you to provide a vision for how you will get the most out of—and give the most to—their schools.

Another place where nonprofit applicants can fall short is in presenting a convincing case that they will be able to blend in and work with consultants, bankers, marketers, etc. While schools will value you for your unique perspective, they want to know that you have enough business sense to be able to contribute to group projects and help move along a class discussion. You can start by showing that you have the intellectual horsepower to stand up to the rigors of the more quantitative subjects. Your GMAT score, past coursework, or pre-MBA courses can help here. Also, you will need to show that you are able to think about broader business concepts, and that you understand their relevance to your career. You can touch upon this subject as you answer the "Why an MBA?" question. Admissions officers will appreciate the candidate who knows what she doesn't know and sees why these skills are important.

Some nonprofit applicants apply to business school in order to change careers, while others want an MBA to help them make a greater impact in their current field. Your game plan won't vary significantly between these two scenarios. The main risk in the case of a career switcher will be in making sure that you have a good understanding of the field that you want to move into. If you plan on going back to the nonprofit sector, then your greatest challenge will be in convincingly spelling out what an MBA will allow you to do that you can't do today. Talking to current MBA students and recent graduates will help you a great deal here.

Recent Graduate

Only a few years ago the trend was for business schools to accept applicants with more and more years of work experience. More recently, however, this trend has been reversed for certain schools, such as Stanford and Harvard. The rationale behind the reversal is that there are some exemplary undergraduate students and recent graduates who've had phenomenal experiences and, as such, shouldn't have to wait to attend business school.

Just to be clear, it is still very difficult to gain admittance directly from undergrad or with less than two years of work experience. Besides, many students maintain the perspective that b-school is most beneficial for students who have significant professional experience. Indeed, top business schools will most likely keep their student population with less than two years of work experience under 5 percent. They will do so in order to preserve the classroom dynamic, in which all students are expected to take on the role of a teacher. Still, there is now a greater window of opportunity for the young and restless.

What you have going for you is clear. Admissions committees are consistently impressed with younger applicants' level of innovation, creativity, enthusiasm, and pure intellectual horsepower. Additionally, younger applicants will often take the academic aspects of business school more seriously than their older counterparts because they're coming directly from academia. Therefore, a higher-than-average GPA and GMAT score are the minimum price of admission for you.

The challenge is also clear: You must emphasize your maturity, leadership, and teamwork dimensions to the hilt. For the most part, you'll know whether you can demonstrate your capabilities in these areas just by flipping through essay questions. If you struggle to come up with experiences to utilize in response to these questions, chances are, you're not yet ready to attend b-school. If you can recall applicable experiences, then your objective should be to discuss them in a way that shows you are multi-dimensional, take initiative, and have great interpersonal skills. These experiences could be related to an entrepreneurial venture that you started, an internship, a study abroad program, an academic achievement, a community service project, a student government position, or a club activity.

You must also be able to demonstrate career focus. The last thing an admissions committee wants to see are staid, unthoughtful career objectives from a profile that it anticipates will produce dynamic, high-impact results. Admissions officers want to know that their young students will one day rock the world, or at least shake it a little bit. More than any other profile, you cannot afford to discuss your career objectives vaguely or without passion. You need to be clear about what skills you will gain from business school and how those skills will translate into a post-business school career. It's just as important that you find a way to emphasize why right now is the perfect time for you to enter b-school as opposed to some time in the future. An example would be an idea that you have for an entrepreneurial venture that requires you to gain the skills provided by the target school and an urgency that requires you to get started immediately on the development of a business model.

In a perfect world, your application would contain an assortment of experiences across the four dimensions. You want to push the admissions committee to the point that it has no reason to ding you other than the fact that you're younger than most applicants. At that point, your propensity to accomplish great things will outweigh what will suddenly appear to be a superficial statistic.

The B-school Classroom: A Diversity of Backgrounds

The sights and sounds of the business school classroom 50 years ago were much different than what they are today. What was once a homogeneous student body in terms of professional experience, age, ethnicity, gender, and career goals, is now much more heterogeneous across every dimension. Today, the legacy of a homogeneous classroom still serves as a deterrent for many potential applicants who imagine that the b-school experience consists of ex-consultants and investment bankers proselytizing the benefits of capitalism. This urban legend is decidedly false.

While consultants and bankers tend to make up a significant portion of an incoming class, they generally represent less than 50 percent of the students. Additionally, the b-school classroom represents a multitude of perspectives from a variety of countries (for U.S. b-schools, international students generally represent 25–40 percent of the class).

The following figures display a typical b-school class distribution of undergraduate majors and professional experience:

Figure 1: Undergraduate majors of students at a typical business school

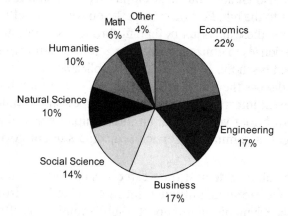

Figure 2: Career backgrounds of students at a typical business school

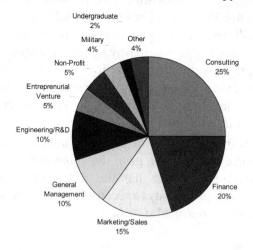

Not surprisingly, in order to maintain or increase heterogeneity, business schools are actively encouraging a diversity of backgrounds in the classroom. Students acknowledge that a variety of perspectives helps to create a dynamic learning environment in which duplication of opinions is rare. For an example of background variety, consider Omari's study group during b-school:

- ❑ A New Zealand physician.
- ❑ A Pakistani economic development analyst.
- ❑ A U.S. military intelligence officer.
- ❑ A Brazilian investment bank associate.
- ❑ A U.S. middle school teacher who taught in Nepal for two years.

So how can these insights help you? First, if you're considering business school and have a non-traditional background, don't buy into the myth of homogeneity. If you have something to add to a school's learning environment, then there is a spot for you. Secondly, you should take some time to reflect on how you can differentiate yourself based on your background and your career goals. Fortunately for you, that's what this book is all about. Finally, once you get to b-school, don't be afraid to share your unique experiences with your classmates. You'll be admitted largely because of your interesting background, so make sure to help those around you benefit from what you've learned along the way.

FAQs

What if the nature of my job makes it difficult for me to draw upon any useful leadership or teamwork examples?

This is a common complaint from people coming from a number of careers. If you feel like you can't come up with any pertinent examples from your experience, try broadening your definitions of leadership and teamwork. You may not have led a group to achieve a major breakthrough, but maybe you helped a colleague develop a skill that he needed in order to perform his job, even though you received no credit for it. This is a more subtle example of leadership, but one that business schools will still appreciate. Similarly, don't think of teamwork as just instances of you sitting in close quarters with a few of your peers, working all night to solve an impossible problem. A good teamwork example could be much broader, such as how you went out of your way to help someone in another department tackle a problem. Think about every person or group with which you've interacted, and consider using instances where you made a difference in helping someone else succeed.

If in my previous job I had a high-flying title, and now I'm applying to business school, won't that look weird?

It will definitely raise some eyebrows. This problem has become more common since the end of the dot-com boom, with some former vice presidents now explaining why they aspire to become junior consultants. If your high-level position came because you were a founding member of a business, then in admissions officers' eyes you are an entrepreneur. This is good, although like all other entrepreneurs, you will need to present a convincing argument for why you want to go back to school now. Also, whether or not your business was a success, keep your application story focused on you. You will ideally have a good number of stories to tell about building a team or a product from scratch, so use them. Focus on your achievements and tie them together with where you want to go—and how business school will help you get there.

How much does my employer's brand name matter when applying to business school?

Having a well-known brand on your resume certainly helps, and business schools do tend to value two years' of experience at McKinsey more than they do experience at an unknown consulting firm. But our advice regarding your undergraduate school's reputation applies here, too. If you come from a relatively unknown organization, spend enough time explaining what the company does, but then move on. You don't need to impress admissions officers with your company's five-year compound annual growth rate. Then, spend the vast majority of your time explaining what *you* did at the company, because that's what admissions officers really care about. Similarly, if you do come from a well-known company, don't plan on coasting on the company's reputation. In fact, if the company is known as a mill that turns out business school students, you will need to work hard to set yourself apart from the pack by selling your unique contributions. Two years "on the beach" at McKinsey isn't going to get you in anywhere, so focus on what you did that makes you different.

I've done something really unique. Do you think that will get me into business school?

The short answer is, "Not by itself." The fact that you did something unique, whether it was professional or personal, will certainly help in setting you apart from the crowd. But that alone will definitely not get you in. Think hard about what your unique achievement says about you, and how it fits into your overall application theme. Spending two years in South America helping locals build a farm is a great story, but it doesn't help you much if you can't relate it to the rest of your story. Also, just like every other experience that you draw upon, simply saying that you were involved in something is not enough. You need to show how you specifically contributed. Finally, a string of interesting experiences can actually hurt you if it is hard for admissions officers to make the connections between them. It is up to you to present your experiences in a way that makes sense to someone getting to know you through admissions essays or an interview.

4

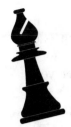

UNDERSTANDING THE
APPLICATION COMPONENTS

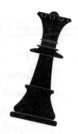

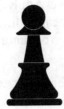

The Process

Now that you have a better understanding of your strengths and weaknesses, and are prepared to differentiate yourself according to your profile, it's time to examine the components of the business school application. So, what should you expect? You should expect to spend an average of 30–50 hours on each application that you complete. Yes, your fourth application may take less time than your first, but be prepared to spend dozens of hours on each application, no matter how many you complete. You should also expect the application process to occupy your life like an attention-starved newborn. Along those lines, don't be surprised if you suffer from a form of "postpartum depression" once the process is completed. If you follow some basic guidelines, however, you can save yourself some frustration and a lot of time.

The Tools

The Internet has drastically changed the way in which business school applications are completed. Imagine calling admissions departments to request applications, filling in data sheets by hand, or agonizing over essays while sitting behind a typewriter. Today, some schools won't even accept paper applications. Thanks to the Internet revolution, you are now faced with two main online options:

❐ **PrincetonReview.com**—In 2001, The Princeton Review purchased the online application services provider, Embark.com. Currently, a large number of business schools use PrincetonReview.com as a portal through which applicants may access their applications. Schools that use this service include: Stanford, Kellogg, Michigan, and Stern. The service provides useful functionality such as:

■ A profile form that retains the data common to all of your applications and automatically enters it into your applications for you.

- Reminder messages for upcoming application deadlines.
- A simple uploading process that accepts your essays in almost any electronic format and translates them into PDF format.

❏ **ApplyYourself.com**—This service powers online applications from such schools as Harvard, Fuqua, and Tuck. The main difference between The Princeton Review and Apply Yourself is that Apply Yourself develops online applications that are tailored for each business school. When you work on an Apply Yourself application, it will appear as though it's the school's own creation. Because Apply Yourself creates school-specific applications, you will see noticeable differences between them. Unfortunately, this means that there is no common data-sharing functionality across Apply Yourself applications.

Some schools, such as Wharton, have created their own online applications. For the most part, these applications reflect Princeton Review's basic functionality, but you'll run into some that fall short. More schools are beginning to develop their own online applications to avoid the fees they incur through the other two options. Fortunately, each new year seems to bring measurable improvements in these options.

Many schools now also accept letters of recommendation via the Internet. This can be a real time-saver, but make sure that your recommenders are at least somewhat Internet savvy before leaving them to their own devices. Also, even though two schools may use the same application service provider, each one may have slightly different rules about how to handle components such as recommendations. Some will accept online recommendations, while others may still prefer paper.

For some schools, you will have more than one online option. In that case we suggest going with PrinceteonReview.com, particularly if you have other applications in process with them. That way you will hopefully save yourself from reentering a lot of redundant information across applications. In either case, online applications are much more efficient than their paper counterparts. The time you will save, the more reliable electronic "paper trail" that you will have in case something gets lost, and the ability to more easily catch and correct errors all make online applications the way to go.

The Components

Business schools essentially all use the same framework in putting their applications together. These similarities allow you to approach each application in a similar manner. Still, don't fall into the trap of thinking that each school is looking for the same type of content. Differences in application strategy by business school are highlighted in Chapter 5.

In general, every business school will request the following information in its application:

❏ Data sheets (for your academic, professional, and personal information).

❏ Transcript.

- ❒ GMAT score.
- ❒ TOEFL score (for international applicants only).
- ❒ Interview.
- ❒ Essays.
- ❒ Recommendations.
- ❒ Resume.

The rest of the chapter will cover each of the application components in depth and provide you with strategies that you should integrate into your MBA game plan.

Data Sheets

Data sheets are pretty consistent from one application to the next. Each application's data sheets will typically ask for:

- ❒ Contact information.
- ❒ Basic biographical information.
- ❒ Education background.
- ❒ Employment history.
- ❒ Extracurricular activities.
- ❒ Awards.
- ❒ Achievements.

The bad news is that this component is often more time consuming than you would think. One reason is that each school usually asks for something slightly different. For example, one school may ask for only one sentence to describe each job you have held, while another may ask for a few bullet points, and yet another will ask for a paragraph of up to 150 words. Also, the "enter once, use over and over" features of sites such as PrincetonReview.com won't always perfectly transport your data from one application to the next. So be ready to devote some manual labor to writing up your background for each application.

The good news is that your work in Chapter 2 will almost directly translate to this section. The grid that you create will give you the opportunity to spell out everything that you have done, making it easy to pluck activities and enter them where needed. Also, the grid will help you think about what dimensions each activity promotes, which is important as you tailor your application for each school. For the most part, the information that you provide in the data sheets for each application will be the same. Even in this apparently dry section, it is important to maintain your focus on demonstrating fit and uniqueness. As tempting as it will be to simply copy and paste, don't pass up an easy opportunity to set yourself apart.

Data sheets often have very short word limits. In many online systems, you simply won't be allowed to go over the limit. Do yourself a huge favor and obey the limits given. Remember that your application will likely be read by a weary-eyed admissions officer who has to work his way through a shoulder-high stack of applications. Even though you will almost inevitably feel that you have more to say than what the application allows, be considerate and keep it concise. Your application reader will appreciate it.

One final tip: Under contact information, make sure to list your cell phone number (if you have one) in addition to your work phone number as the main point of contact. Chances are that the good news will be communicated over the phone, and you won't want to be at work wondering if the phone is ringing at home.

Transcript

Naturally, there is not much that you can do about your undergraduate grades assuming that you are already out of college. Still, there are a couple of things you should know regarding transcripts and how they affect your application.

First, on a logistical note, give yourself plenty of time to receive your transcript(s) from your school(s). It can take anywhere from one week to a month to get a transcript back from a school (some offer rush processing), and you usually need to have a transcript sent back to you in order to be able to send it off to your target business school. Start sending out requests as far in advance as possible. Also, it's fine to send multiple transcript requests to a school at one time, but make sure that you are clear about the directions for each b-school. Some business schools require your college's registrar to not only sign a transcript but also to fill out a form, while others ask for course descriptions to accompany a transcript. You can reduce the chance of error on your college's end by giving them enough time and letting them know exactly what to do for each MBA application.

Now, on to the contents of your transcript. Admissions committees are looking for evidence that you challenged yourself in a wide variety of academic areas (especially in quantitative ones) and came away with at least a 3.0 GPA, preferably higher. Of course, if your undergraduate transcript is stellar, then most of your work is already done. Just make sure to highlight relevant coursework and emphasize your success in order to bring out your innovation dimension, as outlined in Chapter 2. If you can show that you were a dedicated, successful student in college, then it will be easy for admissions personnel to imagine you succeeding in their classrooms.

If your transcript isn't perfect, that's okay. You can usually make up for any apparent deficiencies in other ways. Review the transcript weaknesses section in Chapter 2 for tips on how to address poor grades. In general, poor grades can be addressed with a high GMAT, additional coursework (especially in quantitative areas), and perhaps an additional essay explaining your situation. We'll discuss appropriate usage of the additional essay in the essay section on page 80.

GMAT

There is probably no other aspect of the business school application process that strikes more fear into the hearts of applicants than the GMAT. For most, it is the first step toward applying and the key variable in determining which schools are "accessible." Pressure to perform well on the examination has increased as mean scores have spiked drastically over the last 10 years. While we continue to emphasize the fact that the GMAT score is only one component of the application and should not be overly stressed, it certainly is a key factor in determining your success in applying. It is often said that a great GMAT score alone will never get you into a top business school, but a poor one can most certainly keep you out. We will take a look at the exam and then provide you with advice to help ensure that you don't fall into the latter category.

GMAT background

Graduate business school programs use the Graduate Management Admission Test (GMAT) to help evaluate applicants' analytical writing, mathematical, and verbal abilities. Sponsored by the Graduate Management Admission Council (GMAC), the GMAT is developed, maintained, and administered by the Education Testing Service (ETS). In addition to sponsoring the GMAT, GMAC serves in its role as a nonprofit education association by disseminating information on graduate business education. In looking to augment your knowledge about the GMAT and graduate business school in general, check out GMAC's Website at *www.mba.com*. The Website provides several of the resources that are covered in the "Ace the GMAT" section, in addition to sample problems and information on signing up for the GMAT.

The GMAT and your transcript(s) will be the major criteria used in assessing your academic ability. B-schools evaluate your GMAT score, in addition to your GPA, because it reflects applicants' capabilities in a standardized manner. GPA does not provide the same level of standardization given the large differences across college curricula. Thus, admissions officers use the GMAT as a way to compare "apples to apples" when evaluating candidates' academic aptitude.

The following table displays the format and the content of the GMAT.

Figure 3: Format and content of the GMAT

	Questions	Timing
Analytical Writing Assessment		
Analysis of an Issue	1	30 Min.
Analysis of an Argument	1	30 Min.
Optional Break	-	5 Min.
Quantitative	37	75 Min.
Problem Solving		
Data Sufficiency		
Optional Break	-	5 Min.
Verbal	41	75 Min.
Reading Comprehension		
Critical Reasoning		
Sentence Correction		
Total Time: 3 Hours 40 Minutes		
Score Range: 200–800		

Analytical writing assessment section

Whenever you hear people tossing around GMAT scores, chances are they are not referring to the Analytical Writing Assessment (AWA). In general, schools barely breathe a word about it and many applicants don't even take the time to prepare for it. Nonetheless, you can't get through the exam without first getting through this often-neglected section.

The purpose of the AWA is to test your ability to present a coherent argument and to analyze an underdeveloped one. The section requires you to complete two 30-minute essays, which are divided into two categories: Analysis of an Issue, and Analysis of an Argument.

Analysis of an issue

This section begins with a statement and then asks you to analyze the issue represented by the statement and develop a short essay that takes a position on the issue. You will be evaluated based on your ability to:

- ❑ Dissect the issue and articulate/defend your position on it.
- ❑ Introduce relevant examples and facts.
- ❑ Write an essay that flows well organizationally and meets the standards of grammatically correct English.

Analysis of an argument

This section is almost identical to Analysis of an Issue, but instead of an issue you will be presented with an argument. After reading the argument, which is generally only a few sentences in length, you are asked to write an essay that evaluates the line of reasoning behind the argument, notes the explicit/implicit assumptions, provides ways in which the argument is weak, and cites evidence that would make the argument more compelling. You will be evaluated based on your ability to:

- ❑ Dissect the argument and articulate your analysis of its "rationality."
- ❑ Introduce evidence that could weaken and strengthen the argument.
- ❑ Write an essay that flows well organizationally and meets the standards of grammatically correct English.

Note that in both essays you will be evaluated on your ability to construct and dissect arguments, and not on what arguments you actually make. So, don't worry about picking the "right" side of an issue. Rather, pick a side of the issue that you can argue for most strongly, lay out your reasons in a clear and logical manner, and then move on. Also, no matter what position you take, keep in mind what facts could undermine your position, and demonstrate—at least in a sentence or two—that you have considered these possible weaknesses in your argument.

Quantitative section

The good news about the quantitative section of the GMAT is that it does not test advanced mathematical principles, such as multivariate calculus, differential equations, or multiple regression. The bad news is that the basic mathematical skills that the test does include (arithmetic, algebra, geometry, percentages, fractions, elementary statistics, combinations, and permutations) can appear to be quite complex if you are lacking a quantitative background.

During this section of the exam you will face 37 questions, which will be of two types: Problem Solving and Data Sufficiency.

Problem Solving

Problem Solving questions are generally straightforward in nature, to the extent that you are presented with a mathematical puzzle and are asked to provide an answer. The questions will be very similar to questions that many of us faced on the SAT and ACT. While you most certainly need to spend time bulking up your knowledge of the quantitative concepts tested, very little additional time will need to be spent on understanding how these question types work.

Data Sufficiency

Data Sufficiency questions, on the other hand, are a different story. Contrary to popular belief that these types of questions were devised by a sadist, they are meant to test your ability to determine when there is enough information available to solve a problem. The automatic temptation is to try and actually solve these problems when all that is required is for you to note whether there is sufficient data to solve them.

The problems are comprised of a question and two pieces of information, written as statements and labeled (1) and (2). Your task is to decide whether the statements provide enough information to allow you to solve the stated question. This produces an interesting dynamic in that all answers for this question type are the same. All Data Sufficiency responses look like the following:

A. Statement (1) ALONE is sufficient, but statement (2) alone is not sufficient to answer the question asked.

B. Statement (2) ALONE is sufficient, but statement (1) alone is not sufficient to answer the question asked.

C. BOTH statements (1) and (2) TOGETHER are sufficient to answer the question asked, but NEITHER statement ALONE is sufficient to answer the question asked.

D. EACH statement ALONE is sufficient to answer the question asked.

E. Statements (1) and (2) TOGETHER are NOT sufficient.

If this sounds at all confusing, don't worry, because it takes awhile to get used to this type of question. With practice, though you will learn to like Data Sufficiency questions...or at least hate them a little less.

Verbal section

The Verbal section is the last hurdle of the exam and is composed of 41 questions. By this point in the exam your eyes are blurry from staring at the screen for the last two hours, but it is important to focus because of the large amount of reading and analysis required by this section. In general, the section tests your ability to analyze and draw conclusions about written prose, identify and correct grammatical errors in English phrases, and assess arguments. The section is segmented into three types of questions: Reading Comprehension, Sentence Correction, and Critical Reasoning.

Reading Comprehension

This is another question type that will be familiar to those who have taken the SAT and ACT exams. The problems consist of passages, which can be as long as 350 words, and sets of questions that test your understanding of the passages. Passages are generally focused on natural sciences, politics/economics, and business topics. You can expect to see three to four such passages on an exam.

Sentence Correction

Sentence Correction questions present a statement or a phrase that is to be evaluated on its grammatical and stylistic elements. Part or all of the statement/phrase will be underlined, demarking the portion that you are to assess. You will have the option of selecting from four alternative phrases that would replace the underlined portion or to select the original as the correct phrase. Note that the first answer (answer A) will always be the underlined phrase included in the original statement/ phrase.

When selecting the correct answer, you are to evaluate the possibilities based on the requirements of standard written English. In particular, you should consider grammar, sentence structure, redundancy, word selection, and effectiveness.

Critical reasoning

Critical Reasoning questions are similar to the Analysis of an Argument portion of the AWA section in that you will be tested on your ability to evaluate arguments. Naturally, the major difference between the two is that after you are presented with the Critical Reasoning argument, you must select a multiple-choice response to a question regarding that argument. Specifically, you will be asked questions regarding the arguments' conclusions, assumptions, structure, rationale, and factors that could strengthen/ weaken the argument.

The CAT

The Quantitative and Verbal sections of the GMAT both consist of multiple-choice questions that are presented as a Computer Adaptive Test (CAT). The CAT is designed to dynamically produce exam questions based on your performance on previous questions. These questions, which range in difficulty from low to high, are pulled from a question bank. The result is a unique exam for every test-taker. The CAT begins by providing a question of moderate difficulty. About half of the test-takers are expected to get the question correct and half are expected to get it wrong. If you get the question correct, then your score increases and a more difficult question is supplied. If you get the question wrong, then your score goes down and an easier question is supplied. By the end of the test, the CAT finds your score based on the number of correct answers given to questions at different levels of difficulty. As one might imagine, there is a complex algorithm underlying this process. The algorithm decides the appropriate level of difficulty for your next question, the value of that question, and eventually your score. Because your questions are generated based on previous responses, you may not skip a question and return to it, as was possible on the paper GMAT.

Your GMAT score

So what's the bottom line? The bottom line will be revealed through four scores: Total, Quantitative, Verbal, and Analytical Writing Assessment. The first three scores will be provided to you immediately after you complete the exam. Your AWA score will be sent to you a few weeks later. Here are the details on each score component.

Total score

The Total score is the one that you'll hear thrown around the most. Total scores range from 200 to 800, with students at top schools averaging around 690. In addition to the score itself, schools will take a look at the percentile in which your score falls. The percentiles change on a year-to-year basis as scores go up, but the following table should give you an idea of how competitive different scores are.

Figure 4: Total scores and percentiles of examinees tested from January 1999 through December 2001

Total Score	Percentage Below
750–800	99%
740	98%
720	98%
700	96%
680	90%
660	87%
640	87%
620	81%
600	70%
580	64%
560	57%
540	50%
520	44%
500	37%

Quantitative score

Quantitative scores are placed on a different scale than Total scores and range from 0 to 60. Given the quantitative rigor of business school curricula, most programs will place more of an emphasis on this score than Verbal, especially if you are lacking a quantitative background. The following table provides information on Quantitative scores and their corresponding percentiles.

Figure 5: Quantitative scores and percentiles of examinees tested from January 1999 through December 2001

Total Score	Percentage Below
51–60	99%
50	96%
48	87%
46	80%
44	74%
42	67%
40	62%
38	55%
36	48%
34	41%
32	35%
30	29%

Verbal score

Verbal scores are scaled in the same fashion as Quantitative scores. They, however, are not comparable, because examinee performance on each part of the test differs greatly. Obtaining a score of 40 on the Verbal section is much better than obtaining a score of 40 on the Quantitative section. These differences can be seen by comparing the Verbal score in Figure 6 to the Quantitative score table in Figure 5.

Figure 6: Verbal scores and percentiles of examinees tested from January 1999 through December 2001

Total Score	Percentage Below
45–60	99%
44	97%
42	96%
40	90%
38	85%
36	81%
34	72%
32	67%
30	59%
28	51%
26	43%
24	35%

Analytical writing assessment score

Chances are that no one will ever ask you about your AWA score, because of business schools' heavy dependence on your responses to their own essays. Still, you should be familiar with how this portion of the exam is graded, because it is a criterion that schools consider (albeit to only a small extent). Your AWA score is an average of the scores you receive on the Analysis of an Issue and Analysis of an Argument portions, which are themselves averages of two independent scores. The result is a score that ranges from 0 to 6 in half-point increments, as opposed to one-point increments for the Quantitative/Verbal scores and 10-point increments for the Total score. The following table shows how AWA scores and their percentiles match up.

Figure 7: AWA scores and percentiles of examinees tested from January 1999 through December 2001

Total Score	Percentage Below
6.0	97%
5.5	90%
5.0	79%
4.5	62%
4.0	42%
3.5	24%
3.0	11%
2.5	5%
2.0	2%

Analyzing your score

While it would be nice to score above or at the mean of your target schools, you shouldn't continuously take the exam until you hit that mark. In addition to mean scores, you should consider the 80 percent range of the schools. As mentioned in Chapter 2, it will be very difficult to get into your target schools if your score falls below that range. Indeed, this should be a consideration in selecting your target schools. When you take a look at the GMAT ranges of top schools, you'll notice that they can be divided into three categories: equal to or above 650, below 610 and in between 650 and 610. The table in Figure 8 displays these groupings, sorted by the low-end of the range.

Figure 8: Top business schools' 80% GMAT range

Business School	Middle 80% GMAT Range
Group 1	
Stanford University	675–765*
Columbia Business School	670–750
Harvard Business School	670–755*
INSEAD	660–730
Northwestern University (Kellogg)	660–750
University of Pennsylvania (Wharton)	660–760
MIT (Sloan)	650–760
NYU (Stern)	650–750
University of California at Berkley (Haas)	650–760
UCLA (Andersen)	650–750
Group 2	
Dartmouth College (Tuck)	640–760
Duke University (Fuqua)	640–760
London Business School	640–740
University of North Carolina (Kenan-Flagler)	640–710
USC (Marshall)	640–720
University of Texas	640–710
Yale School of Management	640–740
University of Michigan Business School	630–730
University of Virginia (Darden)	620–740
Group 3	
Carnegie Mellon University (GSIA)	610–730
Emory University (Goizueta)	610–740
University of Chicago	610–750
University of Maryland (Smith)	610–710
Cornell University (Johnson)	600–730
University of Western Ontario (Ivey)	600–720
Purdue University (Krannert)	590–730
University of Rochester (Simon)	590–720
Vanderbilt University (Owen)	588–710
Indiana University (Kelley)	580–710
Michigan State University (Broad)	570–710

* Estimates

Note that these groupings are not meant to serve as some sort of ranking. They are not at all reflective of school quality and are merely one resource that you can use in deciding on your target schools.

Another consideration is your Quantitative/Verbal score split. You'll often hear that top schools look for students who have scored in the 80th percentile on both sections of the exam. While this isn't specifically true, you should be cognizant of your background strengths, your score split, and the emphases of your target programs. Programs that are more quantitatively rigorous will naturally place more of an emphasis on your quantitative abilities. So, if your quantitative score is relatively low, then you will have to show your ability to succeed in that program through other parts of your application.

Submitting your scores

The score submission process occurs immediately after you complete the exam. As part of the $200 test-taking fee, you may submit your scores to up to five schools. Because you have to choose which schools you want to receive the scores before you see the results, you should make an initial selection of target schools before the exam. Naturally, that list can, and, in many cases should, be revised after taking the exam. Once you submit your exam scores, you usually won't have to send any additional GMAT information to the selected schools, other than maybe entering your scores into the schools' application forms. The score report that the selected schools receive will include scores from your three most recent GMAT exams. GMAC holds scores for 20 years, but most schools only accept scores that are less than 5 years old.

After the exam, you can send score reports to additional schools for a $25 per-school charge. The test-taking fee does not cover any post-exam score submissions even if you don't select any schools on exam day.

How to Ace the GMAT

Just like your approach to applications, you should have a strategy in approaching the GMAT that is well thought-out and has some contingencies. Obtaining a good score will help give you confidence as you begin to attack other aspects of the application. This section provides advice on how to tackle the exam and achieve results that broaden your school opportunities rather than limit them.

Start early

There is nothing worse than having to complete applications while studying for the GMAT. Writing essays, managing recommenders, and completing data sheets are time consuming enough, without the requisite hours of GMAT preparation. We suggest that you begin your preparation course or independent studying at least six months before you plan on starting your applications. This will give you ample time to retake the examination if need be. Trust us on this: The faster it's over, the happier you will be.

Once you have your strategy in place, take the next step and sign up for the exam. A lot of applicants don't sign up and lose their focus on studying as a result. If you are like most people, having an actual "D-day" set in stone will help intensify your focus and give you the motivation you need to get ready for the exam.

Know your strengths and weaknesses

You've taken standardized tests before and are familiar with your performance. Additionally, you know your strengths in terms of quantitative skills and verbal dexterity. Finally, you know whether you need a highly structured environment and rigid schedule in order to study effectively or whether you can be successful studying according to your own schedule. Given these considerations, come up with a plan that targets your weaknesses so that you can maximize your performance on exam day. If you historically perform poorly on standardized tests and have trouble calculating tips at restaurants, it probably isn't a good idea to go into the exam after only a couple weeks of preparation.

Despite what you might hear, it is definitely possible to improve your score through concentrated training, so don't get discouraged if you fall into the "can't calculate tips" category. In general, we will focus our GMAT advice to the average to poor test-taker, so make adjustments accordingly if you can pull a 700 in your sleep.

Make a decision on whether to take a prep course

Test preparation companies have become very popular with standardized test-takers across a variety of exams. Despite the cost, which ranges from $1,000 to $1,500, thousands of test-takers flock to test preparation companies each year. It's no different with the GMAT. You should consider a GMAT preparation course if:

❏ **You are a chronically poor standardized test-taker.** Some people are gifted with the natural ability to perform well on standardized exams and don't need any assistance. For the rest of us, the very idea of taking such an exam is disheartening. Enrolling in a GMAT preparation course can be a great way to build confidence and to get a handle on the challenges of the GMAT.

❏ **You need a structured approach.** A big plus of GMAT preparation courses is the fact that they place you on a standard schedule. It can be too easy to fall off the wagon in terms of studying, and taking a course can be a great way to ensure that you stay focused on preparation. Indeed, staying focused is probably the most important part of preparation.

❏ **You would like to maximize your access to resources.** Depending on which GMAT preparation course you select, you will gain access to a number of resources, including books, strategies, sample exams, and of course, teachers.

As the last bullet suggests, all GMAT preparation courses are not created equal. Different courses provide different offerings in terms of teacher training, sample examinations, class size, and general preparation support. Here are the major players:

❏ **Kaplan:** Kaplan (*www.kaplan.com*) is the oldest player in the test-preparation market. In addition to the GMAT, it provides courses for all of the major standardized exams (SAT, ACT, GRE, MCAT, LSAT, etc.). As the first major entrant in the market, Kaplan has made a name for itself through its notoriously grueling exams. In terms of the GMAT, you can expect that your actual GMAT score will greatly exceed the scores you receive on Kaplan exams.

❏ **The Princeton Review:** The Princeton Review (*www.princetonreview.com*) made a dent in Kaplan's market share by offering smaller classes. Princeton Review also offers courses for each of the major standardized exams and, as mentioned earlier in the chapter, has become an application service provider. Similar to Kaplan, Princeton Review practice exams fall short in terms of replicating the actual GMAT exam, as some of the sections are structured differently than those featured on the GMAT.

❏ **Veritas**: Veritas (*www.veritasprep.com*) is the latest incarnation of GMAT preparation courses. Founded by two business school graduates, Veritas focuses strictly on GMAT preparation and has rapidly garnered a large following. Our suggestion is that applicants interested in taking a GMAT preparation course consider Veritas, given its instructors' credentials (all instructors scored in the 99th percentile on the GMAT), extensive in-class training (42 hours), and online and live instructor phone support. Additionally, the Veritas-created exam questions closely replicate those you will see on an actual GMAT. The company currently offers four diagnostic tests and eight CATs that are licensed from ETS and ARCO.

Be aware that taking a prep course does not lift the burden of preparation from your shoulders. You are not paying for a higher GMAT score, you're paying for the resources and training that help you earn a higher score. In order to get the most out of your course, you will need to do at least as much work outside of the classroom as in it. Keep up with the course's brisk pace, and the payoff can be worth the time and money.

Should you decide to pass on taking a GMAT preparation course or decide to take on additional study outside of your GMAT preparation course (which many applicants decide to do), here are some suggestions that successful applicants have found to be helpful.

Become familiar with exam strategy

One of the benefits of taking a GMAT preparation course is the strategies and exam shortcuts that are discussed. The courses do a good job of describing how you should approach the exam. To learn about such strategies and just to get familiar with the exam in general, we suggest taking a look at *Cracking the GMAT* by The Princeton Review. This book, which includes sample exams, is not intimidating and provides solid strategic advice that you will be able to readily apply. We have heard many complaints, however, in regard to the practice exams' ability to replicate a true GMAT in addition to the relative easiness of the questions. We therefore recommend this book as a starter, only to be used to "get your feet wet."

Practice on real GMAT questions

There is no substitute for practicing on actual GMAT questions. There is a certain logic that underlies the questions and their solutions that is uncovered by working on the questions over and over again. As such, we highly recommend *The Official Guide for GMAT Review*, published by the infamous GMAC/ETS coalition. The guide is comprehensive in that it provides more than 1,400 actual GMAT questions, which are accompanied by explanations of the answers. The guide also includes the entire bank of AWA questions, so you could theoretically prepare in advance for every AWA question that it is possible to receive on the day of the exam. While we definitely don't recommend that approach, reviewing a few of the AWA questions to get a feel for the essay topics is helpful.

The other integral part of your preparation should be POWERPREP test preparation software. POWERPREP can be downloaded for free from *www.mba.com* and allows users to take two actual GMAT exams. Placing yourself under actual exam conditions can be extremely beneficial as you get a feel for timing, how the algorithm works, and the overall length of the exam. Unfortunately, POWERPREP questions are drawn from the same bank as questions in *The Official Guide for GMAT Review* were drawn, so you will see overlap. Nonetheless, applicants continuously state that these two resources were invaluable in their GMAT preparation.

One way you can approach the studying process is by labeling the various types of questions as you take them. For example, problem solving problems can be labeled basic algebra, coordinate geometry, fraction, probability, etc. In addition to providing them with a label, give them a difficulty ranking such as hard, moderate, or easy. By assigning labels and difficulty levels to questions, you can track your performance on different problem types and then identify the areas in which you are the weakest. Ideally, after going through enough questions, you will get to the point where you immediately recognize a question's type as soon as you see it, and know how you will approach it. It may seem like the GMAT has an infinite variety of questions, but after enough practice, you will start to see the same types of questions again and again.

Review advanced questions and shore up your weaknesses

One common complaint about the resources offered by GMAC/ETS is that the questions provided are relatively easy as compared to the hardest parts of the GMAT. These complaints are especially directed at the quantitative questions contained in *The Official Guide for GMAT Review*. For additional assistance, take a look at the *GRE/GMAT Math Review*, published by Arco, and *GMAT 800*, published by Kaplan. You can use these guides as supplements to strengthen the areas in which you are the weakest. These guides, combined with the resources provided by GMAC/ETS, should give you ample material from which to prepare. In fact, many applicants will not need all of these resources to attain their target score. Your challenge is to understand the best preparation strategy for yourself, based on your needs, and utilize these materials and courses accordingly.

Don't get discouraged

It can be easy to get discouraged after reading your 15th science-based reading comprehension passage and getting all of the questions wrong. It can be even more discouraging to take the GMAT once or twice and not achieve the score for which you are aiming. It is important in those times to target the areas that are bringing your score down and attack them veraciously. Some applicants have found one-on-one GMAT tutoring to be helpful. Our suggestion is to make sure you've gained a strong understanding of how the exam works and are very familiar with the questions before looking for a tutor. Tutors can be extremely expensive (in excess of $2,000 for 15 hours), so it is in your best interest to learn as much as you can before going down that road.

In general, if you remain dedicated to studying and follow these tips, you should be in great shape on exam day.

Conversation With Chad Troutwine

Chad Troutwine is cofounder of the Veritas GMAT Course, a global GMAT preparation service. Prior to starting Veritas, Chad received his MBA from the Yale School of Management and his J.D. from the University of Missouri. Chad's position within Veritas makes him intimately familiar with the GMAT exam. We had the opportunity to sit down with Chad and get his perspectives on the examination that gives so many applicants sleepless nights.

What exactly is the GMAT supposed to measure?

Business schools seek the best students possible. In an effort to evaluate candidates from a global spectrum of undergraduate institutions, the Graduate Management Admissions Council (GMAC) turned to the Educational Testing Service (ETS) to create an objective measure of the verbal and quantitative abilities of their applicants. While many have roundly criticized the SAT (another ETS-created test) for its racial and socioeconomic biases, the GMAT has remained relatively unscathed for 50 years. Contrary to popular belief, the GMAT has also proven to be a highly accurate predictor of a student's academic success in graduate business school. Still, the GMAT is not a valid proxy for the rest of the application process. Specifically, the GMAT is not particularly helpful in the ultimate task of any admissions committee—assessing an applicant's managerial prowess or leadership potential.

How much of this is innate, and how much can be learned?

Because the GMAT is a test of analytical skill, rather than a subject-based exam, a mythology developed that a test-taker could not dramatically improve her score. Kaplan, and other pioneers in the test preparation industry, exposed the myth—and Veritas has completely shattered it. Applicants who have a history of scoring well on standardized examinations will almost certainly do well on the GMAT. On the other hand, those who do not innately possess those skills can still acquire them. All standardized examinations have patterns. We have completely deconstructed the GMAT and created proven strategies to help our students exploit those archetypes.

What GMAT-related weaknesses do you most commonly see in applicants?

Applicants commonly design flawed preparation strategies. Specifically, we often see industrious students who are convinced that the secret to achieving a high score on the GMAT is simple: Grind through as many practice questions as possible. They are misinformed. The ideal way to prepare for the GMAT is to learn a multifaceted and proven strategy *first*, then perfect that strategy with lots of sample questions. Students who jump right to the second part of the equation typically repeat the same errors, reinforcing their bad habits instead of correcting them.

What are some of the more correctable weaknesses for an average applicant who is preparing for the GMAT? What weaknesses tend to be harder for a typical applicant to correct?

Poor time management is prevalent, but easily corrected. Some students race ahead, leaving valuable minutes unused. Other students move too slowly, sacrificing precious time on early problems and leaving far too little time for later, often more difficult, questions. We offer several practice exams and pacing strategies to help alleviate both weaknesses.

Reading Comprehension takes time to master. Students develop reading skills over a long period of time, particularly non-native English speakers. Other students struggle with esoteric rules of grammar. Still others have rusty (or non-existent) probability skills. The key for any student is to accurately diagnose weak areas and address them during the course of study.

What's a reasonable level of improvement (from an initial diagnostic score to the actual GMAT) that an applicant should shoot for?

Improvement is a function of several different factors, so expectations should vary. If a student starts with a lower score (a 400, for instance), he could reasonably expect a 150–200 point increase. Conversely, if a student starts with a higher score (a 650, for example), she might be thrilled with a 60–100 point increase. A student who has previous exposure to the GMAT will likely begin with a higher diagnostic score, but may not have the same growth potential as her unexposed classmate. Formal preparation should raise expectations, too. According to studies conducted by our biggest competitors, students who prepare on their own suffer with stunted scores (when compared to those who take a full preparation course).

Do you find that applicants who take the test more than once are able to significantly improve their scores?

GMAC statistics indicate that students do not improve much from one test to another. However, we are convinced that many of those repeating students do not take active steps to radically improve their prospects, and their results reflect that apathy. On the other hand, our repeaters are encouraged to adopt Veritas methods before retaking the test. As a result, our students who previously took the GMAT still average a nearly 100 point increase, far above the average for all test-takers.

It seems like top schools' mean GMAT scores keep creeping up. What do you think that's all about?

We have three related theories. First, the pool of test-takers has improved. Raw quantitative scores have surged in the last decade, and the standardization of the GMAT has not kept pace. More students than ever are taking prep courses, so more arrive equipped to score well. Additionally, the number of international applicants has ballooned. According to GMAC, students in several international locales achieve higher average scores than their North American counterparts, particularly on the quantitative section. Tellingly, raw verbal scores have remained relatively flat for the same period. Second, GMAC has verified the predictive ability of the GMAT in several studies with many graduate business schools. Consequently, schools may be relying more and more on the GMAT, shading their means ever higher. Finally, the scores began to climb steadily after ETS switched the GMAT from a paper-and-pencil format to an exclusively computer-adaptive test in 1997–98. Any test that consistently relies on reusing questions is vulnerable.

We hear a lot of rumors that ETS has increased the number of combination and permutation problems featured on the GMAT. What's your perspective?

We hear the same rumors, and they may well be true. Another plausible theory is that, as quantitative scores continue to rise, more students than ever are receiving difficult questions. "Perm/combo" questions typically come from the pool of very difficult questions, so they may be appearing more frequently because the relative skill of the test-takers is rising. We take no chances in our commitment to provide the best GMAT preparation available. As a service to our students, we devote a significant amount of time to probability questions, particularly perm/combo questions, in our advanced quantitative lessons. Our dynamic instructors teach proven Veritas strategies, and the lesson booklets include hundreds of practice problems to help students hone their skills.

Test of English as a Foreign Language (TOEFL)

If the GMAT is the mountain that applicants must conquer before receiving admittance into a b-school program, then the TOEFL is generally considered little more than a speed bump. That's not to say that the TOEFL is wholly insignificant, but an applicant who performs well on the verbal section of the GMAT shouldn't have any problems with the TOEFL.

As the title would suggest, the TOEFL's function is to measure the English proficiency of people whose native language is not English. If your native language is English, you can stop reading this section right now, as you will not be required to take the exam. Many schools will also allow applicants who studied in an English-only curriculum or worked extensively in an English-speaking country to waive the exam. Because b-schools differ on the delineation of who is required to take the TOEFL and who is not, you should check the policies of your target schools.

One of the reasons the TOEFL is not as rigorous as the GMAT is because it is geared toward a wider audience. Indeed, the TOEFL is taken by aspiring students of multiple disciplines at multiple levels, in addition to people applying for scholarships, certifications, and government positions. Like the GMAT, however, the TOEFL has moved to a computer-based exam and is produced by ETS. Although the TOEFL has been offered in a computer format since 1998, applicants still can take the paper-based exam in certain regions. However, unless otherwise stated, we will refer to the computer-based exam.

Format and content

The TOEFL consists of four sections:

☐ **Listening:** Tests your ability to comprehend spoken English, as used in North America. You will hear a conversation, lecture, or classroom discussion and then be asked to answer a question about the conversation's meaning, implications, or supporting details. The content of this section is different from that of all of the GMAT sections, so you shouldn't expect GMAT preparation to help you perform well on this part of the TOEFL. This section is similar to the GMAT, however, in that it is computer-adaptive. As such, you will not be able to go back to a question after you select answer.

❏ **Structure:** Tests your knowledge of formal English grammar. The section consists of two types of questions: Sentence completion and error identification. Sentence completion questions require you to "fill in the blank" with one of four choices that best completes the sentence. Error identification questions require you to select one of four underlined words or phrases that must be changed in order to make the sentence correct. The Structure section is also computer-adaptive, so you will not be able to go back to a question after responding to it.

❏ **Reading:** Tests your ability to comprehend written academic English. You will be asked to read a passage and then answer questions about that passage. Similar to the Listening section, questions focus on the meaning, implications, and details of the passages. Unlike the Listening section, however, the Reading section is not computer-adaptive, so you can go back to previously answered questions.

❏ **Writing:** Tests your ability to write in English on an assigned topic. You will be asked to write a standard English essay that expounds on a topic and provides supporting details. This section is not computer-adaptive, as there is only one essay question to which you must respond.

The following is a summary of the TOEFL's format and content:

Figure 9: Format and content of the computer-based TOEFL

	Questions	Timing	Section Type
Listening	30–49	40–60 min.	Computer –adaptive
Structure	20–25	15–20 min.	Computer –adaptive
Reading	44–55	70–90 min.	Non –adaptive
Writing	1	30 min.	Non –adaptive
Total Time: 2 Hours 35 Minutes–3 Hours 20 Minutes **Score Range:** 0–300			

Scoring

You will receive a separate score for each of the four sections and a total score that represents your performance on the Listening, Structure, and Reading sections. Individual scores for each of these three sections range from 0 to 30, while total scores range from 0 to 300.

When you hear people talking about their "TOEFL score," they are generally referring to their total 0 to 300 score. So what should you shoot for? B-schools tend to be more explicit in stating what their TOEFL requirements are versus their GMAT requirements. While you should definitely find out what your target schools' TOEFL requirements are, top schools generally look for scores close to 260. Figure 10 provides the scores and percentiles of recent test-takers. You should also note that there is a separate scoring system for the paper exam. Figure 11 displays a comparison of the two scoring systems.

Figure 10: Scores and percentiles of examinees tested from July 2000 through

Total	% Below	Listening	% Below	Structure	% Below	Total	% Below
300	99%	30	99%	300	99%	300	99%
280	96%	28	95%	280	93%	280	93%
260	84%	26	84%	260	81%	260	81%
240	68%	24	68%	240	63%	240	64%
220	51%	22	53%	220	47%	220	48%
200	36%	20	39%	200	34%	200	34%
180	23%	18	28%	180	24%	180	23%
160	15%	16	20%	160	15%	160	15%
140	8%	14	13%	140	10%	140	9%
120	4%	12	8%	120	6%	120	5%
100	2%	10	5%	100	3%	100	2%
80	1%	8	2%	80	1%	80	1%

June 2001

Computer-based Score	Paper-based Score
287–300	660–677
273–283	640–657
260–270	620–637
250–260	600–617
237–240	580–597
220–233	560–577
207–220	540–557
190–203	520–537
173–187	500–517
157–170	480–497
140–153	460–477

Figure 11: Computer-based and paper-based score comparison

Similar to the AWA portion of the GMAT, the writing section of the TOEFL is scored separately from the rest of the exam. Scores on the writing section range from 0 to 6 and increase in half-point increments. Most schools don't have a required score for the writing section like they might for the total score. Nonetheless, you should still spend some time practicing a few essays, so that you feel comfortable with the section. Figure 12 provides the scores and percentiles of recent test-takers on the writing section. Most successful applicants score above 4.0.

Figure 12: Writing scores and percentiles of examinees tested from July 2000 through June 2001

Total	% Below
6.0	98%
5.5	92%
5.0	83%
4.5	70%
4.0	50%
3.5	29%
3.0	15%
2.5	7%
2.0	3%

TOEFL preparation

Many applicants find it helpful to prepare for the TOEFL prior to preparing for the GMAT, as it is considered to be less difficult. Additionally, preparation for the TOEFL will help you practice for the verbal section of the GMAT.

Because test-takers' familiarity with English varies so greatly, it's difficult to suggest an appropriate amount of preparation time. On average, applicants generally find about two to three months of preparation to be enough. Similar to GMAT preparation, we suggest first gaining an understanding of exam strategy and then practicing on real TOEFL questions. For exam strategy, we suggest *Peterson's TOEFL Success*. This book will provide you with an in-depth overview of the exam and specific tactics for each section. For practice on real TOEFL questions, you should pick up the *TOEFL Preparation Kit*. In addition to this book, ETS offers PowerPrep software for the TOEFL. You can download TOEFL PowerPrep from *www.toefl.org*. This site contains additional resources in which you might be interested, so check it out when you have a chance.

Performing well on the TOEFL is vital to international applicants' prospects of gaining acceptance to their target schools. By following these simple tips, you should be in great shape to do well on the exam.

Interview

In one sense, your admissions interview will be the fastest part of your entire application process: just 30 to 60 minutes and you're done. Looked at another way, it will be the most stressful part: you need to come out from behind your word processor and face a potential grilling. Neither view is exactly right. The work that you do on your interview will start weeks before it actually happens, as you craft your application. Ideally, by the time you sit down across from your interviewer, your extensive preparation will put you at relative ease. For the most part, your admissions interview will simply be another way in which you communicate the story that you have already constructed. As long as you have your game plan in place, your interview should only help you strengthen your story.

Why interviews?

Believe it or not, interviews are a relatively new phenomenon in the world of business school admissions. While many of the top programs conduct interviews "by invitation only," nearly all of them have a stated goal of interviewing all of the applicants whom they eventually admit. Other b-schools make interviews optional, but highly recommend them. Finally, some b-schools outright require interviews for all applicants. No matter what your target schools' policies are, there is a much greater chance that you will go through this ritual than if you had applied 10 years ago.

Why are interviews becoming a more important part of the admissions process? For one, business schools need more and more mechanisms to separate the great candidates from the good ones, as the admissions process becomes more competitive. What better way to do that than to look an applicant in the eye and ask him why he wants to go to your school? Also, schools have become more and more careful about building strong communities and cohesive student bodies. Because each class is a melting pot of personalities, schools want to personally inspect each one of those personalities before granting admission.

Every school looks for slightly different attributes in its applicants, but you can be sure that the admissions committee will be looking to answer a few key questions about you:

❑ Are you the person you say you are in your application?

❑ How are your communication skills?

❑ Are you someone your classmates would be glad to be around?

❑ Are you ready for business school?

The interview is often the best way to get at these answers. The purpose of an interview isn't to see how well you act under pressure or to try and trick you into revealing something terrible about yourself. Think of it as a way to reinforce what you have already said about yourself in the rest of your application and to help the admissions committee put a face to the name and numbers in your application. Yes, your interviewer may probe around certain weaknesses in your application or resume, but this is your chance to attack those weaknesses head-on and put them to rest.

Types of interviews

There are several different variables that determine exactly what the tone of your interview will be. These variables include: who interviews you, where and how the interview takes place, and how much the interviewer knows about you before your meeting.

Who could interview you:

❑ **Admissions officer:** These interviews tend to be the most formal, and the most specific in terms of what the interviewer is looking for. Admissions personnel will usually have a form from which they work, and will make an effort to cover each area before the interview is over. Beware, though, that if the admissions officer doesn't cover everything in the allotted time and some questions go unanswered, that will be considered your fault. Your main line of defense against this problem is making sure that you don't ramble. Later on we will discuss how you can make sure to cover the most important parts of your story.

❏ **Student:** Some schools train their students to conduct interviews. These students will typically work off of the same forms that admissions officers use. While you may hit it off with some students and end up having an informal conversation, many students tend to conduct interviews "by the book" even more so than admissions officers. Schools tend to use the interview feedback they get from students in the same way as the feedback they get from admissions officers. So, you should treat an interview with a student the same as an interview with an admissions officer.

❏ **Alumni:** Alumni have a reputation for being a little more laid back in terms of how they conduct an interview. They will also have some guidelines for conducting the interview, but tend to be more willing to let it evolve into a natural conversation. Remember, though, that they are still evaluating you. Even more importantly, if there are certain messages that you want to get across and the interviewer just wants to talk about the Red Sox, know that the onus is still on you to cover those messages. Also, keep in mind that alumni interviews tend to be the least restrictive in terms of time. Many alumni will let an interview stretch on for well over an hour if you are both enjoying the conversation. Finally, be prepared for a little more variability in your experience. While most applicants report having great interviews with alumni, there are more than a couple of horror stories of applicants being traumatized by weird, rude, or even harassing interviewers. These types of stories are rare, but know that experiences with alumni interviewers can be less consistent than with other interviewer types.

❏ **Faculty:** While having a faculty member interview you is extremely uncommon, there are some schools (most notably the London Business School) that might have you interview with a professor. These interviews generally feel like a discussion with an admission officer, but tend to be more academic in nature. Therefore, you should go into the discussion having a good understanding of the academic choices you've made in addition to being able to articulate what you want to get out of the curriculum.

Where you could be interviewed:

❏ **On campus:** Most interviews with admissions personnel and students take place on campus. The bottom line is that you should try your best to get to campus to do your interview. It might seem minor, especially because many schools make off-campus interviews readily available, but visiting campus goes a long way in showing your interest in the school (especially if you live far away). Expect your on-campus interview to be conducted in the admissions office, usually in formal attire (although a few schools conduct business casual interviews). While you're on campus, take advantage of the chance to meet with current students, tour the grounds, and sit in on a class.

❑ **Off campus:** Off-campus interviews are usually conducted by alumni, although some schools will do "tours" once or twice a year in which they visit major cities and interview a bunch of candidates at a hotel, or conduct interviews at a GMAC MBA Forum (which is like a traveling job fair, but for business schools). You can expect the format of these interviews to be the same as those of interviews conducted on campus. Interviews with alumni can take place anywhere, from coffee shops to restaurants to the alum's own office. We suggest picking a quiet place, but we advise that you try not to do the interview in the alum's office. Even the best-meaning alum can be easily distracted when surrounded by his work. Also, you will probably feel more comfortable in a more "neutral" setting, so avoid the in-office interview if you can. If your alum suggests his office, reply that it might be nice to get out of the office, and be ready with a few alternatives to suggest. Most alumni will respond positively to this.

❑ **Phone interviews:** Most schools prefer that you meet in person with an admissions representative. However, there are cases in which geographical, financial, or time constraints don't always allow that to happen. In those cases, your interview might be conducted over the phone. Phone interviews are usually with admissions counselors and follow the same format as other interview types. They are given the same weight as other interview types, but given the opportunity, we advocate trying to make it to campus.

How much your interviewer will know about you:

❑ **Resume-based interview:** Most schools' interviews are "blind," meaning that the interviewer has not seen your application before meeting with you. The most the interviewer will know about you is your resume, and some don't even see this before the interview. In these cases, you can expect a lot of general questions to start things off, such as, "Tell me about yourself," or "Walk me through your resume." Because the interviewer knows very little about you in these situations, and you usually have just 30 to 60 minutes to sell yourself, it is critical that you know what messages you want to communicate, and that you hit all of them before time is up.

❑ **Application-based interview:** A few schools have their interviewers read through your entire application before the interview. In this case, the interviewer is generally an admissions officer. After reading your application, the interviewer will develop a picture of you in her mind, and will come to the interview prepared with specific questions. Expect some probing of weaknesses and questions around your motivations for moves that you've made in the past, such as, "Why did you decide to leave Morgan Stanley and go into venture capital?" You can help yourself most by knowing your story cold, anticipating weaknesses, and having reasons for why you've done the things that led you to apply to business school. You should also pay special attention to your career goals, because it is almost certain that you will be asked to expand on them.

Most of the preparation that you do for your interview will be the same no matter where you do it and who interviews you. The differences will mainly be nuances, such as how many specific questions the interviewer prepares ahead of time, how long the interview is, and how many questions you are able to ask. Now we'll dive into specific tips for acing the interview.

Interview preparation

You are the best expert on you. You know why you've made the decisions that have led you to this point, what your strengths and weaknesses are, and (hopefully) where you want to go next in your career. The challenge is in figuring out how to best communicate all of this to your interviewer, and in being ready to tell various stories from your past that illustrate your abilities.

The questions you will get in an interview tend to fall into several broad categories: high-level questions about you, questions about why you want to go to business school (and where you want to go after that), and questions about specific experiences in your background. We will look at each of these question types in turn.

High-level questions about you

These are usually the most open-ended questions. An interviewer who asks these questions is giving you a chance to talk about your own history and traits, and to emphasize the parts of your background that are most important to your application story. Questions of this type include:

- ❏ Tell me about yourself.
- ❏ Walk me through your resume.
- ❏ How would your friends/coworkers/supervisor describe you?
- ❏ What are your biggest weaknesses?
- ❏ What are your biggest strengths?

The first two questions are similar, and are often used to start off an interview. If an interviewer asks you to start this way, this is your chance to take control of the interview and explicitly state the two or three core messages that you want to emphasize. Practice is vitally important. Your goal is to develop an "elevator pitch" of approximately three minutes that describes your background, highlights your strengths, and provides a story above and beyond the simple facts on your resume.

The following is a fictitious example of how someone might answer "Tell me about yourself." The answer to "Walk me through your resume" would be very similar, as you would still be pointing out specific achievements and provide a context for your career path:

Growing up, I was always interested in cars, and I remember helping my dad change the oil in our car when I was as young as 6 years old. By the time I got to high school, I knew that I wanted to become an engineer, so I devoted most of my energy to studying math and science. I went on to attend Ellicot University, where I earned my mechanical engineering degree. I was also very involved in my fraternity, where I was Treasurer, and I am proud to say that I started the Ellicot Racing Club, which has grown to more than 30 members.

After graduating from Ellicot, I pursued my interest in cars by taking a job at Midwest Motor Company. I entered as an Assistant Design Engineer. It was exactly what I dreamed of: I worked on projects that shaped the cars that millions of people drive. In my first year there, I made recommendations for a safer airbag system for Midwest Motor's small passenger cars, which were ultimately implemented. We estimate that at least 500 lives are saved each year thanks to the new system. After my first year, I was promoted to Design Engineer, and I was placed in a team that was charged with redesigning the child safety restraints in Midwest Motor's minivans. It was a tough project because we were given a short deadline and very strict cost controls, but we did a great job of finding creative solutions. I specifically found a way to use new materials that simultaneously increased the effectiveness and reduced the cost of the restraint systems.

After two years, I asked to be moved into the Safety Engineering department, because the safety-related projects that I had worked on had really captured my imagination. The move also appealed to me because it represented my first opportunity to gain experience in managing others full-time. I moved into that group as a Senior Engineer, and was permanently put in charge of a team of four designers. We worked on a series of projects to improve the safety of Midwest Motor vehicles in small but important ways. The achievement I'm proudest of is leading my team to develop a new, safer design for fuel systems in SUVs, which I presented to senior management all the way up to the level of Vice President of our division. The company is implementing the new design this year.

While I still enjoyed the engineering aspects of the job, what I found to be most rewarding was working with people from other functions, including Production, Finance, and even Marketing. For the first time, I realized how much my decisions affected their jobs, and vice versa. It gave me a new appreciation for teamwork. I also learned how to work with people whom I didn't directly influence. Learning how to get things done by influencing others is something that I've been working on for the last year. I'm also working on applying this skill in the Great Lakes Foundation, a nonprofit group that I've been involved with for two years. I do fund-raising for the organization, and have gained a lot of experience in persuading people to donate their time and money to the cause of helping inner-city children find creative outlets for their talents.

Now that I've had a taste of how an entire organization works, I'm interested in one day building my own manufacturing business, particularly one that will help make transportation safer and more fuel-efficient. To do so, I would like to gain an even broader view of how to run a business. While I'll always be an engineer at heart, I now want to learn more about marketing, finance, and how to lead people. From my experience, I see these as the skills that make for the most effective managers. I then want to put these skills to use in running my own business. Given my experiences and my desire to gain new ones, I think now is the perfect time to enter the Johnson School at Cornell.

Your own elevator pitch may be less involved than this one (and you may find that you don't even get all the way through yours if your interviewer hears something interesting and wants to dive right in), but this example gives you an idea of what you want to do. This applicant does a good job of:

- ❏ Communicating his high-level application themes, which are his passion for cars, his experience leading teams to results, and his specific reasons for wanting to go to school.

- ❏ Explicitly naming the results of what he worked on. Many applicants fail here; it not only matters what you did, but also what actually happened as a result of it.

- ❏ Highlighting what he specifically contributed as a member of a team. Applicants also tend to fail here by saying what "we" did, but never explicitly explaining what "I" did.

- ❏ Giving reasons for the moves that he made in his career, and making those reasons consistent with his overall story.

- ❏ Naming some of his extracurricular activities. Remember, business schools don't want someone who is married to his job!

- ❏ Tying together his past experiences into why he now wants to go to business school.

There is a balancing act here. You want to provide enough detail to make your story interesting, but you also don't want it to get too boring or bogged down in details. Develop your elevator pitch with what you feel is an adequate level of detail, and if you find that it's taking too long, then you can start to shave off details (which will likely be covered in other parts of your interview). Whatever you do, keep your high-level themes in there. After all, the main purpose of your elevator pitch is to get all of your main themes "out on the table."

The other questions are designed to see what you perceive your own strengths and weaknesses to be. Be honest when answering about your strengths and weaknesses. Your interviewer won't be impressed if you say that your biggest weakness is that you're a perfectionist who just plain insists on working too hard. One thing you want to do, though, is to focus on skills rather than personality traits when talking about your weaknesses. For example, saying, "I need more experience managing teams and delegating authority," is better than answering with, "I tend to be impatient with others." The former is something that you can clearly improve with time and practice, while the latter is something that will likely never change. You will also win bonus points if you can briefly discuss ways in which you are trying to address your weaknesses. So, if you mention that you haven't had much experience managing teams, mention that you've requested to be placed on a project that would allow you to do so. This shows that you are aware of your growth opportunities and actively try to improve in those areas.

Questions about why you want to go to business school and future goals

These questions include:

- ❏ Why do you think now is the time for you to go back to school?

❏ What do you hope to learn in business school?

❏ What do you think you will contribute that will be unique among your classmates?

❏ Why do you want to come to this school?

❏ Where else are you applying?

❏ Where do you see yourself in 10 years?

Some of these will overlap with the previous questions. Don't be surprised if you cover one of these areas in your elevator pitch, only to have your interviewer dig much deeper later in the interview. Most of these answers will come directly from your application. In your essays, you hopefully will do a good job of explaining your goals and why business school makes sense for you; now it is just a matter of verbalizing these reasons.

In order to answer the "Why do you want to come to this school" question well, you obviously will need to have done your homework on the school. It's amazing that applicants still make the mistake of telling a general management school such as Harvard that they want to go there because they want to become marketing experts. Be ready to list several reasons for wanting to attend the school, including both tangible (curriculum offered, location) and intangible (culture, learning environment). You may be tempted to find the school's curriculum and to rattle off several names of classes in your interview, but be careful unless you can mention more about those courses, beyond their names. Interviewers know that anyone can find a few course names on the Web in a matter of minutes.

When answering the "Where else are you applying?" question, don't be afraid to be honest. The main thing is to have a reason for why each school appeals to you. You don't need to have the same reason for each school, and you may never even end up discussing your reasons, but it helps to have them ready. Admissions officers want to see if the schools you've selected have any commonalities or if you're simply gunning for the highest ranked school that will take you. If you're talking to an interviewer from a lower-ranked school and you rattle off a bunch of top-10 schools, the message can come through that you view the school as a safety. Don't waste your breath in an interview talking about other schools any more than you have to, but be prepared to answer the question if the interviewer presses you on this.

Questions about specific experiences in your background

Some schools will spend most of the interview on these kinds of questions. These types of questions are the ones that famously start with, "Tell me about a time when you...." The idea here is to go deeper than your philosophy on how to manage others, how to prioritize projects, etc., and to hear about how you actually handled these challenges in the past. Your job is to recall experiences from your background that will answer these questions, and to sum them up in tidy two- or three-minute stories that will help your interviewer see exactly what you did in a specific situation and what the result was.

There is a popular technique that successful applicants use to answer these kinds of questions. Most of your answers will ideally be broken down into the situation that you faced, the actions that you took, and the results of your actions. Not surprisingly, this technique is called "SAR," for Situation, Action, and Result. You can start your preparation by building a table that includes questions that you can expect along with your answers, broken down into the SAR format. After a short while, you will likely find that this technique feels very natural for telling your stories.

Below are a few sample questions, with fictitious answers entered into the SAR grid:

Question	Situation	Action	Result
Tell me about a time when you led a team to success despite opposition from others.	I was asked by my company's sales director to develop a version of our software for a new platform. I pulled together a team of developers to produce the product, but the VP of product management resisted, saying that it was a waste of time and effort.	I made a point of understanding why the VP was opposed to the project. I realized he was unhappy that the sales team came directly to the developers to make it happen. He was also dealing with flat sales on his existing products. I addressed each of these concerns, getting him involved in the process and showing him customer feedback that suggested that the new product could boost sales.	The VP gave his support to the project, and we rolled it out in under six months. The new product was a success, and now all of our products are being translated for the new platform. The sales director and prodcut management VP both personally thanked me for making it happen.
Discuss a project that required the use of your analytical skills.	My boss asked me to identify and recommend some new potential sales targets for a product of ours that was facing slow sales. I knew little about the product or its market.	I met with one of our data analysts to identify the common traits among our current buyers. I then dug into market research data to find potential customers who exhibited similar traits. I recommended that we try a direct mail campaign targeted towards a segment that we hadn't previously considered.	The direct marketing test was a success, and we rolled out the campaign nationally. While sales had previously been declining 10 percent per year, this new campaign helped the product see its first double-digit sales gain since it was first launched.
Describe a time when you inspired someone to work harder.	I was running a civil engineering project that consisted fo myself and two engineers. We were asked by a client to design a drainage system for it's property. The unique landscape of the property meant we couldn't apply normal solutions to the problem. However, one member of my team was very busy with other projects and insisted on using a standard solution.	I knew that she was very busy, so I talked to her boss to free her up of some lower-priority projects that were consuming much of her time. Her boss agreed to do so after seeing how valuable this contract was. I then appealed to her creativity. I knew she took a great deal of pride in the work that she did, and I talked to her about how exciting it would be to design a solution that no one had developed before.	Once some of her time was freed up, she became passionate about the project and threw herself into it with the rest of the team. We ended up designing a new system that performed great and saved us and the client a total of $15 million. We couldn't have done it without her intelligence and energy. I made sure she was acknowledged for her had work and we've had a great working relationship ever since.

Each of your answers should take two to three minutes (you can actually tell a pretty in-depth story in this amount of time). Of the SAR components, the situation is the least important. It's critical in that it sets up the next two parts, but don't spend too much time on it. You want to provide just enough background to make the interviewer understand the situation, and ideally to make her care. Err on the side of being brief, and the interviewer will stop you and ask for more depth if needed. For a three-minute answer, less than one minute should be spent on the situation, roughly a minute and a half should be spent on the specific actions that you took, and the remainder on the results.

As mentioned before, two places where applicants often fail are in not stating what the results were, and in failing to mention what they specifically did to help reach a goal. Interviewers will be much more impressed if you can point to tangible results that came about as a direct result of what you did. Saying "We gained $5 million in business because of the ideas I implemented to make the product more reliable," is much more powerful than saying "We gained new business by making the product better." Be specific about what you did, and the results that you created.

This framework will work for nearly any question in which you're asked to describe a situation that you faced and how you resolved it. Ideally, you will be able to prepare for the questions that you are most likely to receive, and to outline an answer for each using the SAR framework. The great thing about SAR, though, is that it also helps you organize your verbal answers to questions that you didn't anticipate. If you find yourself faced with a question like this, take a deep breath, think about an example that could be used to answer the question, and start talking in the SAR format. If you find yourself still talking about the situation after a minute, move on and get to the meat of the story.

With a decent amount of preparation, such surprises should be minimized. Still, it is impossible to prepare for every single question that you will be asked, so being prepared to think on your feet is as critical as preparing for specific questions. The following is a list of common questions that you might expect to get in a business school interview. Plug these into your own SAR grid and try to develop real-world stories from your own experiences:

Leadership

- ❑ Discuss a time when you successfully supervised a diverse group of people toward a difficult goal.
- ❑ Give an example of when you accomplished something significant that wouldn't have happened if you hadn't been there.
- ❑ Tell me about a situation where you had to persuade someone to agree with your point of view.
- ❑ Describe a time when you had to gain upper management's support for an idea/proposal.
- ❑ Name a time when you had to convince someone who didn't report directly to you to do something they didn't want to do.
- ❑ Describe a situation in which you identified key problems early on in a project and were able to avert a crisis.
- ❑ Tell me about a time when you led a team to a goal even though the individual team members were skeptical that it could be accomplished.
- ❑ Discuss a time when you had to make an unpopular decision.

Teamwork

- ❑ Tell me about the toughest group that you ever worked in. What made it so tough, and how did you handle it?

- ☐ Describe a time when you had a conflict with another person in a corporate or school setting.
- ☐ Tell me about a time when you worked with someone who didn't follow through. What did you do?
- ☐ How have you dealt with a person who was difficult to work with?

Ethics

- ☐ Describe an ethical dilemma that you faced in your career. How did you resolve it?
- ☐ Give me an example of when you pushed back against doing something.
- ☐ What is the hardest decision you have ever had to make on the job? Outside of your job?

Innovation

- ☐ Name a time when you developed a unique and resourceful solution to a problem.
- ☐ Describe a situation when you had to make an important decision without having all of the necessary information at hand.
- ☐ Tell me about a time when you had to analyze facts quickly, identify the issues, and develop an action plan.
- ☐ Give me an example of when you thought out of the box.
- ☐ Tell me about a time when you took a smart risk.
- ☐ Have you ever had to bend a rule to get your work done more efficiently?

Maturity

- ☐ Tell me about your most spectacular failure. What happened? What did you learn?
- ☐ Discuss a time when you didn't succeed on the first try.
- ☐ What is the worst professional decision you have ever made?
- ☐ Tell me about a time when you weren't very pleased with your performance.
- ☐ Describe a situation in which you wish you had acted differently with someone in your group.

One note: For "failure" questions, don't be afraid to admit your failures. The most important thing that an interviewer is looking for with these kinds of questions is evidence that you learned from your past mistakes. Ideally, your answer will consist of what happened, what went wrong, what you learned, and how you applied that lesson in a later situation.

How to carry yourself in interview

In your admissions interview, you want to come across as personable, confident, interested, interesting, and sincere. For everyone one of these descriptors, think of the opposite. No one would want to be surrounded by arrogant, tentative, indifferent, dull, or phony people. In short, you want to convey that you are who you said you are in your application, and you want to show the interviewer that you're someone who would make a great classmate in business school. Yes, this may seem daunting, given the application themes that you already want to communicate. Most of these personality traits, though, should come through if you can relax and simply be yourself.

For the most part, your interviewer will set the tone of the discussion. As described earlier, some will be laid back and interested in getting to know you personally, while others will want to drill down on specific parts of your resume or application. Obviously, how serious or informal you are will largely depend on the person across from you. Your job is to make adjustments accordingly, and to answer the questions that they ask. But you must make sure that by the end of the interview you have covered the main themes that you came in with. For instance, you may have a laid-back, "get to know you" kind of interviewer who doesn't ask you the kinds of pointed questions that would allow you to talk about your strengths. If this is the case, it's perfectly appropriate to say, "By the way, there are a couple of things that I think make me a good fit for this school. I'd like to talk about them and hear your thoughts," before the interview is over. You don't want to be too transparent, but all but the most inept interviewers will appreciate the fact that there are certain ideas that you're trying to get across before the discussion is over.

If you have a stone-faced interviewer who won't laugh at your jokes, don't press the matter. Act professionally, answer the questions that are asked, and make sure to hit your main themes. In a way, these interviews can sometimes be easier because the interviewer's business-like questions will more likely give you a chance to strut your stuff. If you have a downright hostile interviewer (which happens from time to time), don't let yourself get flustered or goaded into an argument. Relax, think of it as the interviewer's half-baked way of testing your mettle, and answer the questions as they come. Don't be argumentative, but don't be afraid to be assertive, either. A hostile interviewer may be looking for poise and confidence more than anything else, so make sure to demonstrate these.

At the end of the interview, ask a couple good questions. Good questions don't have answers that you could have gotten from the school's Website or brochure. If you are interviewing with an alum or a student, asking about her experience is always a good place to start. Similarly, if you are interviewing with an admissions counselor or a faculty member, asking about the direction of the curriculum will generally generate an interesting response.

Interview etiquette

It is considered appropriate to send your interviewer a short thank-you note after the interview. There is a small debate over whether that thank-you note should be e-mailed or handwritten. The benefit to e-mailing a thank-you note is that the interviewer is likely to receive it prior to submitting the evaluation report. A well-written note can reinforce your message and leave the interviewer with a positive feeling about your candidacy. The handwritten note, however, adds a personal touch that some applicants insist outweighs e-mail's "speed factor." The bottom line is that this is not a decision worth losing sleep over, as it won't have an impact on the school's decision to admit you. You should choose the method with which you feel most comfortable. Regardless of the communication method, keep it brief and try to echo one or two topics that were discussed during the interview.

Our view is that interviewing will continue to become a more important application component with time. Schools consistently mention that it is a great way to differentiate applicants. It is important that you understand how to make your story come alive during the interview. Just as important, you should communicate a distinct passion for the school and its mission. Demonstrating this level of fit and desire will get you one step closer to acceptance.

Essays

After GMAT preparation, writing your essays will likely be the most time-consuming part of the application process. Admissions directors often cite essays as the most important part of the application. The combination of these two factors means that you should dedicate a significant amount of time (15–25 hours per application) to producing powerful and persuasive essays that are succinct in style.

Your essays should be the base upon which all other application components are built. You can think of your essays as a platform that can be used to tell your personal and professional story. You have flexibility in terms of tone, so feel free to utilize a professional, informal, or humorous voice in establishing your story. The other components (recommendations, interview, resume, and data sheets) should substantiate that story. The more aligned your components are around common themes, the more positive the impact on your application. We will discuss putting together a game plan that links all of the components in Chapter 6.

As part of the storytelling process, you should try to augment your strengths and anticipate your perceived weaknesses. Use the analysis from Chapter 2 and the profiles in Chapter 3 in identifying and addressing both. In sum, your essays should effectively communicate your differentiated position, your embodiment of the four dimensions, and your fit with the school. As frustrating as the essay-writing process may seem, ultimately it helps crystallize your reasons for wanting to go to b-school and some of your career objectives.

The rest of this section will review what admissions committees typically look for in essays, essay types that candidates predictably come across, samples of successful essays, and a prescription for how to approach the writing process.

What are admissions committees looking for in the essays?

There are essentially three aspects of your essays that will be explicitly or implicitly evaluated by admissions officers:

- ❏ **Content:** In response to the question, "What mistakes do applicants commonly make?" admissions officers often respond that many applicants fail to adequately address the essay's questions. Seems like a stupid mistake to make, but many applicants "copy and paste" an essay that doesn't quite fit, try to "shoehorn" responses that don't answer all of the questions' elements, or just completely miss the point of the essay. Regardless of the reason, not succinctly answering essay questions is an easy way to win your application a quick trip to the "ding" pile. Many other applicants are guilty of simply rehashing their resumes, offering nothing new in their essays that lets the admissions committee know who they really are. In general, you need to answer the questions asked, and do it in a way that helps the admissions committee see you as a person, not a GMAT score and a data sheet.

❐ **Grammar:** It doesn't matter how strong your story is if your essays are riddled with grammatical errors. Poor grammar dilutes essay responses and can ruin the best applicant's chances. You should focus on ensuring that you are using appropriate syntax, idioms, and sentence structure. Additionally, beware of run-on sentences, as they often lead admission counselors to confusion. Being concise and clear will always benefit your cause. Grammar is usually the area of essay-writing where having a second, third, and even fourth set of eyeballs can provide the most immediate help.

❐ **Structure and parameters:** Maintaining an organized structure and a logical flow of ideas will help increase the impact of your statements. Consider, especially for longer essays, using headers to help guide the reader. Another consideration in terms of structure is word usage. While you certainly want to be descriptive in your writing, stay away from esoteric vocabulary. Your goal is to effectively communicate ideas, not to show off your knowledge of the English language. Finally, make sure that you observe word limits. As a rule, you shouldn't surpass word limits by more than 10 percent. Going beyond that can be an easy way to buy a "ding." Remember that admissions counselors are reviewing thousands of applications, so they can be very sensitive to applicants who don't respect word limits.

Essay types

As you move from one application to another, you will encounter many essay questions that are similar in nature. We've found that there are basically 10 different types of essays that you will come across:

- ❐ Future goals and school fit.
- ❐ Leadership and initiative.
- ❐ Teamwork.
- ❐ Ethics.
- ❐ Personal philosophy.
- ❐ Personal evaluation.
- ❐ Hobbies.
- ❐ Diversity.

❐   Professional experience.

❐   Failure.

The types of essays that a school includes on its application are a reflection of that school's approach to learning and the sort of applicant for which it looks. Therefore, it is imperative for you to understand the implications that underlie the essay questions. While we will cover the implications, it is important to note that essays don't always fall into one of these discrete buckets. For example, a question might ask about your approach to leading teams, which obviously touches upon both the teamwork and leadership themes.

The sample essays express ways in which successful applicants have played on those themes. The applicants received admission to at least one of the schools reviewed in Chapter 5 and their backgrounds are diverse in terms of work experience, gender, academic background, ethnicity, nationality, GMAT scores, GPA, etc. For each essay, we provide some commentary on the applicant's perspective and highlight the attributes that resonated positively with the admission committee. While no essay is necessarily perfect, these essays should help you in creating ideas for your own approach. And crafting your own approach is the key. This is *your* MBA game plan, after all.

Future goals and school fit

This type of essay is almost universally used in applications. Of the 30 schools reviewed, 28 included this essay type in their applications. This should give you an idea of how important fit is to schools.

For the most part, this question type is trying to drive at whether now is the best time for you to get your MBA. Additionally, schools want to know how they fit into your long-term plans. Lastly, the school wants to know how you envision yourself having an impact, either in your career, or more broadly, on society. Most schools are not looking for you to state an exact position in which you envision yourself, but rather where and how you see yourself having an influence. Many applicants fall short in this essay by providing a very generic response in terms of their future goals. Simply stating that you want to move into private wealth management is not enough. You must go a step beyond that, explain how you see yourself having an influence in that field, and explain how the school fits into the picture.

Many times this question type will ask for a summary of your professional background and then ask you to relate it to the school and your career goals. Be careful not to simply rehash your resume. Rather, provide some context as to why you've made the choices that have led you to where you are today. The three components (professional background, school, future goals) should be linked in a fluid manner. You should highlight your strengths, outline your future goals, and then underscore how the school will help you build additional strengths in order to achieve those goals.

Some examples of questions that fall into this type:

❐   *Why have you decided to pursue an MBA?* (Dartmouth College—Tuck)

❐   *Discuss your career goals and why you want an MBA degree. How will the skills you have developed to date contribute to your effectiveness in fulfilling your post-MBA career objectives?* (UCLA—Anderson)

❑ *What are your short-term and long-term post-MBA goals? How will Columbia Business School help you achieve those goals?* (Columbia Business School)

❑ *Describe your short-term and long-term career objectives after completing your MBA. What experience and attributes do you possess that would make you a good fit for that position?* (Emory—Goizueta)

Sample essay

Briefly assess your career progress to date. Elaborate on your future career plans and your motivation for pursuing a graduate degree at the Kellogg School.

Where I've been

I joined Withers Incorporated after graduating from Dawson University in order to experience numerous business practices across multiple functions. During my tenure at Withers, I have made substantial contributions on both a global and local level to our customers and internal initiatives. Operations and corporate finance are the primary areas in which I have practiced.

Over the last year, I have narrowed my focus to financial cost analysis. As a leading contributor to a $32 million cost reduction effort, I have expanded my knowledge of finance beyond the surface level. In order to expedite an assessment of the Firm's financial situation and gain an understanding of primary business drivers, I created financial models for four major business units whose yearly technology expenditures exceeded $400 million. I provided my expertise to over 20 individual business and technology partners to validate cost reduction opportunities, and implement cost reduction plans. By developing and honing cost reduction skills and understanding how to create strategies oriented towards reducing the bottom line of a company's budget, I have become a valuable asset to the Firm, even in an unstable economy. _____

> The applicant does a good job of quantifying the impact he had on the organization. By showing his ability to work in a numbers-oriented environment, he helped "make up" for a quantitative GMAT score that fell a little bit below Kellogg's mean.

Exemplary results and the exhibition of strong management capabilities in Firm initiatives led to my appointment to the Global Finance Advisory Council (GFAC), a premier leadership group within the Firm. The primary function of the 10-member GFAC is to proactively shape and influence the direction of Withers' financial position from a macro level.

In an effort to provide consistency and standardize business units' approach to financing operations, I am leading an effort to create protocols for over 2,000 managers globally. Developing standard protocols for the entire Firm has required me to adjust my communication style according to the business unit and geographical region. _____

> Clearly a demonstration of the leadership dimension. The applicant's strategy was to emphasize leadership in this essay, and the teamwork dimension in the interview and in a separate essay.

Where I'm going

As a result of working closely with multiple business units, I've gained a strong interest in initiating my own venture. — — —

> Nice transition. Coupled with the header, it makes the direction of the essay clear.

This ambition drives me toward my professional goal: to redefine American fashion by developing an import business that specializes in a mélange of South American and North American clothing. In my travels and research, I have observed a growing interest in multi-ethnic clothing that uses fabrics, prints, and styles that are not indigenous to the U.S. Market studies have shown a strong demand on the West Coast for clothing and articles with South American motifs. Although these types of products exist in the United States, they are generally not marketed or distributed adequately, and are not tailored to the average American. I believe there is opportunity to promote a new line of fashion that fuses the cultures of the North and the South. Although at first glance this might appear to be a complete departure from my current career path, it will actually build upon the fundamental skills that I've acquired in the analysis of business models. Indeed, the ability to achieve operational efficiencies would be a key success driver in this mid-to low-margin business. — — — — — — — — — — — — — —

> Good discussion of future objectives. The applicant adds a nice touch by showing insight into the business and how his background could help him be successful.

The flexible Kellogg learning model would allow me to build upon these skills through its concentrations in entrepreneurship and marketing. Courses such as Entrepreneurship and New Venture Formulation, Managing Entrepreneurial Growth, Marketing Strategy, and Sales Promotion and Retailer Behavior would be vital assets in the development of my business model. During my visit to Kellogg, I was impressed by the way in which faculty actively show how theory works in practice. Being able to make that transition will also be vital to my success. — — — —

> Excellent work in terms of providing Kellogg specific information that would clearly be of benefit in achieving his career goal.

As a member of the Kellogg community, I would actively engage in the diverse range of global forums, club activities, and business plan competitions. All of these opportunities would bolster my efforts in becoming a successful entrepreneur. — — — —

> Could make the essay a bit stronger by providing some more Kellogg-specifics in this section.

Leadership and initiative

B-schools' increased emphasis on leadership is reflected in the large proliferation of this essay type. Many schools even have more than one question of this type on their applications. Questions will generally ask you to describe a situation in which you displayed leadership, initiative, and/or creativity. Schools are trying to gain an understanding of your approach to leadership and the style(s) you employ when the situation calls for it.

These are great questions for utilizing the SAR framework, which was discussed in the interview section. It is important that you cover each component of SAR in order to maximize the impact of your essays. We suggest that you try and dedicate approximately 30 percent of the word limit to the situation, 50 percent to your actions, and 20 percent to the result. While there is no hard and fast rule, this is just a guideline that can be helpful in evaluating whether you have dedicated enough time to each part. While b-schools are most interested in your actions and the result of those actions, setting the context of the situation is vital to understanding the other components. The takeaway is that, although you might write more for one component than another, they are all key to writing a solid leadership and initiative essay.

In many cases, schools will focus a portion of the question on teamwork, so don't think of the two as mutually exclusive. Indeed, showing that you have the ability to lead in a team environment is probably more important than showing your ability to lead on an individual level.

Some examples of questions that fall into this type:

- ❏ *Part of leadership is the ability to make a difference under difficult circumstances. With this in mind, describe a situation in which you exhibited such leadership.* (Yale School of Management)

- ❏ *Describe a situation where leadership and teamwork were critical to the outcome of a project in which you were directly involved. What did you learn from the experience and how have you applied what you learned to other situations?* (University of Pennsylvania—The Wharton School)

- ❏ *Please give an example of when you had an impact on a person, group, or organization. Please describe the situation, your actions, and the results.* (MIT—Sloan)

- ❏ *Describe a situation in which you used your leadership skills to assist a team in successfully completing a project or achieving a goal.* (University of Western Ontario—Ivey)

Sample essay

What makes work fulfilling? Describe a situation where, as a team member or project leader, you have made work more interesting or enjoyable for your group. (University of Michigan Business School)

The thing I remember most about my first day as a Regional Manager at Global Rent-A-Car is that no one else wanted to be there. In fact, one of my new employees mentioned that he did not enjoy coming to work because he had nothing to show for it. I understood what he meant: The office was last in every category—profit numbers, customer service, and fleet growth. Even more interesting to me was when he mentioned that he did not trust the other employees in the office because he felt like no one wanted the office to be a success. I began to realize that the negative attitude in the office was not due completely to our poor performance, but to a lack of teamwork between the employees.

Great details in here. Gives the reader the feeling that the applicant has his work cut out for him.

That day I made it my mission to make the office a more desirable, fun place to work. I started by doing the least desirable activity myself—washing cars. By doing the job everyone liked least, I hoped the employees would begin to trust me. Indeed, my employees told me that when they saw me washing cars, they realized that the goals of the office were more important to me than keeping my suit clean and that I had proved to them that the team took priority over the individual. To encourage them to get to know each other better, I started to take them out, as a group, every Thursday evening for drinks and appetizers at a nearby restaurant. Soon the employees were joking with each other and I could see that they were becoming closer.

As our team began to trust each other on a personal level, they began to trust each other on a professional one. I encouraged one employee who felt "trapped" in the office all day, to take donuts to the corporate accounts in our area. At the end of the month we sat down and counted the number of referrals we had received from her sales calls. When she saw the increase in referrals from the month before, she began to realize that she was truly making a difference in our profits. She began to encourage the other employees to become involved in the marketing plan. Within six months we had increased our corporate business by almost 100 percent, and it was directly attributable to the team marketing effort. —————————————

> Great discussion of the actions taken to resolve the issues the organization was facing.

Under my leadership, we began to see our income and profit numbers skyrocket. I am now convinced that leadership cannot simply be an order from a supervisor, it must come from dedication to a vision that is greater than any individual. Our success was due in part to the fact that the employees began motivating each other. I now know that what makes work fulfilling is being part of something that you have helped create, and knowing that your efforts on the team are making a positive impact. My washing cars was a small price to pay for the kind of turnaround my team achieved in nine months and the dividends that accrued from working together. —————————

> The applicant does a nice job of stating the results and then mentioning what he learned. He is also careful to make sure to answer the first part of the essay question.

Teamwork

While many essays on leadership dedicate a portion of the question to teamwork, there are some that focus purely on the interactions and relationships that you have with others. We consider these "genuine" teamwork questions. The admission committee is looking to see how you communicate and cooperate in a group environment. Therefore, expressing your interpersonal skills is an essential part of answering these types of questions.

Similar to questions on leadership, teamwork questions sometimes ask you to reflect on a situation. As such, using the SAR framework for these question types can be a great way to respond to them. Although SAR can be a great framework to use, don't feel chained to it. If you have a more creative and powerful way to get your points across, then go for it. Remember, SAR is just a framework to help you organize your thoughts.

Some examples of questions that fall into this type:

❐ *Using an example from your work experience, describe what factors contribute to a dysfunctional team experience. What steps can the individual or group take to help alleviate this situation and help develop a constructive team environment?* (Michigan State University—Broad)

❐ *Please give us an example of a difficult interaction you had with someone. Please describe the situation, what was difficult about it, and how you resolved it.* (MIT—Sloan)

Sample essay

Describe an experience in which the relationships you developed enhanced the outcome of a team effort. (Columbia Business School)

A few years ago, I participated in a cross-continent choir that was composed of members from France and the United States. As a part of the American contingent, I traveled to Paris for vocal training and performances.

Arriving in Paris, we met our French counterparts for the first time and were immediately overwhelmed. Although we had considerable talent, and had performed several times together in the States, our French team members were well-known throughout the European continent. We felt additional pressure, as most of the songs we were to sing together were to be sung in French. For months prior to the trip we practiced the inflections and intonations that were to be used while singing the French compositions, but it became immediately apparent that we were far from meeting their standard.

Initially, the choir was fragmented based on citizenship. The cultural environment and the skills of the French team members intimidated us. In order to counteract the intimidation factor, I asked the choir director if each U.S. choir member could partner with a French choir member. The director agreed that having us pair off would be a good relationship builder and I was soon chatting it up with my partner, Serge.

Nice description of why the team was initially fragmented.

I asked questions as they came to mind in an attempt to understand the French language, culture, and music. Serge often responded with his own questions and a dynamic dialogue ensued. Outside of the formal choir practices, Serge and I held sessions that focused on the proper pronunciation and delivery of the songs. In addition to learning more about the music, I began to learn more about the culture and the language.

Over the next few weeks, Serge and I became inseparable. I learned that despite the initial surface differences that existed, we were very similar at the root. We both wanted respect, under-standing, and the opportunity to succeed. Furthermore, I was amazed at the new perspectives and insights on life that I gained from him. The result was that I not only developed my vocal talents, but also realized a new appreciation for other cultures and the possibilities for improved communication across geo-graphical borders. — — — — — — — — — — — — — — — —

> Terrific explanation of the actions taken to build the relationship.

My American compatriots had experiences similar to mine and we found that as a result of our newfound relationships, we performed on an entirely higher level. When we first practiced as a unit, one could easily distinguish our voices. Now we truly sounded like a single unit. The audiences were extremely recep-tive to our performances and unanimity. In fact, we went on to win first place in a regional competition.

This experience taught me the power of relationship build-ing. No doubt our choir would still have been successful with-out partnering up. Still, I don't think our harmonies and melodies would have sounded as pure and I know that we wouldn't have had as much fun. Now I always look to build an understanding with my colleagues in order to enhance team dynamics. — — — — — — — — — — — — — — — — — —

> The applicant does an excellent job of relaying the results of the actions and what she learned from the experience.

Ethics

Many applicants struggle in coming up with examples to use for essays that ask about ethics. If you think about it long enough, however, you can certainly come up with an example in which your sense of ethics was tested. A relevant story doesn't need to be as intriguing as a corporate scandal; many of the best ethics essays deal with subtle issues, such as making a tough decision when you could have gotten away with less. For many questions, your response doesn't necessarily have to reflect on a professional situation.

Admissions committees are most interested in understanding your thought pro-cess in approaching ethical situations, so you should dedicate a good portion of your essay to that. Just like with other situation questions, you can use the SAR framework for most of these question types. Discussing your thought process generally would fall under the "Action" section.

Some examples of questions that fall into this type:

❏ *Please describe an ethical issue that you have faced in your professional life, how you dealt with the situation, and what the outcome was.* (Carnegie Mellon University—GSIA)

❑ *Describe an ethical dilemma that you have faced and how it was resolved.* (Northwestern University—Kellogg)

Sample essay

Discuss an ethical dilemma that you experienced firsthand. How did you manage and resolve the situation? (Harvard Business School)

It's funny how powerful the desire to receive accolades can be. As far back as I can remember, I've always sought approval from my superiors; whether they've been my parents, teachers, or managers. That's why it was so difficult for me to not fulfill my manager's request.

The request came two months after I started working for Ong Semiconductors as an economic analyst. My manager asked me to conduct a comprehensive market analysis for a new product we were planning to release in the next year.

Eager to prove myself, I dug right into the analysis. I estimated the • 450 million market potential by hosting discussions with potential customers, analyzing research reports, and speaking with analysts. Working with engineers, I calculated the manufacturing costs at different production levels. Finally, I completed a competitive analysis that highlighted other companies' abilities to compete in the market. After working four 70-hour weeks, I submitted a draft of my analysis to my manager. — — — — —

> Nice details in this paragraph. The applicant does a great job of providing the details of her hard work, highlighting her capabilities even in an "ethics" essay.

Apparently, it wasn't good enough. The competitive analysis didn't reach my manager's expectations. He began to press me to include more details, specifically details regarding my former employer. My manager requested that I include proprietary information on a potentially competing product on which my previous firm was working. The information request included: technical specifications, cost data, and the product launch date. It was clear that I was being asked to break a good faith understanding I had with my old firm not to reveal proprietary information.

I could've easily provided all of the information and satisfied my manager's request. I probably would've received major accolades for the insights. Indeed, I'm confident that there wouldn't have been any direct ramifications for revealing the information. Still, based on my sense of ethics, I simply could not break the understanding I had reached with my old company. I did my best to explain this to my manager. — — — —

> The applicant effectively conveys the ethical dilemma and takes the reader through her thought process.

Needless to say, he wasn't pleased with my stance. A short time after our discussion, I was removed from the project. Over time, I discovered that the company had a history of conducting competitive analyses that bordered on corporate espionage. Three months after being removed from the project, I put in my notice and subsequently left the firm. A year later, several executives were investigated for illegal competitive practices. — — —

> This paragraph shows that the applicant is willing to take action based on her convictions. She also subtly explains her five month stint with the firm; something that would otherwise be viewed negatively.

Reflecting on my experiences, I'm proud of the way I acted. While compliance would have allowed me to satisfy my manager's request, it would have also placed me on an ethical "slippery slope." I've reached the conclusion that before I seek approval from my superiors, I must first seek approval from myself. This continues to be a personal philosophy that I actively practice. — — — — — — — — — — — — — — —

> As all applicants should, she explains what she learned from the experience. The closing is also very effective in that it ties back to the introduction.

Personal philosophy

Personal philosophy essays focus on your overall perspective on life. They often ask you to reveal "life-changing" experiences or to discuss something that is extremely important to you. Here, the admissions committee is really trying to get to know you and find out what drives you. A portion of the essay will often ask you to describe what you've learned from the experience. Responding to that is imperative because it provides insight into how you learn and what you value.

You will run into at least one personal philosophy essay on most applications, so you should spend some time thinking about the message you want to send. Once you've identified your message, it is important that you communicate it with passion. While passion should be threaded throughout your entire application, it should ooze out of this essay.

Some examples of questions that fall into this type:

❒ *We all experience significant events or "milestones" that influence the course of our lives. Briefly describe such an event and how it affected you.* (USC—Marshall)

❒ *What unique personal qualities and/or life experiences distinguish you from other applicants?* (University of Rochester—Simon)

❒ *Imagine that you will be taking a 72 hour car ride with two other individuals. If you could choose your travel companions, whom would you choose and why? (These individuals can be living or deceased.)* (University of Maryland—Smith)

❒ *What matters most to you, and why?* (Stanford)

Sample essay

Please tell us something else about yourself that you feel will help the Admissions Committee know you better. (University of Pennsylvania—Wharton)

My name

My middle name is Carlson. Carlson is a family name, passed on to me from my grandfather Michael Carlson

Stevenson. It is a representation of the heritage and the legacy that I have been bestowed. It is also a reflection of the standard to which I will be held. In every facet of his life, Grandfather has been a visionary striving for excellence. He has extended his vision through education and servitude. Expanding the legacy of my Grandfather is extremely important to me, because failing to do so would be to dishonor the very name that I bear.— — — —

> Interesting introduction, which speaks to the applicant's motivations.

My grandfather

Grandfather has six sons, all of whom have either an M.D. or a Ph.D. Success in education was always emphasized in his household. Grandfather views education as a key that is necessary for achievement. If one is educated, Grandfather says, than he can effectively decide his own fate and help positively impact the fate of others. Grandfather himself holds a B.A. and an M.A. in education administration. After earning his degrees, Grandfather went on to start his own private school for pre-school to middle school students. He feels that if children are shown the value of education while they are young then they will not depart from that teaching as they grow older. As a result, he not only educated his own children, but also hundreds of children in his surrounding neighborhoods. He has provided education support through his own teachings, the establishment of scholarships, and career counseling.

As a public servant, Grandfather is well-known both domestically and internationally. In addition to his education initiatives, Grandfather has served his local community through the church that he pastors. Community service functions have included: Feeding and clothing the needy, and supplying financial support for area building projects. At an international level, Grandfather has provided support to initiatives in more than five nations, such as Haiti, Ghana, and Liberia. On several occasions, he has personally traveled to these emerging markets and directly assisted with the projects. The projects have ranged from the construction of schools, to the dispersion of food, to the building of churches.— — — — — — — — —

> Family is clearly important to the applicant. The discussion of education provides some insight into his motivation for applying to b-school.

My turn

I have found truth in Grandfather's beliefs on education and servitude. My successes have mainly been a result of effective preparation, which equates to proper education. Once knowledge has been obtained, I believe that it should be freely shared. As such, I am intrigued with the persuasive power inherent to speaking and writing. Whether it is delivering the commencement address to my graduating college class, writing editorials for the local newspaper, or leading a discussion on career success with indigent populations, I enjoy speaking and writing into the lives of others with candor and truth. Communication contains the possibilities of inspiration, reconciliation, and illumination. To communicate well is to be understood. To communicate powerfully is to effect change. I will effect change. My middle name is Carlson.— — — — — — — — — — —

> This paragraph gives the admissions committee good examples of the applicant's commitment to education, communication, and community service. This essay really aligned well with the applicant's career objectives to start a nonprofit organization. The applicant also expressed an interest in starting a magazine that focuses on global community service opportunities.

> The closing is nicely linked back to the opening.

Personal evaluation

This essay type calls for applicants to provide a perspective on themselves. That perspective is often asked to be given in an evaluation style. The admissions committee is looking to see how you view yourself in terms of strengths and growth opportunities. Although you certainly don't want to cast yourself as inept, describing one or two areas in which you can develop is as important as depicting your strengths. It is important because the committee is interested to know how you can benefit from its learning model, so make sure you describe a connection between your growth areas and the school's strengths.

The most effective personal evaluation response supports your overall story in addition to displaying fit with what the school has to offer. It is also important that your response doesn't contradict what your recommenders are saying. In other words, if you state that your interpersonal skills are some of your greatest assets and one of your recommenders writes that it's an area in which you need improvement, then the rest of your evaluation might be called into question. This is just one more reason why creating a game plan for yourself and for your recommenders can be such an effective tool.

Finally, as mentioned in the interview section, the weaknesses that you present will ideally be skill-based, more than personality-based. After all, there is no MBA course that can change someone's personality. Keep this in mind as you choose which weaknesses to discuss.

Some examples of questions that fall into this type:

❑ *Is your academic performance to date an accurate predictor of your potential for success at London Business School? If so, why? If not, why not?* (University of London—London Business School)

❑ *You have been selected as a member of the Kellogg Admissions Committee. Please provide a brief evaluative assessment of your file.* (Northwestern University—Kellogg)

❑ *If you could change one characteristic about yourself, what would it be?* (UC Berkeley—Haas)

❑ *Creatively describe yourself to your MBA classmates. You may use any method to convey your message: words, illustrations, etc.* (NYU—Stern)

Sample essay

Give a candid description of yourself, stressing the personal characteristics you feel to be your strengths and weaknesses and the main factors which have influenced your personal development, giving examples when necessary. (INSEAD)

Kaizen

The Japanese have a concept known as "kaizen," which roughly translated means continuous improvement. In recent history, this term has become most closely associated with the improvement of manufacturing operations and adopted as a mantra by several companies. However, the original meaning of the word kaizen carries an even more noble intent than business success—its intent is a successful life. A person adopting the philosophy of kaizen knows that human perfection is unattainable, yet strives to achieve it every day. Following this philosophy means always acting in a manner that increases knowledge and leads to personal development. Having always been a highly motivated person, this concept struck a chord with me and I adopted the philosophy of kaizen, making self-improvement a daily goal.

Over time, the adoption of this principle has allowed me to build strengths in several areas. While I realize I still have several areas in which I can grow, I know my belief in kaizen will help to address those areas.

> This section sets up a nice context for why the applicant is strong in certain areas and how she is able to identify the areas in which she needs to improve.

Strengths

My leadership skills, broad educational and professional experiences, analytical abilities, and strong personal presence are all strengths on which I continually rely.

The leadership skills I first developed playing team sports have allowed me to become a leader in my educational and professional endeavors. At Carella College, I was a founding member of the Investment Club and delivered presentations at most club meetings. While working for Amariglio Financials, I supervised a 35-employee department of mostly first and second generation Americans. With Taverna Holdings, I led client training sessions for over 50 employees, and have also served as a mentor to newly hired Taverna Associates.

> Rather than stating that leadership is a strength, the applicant goes a step further and provides nice examples of how she displayed leadership.

My broad educational and professional experiences developed my unique perspectives into business. Having examined companies from both an external shareholder view as a securities analyst and from an internal management perspective, I have insight into both the challenges faced by companies in developing and implementing strategic direction and the shareholder perception of strategy's value, something every executive should evaluate. My global experience, resulting from work experiences in the United Kingdom, Germany, France, South Korea, and Canada, have provided insights into the unique challenges of competing internationally and of growing a company through international acquisitions. — — — — — — — — — — — — — —

> The applicant clearly understands how much INSEAD values global professional experience and displays fit by highlighting her exposure to international business.

Some of my strengths are inherent. My ability to read and comprehend information at a rapid pace began when I first started reading the newspaper's sports section at age 3. My calm demeanor has also been a constant in my life, allowing me to remain composed and positive in challenging situations. This translates into a strong personal presence, often noted by managers as making me seem older than my years.

Weaknesses

I also recognize my development needs. In pursuing the goal of owning a successful large venture capital firm, my prior focus on large corporations has limited my knowledge of how to start and manage a small business. By pursuing an MBA at INSEAD, I hope to increase my knowledge of small business financing and development.

From a skills perspective, I need to work on reigning in my strong perspectives. While being willing to debate a position is an attribute, at times I defend my point so strongly that I may miss the value in my opposition's argument. One of INSEAD's appeals is the opportunity to debate viewpoints with a group of incredibly intelligent people, learning from their experiences while sharing my own. — — — — — — — — — — — — —

> The stated weaknesses align well with INSEAD's strengths.

I hope to be able to build upon my strengths and address my weaknesses over the next year at INSEAD, as I continue to live by the kaizen philosophy. — — — — — — — — — — — — —

> Nice job of connecting the closing back to the opening.

Hobbies

Another way that b-schools sometimes try to find out more about you is by asking about activities in which you're involved outside of work. These questions provide you with a great opportunity to convey your interests outside the professional environment. You can use the opportunity to express one of the dimensions that wasn't as strongly articulated in other parts of your application.

Some examples of questions that fall into this type:

❑ *Outside of work I...* (Northwestern—Kellogg)

❑ *Please explain if you have been involved in charity/volunteer and/or entrepreneurial activities, giving examples of your involvement, the amount of time you gave to each activity and why you chose to get involved.* (University of London—London Business School)

Sample essay

People maybe surprised to learn that I... (USC—Marshall)

People maybe surprised to learn that I enjoy acting as a dance choreographer. I have found cultural dance to be an outlet that allows me to utilize innovation and imagination through graceful moves, balanced by synchronized music.

Over the last 10 years I have choreographed numerous folk dances for audiences of over 5,000 people. Each performance is significantly different. Two years ago, I choreographed a dance for 16 women. Each of us carried candles throughout the performance, adding effervescence to execution. The following year, I modified a traditional Swedish dance that manipulates pieces of ribbon on a central pole. As part of a grand finale act, I, along with 11 other participants, performed the ribbon dance in a manner that reflected a classic Norwegian drama. — — — — —

> Shows a combination of creativity and dedication.

In addition to the energy and creativity that is required by choreography, I also enjoy the teaching aspects of it. Teaching participants how to move with harmony and style are key to the successful implementation of any dance. It is satisfying to be able to not only see the participants learn the components of the dances, but also to watch them as they add their own personality to the movements. I will continue to choreograph dances, because it provides me with an avenue through which I can celebrate my culture, spirit, and life. — — — — — — — — —

> The applicant's interest in teaching certainly would benefit Marshall's active learning model. The applicant successfully raised that point during her interview.

Diversity

Diversity essays can be similar to personal philosophy essays in that they are asked in an attempt to find out how you are unique. However, diversity essays differ in that they will frequently ask how your uniqueness will contribute to the classroom.

It is important to understand that admissions committees have a broad definition of diversity, and that isn't limited to culture or ethnicity. Diversity is defined as unique experiences or background, so it applies to professional roles that you've played, perspectives that you have, hobbies in which you participate, topics that you've studied, and so on. Regardless of how you are unique, make sure to bring it out in response to this type of question in order to show that you have something different to bring to the classroom dynamic.

Some examples of questions that fall into this type:

☐ *Describe any meaningful cross-cultural experiences you have had that highlight your awareness, understanding, and appreciation of interacting with people from diverse backgrounds. How have these experiences influenced your interpersonal, communication, and team skills and your desire to pursue a management career?* (Vanderbilt University—Owen)

❑ *The Darden School seeks a diverse and unique entering class of future leaders. How will your distinctiveness enrich our learning environment and enhance your prospects for success as a leader?* (University of Virgini—Darden)

❑ *Describe how your skills, knowledge, and life experiences could benefit potential classmates.* (Purdue University—Krannert)

❑ *Fuqua's culture values the individual contributions that each student brings to the community. What qualities and life experiences will you bring to Fuqua, and how will they enable you to contribute?* (Duke—Fuqua)

Sample essay

Describe any experiences you've had that highlight the value of diversity in a business setting. (University of Michigan Business School)

Diversity of talents on the court

Over the course of my basketball-playing career, I have captained my high school and college varsity basketball teams, represented the state of California in a national invitational, and led the country in free-throw shooting accuracy. These individual successes came as a result of hard work, personal sacrifice, and commitment. However, as I matured as a person and leader, I recognized that these individual accomplishments meant nothing when compared to team victories and championships. I learned an early lesson in teamwork, and the potential for team success when a group of uniquely skilled individuals was well-managed and integrated appropriately. In looking back at our team successes, I realize our victories and championships could not have been accomplished without the collaborative efforts and diverse talents of those around me. — — — — — —

> The applicant does a nice job of setting the context of the essay by discussing his previous experience with the power of diversity and teamwork. He also is able to discuss some past accomplishments that might not have otherwise come out.

Diversity of talents off the court

Since beginning work, my lesson in diversity has logically translated to my life in the business world. Early in my career, I worked on a project with an information systems expert from mainland China and a business major from a small Midwest town. Although we made up a relatively small project team, each of us had very unique backgrounds and project experiences. These backgrounds and experiences contributed to individual strengths, as each of us led the portions of the project that most accurately aligned with these strengths. Additionally, due to the size of the team, we actively participated in all engagement stages, ultimately learning a great deal from each other. The project was an eventual success, and it helped to equip me better for future engagements in which I could maintain larger management responsibilities.

My current project team also exemplifies the value of diversity. From a cultural standpoint, my team has members from nine different countries. As each practitioner has gone through different educational and cultural experiences, they are able to bring a unique perspective in attacking project issues and creating business solutions. In a professional sense, my team is made up of practitioners with backgrounds in technology implementations, Oracle database design, business process, system testing, and user training. The complex technology and business aspects of the project require a constant interaction among these different professionals. There is no doubt that this effective integration of individual contributions has directly led to our successful project completion. — — — — — — — — — — — — —

> These two paragraphs transition nicely into how diversity can be an asset in the professional environment.

In each of these engagements, my challenge as a leader and team member was to evaluate and capitalize on the diverse abilities within my team. I have benefited from these challenges, as I have been able to cultivate new functional expertise and business perspectives. However, in a much larger sense, these engagements were successful due to the diversity of talent that we maintained as a team. Although the merging of talent is sometimes challenging, the benefits achieved in effectively doing so can be as substantial as winning a team championship.

Looking ahead toward future growth

As I grow through personal and professional experiences, I have come to realize that diversity can be an extremely valuable part of a successful team. I look forward to the learning opportunities that will come with interacting with the unique students that make up UMBS, and will enjoy the challenge of merging our diverse perspectives as we grow into business leaders of the future. — — — — — — — — — — — — — — — — — — —

> Nice closing The admissions committee gets the sense that the applicant understands the value of diversity and that he personally would have a lot to add to the diversity of UMBS.

Professional experience

With the large emphasis that b-schools place on work experience, it isn't surprising that a number of them have essays dedicated to discussing a professional accomplishment or experience. Admissions committees are interested in seeing how you perform in a professional environment and how you learn from work experiences. This is your opportunity to display innovation, leadership, and teamwork abilities, so take advantage of it.

Some examples of questions that fall into this type:

❒ *List one of your most significant professional or organizational accomplishments. Describe your precise role in this event and how it has helped to shape your management skills.* (Emory University—Goizueta)

❒ *Describe the most significant lesson you have learned in your full-time employment and how this influenced your personal development and career aspirations.* (University of Western Ontario—Ivey)

❑ *Discuss three professional accomplishments which demonstrate your potential for a successful managerial career.* (University of Rochester—Simon)

❑ *What is the most significant change or improvement you have made to an organization with which you have recently been affiliated? Describe the process you went through to identify the need for change and manage the process of implementing change. What were the results?* (Indiana University—Kelley)

Sample essay

Describe your professional work experience since earning your bachelor's degree and discuss how you chose your career path. (Duke University—Fuqua)

After graduating from Coggins University with a Bachelor's degree in business, I took a job with Gardner Technologies, a company that sells data analysis tools for large businesses. All new Gardner employees must pass an intensive six week database "boot camp," and I came away from my training with a deep understanding of database technology and an appreciation for how it can be used in business. My specific interest was in the intersection of technology and marketing, and in my first year at the company I further familiarized myself with database technology while I served in a corporate marketing role. — — —

> Succinct statement of professional interests. Shows the rationale behind decisions that the applicant makes later on in his career.

I developed and executed marketing campaigns with the company's partners and represented the company at industry events. Over time I took a greater interest in how the company was marketing its individual products, and I was able to pursue this interest by working with the product management team to develop a marketing plan for each of the company's four main product lines.

During this time, I reported to the vice president of marketing. After my first year, he asked me to join a newly formed group, Marketing Technology Solutions (TSM). TSM's goal was to develop deep expertise in each industry that Gardner served, including Healthcare, Telecommunications, and Finance. The group's role quickly turned into a strict business development function as we pursued large e-commerce deals with a handful of prospective partners. It was an exciting opportunity for a 23-year-old because we were negotiating deals worth over $10 million each. However, I found that I was drifting away from the application of technology in marketing, and I wanted to reverse that trend. — — — — — — — — — — — — — — — — — — —

> Nice example that shows the reader that the applicant had a significant level of responsibility even in the early period of his career.

That's when the opportunity at The Source presented itself. The Source operates one of the most popular personal finance and investing sites on the Internet (FinSource.com). Most of the Website was free when I joined in 1999, but the company did sell some products on the site, mainly investing books and stock research reports. I was hired into the product management group to improve how we marketed our products to our users and to turn more of them into paying customers. It was a great opportunity in that the company's large database of users allowed me to put my database skills to use. — — — — — — —

> The last sentence of this paragraph shows that the applicant searches for background fit in making career decisions. This is subtle, but important to the admissions committee.

In my first year, my team had some great successes, including improving our promotion conversion rates by 50 percent through the use of new database targeting techniques. We also introduced a successful new line of online seminars that teach paying customers about a range of personal finance topics. My most satisfying personal accomplishment was leading the market research for and launch of a new investment newsletter, which is now our most profitable premium service.

Earlier this year, I was promoted to the role of senior marketing manager, and I now report to the company's vice president of marketing. With the title have come new responsibilities, including the goal of generating $2.3 million in revenue for our existing products, and leading the marketing launch of a new financial advisory service that is expected to generate $5 million in its first year. I am currently the only person in the company without an MBA who has revenue-generating responsibility. —

> Great details provided in these two paragraphs.

It's a challenging role, especially because we are like many "dot-coms" and have had to figure out how to reach our goals with a reduced staff. Even more importantly, I don't have any direct reports and must therefore manage people in other departments through indirect influence. Over the last two years, I have learned how to influence and cooperate with others to get things done, learning a great deal about leadership and teamwork in the process. I have found this aspect of my professional development to be most rewarding, and I plan on further developing these skills at Fuqua and in my future career. — — — —

> The last paragraph serves as a nice summary. The applicant does an excellent job of relating his professional experience to Fuqua's strengths.

Failure

Similar to essays on ethics, many applicants struggle in coming up with responses to these types of questions. Failure essays will typically ask you to describe a situation in which you did not meet an objective or you made a mistake. Applicants often wonder if they should actually write about a true lapse in judgment, or simply disguise an accomplishment and call it a "failure."

What admissions committees are really looking for here is how you learn from your mistakes. They want to hear about a situation in which you truly did fail, not a cloaked accomplishment. This is another essay type that lends itself to the SAR framework. The difference here is that you should focus a majority of the essay on the "Results" section, telling the admissions committee how this experience has impacted your outlook. To a certain extent, the greater the failure, the more learning you can discuss. That's not to say that you should reveal some sort of fatal flaw, such as a tendency toward criminal behavior, but admissions counselors know that we've all "messed up big time." This essay is really one in which you should discuss such an event, and more importantly discuss what you learned and the steps you've taken to ensure that it won't happen again.

Some examples of questions that fall into this type:

- ❏ *Describe a failure or setback in your life. How did you overcome this setback? What, if anything, would you do differently if confronted with this situation again?* (University of Michigan Business School)

- ❏ *Recognizing that successful leaders are able to learn from failure, discuss a situation in which you failed and what you learned.* (Harvard Business School)

Sample essay

Describe a situation taken from school, business, civil, or military life, where you did not meet your personal objectives, and discuss briefly the effect. (INSEAD)

It's one thing to fail to meet your objectives in the business world, but quite another to fail to meet them while serving in the military. In the business world not meeting personal objectives could mean revenue goals are not met, a transaction falls through, or in a worst-case scenario that colleagues lose their jobs. In the military, however, not meeting personal objectives could mean that people lose their lives. The magnitude of that difference translated into a powerful learning from an unfortunate experience. — — — — — — — — — — — — — — — —

> This opening paragraph sets the tone for the situation and certainly makes the reader realize that the discussions that follow will not be trivial.

When a military coup ousted an inspection team to prevent the discovery of weapons of mass destruction, I went to Eastern Europe to plan subsequent air strikes. Despite my personal objectives to exceed the expectations of my senior officers, I made a colossal mistake on my first assignment. — — — — — — — —

> Very succinct explanation of the situation, which allows the applicant to quickly get to the other parts of the essay.

I was charged with investigating the appropriate approach to taking out a bunker that housed some of the illegal weaponry uncovered by the inspection team. Eager to prove myself in a new environment and uncomfortable asking for assistance, I went to work. Using modeling software, I created a blast pattern to depict the strikes' destructive radius. Simply following the step-by-step training that I received, I did not acknowledge the fact that this pattern partially covered a nearby building. This was a glaring error that became evident later that night.

Standing before tense pilots, my briefing lasted 30 seconds before whispers grew into an agitated roar. The senior officer leading the strike proceeded to "dress me down," pointing out that the structure alongside the bunker was housing for the coup's families. The strike approach that I chose would have easily damaged this building, injuring or even killing civilians in the process. Because my training had never accounted for this sort of risk, I never considered threats to non-military structures. My inexperience and narrow reliance on procedure almost cost innocent lives. Because our jets were about to launch, the assault on the bunk was eliminated. _ _ _ _ _ _ _ _ _ _

> The imagery in this paragraph is very effective.

I was relegated to observer status for my remaining week on site, making the lesson stick, and turning me into a better officer and person. I learned that computers and procedures are simply tools, but teamwork and inter-personal communication lead to real understanding. By performing my analysis alone rather than engaging the experts around me, I hampered the mission. Furthermore, I learned that by asking questions of the people around me I can gain access to a wealth of information that otherwise remains underutilized. Six months later, when I ran my own team in Bosnia, I turned these realizations into meaningful action by instituting information sharing in a formalized manner.

Ironically enough, despite the magnitude of difference in impact, these are all lessons that easily translate back into the business environment and that I certainly intend to employ as I switch careers. _ _ _ _ _ _ _ _ _ _ _ _ _ _ _ _

> The applicant does a nice job in these two paragraphs of covering what he learned as a result of the experience. Additionally, he touches upon how he's focused on building skills for which the admissions committee looks. Finally, his closing is very effective in that it ties back to the first paragraph.

Additional information

In addition to the 10 main types of essays, most schools also allow applicants to respond to an optional "catchall" essay that basically asks whether there is any additional information that the applicant would like to share with the admissions committee. Most applicants who respond to this essay abuse it by either pasting in an essay written for another school or by simply writing about every topic that comes to mind. Neither of these approaches matches this essay's purpose.

The purpose of the essay is to allow applicants to discuss any evaluation criterion for which they might appear to be an outlier. The essay allows the applicant to attack the glaring weakness head on and provide additional information as to why it really isn't a weakness, or how the applicant is addressing the weakness. Good reasons for using this essay include addressing a GMAT that falls below the school's 80 percent mark, pointing out that you worked 30 hours a week to pay for your undergrad tuition (which affected your GPA) or explaining some other extraordinary circumstance.

If, however, there is no exceptional aspect of your candidacy that hasn't already been addressed in some other aspect of the application, then it would be in your best interest to skip this essay.

Some examples of questions that fall into this type:

- ❏ *Is there anything else about your background you think we should know as we evaluate your application? If you believe your credentials and essays represent you fairly, you shouldn't feel obligated to answer this question.* (Indiana University—Kelley)

- ❏ *Please provide additional information about whatever else you would like the Admissions Committee to know.* (MIT-Sloan)

Sample essay

Please use this opportunity to present any additional information that would assist the Admissions Committee in the evaluation of your candidacy. (University of Virginia—Darden)

The failure of regression analysis

My favorite aspect of regression analysis has always been the "outliers." These anomalies defy logic by refusing to conform to their destiny, outlined by defined variables.

Over the years, standardized tests have been touted for their ability to predict academic and career success. Several econometric analyses have been created to support these contentions. For every one of these models, however, there are a few instances in which the predicted result of low standardized test scores deviates from the line. I am the deviation. — — — — — — — — —

> This applicant takes an unconventional approach to this essay type by referencing an analytical tool. In doing so, he's able to show off his strength in an area of perceived weakness and also subtly present a potent argument for looking past what otherwise would have been a "game-breaking" GMAT score. It turned out to be a "game-winning" approach.

The GMAT experience

The disappointment I felt when I pressed the "enter" button and saw my 550 GMAT score flash across the screen is indescribable. How could I receive such a low score after months and months of tireless study? The fact that it was my third attempt at the exam made the failure all the more painful.

Still, my experience with the GMAT exam is reflective of my history with standardized tests. Throughout high school and college, I have always underperformed on these exams. I have learned that my "standardized test anxiety" does not have to limit my academic or career success; rather I use these "failures" as motivating factors to succeed inside and outside the classroom. — — — — — — — — — — — — — — — — — — —

> The applicant is very effective in setting the stage for a deeper argument as to why his GMAT score does not accurately reflect his abilities.

The experience of an outlier

Throughout my undergraduate career, I was able to balance a rigorous course load in the business engineering (BE) program and multiple extracurricular activities. Earning a 3.87 GPA in the BE program allowed me to gain a strong foundation in business operations, procurement, and logistics. The BE program at Kuziev University was recently ranked as the second best program in the nation and focuses on the student's ability to apply quantitative analysis to business case scenarios.

Early success in quantitative courses such as Economics and Applied Calculus allowed me to serve as a tutor for three of my four years. As a tutor, I trained students in fundamental mathematic and economic concepts, through review sessions and challenging practice examinations. Building upon my tutoring experience, I developed a new academic coaching program within the College of Engineering. The coaching program allowed me to assist over 70 students through resume and networking workshops, test-taking strategy sessions, and time management analysis. In recognition of stellar academic performance and my representation of the College of Business, I was named as Kuziev University's "Most Outstanding Business Student" for the graduating class of 1998.

> The applicant shows that he clearly has the academic background and quantitative ability to succeed in an MBA program.

These victories did not, however, preclude my attempts to succeed on the GMAT examination. In fact, I modified my approach to the exam several times, dedicated over a year to studying, and even worked with a tutor for a four-month period. Taking over 20 practice exams and mastering more than 4,000 practice problems, I tried to push beyond my standardized test anxiety and surpass my historical performances. I certainly feel that I have a good grasp of the exam material, as I consistently score in the high 600s on practice exams.

> This paragraph demonstrates that the applicant has given the GMAT his all and that he didn't merely take the GMAT one time without preparing.

Although I fell short in this area, my "failure" only further motivates me to prove that I am the exception to the rule. I continue to manage these "failures," because I refuse to be defined by them. Indeed I succeed in spite of them, as I am an aberration. I am the outlier.

> Great closing. The last sentence connects well with the introduction.

Final thoughts on essays

There's no doubt that your essays will be your greatest point of differentiation from the rest of the applicant pool. It's incredibly important, therefore, that you are able to write your story in the most effective manner possible. Again, Chapter 6 will help with the assembly of the full game plan package.

Here are a few last tips that should help you put together the best essays possible:

- ❑ **Make edits to your essays in several rounds.** You will constantly make revisions to your essays as you find better ways to express yourself and different methods for highlighting your attributes. As such, you should look at essay writing as an repetitive process that ultimately results in a masterpiece. You should never submit an essay with which you are unsatisfied.

- ❑ **When you are done with your essays, set them aside for a of couple days before submitting them.** Sometimes applicants get caught up in the writing and editing process and simply want to get the essays out the door as soon as possible so that they can check that task off the list. This mentality is certainly understandable, but can be detrimental as in many cases it leads to essays that have been rushed. By leaving completed essays alone for a couple of days, you will be able to read them with a fresh perspective, and will most likely be able to evaluate them better.

- ❑ **If possible, provide your recommenders with a sample essay.** In addition to providing your game plan to your recommenders, consider giving them a sample essay that discusses your career goals. This will bring out some details of your story that they are less likely to have a handle on, and will help create an application with messages that are fully aligned.

Recommendations

If your essays are the most important embodiment of the core messages that you want to communicate, then your recommendations are a close second. There is no more powerful way to reinforce the image that you're trying to present to an admissions committee than by having a former supervisor or coworker corroborate it. Think of each recommender as a character witness who is ready to illustrate your strengths with unique examples from your past. Just as in a court case, you can't afford to have a witness who is lukewarm. Your recommenders need to exude passion about you as a person, confidence about your career potential and your ability to succeed at business school.

Most schools ask for two or three recommendations, with a few asking for just one. Some leave open the option of submitting an additional recommendation. Consider this extra recommendation *only* if it would add something new to your application story. If your first two recommenders tell the admissions committee that you're a great team player, then you don't need a third person telling them that, too. If you do have one recommender in mind who has seen strengths of yours that no one else has seen, though, then adding that extra letter to your application will certainly help.

Who should write your recommendations?

More than anything, your recommenders need to know you well. You may be able to get a letter from your Executive Vice President and CEO, but if they haven't worked with you much, it will be very apparent in your recommendations. Admissions officers evaluate a recommendation based on its content much more than on the name signed at the bottom of the letter, so keep that in mind.

Also, in an attempt to provide variety, choose recommenders who can give examples covering a wide range of work experiences. If your boss will be most able to cite examples of your leadership abilities, then get your second recommendation from a coworker who has seen how well you work in teams. Ideally, each recommendation that you submit will present a well-rounded picture of you. But it is acceptable to have recommendations that each emphasize a particular dimension, if each of your recommenders has mostly seen you perform in certain types of situations.

Most schools want at least one of your recommendations to come from your immediate supervisor. This person should know you best in terms of your working style, your ambitions, and your strengths and weaknesses. If your current supervisor doesn't know you particularly well (perhaps you've just moved into your current role), then make sure to also get a recommendation from the person who knows you and your capabilities best.

Of course, it may be possible that you don't want your boss to know that you are applying to business school. This is fairly common, especially in disciplines outside of the traditional "feeder" industries of consulting and investment banking. Schools understand this, and most have a provision stating, "If you cannot get a recommendation from your supervisor, please attach a note explaining why." In this case, consider approaching a former boss (within your company or in a past job) or someone else with whom you have worked closely. Admissions officers prefer to hear from someone who supervised you or someone who was above you on the organizational chart, so start with those people first. The recommender needs to be more than a buddy, but a colleague who has seen you in a variety of situations can still write a good recommendation if he can provide strong examples of your leadership abilities, teamwork skills, etc.

A few schools also ask for a recommendation from a professor or advisor from your undergraduate school. In general, unless a school asks for a recommendation from an academic source, concentrate on just professional recommendations. The one exception is if you had an exceptional achievement in college that will bolster one of your application dimensions (something more than great grades or run-of-the-mill lab work). If this is the case, a recommendation from this source is worth the effort, particularly if it can emphasize any leadership traits or maturity that you haven't been able to express as much in the office.

What should they say?

Your recommendations should support the position you establish for yourself in your other application components. They should add depth to this position by citing examples that go beyond what you cover in your own essays.

Start with the grid that you built for yourself in Chapter 2. Odds are that you covered many of the Xs in your essays and data sheet, but not all of them. Your recommenders can help cover more of these examples, most often the ones pertaining to professional experience. Each example that they bring up will ideally complement what you have said about yourself in the rest of the application. A little bit of redundancy isn't damaging, but you need to make sure that your recommendations aren't simply rehashing what you have already said about yourself.

As for how they deliver the message, the advice that applies to your essays applies here as well. As the old writer's adage goes, "Show, don't tell." It is far more powerful for a recommendation to illustrate your abilities by describing concrete examples than to simply say that you are a good leader, strong analytical thinker, etc. The stories of what you did in specific situations are what admissions officers are looking for. Next we will discuss how you can arm your recommenders with the stories they can use as support for their opinions of you.

How can you make sure they're saying the right things?

Ah yes, the time-honored question. How much coaching is too much, and what do you do if you're afraid that your manager can't write an effective recommendation? It depends on several issues.

First, the ethics of the matter. Everyone would agree (we hope) that you shouldn't write your own recommendations. Outside of the ethical reason not to write your own recommendation, chances are that you'll struggle to write a letter as well as a good recommender would. We've found that recommenders come up with examples that we've long since forgotten. Also, avoiding the self-written recommendation allows you to avoid the "how positive sounds too positive?" dilemma. As such, we think it's best when the recommendation is in your recommender's own words. But what if your boss says, "I'm too busy. You can go ahead and put it together and I'll be happy to sign it," leaving you to write it on your own? One option is to simply find another recommender, but odds are that you picked that person for a reason. Your other option is to try to make the process as easy as possible, and you can do that by providing the recommender with substantial background information.

Next, it's a question of how comfortable you are coaching your recommenders. Again, it needs to be written in their words, but you can help your chances a lot by at least suggesting some stories from your work history that can illustrate your key application dimensions. Even better, create a game plan, as shown in Chapter 6, and provide that to your recommenders. Also, try to provide them with a sample essay or two that provides additional details on your career goals. Review the plan with them and discuss how important the recommendation process is. In those discussions you will inevitably end up doing a lot of self-promotion, so take some time now to get comfortable with the fact that you will be tooting your own horn, or at least asking others to toot it for you. It can also be helpful to provide your recommenders with a sample recommendation, such as the one shown below, to give them an idea of the level of quality that you are expecting.

You can decide for yourself how much detail you want to include in the game plan you share with your recommenders. The idea is to give each recommender enough information so that she can make a statement about you and then back it up with a short, illustrative story. Ideally, you will give each recommender a different set of stories, so that you don't have three people all writing about the same things. This requires some extra coordination on your part, but is an important step to ensure that each recommendation adds something new (and that they don't all sound like they were written from the same template).

Of course, if you find that you can't provide multiple types of stories to each recommender, that's okay. As mentioned above, not every recommendation needs to sell 100 percent of your skills; it is most important that your recommendations all work together to present a complete picture of you as a well-rounded applicant. So, if one really stresses your teamwork skills and one puts more emphasis on your leadership skills, that's fine. Of course, you may never see what each of your recommenders writes, but you can definitely influence their output by carefully controlling the inputs that you give them.

Sample recommendation

The following is a sample recommendation that includes typical questions found on numerous applications. Note the recommender's style, as she illustrates the applicant's strengths and doesn't merely state them. We've highlighted the aspects of this recommendation that we feel are especially strong.

Top Business School Recommendation

Dear Members of the Admissions Committee:

I have had the pleasure of working with Shannan on several projects over the last 20 months, both directly as a Project Manager, and indirectly as a member of Kramer-Dover Consulting's Outsourcing Business Unit. I have had the opportunity to get to know Shannan both professionally and personally, and I believe that I can fully evaluate and recommend Shannan for enrollment at Top Business School.

I am a Project Manager in the San Francisco office of Kramer-Dover, having worked here for 12 years. I have seen many professionals over that time frame, and Shannan is clearly one of the best I have ever seen. This is no small accomplishment as Kramer-Dover hires only the best and brightest people, and Shannan is consistently in the top 15 percent of that group of people in terms of professional capabilities. In addition, she rounds out her professional expertise with many personal activities and pursuits. Consequently, the phrase that comes to mind when I think of Shannan is "Renaissance Woman."

Shannan would be a great asset to Top Business School and any future employer. Specific answers to your standard questions are included below. — — — — — — — — — — — —

> The introduction letter to the recommendation adds a professional touch and allows the recommender to summarize her thoughts before answering the specific questions.

Sincerely,

Cindy D. Peterson

Project Manager

Kramer-Dover Consulting

1.   Define your relationship to the applicant and describe the circumstances under which you have known him or her.

I first met Shannan on a project we worked on together at a telecommunications client approximately 20 months ago. As a firm, we had just begun to develop a new Outsourcing Business Unit. The first project that Shannan and I completed was the first engagement of its kind for our firm, and we believe one of the first of its kind for anyone in the industry.

I was the Project Manager on this engagement, responsible for the success and deliverables to the client for the project. Shannan was a lead consultant, reporting directly to a manager who reported to me. This engagement lasted approximately four months. During this time, Shannan and I had daily interaction in developing the methodology and deliverables associated with this new Business Unit. Because of the complexity and uncertainty of determining how this methodology applied to our client, there were numerous late night meetings and discussions that we used to refine our approach and thought process.

Over the next eight months, as I moved on to another client, my interaction with Shannan was less frequent. Our contact was mainly during meetings when our Business Unit professionals met to further our thinking and better develop our deliverables that we used at our clients. Shannan took a lead role in helping develop many of our tools, which I subsequently used for other clients. At one time, I had Shannan come to my client site for a few weeks to help "kick-start" our engagement by training other consultants on our tools. The client was so impressed by Shannan's expertise that he begged me to place her on the project. Shannan continued to play an advisory role and we completed the project in record time. The client was able to reduce operational costs by more than $100 million, due in large part to Shannan.

For the past eight months, Shannan has been reporting directly to me in another Outsourcing engagement at another large telecommunications client. We interact several times a day due to the complexity and sensitivity of the client and Shannan's key leadership role on the team.

2.   What do you consider the applicant's primary talents or strengths?

I believe that Shannan has several significant strengths that enable her to be successful as a consultant. A few of her exceptional strengths include:

❑ ***Leadership:** Shannan has the unique quality of commanding respect from her peers, clients, and leaders.*

Although Shannan would be considered a junior member of the team in her current assignment based on age or years of experience, she became the leader of the team. This was due to her grasp of the details, with the foresight of being able to articulate the activities required to complete the project successfully.

☐ *Client Relationship: Our current engagement started as a small assignment with a minimal span of influence. Largely due to the development of solid relationships with our client, we were able to create a significant role with the client in one of its key strategic areas. Shannan played a major role in developing that relationship. There was actually a time when I was telling the client to hire a less expensive consulting firm, and they refused because they trusted and believed in our consultants, namely Shannan.* — — — — — — — — — —

The recommender does a good job of giving a specific example of how Shannan's relationship with the client played a crucial role in the success of the project.

☐ *Teamwork: Shannan is everyone's favorite consultant to ask questions of. Many consultants and clients refer to her on a wide range of issues including finance, industry information, regulatory interpretation, and consulting tools. Everyone feels comfortable going to her, because she is very approachable, friendly, articulate, knowledgeable, and goes out of her way to help.* — — — —

These bullet points really highlight Shannan's strengths and position her as a leader who is great to work with and for.

3.   What do you consider the applicant's weaknesses or developmental needs?

Shannan's development needs revolve around gaining more high-level experience in the consulting profession. These types of experiences include:

☐ *Conducting formal performance reviews and career development discussions with subordinates within the firm.*

☐ *Having a significant role in the selling of our professional services to our clients.*

☐ *Developing a broad base of client roles, relationships, and engagement experiences.*

☐ *Presenting in more formal settings to high-level client or firm leadership.*

4.   What did you like best about working side-by-side with the candidate?

Shannan is a very well-rounded individual, professionally and personally, which makes working with her enjoyable. She is not one-dimensional, and always has some insight or anecdote to share with a team. She epitomizes Kramer-Dover's core attributes of integrity, teamwork, flexibility, leadership, reliability, and professionalism.

Outside of her demonstrated professional capabilities, one aspect of Shannan's character that greatly impresses me is how she is just all-around a great person—a "Renaissance Woman." On top of her professional talent (and related time commitment), Shannan still finds time to be a Big Sister through the Big Brothers Big Sisters Program. This is a relationship that she has developed over several years, not a "try it and see if I like it" kind of relationship. Shannan is also active in fund-raising and recruiting at her undergraduate alma mater. — — — — — — —

This section demonstrates Shannan's desire to get involved with the community and her initiative. The school's takeaway is that Shannan is multi-dimensional.

5. Comment on the applicant's personal integrity.

I rate a person's integrity and behavior based on how their peers and clients perceive them. Shannan has an enormous amount of respect. People enjoy being around her. They can "bank" on her answers to their questions as being accurate. Shannan conducts herself in a very professional manner under very stressful conditions. She is a role model for new consultants in our firm. I trust Shannan to perform with the utmost integrity and accountability in all aspects of her profession.

6. Please discuss observations you have made concerning the applicant's leadership abilities, team, and/or group skills.

I believe the largest change in Shannan over the past 20 months is the growth she has exhibited in the leadership area. When I first worked with Shannan, she was very effective at doing what she was told. Now, she clearly goes beyond performing tasks and seeks out ways to increase the performance of the entire team, not only her own work. Shannan is the leader of the team, and also shows an active interest in several of the other teams by inserting herself in areas that she can help to resolve issues, answer questions, and overall contribute to their progress.

7. What impact has this person had on the organization in which he or she works?

Shannan has had a major impact on Kramer-Dover. On an individual level she has been responsible for generating well over $25 million for the firm. From a client perspective, she has been directly responsible for improving profitability by almost $250 million. When you take into consideration how much she has trained internal employees and external staff in addition to the benefits of having her in a team environment, Shannan is responsible for having an even much greater impact.

Additionally, Shannan has helped create a lot of internal interest for the telecommunications industry in general and specifically our Outsourcing Business Unit. Although I am not part of her region, it is my sense that Shannan is very popular within her peer group. I receive many phone calls from consultants in her region who would love to be part of our projects. We have been able to staff some of those consultants in large part due to Shannan's influence. Her presence is a signal to others that it must be interesting to work on our engagements. This impact has resulted in large growth in terms of the number of projects we sell in addition to the number of consultants we have been able to staff.

8. What will this individual be doing in 10 years? Why?

I'm not even sure what I'll be doing in 10 years, but my guess is that Shannan will be a successful partner in our firm. She has indicated to me that she would like to come back to our firm post-graduation and practice in our growing Mergers and Acquisitions Business Unit, focusing on the telecommunications industry. She enjoys the challenge that consulting brings, and possesses all of the major attributes required to be successful. I'm convinced that she will not only be a partner, but a global leader within our firm. I'm convinced of this because Shannan has been successful in everything she has been determined to do. — — — — — — — — — — — — — — — —

> The game plan that Shannan provided to her recommenders helped make sure that this message aligned with her essays on career goals.

9. If you have additional comments that you think would assist the Admissions Committee in making this decision, please add them here.

Shannan is the best all-around consultant I've had the opportunity to work with. She has become an invaluable resource to numerous employees in our firm, and to our clients. She has managed to do outstanding work in our difficult working environment through the use of her leadership, teamwork, analytical, personal, social, and all-around consulting skills. She has managed to meet the ultimate professional challenge—earn respect through outstanding professional effort and achieve outstanding results. She has also become a personal friend whom I trust and hold in high regard. I believe Shannan would become a welcome addition to Top Business School. — — — — —

> Strong closing that again touches upon Shannan's main strengths.

Logistics

This mostly boils down to one concept: Give your recommenders enough time to do their thing! You should plan on giving each recommender at least two months to go from start to a finished recommendation. Right about now you may be asking, "But what if I don't have two months?" If that's the case, then start immediately, but realize that you may already be making tradeoffs in terms of recommendation quality. Just like essays, very few great recommendations are written overnight. Even if you're particularly close with someone and think that you can get a week's turnaround from him, you still risk getting a rushed recommendation. Unfortunately, the admissions committee will likely translate this into either you being disorganized or your recommender not particularly caring about whether or not you get in (which also reflects badly on you). Ideally, your recommender will have enough time to digest your game plan, write her piece, let it sit for at least a few days, then revisit it and make improvements where needed—again, very similar to the essay-writing process.

Also, make sure that you know what your recommenders need to do once they're done writing their letters. Some schools ask that the recommenders submit the letters via mail by themselves, some ask that they submit them online, and others want you to send them with the rest of your completed application. Again, build enough time into your planning to account for this "back-end" part of the process. If a recommender fails to get her letter to the school in time, the admissions committee will consider it to be your fault.

Some of your recommenders may want to write a single letter that you can use for multiple schools. While most schools' recommendation forms are quite similar, there are enough subtle differences that you should try to avoid this as much as possible. Some schools (Stanford is one example) expressly discourage this practice. If a really valuable recommender insists that she can't write you multiple recommendations, make sure to start by getting a recommendation for your most selective school, and then weigh the benefits of recycling that recommendation for another school versus getting an entirely new letter for a different school. Again, you should think about your recommendations in totality. So, if you already have a strong, specific recommendation for a particular school, then having a second one that is somewhat recycled is more acceptable. This is another reason to limit the number of schools that you target. Naturally, as this number grows it becomes more difficult to receive a letter that is written specifically for each school. In general, you should avoid asking a potential recommender to complete more than three recommendations. This will help ensure that you receive specific responses for each recommendation.

Overall, we advise erring on the side of choosing recommendations that were written specifically for a given school. But this isn't always feasible, so you can afford to get some mileage out of an existing recommendation if you feel that it still adds something to your application that your other recommendations don't, and that it actually answers the questions that the admissions committee asks (which is obviously important!). If you can't get specific recommendations written, ask your recommenders to write a single recommendation that covers all of the questions for which your target schools ask.

Resume

In many ways, preparing a resume or curriculum vitae for your b-school applications seems redundant. After all, you are already required to report your employment history in the data sheets and expound on your professional experiences and career goals in the essays. So what's the point of requiring the resume? For one, the resume summarizes your background into one page. This allows the admissions committee to get a high-level understanding of where you're coming from and what you've accomplished. Secondly, your resume will often be the only reference point that your admissions interviewer has on you. For those two reasons, it's important that you prepare a resume that reflects your story from both a background and a career goals standpoint.

Format

We suggest that you follow the standard one-page, reverse-chronological order format. Producing a resume that is longer than one page shows an inability to state concisely the important aspects of your background. Given the fact that admissions representatives probably won't spend much more than two minutes reviewing your resume, your goal should be to make your points succinct yet effective. Writing your resume in reverse chronological order allows you to display your progress over time. Additionally, the admissions representative will probably spend the majority of her time concentrating on the top of your resume, so you want your best stuff to come across first.

One way that you can make sure that your format fits well with your target schools is by using your target schools' formats in creating your resume. Many business schools have standard formats that their students are required to follow. Using those formats can be a simple way to show that you've done some due diligence on the school and ensure that your format works. You should be able to gain access to a school's format through a friend, colleague, or a quick search on *www.google.com*. Going with a business school's standard format gives you the added benefit of having a pre-formatted baseline resume from which you can work once you start classes.

In general though, your resume should consist of three sections: education, experience, and additional. The commonly followed rule is that if you are coming out of school, you should place the education section first, but in other cases, the experience section should be placed first. The placement of one in front of the other is supposed to reflect their level of relative importance based on where you are in your career. In terms of business school admissions, your academic background is just as important as your professional background, so you have some flexibility here in terms of placement. If you follow a business school's format, then the education section will almost certainly come first.

Content

It's easy to get wrapped up in figuring out what format you want to use for the resume, but don't let that overshadow the more important task of creating your resume's content. As much as possible, you should try to make sure that your resume reflects the four dimensions: innovation, maturity, leadership, and teamwork. You should also make sure that progression in responsibility and achievements are highlighted. Finally, it should be clear that your career goals are achievable in light of your background, and that the target school is a good place for you to develop the skills you need to achieve those goals. This means emphasizing the experiences that are relevant to your career goals and deemphasizing those that are not.

In covering your experiences, you should focus on your actions and their result, not on your job descriptions. Provide tangible figures as much as possible. This is probably the biggest mistake that applicants make in regard to the resume. They make subjective statements, such as "Interfaced with Sales and Marketing in order to evaluate product potential." This statement is of little value to the resume reviewer and basically just takes up space. Your focus should be on providing the reviewer with hard numbers, so that she can see how your actions translate into success. Let's take another look at how this statement could be phrased: "Worked with seven members of Sales and Marketing in evaluating a new product with $125 million revenue potential. Evaluation led to eventual launch and 35 percent market share." Certainly this approach takes up more room, but it is more effective than wasting space with esoteric statements about your contributions.

To serve as an example, consider the case of a fictitious applicant named Stephen Pearson. Stephen's career goal is to work for a venture capital firm, focusing on high-tech investments. Take a look at Stephen's resume and pay particular attention to how he focuses on actions and results. His resume certainly isn't perfect, but it does do a nice job of touching on each of the four dimensions while showing fit with his career goals. We've added some commentary to stress the aspects of the resume that we feel are truly solid.

STEPHEN PEARSON

2220 Tenth Street, Apt. 320

New York, NY 10027

(212) 555-1234

spearson@coldmail.com

EDUCATION

CARELLA UNIVERSITY   **Washington D.C. May 1999**

Bachelor of Arts degree in Mathematics and Economics, Honors

- ❏ Honors thesis in Economics.
- ❏ Elected Economics Student Association Representative.
- ❏ Co-Founder of student investment fund.
- ❏ Co-Chaired Big Brother/Big Sister Program. _ _ _ _

> Stephen immediately comes across as someone who is intelligent, well-liked, willing to get involved, and takes initiative.

CHARTERED FINANCIAL ANALYST (CANDIDATE)

Passed all three levels of CFA exam and completed 18 of 36 months investment-related work experience.— — — — — —

> Don't hesitate to show accomplishments that are in progress. For example, if you are learning a new language, taking a statistics course, or participating in a public speaking class, try and mention it somewhere.

PROFESSIONAL EXPERIENCE

EISENBERG WEXLER-MERGERS & ACQUISITIONS GROUP   New York, NY

Associate   **2001-2003**

Constructed more than 100 financial models including discounted cash flow, comparable company and accretion/dilution analyses. Evaluated more than $4.5 billion potential transactions including leveraged buyouts, acquisitions, and spin-offs. Worked with more than 10 advisory teams composed of company executives, attorneys, investment bankers, and accountants. Received highest rating among the associate class.

> Nice summary. Shows Stephen's ability to stand out even in a highly-competitive environment.

- ❏ Lead associate in the $145 million leveraged buyout of Stapleton International, manufacturer of semiconductors.

- ❏ Structured the $900 million sale of Seeber Trust, software development company. Conducted benchmark, competitor, and valuation analyses, assisted in bid evaluation, and oversaw auction processes. Led due diligence process, which included more than 75 hours of dedicated company analysis.

- ❏ Researched more than 40 companies in the high-technology sector to identify potential clients whose combined market capitalization was over $70 billion. Led more than 20 meetings with clients to discuss financing needs and strategic objectives.

> Displays deep industry knowledge that certainly would be used in his desired career.

- ❏ Assisted in business development efforts, including the hosting of M&A seminars that more than 150 executives attended and resulted in more than $75 million in business.

- ❏ Created financing strategy and raised more than $70 million for Schudmak Incorporated through debt and equity offerings.

- ❏ Developed training materials and oversaw training of 35 new analysts and summer MBA associates.

> Shows willingness to perform "extracurricular" activities and an ability to work with others.

SANNI MUTUAL FUNDS   **San Francisco, CA**
High-Yield Bond Analyst   **1999-2001**

- ❏ Researched high-tech and aerospace industries to determine trends and develop outlook on industry opportunities and threats.

- ❏ Made buy/hold/sell recommendations to portfolio managers for $150 million in industry holdings based on industry outlook and analysis of the underlying companies' financial information and business strategies.

- ❏ Analyzed Japanese economy, specifically banking industry, and recommended the sale of $30 million of Japanese bank preferred shares 10 months prior to Japanese sovereign credit downgrade by rating services.

Management Trainee

❏ Supervised a diverse department of 35 employees, mostly 1st and 2nd generation Americans from 7 countries.

WALLER SECURITIES Washington, D.C.

Brokerage Intern **Summer 1998**

❏ Created a database that segmented 45 brokers' accounts according to sales potential.

❏ Completed the Series 7 exam and received license to buy and sell financial securities.— — — — — — — —

> Displays fit with future career goals and profession from here to the point he achieves CFA status.

ADDITIONAL INFORMATION

❏ Languages: Conversant in Spanish, working toward fluency. — — — — — — — — — — — — — — — —

> Language capabilities are always an added bonus.

❏ Community: Teach economics through Junior Achievement to a 27-student class and helped establish two new Junior Achievement programs in the local community.— — — — — — — — — — — — —

> Nice job of showing community involvement. He doesn't simply list community service activities.

❏ Hobbies: Traveling, personal investing, golf, chess, deep sea diving.— — — — — — — — — — — — —

> Shows he has a life outside of work.

The Admissions Consultant Question

It's a question that many business school applicants ask at some point in the process: "Should I spend a couple of thousand dollars on an admissions consulting service?" No matter how excellent your experiences are or how sharp your story is, the intimidating odds of getting into the top schools means that this question will likely cross your mind somewhere along the way. The short answer is...it depends.

First, let's look at what an admission consultant can do for you. Typical service offerings provided by admissions consultants include:

- ❏ An end-to-end service that starts with an in-depth interview, where the consultant will get to know you and learn about your experiences, your goals, and your strengths and weaknesses. The consultant will then help you develop a compelling application story (this is usually the most valuable part of the consultant's offering), and work with you to weave it through every part of your application, especially your essays and your recommendations. The consultant will also coach you on how to handle the interview. Admissions consultants tend to know the top business schools quite well, and they will give you a professional second opinion on which schools you should consider based on your profile.

- ❏ A more limited offering that covers certain parts of your application, most often your essays. These services appeal to applicants who are confident that their application stories are sound, and want some help in fine tuning their message. Some consultants offer this "stripped-down" service as an alternative to an end-to-end service, while others strictly offer essay editing services.

In terms of pricing, you can expect that access to such services will set you back anywhere from $50 to $4,000. Naturally, the more a consultant does for you, the more you will pay. Some will charge you a flat fee for their services, while others will charge you on a per-application or a per-essay basis.

Once you hire a consultant for the "full-service" treatment, he will first take an in-depth inventory of your career up until this point. He will quiz you on:

- ❏ What extracurriculars you did in college.
- ❏ Why you chose your major.
- ❏ Your grades in college.
- ❏ Why you chose your current employer.
- ❏ Evidence of success in your job.
- ❏ Your extracurriculars outside of the workplace.
- ❏ Your future career goals.
- ❏ Your GMAT scores (if you have taken the exam).
- ❏ What you're looking for in a business school.
- ❏ Which schools you are targeting.

He may also ask for writing samples, including any application essays that you have already written. All of these questions will help him answer the question of, "How good are this applicant's chances?" He will evaluate you using the same criteria that admissions committees use, and will be pretty frank about your chances at each of your target schools, possibly suggesting that you narrow or broaden your scope.

Once your admissions consultant knows you better, he will work with you to develop an overall application story. This will be the high-level "Here's who I am, and this is where I want to go" theme, similar to the story that this book helps you create. Once that is in place, he will work with you on each of the application components. Most consultants will spend the majority of their time on your essays, followed by your recommendations and your interview. If your GMAT score is too low, an admissions consultant can help point you to the right resources.

The most value that admissions consultants provide is usually in helping you present your story in a coherent package and in supplying you with third-party insight. They usually have a good idea of what each school is looking for, and are usually on top of the trends in business school admissions. Some even offer post-admissions advice, such as which courses to take once you get to school, although most applicants mainly pay for the chance to improve their admissions odds.

So, cost aside, admissions consultants do tend to help people get in. Similar to GMAT prep courses, at the very least these services tend to provide a good kick in the pants for applicants who need someone looking over their shoulder, prodding them to get their recommendations in on time, etc. They're also usually good essay editors, and they generally do know what admissions committees are looking for. But know that no admissions consultant (at least not any scrupulous one) will write your essays for you. He will push you, stretch your thinking, and help you remember accomplishments that you didn't think would matter in your application, but he will not simply take your resume and spin it into a golden application. The bottom line is that only you can write your own story. Admissions counselors can help you discover it, but you'll have to tell it.

Now let's return to the big question of whether or not you should hire an admissions consultant, first by answering an easier question: Do you need these services? Almost always, the answer is no. Given enough time and the right resources (all of which add up to far less than the price of a consulting service), nearly anyone can research a school in depth, craft a compelling story, develop a strong set of essays, perform well on the GMAT, get glowing recommendations, and nail the interview. In short, you can most likely do on your own all of the things that you would hire an admissions consultant to help you do. It's just a matter of time, motivation, and resources (this book will play a large role in the last one).

Finally, you have to take these service's success records with a grain of salt. There is likely some selection bias going on. We believe that admissions consultants are telling the truth when they boast that most of their clients get into at least one of their target schools, but we don't know much about who their clients are. Even if they don't have GMAT scores hovering somewhere above the stratosphere, they are probably among the more motivated applicants you will find. We don't doubt that admissions consultants have helped all of these applicants to some·extent, but you have to wonder how many of these applicants would have gotten in on their own.

Okay, so who does use these services? Someone must be paying money to these consultants if they're still around, right? There are definitely situations in which a b-school candidate would benefit from an admissions consultant, more than the average applicant would:

❐ **No business experience:** We discussed these kinds of applicants in Chapter 3. They absolutely can get into business school, but they may have an unclear understanding of how to communicate their experiences in a way that admissions officers will respond to. Also, unlike bankers or consultants, they likely know far fewer people who can give them advice throughout the process. Thus, admissions consultants can often add insight to which they might not otherwise have access.

❐ **A glaring weakness:** Some people will never get above a 600 on the GMAT, no matter how hard they try. In instances like these, an admissions consultant can help applicants bolster their perceived analytical abilities (often by encouraging them to do the things that we advise in this book), and help them overcome weaknesses with an application that shines in every other way. More generally, consultants can sometimes help an applicant rise above a shortcoming that would otherwise keep him out of his target school.

❐ **International applicants:** Similar to the "no business experience" crowd, some international applicants may have a harder time getting their hands on sound application advice and information on their target schools, in which case admissions consultants can help. Also, consultants can help them with simple language barrier issues that could keep them from gaining admission.

Lastly, some applicants enroll the help of an admissions consultant because they simply lack the confidence that they can get in on their own. If you've read this book, have evaluated your own background, and still feel that you don't stand a chance, then it's okay to look into hiring a consultant. But don't fool yourself into thinking that the competition walks on water, and that the only way you stand a chance of getting in is by hiring a professional. It's easy to get caught up in an imaginary arms race in which everyone else is taking GMAT prep courses and buying books on how to get in, so you need to do them one better by hiring a full-blown admissions consulting service. The reality is that most other applicants are just like you—they have some good experiences, are bright, can communicate pretty well, but also have a weakness or two. Some have GMAT scores above yours, and some have more impressive professional experiences, but none of them is any more entitled to a top-tier MBA than you are. So relax and let your personality and your strengths come through in every part of your application. Using this book will help you do exactly that.

FAQs

Does it matter which round I apply in?

The old adage is, "the earlier you apply, the better." Generally, admissions officers state that there is very little difference between the first and second rounds. Beyond round two, however, many schools fill just a handful of remaining seats, so your odds of getting in plummet dramatically. We recommend not even considering applying after the second round, unless you find yourself in an extreme circumstance. We recommend the first round above the second round for a couple of reasons. First, more applicants apply in round two than in any other round, meaning that you will have a better chance (even if it's a slight one) of standing out in round one. Also, applying early helps to communicate your interest in the school, which is always a plus. Finally, applying in the first round means that you will probably receive responses from your schools in the January time frame. This is advantageous from a planning standpoint. After all, there is plenty of work to be done after you receive an admittance.

If you are confident that waiting to apply in the second round will give you time to take your application from good to great, then that is definitely a tradeoff that is worth making. You want to make sure to put your best foot forward even if that means waiting a round.

As an international applicant to U.S. b-schools, how do I translate my GPA?

For the most part, you shouldn't need to translate your GPA. In general, international applicants (defined as an applicant who is neither a U.S. citizen nor a U.S. permanent resident) are required to submit their official academic records in their original language along with literal English translations prepared by the academic institutions. Most schools will also accept translations from the consulate, embassy, or other such organizations of the institutions' country. Business schools are very familiar with the various grading policies across countries and are very aware that the 4.0 scale used in the United States is not universal. For that reason, U.S. b-schools take a close look at your academic standing relative to your classmates in assessing your performance. You should follow up with your target schools in order to understand their specific policies.

Do my AWA scores really matter?

In comparison to the base and individual GMAT scores, the AWA doesn't matter much at all. When was the last time you saw a b-school publish its average AWA score? In judging applicants' writing ability, schools tend to emphasize their own essays much more than the AWA and pretty much glance at the score as an afterthought. With that said, you shouldn't totally blow off the AWA. There are some cases in which the school will take a closer look at the score; most notably in a situation where admissions counselors suspect someone else other than the applicant responded to application essays. That alarm can be triggered when the applicant comes from a highly technical or international background, has the essays of a literary genius and an AWA score below 4.0. Therefore, you should become familiar with this portion of the exam and attempt a few sample essays, but you shouldn't spend nearly as much time preparing for it as you do preparing for the main sections of the GMAT.

Is it possible to increase my GMAT score more than a few points?

As a business school applicant, you will most likely run into some people who will insist that the GMAT exam is like an IQ test in that you can't improve your score. This is definitely not the case. While you may never be able to hit 800, you can definitely improve your score by a significant amount. There are a number of applicants who were able to increase their score by well over 100 points. The key is to remain diligent in preparation and to not develop a psychological apprehension towards taking the exam.

What do schools do if I retake the GMAT?

Schools almost universally take your highest total score into consideration if you retake the GMAT. This is in the school's best interest because it allows the school to report higher average GMAT scores to periodicals for their rankings. Indeed, as average scores have increased, applicants have begun to retake the exam more often. You shouldn't, however, take the examination over and over again indiscriminately. Schools that see such behavior will question whether you understand what the purpose of applying is. Taking the exam more than three times may raise some eyebrows, so you should put your best foot forward on each attempt.

How early in the process should I interview?

Just like everything else in the application process, scheduling an interview earlier rather than later should only help your chances (when it is actually up to you to schedule the interview). From a logistics perspective, scheduling early is beneficial because spots are taken very quickly. Friday interviews can be especially difficult to lock down. We recommend spending a great deal of time on your application, getting it done early, and then doing your interview shortly thereafter.

Should I always do an interview, even if it's optional?

Yes, you should make every effort to interview with your target schools. It will demonstrate your interest and help the admissions committee put a face to a name. If it's difficult for you to arrange an interview (such as for geographic reasons), then going through the process of setting one up is all the more impressive. If you can't do one in person, try to at least arrange a telephone interview, which is better than nothing.

What should I do if the interviewer is rude or late?

If your interviewer is considerably late but it doesn't affect the amount of time that you have for the interview, let it go. Focus on being positive and getting your main points across once the interview begins. If your interviewer's late arrival does cut into the amount of time that you have, then consider requesting a follow-up interview. Few interviewers will put you in this situation (the ones that do are typically harried alums), but if they do, be positive and polite, but firm.

If your interviewer is just plain rude (again, this tends to happen with alumni more than with admissions personnel), keep your cool. They may very well be testing you, so the worst thing you can do is try to fight fire with fire. Stay calm and confidently answer the questions that they ask. Remember, it's up to you to emphasize your main points. It's not up to the interviewer to get you to bring them out. If you are asked an inappropriate question (it's been known to happen), know that you don't have to answer it. Stay positive and professional, but let the interviewer know that you won't get sucked in.

After the interview, if you feel that the interviewer behaved unprofessionally and that you weren't able to make your case because of it, consider contacting someone in the admissions office to request a new interview. Again, keep it as positive as possible and remember that the goal is to get yourself into business school, not to get back at your interviewer.

Some candidates are tempted to contact the admissions office after they have a bad interview, even if the interviewer did nothing wrong. Don't do this. It will sound "whiny," and will most likely only hurt your chances. Also, a lot of applicants feel that they bombed their interview when they actually get a positive evaluation. In that case, calling undue attention to the interview can only hurt your cause. Only contact the admissions committee if the interviewer behaved rudely or unprofessionally in some way.

What if I freeze up?

If your interviewer asks you a question and your mind goes blank, it's entirely okay to take a moment to collect your thoughts. In fact, most interviewers appreciate it when an applicant says something like "Let me think about that for a moment" or "That's a good question." Silence is okay. In fact, silence is considered to be one of the most effective communication tools there is, so learn to get comfortable with it. Pausing shows that you're giving a question a lot of thought, which is good. Whatever you do, don't just start talking and hope for something good to come out. Many applicants do this, but they end up doing more harm than good. If you are at a loss, simply take a deep breath and take a few moments to gather your thoughts before speaking. It will only help you.

If I'm intending to return to my present company after graduation, what message should I convey?

This is something at which many applicants fail miserably. Uninspired by the fact that they will return to their present employer after business school, applicants who fall into this category tend to write about their career goals in a dispassionate manner. If you intend to return to your current company, then say so. It's fine to acknowledge the fact that it's the career path you would like to follow. However, you need to be very specific in demonstrating how an MBA will help improve your skills. Additionally, you need to demonstrate how you intend to have an impact on the future direction of the company. This doesn't mean listing the titles you hope to achieve, but rather stating the problems you want to address and some form of innovation that you would like to use in addressing them. Simply highlighting the fact that you intend to return to XYZ consulting firm will make you sound just like 95 percent of your direct competitors. Go the extra step, and be explicit about what you will do that you can't do without an MBA.

Who should I have review my essays?

Ideally, among the people who review your essays will be a good writer/editor, one person who knows you really well, and someone who is familiar with the business school application process (such as a current student, alum, or fellow applicant). You obviously want a good writer to read your essay to check for grammatical errors and ways in which you can improve the structure of your essays. You would also like someone who knows you well enough to read them, as a sort of litmus test to make sure that the essays actually sound like they came from you. After all, your own voice should come through in your essays. Finally, someone who has navigated the admissions process will be able to provide other insights as to how well your essays help your overall application story. One person may very well fit all three of these descriptions, in which case you don't need too many people reading your essays. However, showing your essays to at least one person who doesn't know you too well can help, because that person is better able to flag areas that are confusing to someone who isn't familiar with your background. Plus, having an extra set of eyeballs to catch typos is always a good thing.

One note: It is possible to get too much feedback. Some applicants try to incorporate so much feedback into their essays that the final product sounds nothing like what they started with. As a result, the application no longer sounds as though it were written by the applicant. Remember that you have the final say on everything that goes into your essays. Don't feel obligated to include every last bit of advice that you receive.

How many recommenders should I recruit?

You may only need two or three recommenders total, but it depends on how many schools you apply to, and on how busy your recommenders are. Start by recruiting your immediate supervisor or, if this isn't possible, another coworker who knows you well and can comment on your professional abilities. You'll then want to add one more colleague from your work, and perhaps someone who can comment on your abilities in another light, such as someone whom you know from an extracurricular activity. You can reasonably expect each person to complete at most three or four recommendations. More is possible, but you'll risk spreading each recommender too thin. So, be ready to recruit more recommenders as needed, assuming that each additional recommender is also qualified to comment on your strengths and weaknesses. Ideally, though, your immediate supervisor will complete a recommendation for every one of your target schools. Because most schools ask that one of your recommendations come from your supervisor, do everything in your power to make it easy for her to complete a recommendation for each one of your applications.

My supervisor's writing is horrendous. What should I do?

This can be a delicate situation, depending on how close you are with your supervisor, but there are ways to deal with it. If you know ahead of time that your supervisor's writing isn't strong but don't feel comfortable reviewing her recommendation, then consider recruiting a capable third party to serve as an editor. Ask your boss, "Would you mind having Jane give it a read-through before you submit it?" Most bosses will respond positively, or they may even suggest that you review it yourself, but few will balk at the suggestion. After all, they want to help you get in (unless they hate you, in which case you should ask someone else for a recommendation). Once you or someone else is able to review it and make changes, pick your spots carefully. Don't obsess over every word or punctuation mark (although you want to catch all obvious typos), but rather focus on making sure that the recommendation is readable, is well-organized, and makes the points that you want emphasized. Don't be afraid to make the changes that need to be made, or at least suggest them. When you go back to your boss with the revisions, keep everything very positive, and give reasons for your suggestions. Most supervisors will appreciate the help. If yours doesn't, and you know that the final product is destined to be terrible, then start looking for a Plan B. After all, how intelligent your recommenders come across in their written work will reflect upon you, too.

How do schools use the evaluation grid that recommenders are required to fill out?

Admissions officers know that most recommenders feel that they need to give "Outstanding" ratings for each trait in the evaluation grid, lest they hurt their applicant's chances. They therefore don't place too much emphasis on the grid, and instead spend most of their time reading the recommendation letter. Still, the grid communicates a good amount of information very quickly, and application readers will scan it to get an idea of what your strengths and weaknesses are. If your recommender gives you the absolute best rating in each category, then that actually doesn't give the admissions committee much to go on (other than the fact that you're amazing, which the rest of your recommendation had better support). If you receive "Outstanding" ratings for four categories and receive "Very Good" for the other two, then the admissions committee will think about those two a bit more, and see what your recommender has to say about those traits elsewhere in the recommendation. In any case, what the grid says is less important than the supporting evidence that is presented in the written recommendation. Nonetheless, you probably don't want your recommender giving you anything lower than the second rating. Anything below that will likely catch an application reader's eye and cause him to dig deeper. Your main focus should be on arming your recommenders with examples that illustrate each of the traits in the grid will help you the most.

What is an appropriate gift to get my recommenders for their assistance?

Writing recommendations is a difficult job; especially when you consider the busy schedules of those who are often asked to do it. After it's all said and done, your recommenders definitely deserve some recognition for their efforts. Giving each recommender a token of your appreciation is the least that you can do as an applicant. Depending on how well you know your recommenders, there are a number of great gifts with which you can provide them. Common examples include: a gift certificates to a nice restaurant, fresh flowers, or wine. Some applicants wait until they receive their admittances and then give their recommenders a memento from their chosen school, such as a shirt, sweatshirt, or coffee mug. Naturally this strategy can backfire if you don't get admitted. Regardless, there is only one simple rule that you should follow: "Don't be cheap!" In addition to a thoughtful gift, a handwritten thank-you card is also always a nice gesture. Outside of common courtesy, showing your gratitude is a good idea because you never know whether you might have to call on your recommenders again to serve as your champions (for job references, etc.). Making them glad that they helped you now will only make it easier for you to ask for their help again in the future.

How should I structure my resume if I'm a recent college graduate or have no professional work experience?

As mentioned in Chapter 3, if you're in this situation, you should try to emphasize your leadership, maturity, and teamwork dimensions. Because you don't have much professional experience, the education section should come first. Here you should discuss as many extracurricular activities as possible that display those dimensions. Additionally, this is a case in which you should include your GMAT score and your GPA, assuming that they're high, to show your intellectual capacity. If you have any work experience, including internships or entrepreneurial ventures, make sure to include them.

5

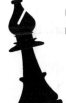

Developing Strategies for
the Top Programs

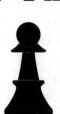

You've demonstrated your strengths and addressed your weaknesses. You have multiple examples that demonstrate your leadership and problem-solving capacity. Your differentiated position will leap off the page as the admissions committee pores over your application.

Great. You're halfway there. Now comes the other—equally important—part: demonstrating how you and your skills are a good fit for each of your target schools. Applicants sometimes forget about this part of the process. After all, a lot of schools' essay questions seem pretty similar. No harm in just copying and pasting, changing the school's name, tweaking a few lines, and moving on, right? In reality, most applicants have done this with at least one application, but doing so means possibly missing what each school is really looking for.

Researching Schools

So how exactly do you determine what a school wants in its applicants? Start with the usual suspects:

- ❑ **The school's Website:** This is a no-brainer these days. Here you can get high-level information on the school, learn about its curriculum and faculty, and start to get a sense for what it's known for (or what it wants to be known for, which is sometimes more important).

- ❑ **Third-party Websites:** For different perspectives on business schools and the application process, check out Websites that dedicate content to the b-school applicant audience. Some of the more popular sites include: BusinessWeek Online (*www.businessweek.com/bschools*) and MBA Jungle (*www.mbajungle.com*).

- ❑ **Brochure and application:** These are readily accessible on any school's Website. It can be painful to look at brochure after brochure of what seems to be the same material, but you should really spend some time with these. Think about how long each admissions officer will spend getting to know your application, and spend at least twice as much time with the school's material. More than many applicants realize, schools are fairly explicit about what they are looking for, and these materials are a natural starting point for finding this information.

❏ **Rankings:** Rankings are notoriously overused, but they can give you a good high-level flavor for each school. While the brochures may tell you what the schools want to be known for, the rankings issued by periodicals are sometimes a good reality check that let you know what a school is actually good at.

❏ **Campus visit:** Whether or not you interview on campus, you should plan on visiting each school in which you're truly interested, unless geography makes it impossible. Walk around, meet some current students, sit in on a class, and at least visit the admissions office to let the school know you came. Odds are that the office will probably blow you off, but it's worth a shot. Whether or not you get any good face time with an admission officer, make sure to mention your visit somewhere in your application to show your sincere interest in the school.

❏ **Current students:** Students are probably the most underutilized resource. Even if you don't visit the campus, it's easy to find business school students' contact info on the Web. Find one with whom you have something in common and send her an e-mail. Some students are just too busy to have a real heart-to-heart with you, but odds are that you'll easily find someone who's willing to give you the skinny on the school. Think of a few things you want to know about life at the school and fire away. This is a safe way to ask candid questions about the school.

❏ **Alumni:** Alumni are especially helpful in answering questions about what life will be like after business school. Ask them about their experiences in school, but realize that schools evolve over time, so realize that someone who graduated 15 years ago probably had a pretty different experience than what you would face.

❏ **MBA Forums:** MBA Forums, hosted by the GMAC, provide applicants with an informal environment in which they can learn more about business schools and the admissions process. Over 200 b-schools typically attend these forums, which take place in cities around the world. In addition to opportunities to speak with b-school representatives, MBA Forums host workshops that assist applicants in selecting their target schools and in exploring their career options. For more information on MBA Forums, check out *www.mba.com*.

Understanding the Rankings

The periodic ranking of top business schools has become one of the most discussed aspects of the application process. Since 1988, when *BusinessWeek* released its first biennial ranking, multiple other media outlets have also taken a cut at evaluating business schools including: *U.S. News and World Report, Financial Times*, and more recently, *The Wall Street Journal*. Currently, each outlet claims to have the most precise, and therefore applicable, ranking methodology and has earned numerous sales as a result of their claims. Indeed, the rankings are generally the first place aspiring applicants look when deciding whether and where to apply. No doubt you will evaluate the ranking that rates your favorite school the highest as the most "fair."

Not many people would have expected it 20 years ago, but the rankings have gained a lot of power in influencing both applicants and schools themselves. Here is a quick look at what some of the major issues surrounding the rankings are.

Impact

Rankings have had a powerful effect on the business school world. Recruiters, admissions directors, faculty, students, and applicants all keep a close eye on them. Over time, most schools have made positive changes to their facilities, curricula, and recruiting processes as a result of issues that the media outlets have uncovered. If a business school makes a jump in the rankings, then the dean will most likely trumpet the success. Should a business school slip, however, then crisis management techniques often kick in. It is not unheard of for members of the business school community to be fired over a poor ranking.

Controversy

The power of the rankings has also become the center of controversy. An underlying, inherent goal of media outlets is to sell newspapers, magazines, and books. Their core competency is probably not to provide suggestions for business school improvements. Nonetheless, this is often the result of their insights. Many would argue that the rankings' ability to affect business school change has become too great and needs to be curtailed. Your challenge is to understand the rankings and their methodologies so that their impact on your decision-making is not overstated.

Methodologies

BusinessWeek

The oldest and perhaps the most publicized modern ranking of business schools comes from *BusinessWeek*. Its ranking methodology focuses on three components: student evaluations (45 percent), recruiter evaluations (45 percent), and the schools' intellectual capital (10 percent). *BusinessWeek*'s perspective is that customer evaluation (in this case students and recruiters) is what matters most in evaluating a business schools' abilities. The rankings are mainly based on responses to surveys taken by recent business school graduates and a majority of the recruiters who hire them. Because of the survey format, *BusinessWeek*'s rankings are always accompanied by detailed anecdotal information.

The *BusinessWeek* rankings are often criticized, however, for their high degree of subjectivity. Using recent graduates' perspectives as a heavily weighted component of the rankings is the aspect of this subjectivity that is most often denounced. These criticisms definitely carry some validity, as it seems a bit contradictory to create a relative ranking using input from students who have only attended one business school. That contradiction is compounded by alumni's incentive to inflate the scores that they use in evaluating their schools. Why would an alum give her school a low evaluation when she has such a vested interest in the school's status? Another apparent weakness of the *BusinessWeek* rankings is the time at which the students are evaluated. Because they have only recently graduated, it is difficult to imagine that they have more than a limited view of the value of their MBA.

Financial Times

The rankings released by *Financial Times* are undisputedly based on the most complex methodology of all of the media outlets. First released in 1999, in response to *BusinessWeek* and *U.S. News and World Report*'s omission of international programs, *Financial Times* uses 20 criteria in its evaluation of business schools. These criteria can be segmented into three groups:

- ❏ **Employment:** Salary increase over three years, return on business school investment, career progress, achievement of post-MBA goals, job employment success, and recruiter recommendations.

- ❏ **Diversity and International:** Women faculty, students, and board members; international faculty, students, and board members; international mobility and curriculum.

- ❏ **Faculty and Research:** Faculty with doctorates, number of doctoral graduates, and faculty publications.

The *Financial Times* differentiates itself from the others by taking into account graduate performance a few years after graduation and by evaluating the schools' international and research foci. However, only 2 percent of the weighting in the ranking takes the recruiters' perspectives into account and there is no formal evaluation of curricula outside of the international and research components.

U.S. News and World Report

U.S. News and World Report releases an annual ranking of the top business schools along with rankings for advanced degree programs in education, engineering, law, and medicine. Its rankings first appeared on the scene in 1990, using a mixture of subjective and objective criteria for its evaluations. This mixture creates a straightforward balance that is absent in the other rankings. The methodology is composed of eight criteria including: dean and program director evaluation, recruiter evaluation, starting compensation, job placement, GMAT score, undergraduate GPA, and percentage of application rejections.

Many would argue, however, that the methodology has contributed to selection bias. By heavily weighting the GMAT score and undergraduate GPA, *U.S. News* may encourage admissions committees to turn away applicants who might cause them to slip in the rankings. The academic peer evaluations have also raised eyebrows, as deans and program directors have an incentive to discount other business schools in their ratings.

The Wall Street Journal

In 2001, *The Wall Street Journal* shook up the rankings world by introducing a methodology that is based solely on the perspective of recruiters. The survey-based methodology is subjective in nature and asks recruiters to evaluate business schools and their students according to 26 attributes. The results of the surveys have been drastically different than any of the other three rankings, as some of the historically top schools were shuffled to the bottom and many schools normally neglected were pushed to the forefront.

Similar to the *BusinessWeek* rankings, a great deal of anecdotal revelations have resulted from the rankings, but the methodology has several contradictions from the perspective of applicants. Because recruiters and students sit on opposite sides of the negotiating table, there are some attributes that benefit recruiters when students are disadvantaged. For example, one of the attributes of the survey has been "past acceptance rate of job offers from a student at this school." Naturally, from a recruiter's perspective, the higher the acceptance rate, the better. From a student's perspective, however, higher acceptance rates can mean less job opportunities. Aspiring applicants should therefore keep in mind that students' perspectives are not accounted for in this methodology. Many applicants have completely written this methodology off for that reason. Between the first release of the rankings and the second release, *The Wall Street Journal* made some adjustments to the survey questions to minimize some of those contradictions. Our understanding is that more adjustments are forthcoming.

Usage

So the big question remains, *"How should I view the rankings?"* The rankings should be viewed as another source of information, but definitely not as the be all, end all. If you decide to apply to the schools ranked 15–20 based on the assigned number alone, then you are probably making a bad choice. The high variation of where schools fall in the different rankings alone indicates that different schools will be better for you based on what you value. As such, rankings are a good starting point for researching schools, but shouldn't be the focal point.

If you find yourself obsessing over the rankings (most of us do at some point), use your gut. Ask yourself: "Is there really a huge difference between the 10th-ranked school and the 15th-ranked school?" Probably not. There are differences, but they will be in the details, which you will uncover through your own research.

The question you should really ask yourself is: "What school(s) can meet my academic, professional, social, geographic, and financial needs?" Naturally, the answer to this question will be different for every person. That is why no single set of rankings really works for everyone. It is a question that you must answer based on all the information available. No methodology will simply produce it for you.

The rankings of the four media outlets are listed on page 130.

Financial Times 2003 Business School Rankings	
School	Rank
University of Pennsylvania (Wharton)	1
Harvard Business School	2
Columbia University	3
Stanford University GSB	4
University of Chicago	4
INSEAD	6
London Business School	7
New York University (Stern)	8
Northwestern University (Kellogg)	9
MIT (Sloan)	10
Dartmouth College (Tuck)	11
Yale School of Management	12
IMD	13
University of Virginia (Darden)	14
Duke University (Fuqua)	15
University of California-Berkeley (Haas)	15
Georgetown University (McDonough)	17
Iese Business School	18
Cornell University (Johnson)	19
University of California-L.A. (Anderson)	20
University of Toronto (Rotman)	21
University of Western Ontario	22
Carnegie Mellon University	23
University of North Carolina (Kenan-Flagler)	23
University of Michigan Business School	25
Instituto de Empressa	26
York University (Schulich)	26
Rotterdam School of Management	28
Emory University (Goizueta)	29
University of Cambridge (Judge)	30

U.S. News 2003 Business School Rankings	
School	Rank
Harvard University	1
Stanford University	2
University of Pennsylvania (Wharton)	2
MIT (Sloan)	4
Northwestern University (Kellogg)	4
Columbia University	6
Duke University (Fuqua)	7
University of California- Berkeley (Haas)	7
University of Chicago	9
Dartmouth College (Tuck)	10
University of Virgina (Darden)	11
New York University (Stern)	12
University of Michigan	13
Yale University	14
Cornell University (Johnson)	16
Carnegie Mellon University	17
University of Texas-Austin (McCombs)	17
Ohio State University (Fisher)	19
University of Southern California (Marshall)	20
Emory University (Goizueta)	21
University of North Carolina (Kenan-Flagler)	21
Indiana University (Kelley)	23
Georgetown University (McDonough)	24
Purdue University (Krannert)	24
University of Minnesota (Carlson)	26
Rice University (Jones)	27
University of Florida (Warrington)	27
Brigham Young University (Marriott)	29
University of Iowa (Tippie)	29
University of Notre Dame (Medoza)	29
Washington University-St. Louis (Olin)	29

BusinessWeek 2002 Business School Rankings	
School	Rank
Northwestern University	1
University of Chicago	2
Harvard Business School	3
Stanford University	4
University of Pennsylvania (Wharton)	5
MIT (Sloan)	6
Columbia University	7
University of Michigan	8
Duke University (Fuqua)	9
Dartmouth College (Tuck)	10
Cornell University (Johnson)	11
University of Virginia (Darden)	12
University of California-Berkeley (Haas)	13
Yale University	14
New York University (Stern)	15
University of California-L.A. (Anderson)	15
University of Southern California (Marshall)	17
University of North Carolina (Kenan-Flagler)	18
Carnegie Mellon University	19
Indiana University (Kelley)	20
University of Texas-Austin (McCombs)	21
Emory University (Goizueta)	22
Michigan State University (Broad)	23
Washington University (Olin)	24
University of Maryland (Smith)	25
Purdue University (Krannert)	26
University of Rochester (Simon)	27
Vanderbilt University (Owen)	28
Notre Dame (Mendoza)	29
Georgetown University (McDonough)	30

Wall Street Journal 2003 Business School Rankings	
School	Rank
Dartmouth College (Tuck)	1
University of Michigan	2
Carnegie Mellon University	3
Northwestern University (Kellogg)	4
University of Pennsylvania (Wharton)	5
University of Chicago	6
University of Texas-Austin (McCombs)	7
Yale University	8
Harvard Business School	9
Columbia University	10
Purdue University (Krannert)	11
University of North Carolina (Kenan-Flagler)	12
Michigan State University (Broad)	13
Indiana University (Kelley)	14
University of California-Berkeley (Haas)	15
University of Maryland (Smith)	16
Emory University (Goizueta)	17
Cornell University (Johnson)	18
University of Virginia (Darden)	19
IMD International	20
University of Rochester (Simon)	21
Wake Forest University (Babcock)	22
New York University (Stern)	23
Duke University (Fuqua)	24
Vanderbilt University (Owen)	25
ITESM	26
IPADE	27
Southern Methodist University (Cox)	28
MIT (Sloan)	29

The school selection process

Wouldn't it be great if schools had to submit an application for you to review and then you had the opportunity to accept or reject them? Selecting which school(s) to which you will apply is about the closest you'll come to this. In selecting your schools, you must make a decision on how many to focus on. In general, there seems to be two divided camps on this decision.

The shotgun camp

Members of the shotgun camp believe that applying to top business schools is like shooting in the dark, so they use the biggest gun possible. They claim that the applicant selection process is essentially random, and they therefore target as many schools as possible. The thought is that in doing so, they will raise their overall chances of admittance. It can be easy to be seduced by the theory that the process is entirely random when you look at the low acceptance rates and hear stories of people getting into Stanford, but getting dinged by Samford. Although no one will deny that there is a certain level of "randomness" in the selection process, basing your application approach on that premise can have disastrous results. The more applications you add to the pile, the more difficult it will be to tailor them to your schools. You have to conduct more research, solicit more recommendations, and produce more essays; not mention shell out more cash (application fees can cost up to $200 each).

Ultimately this approach generally leads to a bunch of applications that all look the same. Because of schools' concerns with fit, this approach can lead to several rejections and just as bad, admittance into a school you don't want to attend. Because of these pitfalls, successful applicants tend to be members of the sniper camp.

The sniper camp

Members of the sniper camp maintain that by utilizing application strategy you have a much better chance of hitting your targets. The key here is for the applicant to perform due diligence on the schools that interest her and then conduct even more research after the target schools have been selected. By limiting the number of target schools based on their fit with your needs and objectives, you will be able to create a better story that fits with those schools rather than under the shotgun approach. Additionally, you will have more time and resources to show the requisite interest in your target schools by visiting campuses, talking to students and alumni, and investigating interesting program-specific opportunities.

You will find some applicants who succeed using the shotgun approach. But overall, taking a strategic approach will allow you to have a better chance at gaining acceptance and will allow you to get to know your target schools better.

How many schools should I apply to?

So the analogies are great, but where are the tangible numbers? We suggest that the average applicant apply to three or four schools. This allows you to target one stretch school, one safety school, and one or two schools that seem right within your range. Naturally, many external factors such as significant others, or financial or geographical constraints can present situations that call for applying to a different number of schools, but in general, three to four will allow you to perform an adequate amount of due diligence and still give you enough coverage to maximize your probability of acceptance. When you apply to more than four, you risk diluting your applications' content and limit your ability to establish fit with each target school.

Differences across schools

As you explore potential target schools, you will notice that many of the brochures look and sound the same. Indeed, there are several business school trends that have pushed schools to adopt similar learning models. Once you visit the schools, however, and dig a little deeper, you will begin to notice that there are larger differences across schools then you initially thought. Three differences across schools that you should pay special attention to are the learning model, typical career paths of graduates, and the culture.

The learning model

Most business school curricula are composed of a combination of three pedagogical methods:

❐ **Case study:** The case study method is an integral part of most students' business school experience. Cases are two to 50 page documents that focus on real-world management situations and generally place the reader in the shoes of a decision-maker. Each case generally focuses on a single topic within a course and can be written for any class from Marketing to Finance. Class discussions based on the case method are consistently dynamic and rarely conclude in a single solution. The professor generally begins class with a dreaded "cold-call." A cold-call is a business school tradition, whereby an unsuspecting student is asked to introduce the case and provide his perspectives on how the decision-maker (referred to as the case protagonist) in the case should respond to the challenges described by the case. After the student has provided his perspectives, the professor invites other students to participate and a dialogue ensues. Generally, students speak for more than 80 percent of the class with the professor directing the conversation flow. Sometimes, the case protagonist is even present and provides concluding comments on the class's dialogue.

❐ **Lecture:** We're all familiar with this teaching method. Most schools use the lecture format to teach the more technical aspects of their curricula.

❐ **Experiential:** Experiential teaching methods, which include business simulations, consulting projects, business plan development, and group activities, are becoming more popular among business schools. Many students enjoy the opportunity to put the knowledge that they've gained in the classroom to work.

As you research schools, you will discover that they all place different emphases on these three approaches. When reviewing the learning models, consider the type of academic environment from which you will benefit most. Also, know that business schools differ in terms of the amount of work (inside and outside of class) that students typically must complete. You should be able to get a decent feel of a b-school's workload by speaking with students and reviewing curriculum requirements. Beware, however, of asking students to compare the workload at their school to that of other schools, as students are notorious for exaggerating cross-school differences.

Typical career paths of graduates

Business schools probably focus on recruiting more than any other type of graduate school program. As soon as students begin classes, there is a strong emphasis placed on career selection and development. Most business school graduates evaluate their alma maters, to a large degree, based on the schools' ability to help them meet their career objectives. It only makes sense, therefore, to examine the career opportunities that different b-schools provide. What you will find is that different companies recruit at different schools generally because of geographical or skill and experience requirements. Many students find themselves in a situation where they decide to attend a school only to find out that many of the companies in which they are interested do not recruit from that school.

Most programs release an annual career guide that provides a wealth of recruiting information, which should give you an idea as to whether that program aligns well with your career goals. Keep in mind, however, that schools can sometimes be generous when they list who their "recruiting partners" are. They often lump all companies who hired any graduates—whether the company came on campus and hired a dozen people or hired just one person who got the job on her own—into one list in their brochures. So, pay attention and make sure that the companies in which you are really interested actually have a presence on campus. One good measure is learning how many alumni from your school are at a given company. Additionally, you should consider speaking with current students and alumni to see if your career goals fit well with the recruiting support that the school provides. Finally, consider the overall level of support that the career center provides students and what its relationship with recruiters is like. Career centers can differ drastically in terms of their performance and you certainly want to be at a school that offers a broad level of support and that maintains close relationships with recruiters.

Culture

While the learning model and recruiting opportunities may be the most obvious areas to research prior to selecting your target schools, examining schools' cultures is just as important. The best way to get a feel for a school's culture is to visit the campus, chat with students, and check out a class. Each school has its own mission, values, and norms. This has a powerful effect on the student experience, and you should take the time to gain an understanding of the type of culture with which you best fit prior to deciding on your target schools. Also, don't forget that any school's culture is the sum of the individual personalities at the school. When you visit, make sure to meet students and ask yourself "Do these seem like the kind of people I'd want to study with at 2 a.m.?"

Application Strategies for 30 Top Business Schools

Now that you have an idea of how to approach the school selection process, we will delve deeper and provide specific strategies on how to get into 30 top schools. While we provide insights for each of these schools, the techniques we've outlined in previous chapters are applicable to all business schools. There are dozens of other good schools (in the United States and abroad) that we don't cover here.

The purpose here is to apply the dimension framework described in Chapter 2 to 30 schools and to give you some school-specific information that you can utilize in developing application strategies for your target schools. These 30 business school application strategies each provide application requirements, school background information, and advice on how to approach the school's application. The application strategies also feature a section called "insider information," which highlights a trend that you can leverage in your application or a key insight that insiders say should be featured in your approach. Finally, we've selected up to four other schools that call for a similar application strategy. Please note that this is not to say that the schools are exactly alike, but rather that applicants have been successful in employing similar strategies across those schools.

Don't read too much into the 30 schools we selected. We reviewed all of the major rankings and picked 30 schools, both domestic and international, that received broad support as top business schools.

Without further ado, here are individual application strategies for 30 top business schools.

Carnegie Mellon University Graduate School of Industrial Administration
www.gsia.cmu.edu
Pittsburgh, PA

Application at a glance

Application due dates (first, second, third, and fourth round): Nov. 15, Jan. 15, Mar. 31, Apr. 30.

Requirements

- ❏ Essays: Three essays (two pages each).
- ❏ Interview: By invitation only.
- ❏ Recommendations: Two, with one preferably coming from your direct supervisor.
- ❏ Resume.
- ❏ Application fee: $100.

School at a glance

Dean (start of tenure): Kenneth B. Dunn (2002)
Admissions director: Laurie Stewart
Program size: 469 full-time
Acceptance rate: 26 percent

Yield: 54 percent

Mean undergraduate GPA: 3.3

Mean GMAT: 672

Middle 80 percent GMAT: 610-730

Average years of work experience: 5.5

International: 34 percent

Women: 23 percent

Minority: 22 percent

Your Carnegie Mellon application strategy

Carnegie Mellon's MBA program is highly analytical, as quantitative rigor is integrated throughout the entire curriculum. The school's proper name—Carnegie Mellon Graduate School of Industrial Administration—invokes images of a program turning out leaders for the manufacturing sector. Although this is partially accurate, the school is also well known in finance circles, where Carnegie Mellon grads' quantitative skills are also highly prized.

While many schools have a minimum math requirement for applicants, Carnegie Mellon expects its applicants to have at least completed one college-level calculus course along with another high-level course in calculus, statistics, or linear algebra. Don't worry, you can take a course part-time before enrolling, but realize that quantitative skills are something that will have to come through in your application no matter what discipline you want to pursue. Also, more than half of each full-time class holds an undergraduate degree in a technical major. Make sure that you're capable of keeping up with applicants that have computer science and engineering backgrounds (if you don't have one yourself). This capability will mostly be represented in your GMAT score, your undergraduate studies, and your previous work experience.

The school's emphasis on analytical abilities is apparent in its core curriculum. Required courses in Probability and Statistics, Decision Models, and Operations Management have the usual dose of quantitative lessons. But classes such as Finance and Economics also have a heavy dose of analytics. One unique feature of the program is its mini-semester system. Students have four mini-semesters a year, instead of the more typical two-semester system. Starting in the spring semester of their first year, students can begin taking electives at the business school as well as at Carnegie Mellon's other schools. If you are interested in expanding your knowledge in such fields as biotechnology or computer science while earning your MBA, explore and consider discussing these opportunities. They provide great ways for you to demonstrate fit and enthusiasm for the flexibility of Carnegie Mellon's program.

Carnegie Mellon also touts its practical, hands-on approach to learning, exemplified by its Management Game, a highly involved computer simulation that runs from the last mini-semester of the first year through the first semester of the second year. Student teams each run their own simulated business, making decisions affecting operations, finance, marketing, and labor relations. Adding a level of realism to the game, each team is assigned a board of directors, comprised of local business leaders.

Teams also practice contract negotiations with local labor leaders and consult with law students at the University of Pittsburgh.

The Management Game requires not only superior quantitative skills, but also strong communications and teamwork abilities, both of which the school also looks for in its applicants. If you are an applicant coming from engineering or an otherwise technical background, be sure to bring out the teamwork dimension in you application. Carnegie Mellon values strong thinkers, but values most those strong thinkers who can turn insights into action.

Nearly half of the 2002 graduates pursued careers in finance, especially corporate finance in the manufacturing sector. Healthcare is also a popular choice for graduates (including pharmaceuticals and biotechnology). Carnegie Mellon alumni are also active entrepreneurs, and the school looks for entrepreneurship traits in its applicants. If you have entrepreneurial aspirations, discussing them in your essays and during your interview can be a great way to establish fit with what the school looks for in its applicants.

Insider information

You won't find any majors at Carnegie Mellon, or any academic departments for that matter. The school promotes an interdisciplinary approach to learning, encouraging faculty members from different fields to teach courses together. The result is a fairly broad approach to management education. While students can choose from concentrations in 12 different subjects, most tend to choose multiple concentrations, further broadening their learning. While Carnegie Mellon's deep analytical focus makes it very different from other general management programs such as Harvard or Darden, keep the school's interdisciplinary philosophy in mind as you build your application story.

Schools that call for a similar approach

- ❐ MIT (Sloan).
- ❐ Purdue (Krannert).
- ❐ University of Chicago.
- ❐ University of Rochester (Simon).

Columbia Business School
www.gsb.columbia.edu
New York, NY

Application at a glance

Application due dates (Early Decision, International, Domestic): Oct. 15, Mar. 1, Apr. 20 (rolling admissions).

Requirements

- ❐ Essays: Four (one of 1,000 words, two of 500 words, and one of 250 words).

❐ Interview: By invitation only.

❐ Recommendations: Two, with one preferably coming from your direct supervisor.

❐ Resume (professional resume and activities resume).

❐ Application fee: $180.

School at a glance

Dean (start of tenure): Meyer Feldberg (1989)

Admissions director: Linda Meehan

Program size: 1,200 full-time

Acceptance rate: 11 percent

Yield: 72 percent

Mean undergraduate GPA: 3.5 (estimate)

Mean GMAT: 705

Middle 80 percent GMAT: 670-750

Average years of work experience: 4.0

International: 28 percent

Women: 35 percent

Minority: 20 percent

Your Columbia application strategy

Make no mistake, Columbia is a finance school above all else. Students rave about the school's finance faculty and the access that they have to top Wall Street executives. The alumni network doesn't hurt either—nearly every Wall Street firm is stacked with Columbia alumni. The result is that most finance-minded applicants consider Columbia. If you are one of them, you will need to especially focus on differentiating yourself from a large pool of similar-sounding applicants. Therefore, start thinking now about what makes you different from the rest of the investment bankers (and aspiring bankers) who apply to Columbia. Chapter 3 should help in that regard.

As you might expect, Columbia's core curriculum is heavy in finance and related courses. First-years take required courses in Financial Accounting, Corporate Finance, and Global Economics, among others. Non-finance topics such as Marketing and Strategy, however, are studied in half-term courses. While these courses are also strong, be aware that much of your time will be spent on finance-related topics. Of course, you will therefore need to demonstrate an ability to handle a quantitative workload, ideally through your GMAT score and relevant work experience.

One academic area that Columbia emphasizes outside of finance is entrepreneurship. Some of the school's most popular electives include "Introduction to Venturing" and "Launching New Ventures." Entrepreneurship is also studied and pursued outside of the classroom. Launched in 1996, the Eugene Lang Entrepreneurial Initiative Fund provides seed capital to worthy business plans crafted by Columbia students.

The Fund acts less like a traditional business plan competition and more like a venture capital firm, taking an equity stake in any Columbia start-up with promise (with the school benefiting if the venture takes off). For students looking for a more conventional business plan competition, Columbia has joined forces with UC Berkeley's Haas School of Business to run the Social Venture Competition, which provides seed money to promising start-ups whose goal is to have a positive social impact. The bottom line is that if you are interested in an MBA for entrepreneurial reasons, let the Columbia admissions committee hear about it in your essays and your interview.

Columbia also emphasizes the international aspect of its curriculum. Each semester, the school's Chazen Institute of International Business offers fellowships to up to four students for their work in advancing Columbia's global approach both inside and outside of the school. The Chazen Institute also runs an exchange program that gives students the opportunity to study abroad at one of 22 partner schools, as well as participate in international study tours. Keep this in mind as you craft your story for why you will fit in at Columbia.

Although they acknowledge that their peers are competitive, students and grads emphasize that Columbia is not a cutthroat environment. Most consider Columbia to be a competitive but respectful and helpful community. Students spend their entire first year in the same "cluster" of 60 students, taking their core classes together. Like other schools, Columbia encourages cooperation and trust within these clusters. As such, you will need to demonstrate the ability to get along with your peers. Also, like other schools in big cities, Columbia sometimes has to battle the reputation that its students spend less time on campus with each other. Demonstrating your enthusiasm for the program and a willingness to get involved in extracurricular activities will help show that you don't fit this stereotype.

Insider information

Columbia's other departments aren't as well known as its finance department, and some grads have commented that these other departments take a backseat to finance. However, the school's administration has a reputation for going out of its way to respond to students' concerns. If you are interested in an area outside of finance, particularly something as far as removed such as organizational behavior or nonprofit management, Columbia may be worth a look. Your interest outside of finance alone will help you stand out, provided that you can prove that you have the quantitative skills and business acumen to learn alongside the finance crowd.

Schools that call for a similar approach

- ❏ NYU (Stern).
- ❏ University of Pennsylvania (Wharton).
- ❏ University of Chicago.
- ❏ University of London (LBS).

Cornell University (Johnson Graduate School of Management)
www.johnson.cornell.edu
Ithaca, NY

Application at a glance
Two Year Program application due dates (first, second, third round): Nov. 15, Jan. 15, Mar. 15.

Requirements
- ❐ Essays: Four (400 words each).
- ❐ Interview: By invitation only.
- ❐ Recommendations: Two, both should come from people who are familiar with your professional capabilities and at least one from a direct supervisor.
- ❐ Resume.
- ❐ Application fee: $200.

School at a glance
Dean (start of tenure): Robert J. Swieringa (1997)
Admissions director: Natalie M. Grinblatt
Program size: 560 full-time
Acceptance rate: 22 percent
Yield: 57 percent
Mean GPA: 3.3
Mean GMAT: 680
Middle 80 percent GMAT: 600-730
Average years of work experience: 5.0
International: 23 percent
Women: 28 percent
Minority: 23 percent

Your Johnson application strategy
Johnson is a quintessential small MBA program. With less than 300 members in each class, students receive a high degree of attention from faculty and from the dean. Perhaps no other top business school program emphasizes professor accessibility as much as Johnson does. Professors at Johnson literally open their homes to students and go the extra mile to ensure that opportunities to learn course concepts extend beyond the classroom. Indeed, joining the Johnson program is more like joining the Johnson family. Your application should echo that sentiment in addition to reflecting the core values upon which the Johnson program has built its reputation.

The values that are central to the Johnson program include: a dedication to analytical rigor, an action-oriented approach to learning, and a collaborative learning environment. Your application should highlight your ability to think in an analytical manner. This could manifest itself through a discussion of how you focus on developing solutions, your approach to analyzing problems, or an analytically driven business idea that you have. Analytical in this sense doesn't purely mean numbers oriented (although Johnson will take a close look at your quantitativeitativeitative GMAT score), but rather it means based on rational and in-depth thought and examination. Examples you can provide along those lines will help you establish fit with the analytical strength Johnson values in addition to its application-focused learning model. As a member of the Johnson family, you will be expected to contribute to your classmates' learning and to the school as a whole. Said in another way, Johnson is looking for applicants who are team players. While you definitely shouldn't shy away from publicizing your accomplishments, be careful not to come across as arrogant in tone and be sure that your recommenders reflect positively upon your teamwork skills.

Although Johnson is a general management program in that there are no majors and a majority of courses that students take are electives, the program's strength lies in its finance curriculum. Johnson even offers a financial engineering program that focuses on subjects such as: derivatives, portfolio analysis, stochastic processes, and computer-based modeling. Another alternative for those who are interested in technical training is the Twelve Month Option MBA program. This program requires an advanced scientific or technical degree and is perfect for those applicants who don't want to be out of the workforce for two years.

Like many other b-schools, Johnson has jumped on the "leadership bandwagon." However, leadership potential is not merely a criterion listed in brochure material; it is one of the most important applicant characteristics by which you will be evaluated. In fact, Johnson offers up to 30 two-year full-tuition scholarships to students who have demonstrated exemplary performance in the area of leadership. The admissions committee will look to see whether you take initiative on a regular basis and will specifically assess how you have an impact on your professional and personal environments. Writing about leadership roles that you've taken on and how those roles have progressively increased in level of responsibility is a great way to implicitly state your further leadership potential. Your interview is another proving ground on which leadership will be discussed. You should anticipate that you will receive several questions on leadership, especially questions asking you to provide examples of displayed leadership. You should also anticipate being asked a question on current business events, so make sure you have a decent understanding of what's going on in the business world before your interview. Respond to "situation"questions using the SAR interview framework discussed in Chapter 4. Chapter 4 also contains a comprehensive set of interview questions on leadership that will serve as great preparation.

Similar to its learning model, Johnson's application offers more flexibility than most. This becomes most apparent in its essay requirements, which allow you to select from a great number of options. Utilize this flexibility to cover all four dimensions discussed in Chapter 2. Your emphasis, however, should be on the leadership and innovation dimensions. Your ability to establish fit along these lines will help grant you entry into the Johnson family.

Insider information

The Immersion Learning curriculum is probably the best example of Johnson's action-oriented approach to learning. Immersion Learning, also referred to as "the semester in reality," is an experiential method that allows students to take a hands-on approach to functions such as: Managerial Finance, Investment Banking, Brand Management, Manufacturing, and e-business. Students visit companies, work on actual business challenges, and are evaluated based on the solutions that they develop in response to those challenges. Discussion of Immersion Learning can be a great way to display your knowledge of the Johnson learning model.

Schools that call for a similar approach

- ❏ Dartmouth College (Tuck).
- ❏ University of Michigan Business School.
- ❏ University of North Carolina at Chapel Hill (Kenan-Flagler).
- ❏ University of Virginia (Darden).

Dartmouth College (Tuck School of Business)
www.tuck.dartmouth.edu
Hanover, NH

Application at a glance

Application due dates (Early Action, first, second, third round): Oct. 18, Nov. 1, Jan. 3, Apr. 18.

Requirements

- ❏ Essays: Five (four of 100 words, one of unlimited length answering a mini-case question).
- ❏ Interview: Required.
- ❏ Recommendations: Two "Confidential Statements of Qualifications," with one preferably coming from your direct supervisor.
- ❏ Application fee: $180.

School at a glance

Dean (start of tenure): Paul Danos (1995)

Admissions director: Kristine Laca

Program size: 470 full-time

Acceptance rate: 14 percent

Yield: 51 percent

Mean undergraduate GPA: 3.4

Mean GMAT: 698

Middle 80 percent GMAT: 640–760

Average years of work experience: 4.8

International: 29 percent

Women: 32 percent

Minority: 17 percent

Your Tuck application strategy

Think small. Think intimate. Think great outdoors. That's exactly what life at Tuck is all about. The country's first graduate school of business offers one of the smallest programs among the top 30 schools, with fewer than 250 students in each class. The small class size—coupled with the school's location in rural Hanover, New Hampshire—results in a close-knit community in which everyone knows everyone else.

Academically, Tuck's MBA program focuses on turning out competent general managers. Most of the first-year curriculum consists of core courses in the main management disciplines (including Finance, Marketing, Strategy, and Economics), with the second year left open for electives. No specific majors are offered. First-year students complete most of their coursework in the same study group, which Tuck emphasizes as a way for students to grow closer and develop their teamwork skills. More than the average top program, Tuck is looking for students who demonstrate strong teamwork skills, so make sure that this is a main theme in your Tuck application.

Tuck is also serious about leadership, and one unique part of the first-year experience is the Tuck Leadership Forum, which runs throughout the first year. The Forum is a series of mini-courses in topics such as management communication and entrepreneurial management, all designed to help improve students' leadership skills. Students then complete a team project, such as creating a business plan or doing consulting work for an existing business. The program also provides students with a chance to work closely with faculty and plug into Tuck's alumni network while still in school.

Speaking of the alumni, what Tuck lacks in size is made up for in devotion. Tuck's alumni have been described by some as "fierce" in their loyalty to the school and to each other. Tuck touts its alumni's 60 percent plus annual giving rate as further evidence of this dedication. While the school may not have an alum in every company, Tuck students are known to get good results from the alumni they do call upon. In your own application, make sure that you can provide convincing proof that you, too, will be an active alum, preferably by demonstrating loyalty to your undergraduate school.

Tuck's remote location means that it's not for everyone. Some applicants, especially those with spouses, often find it difficult to relocate to Hanover. To its credit, Tuck goes out of its way to make the transition a smooth one, often providing spouses and partners with full-time work around campus. Still, only slightly more than half of Tuck's admitted applicants actually enroll in the program. This means two things for you: (1) Make sure that you really want to attend Tuck before you apply. It's a great school, but its size and location sometimes turn people off. Save yourself a lot of time if you think these aspects of the program will be a problem for you. (2) Even more importantly, you really need to demonstrate why Tuck is for you. Tuck's students tend to be passionate about their school, and you need to demonstrate this same passion in your application. Visiting the school—especially for your interview—can go a long way toward helping you make your case. Also, think about applying in Tuck's Early Action round (with applications due in mid-October) if you are sure that Tuck is where you want to be. This relatively new program is a great chance for you to show your commitment to the school.

Insider information

Tuck isn't the household name that Stanford and Harvard are, but its general management program is known to be one of the best in the country. Tuck graduates have a strong reputation in consulting and financial services, particularly on the East Coast, where nearly two-thirds of its graduates end up living after school. If you are considering a career in general management, or are interested in consulting or banking, don't overlook Tuck. If you can demonstrate that the school's environment is right for you, and make a case for why the general management approach is what you want out of business school, then Tuck will give your application strong consideration.

Schools that call for a similar approach

- ❏ Cornell University (Johnson).
- ❏ Duke University (Fuqua).
- ❏ Emory University (Goizueta).
- ❏ University of Virginia (Darden).

Duke University (Fuqua School of Business)
www.fuqua.duke.edu
Durham, NC

Application at a glance

Application due dates (first, second, third, fourth round): Oct. 31, Dec. 16, Jan. 30, Mar. 13.

Requirements

- ❏ Essays: Three essays (one of 250 words, one of 400 words, and one of 500 words).
- ❏ Interview: Highly recommended.
- ❏ Recommendations: Two, with one preferably coming from your direct supervisor.
- ❏ Resume.
- ❏ Application fee: $175 online, $200 paper.

School at a glance

Dean (start of tenure): Douglas T. Breeden (2001)

Admissions director: Liz Riley

Program size: 700 full-time

Acceptance rate: 19 percent

Yield: 57 percent

Mean undergraduate GPA: 3.6

Mean GMAT: 701

Middle 80 percent GMAT: 640–760

Average years of work experience: 5.0

International: 34 percent

Women: 34 percent

Minority: 21 percent

Your Fuqua application strategy

No school has come as far as Fuqua (pronounced: "FEW-kwa") has in the last 20 years. Duke opened its business school in 1969, but things really started to happen after the school took J.B. Fuqua's name (and his money) in 1980. What was once a well-regarded school with mostly regional appeal has grown into one of the top business programs in the world.

Young and small, Fuqua has an advantage over the business school competition with its innovative curriculum and approach to learning. Students have four terms (of six weeks each) per year, meaning that they get a taste of many more subjects than students at most other schools. Fuqua's emphasis has traditionally been on turning out general managers, although recent graduate classes have skewed more towards marketing. The only concentration that the school offers is its Health Sector Management (HSM) program, which takes advantage of the school's location in Research Triangle Park in North Carolina. If you are interested in biotech, pharmaceuticals, medical devices, or healthcare management, take a close look at this program.

Fuqua has also been aggressive in giving its students opportunities to study abroad, and currently has reciprocal exchange programs with 25 international business schools. Its Global Academic Travel Experience (GATE) program provides students with the opportunity to travel abroad for a shorter period of time. GATE is extremely popular with students, with close to half of the class participating in the program for two weeks each year. Fuqua's push to build its brand around the world means that it looks for applicants with global perspective. If you have international experience, be sure to emphasize it in your application. If you haven't worked abroad, that's okay. You definitely don't need to lie about wanting to spend your next five years in Hong Kong. Just demonstrating a willingness to work with people of other backgrounds (and any experience that you might have in this area) is a great start.

Work in most classes is done in teams, and Fuqua's graduates have gained a team-ready reputation that rivals that of Kellogg's graduates. Students often refer to themselves as "Team Fuqua," and they mean it. They also have a reputation for being some of the most energetic and close-knit students at any business school. This is reinforced by the fact that Fuqua is a smaller school—approximately 700 full-time students in 2003. When you apply to Fuqua, make it clear that you understand what it means to be part of a smaller community, and spell out why it appeals to you. Along those lines, Fuqua students are heavily involved in everything going on at the school. If you apply Duke, make sure that this is what you want out of your business school experience. Even more importantly, make sure to make that clear in your application through multiple examples of teamwork and involvement.

Fuqua's focus on excellence in general management will definitely come out during the interview. Most interviews are conducted by students who are members of the admissions committee. It is therefore important to position yourself as a prospect that your interviewer would like to have as a classmate. This means you should provide examples of professional excellence, but do so in a non-arrogant tone. In the back of his mind, your interviewer will be evaluating you as a potential team member in addition to evaluating you as a leader. If you have three years professional experience or less, you should also expect to receive questions on your ability to contribute in the classroom. Have a response prepared as to why "now" is a good time for you to attend Fuqua.

Insider information

Fuqua has built a strong reputation, and it now attracts many of the same people who also apply to the Harvards and Whartons of the world. The downside for Fuqua is that some top applicants still view Fuqua as somewhat of a backup school, even though Fuqua's acceptance rate is below 20 percent. This is evident in the school's yield (percentage of accepted students who enroll), which was 57 percent in 2001, more than 10 percent below that of other top schools. The school therefore looks for applicants who are interested in Fuqua for what it offers, not just because it's listed next to the other big names in the rankings. In other words, the admissions committee wants to be sure that if they accept you, you will enroll. If you can demonstrate that you truly want to attend Fuqua—and *why* this is so—you will greatly improve your chances.

Schools that call for a similar approach

- ❐ Northwestern University (Kellogg).
- ❐ Dartmouth College (Tuck).
- ❐ University of Michigan Business School.
- ❐ University of California at Berkeley (Haas).

Emory University (Goizueta Business School)
www.goizueta.emory.edu
Atlanta, GA

Application at a glance

Application due dates (Early I, Early II, Final): Nov. 1, Jan. 2, Mar. 15 (rolling admissions).

Requirements

- ❏ Essays: Four (two of two pages, two of one page).
- ❏ Interview: Highly recommended.
- ❏ Recommendations: Two required, three recommended, preferably from supervisors or coworkers.
- ❏ Application fee: $100.

School at a glance

Dean (start of tenure): Thomas S. Robertson (1998)

Admissions director: Julie Barefoot

Program size: 390 full-time

Acceptance rate: 24 percent

Yield: 46 percent

Mean undergraduate GPA: 3.4

Mean GMAT: 675

Middle 80 percent GMAT: 610–740

Average years of work experience: 5.5

International: 31 percent

Women: 22 percent

Minority: 9 percent

Your Goizueta application strategy

Emory University's Goizueta (pronounced: "goy-SWET-uh") Business School is one of the smallest of the nation's top programs, with just 170 entering the school's traditional two-year MBA program each year. Like other small programs, Goizueta is noted for its close-knit culture and high student involvement in every aspect of the school. Student Action Groups give students a strong voice in many of the school's departments, including admissions, curriculum development, marketing, and facilities planning. Not surprisingly, the school expects that each of its students will get involved in at least one opportunity to leave a mark on the school.

Goizueta promotes its own flavor of leadership training, which it calls Leadership in Action. The school believes that effective leadership requires seven important traits—courage, integrity, accountability, rigor, diversity, teamwork, and community—which it has deemed its "Core Values." Goizueta students are immediately introduced to the school's Core Values during their orientation week, with one activity devoted to each of the school's core values. Students participate in ropes courses and skydiving to learn courage, perform service projects to gain a sense of community, etc. In other words, the school expects each student to embrace its Core Values, and you should be prepared to explain what these values mean to you.

Before the start of each semester, Goizueta students take part in a pre-term course called Lead Week, an intense program that gives them exposure to real-world business issues. Before the start of the first-year fall term, students study a series of cases focused on a single company. Each case emphasizes an academic discipline, such as operations, strategy, finance, or marketing. Students compete in teams to prepare analyses and recommendations for the subject company, and the winning team gets to present its findings to the company's executives. To start the second year, student teams compete in a business plan competition, with each team preparing a business plan from scratch and pitching it to a panel of venture capitalists. Lead Week programs in the winter and spring give students opportunities to focus on topics of their choosing, and even study issues abroad. Additionally, Goizueta Plus is a series of seminars that students take in their first year, giving them the opportunity to explore their own personal interests, their leadership traits, communication skills, and larger issues in business ethics. Although these programs are constantly evolving, they remain a centerpiece of the Goizueta program, and expressing an understanding of how they embody the school's Core Values will help strengthen your application.

The annual Goizueta Marketing Strategy Competition gives student teams another chance to tackle real-world business challenges. Students work with executives from partner corporations in developing solutions for real marketing challenges that these businesses face. While performing their analyses and developing their recommendations, students are coached by faculty members and receive additional training through a series of training seminars. A panel of executives and Goizueta faculty judge each team's output, with the winning team taking home $10,000. Especially if you are interested in marketing, be sure to express your enthusiasm for the competition and hands-on experience that it provides.

While most schools prefer students with some amount of work experience, Goizueta explicitly states that students need at least a year of work experience in order to apply. It is therefore not surprising that its student body tends to skew slightly older than those of other top schools. Although all schools look for maturity in their applicants, Goizueta is clear about the importance of this dimension of your application. It is therefore important to choose essay and interview stories that emphasize your own professional maturity.

Insider information

Perhaps Goizueta's most important espoused Core Value is courage, which the school defines as a willingness to take risks and push yourself out of your comfort zone. The school believes that this is an important component of leadership, and you can therefore expect the Goizueta admissions committee to look for examples of this trait in your application. The school is most interested in the applicant who takes the road less traveled and is willing to take some risks. Any way in which you can demonstrate this trait in your own past—and what you learned from it—will help the admissions committee see how you fit in at Goizueta. Think about how you can weave these stories into your application, particularly in the essays.

Schools that call for a similar approach

- ❏ Cornell University (Johnson).
- ❏ Dartmouth College (Tuck).
- ❏ UNC (Kenan-Flagler).
- ❏ USC (Marshall).

Harvard Business School
www.hbs.edu
Boston, MA

Application at a Glance

Application due dates (first, second, third round): Oct. 17, Jan. 7, Mar. 11.

Requirements

- ❏ Essays: Six (five of 400 words, one of 600 words).
- ❏ Interview: By invitation only.
- ❏ Recommendations: Three, with one preferably coming from your direct supervisor.
- ❏ Resume.
- ❏ Application fee: $190.

School at a glance

Dean (start of tenure): Kim Clark (1995)
Admissions director: Brit Dewey
Program size: 1,800 full-time
Acceptance rate: 10 percent
Yield: 89 percent
Mean GPA: 3.6
Mean GMAT: 705
Middle 80 percent GMAT: 670–755 (estimate)
Average years of work experience: 4.3
International: 32 percent
Women: 35 percent
Minority: 24 percent

Your Harvard application strategy

Leadership is unquestionably the most emphasized dimension at Harvard Business School (HBS). The school's mission is to "develop outstanding business leaders who contribute to the well-being of society." This mission, along with the school's community standards, can be found posted in every classroom on campus. Candidates' potential as leaders should therefore permeate every aspect of the HBS application. Leadership should be projected on multiple levels; professional experience, academic experience, extracurricular activities, hobbies, and community service can all be used to highlight leadership capabilities. Good examples demonstrate your ability to have positive influence over the actions of others. A focus on leadership should also play a role in describing your career goals. More than most schools, HBS will closely evaluate your career goals based on their level of impact on society. Finally, remember to describe your leadership style and how it has changed over time. The admissions committee is really interested in what you have learned along the way and will be impressed with reflections on your "leadership evolution."

HBS is known as the quintessential general management program. In line with the mission of the school, students' decision-making ability across multiple business disciplines is the constant focal point. Students do not formally specialize in a particular aspect of business, as they do at most schools, and take the first year required curriculum in sections of 80–90 students.

The section experience is one of the defining aspects of the HBS learning model, as each student is expected to take on the responsibility of teaching her classmates. Students constantly draw from their own background and experiences, creating a dynamic atmosphere that is supplemented by the faculty's insights. To ensure that classrooms are filled with numerous perspectives, students' backgrounds are extremely diverse in nature. It is not uncommon for most sections to contain, lawyers, teachers, investment bankers, doctors, consultants, brand managers, professional athletes, military officers, and entrepreneurs. The required curriculum in the first year is followed by an entirely elective curriculum in the second year. Students utilize this year to further hone their decision-making abilities in areas that they believe will be the most beneficial for their careers.

Applicants should be aware that their undergraduate school's reputation will be factored into the selection process at HBS. The undergraduate schools that are most densely represented are Harvard University, University of Pennsylvania, and Stanford University. This, however, should definitely *not* be a deterrent to applicants from lesser known schools. Indeed, more than 150 undergraduate institutions are represented in a typical HBS class. Nonetheless, applicants who graduated from schools with less brand strength than most should make a concerted effort to highlight the strengths of their school and their accomplishments at the school. One way to do this is through the recommendation process.

HBS is one of the few business schools that doesn't mind recommendations from former professors. While your recommendation approach should primarily focus on your professional experience, a recommendation that highlights your academic prowess can help augment your position as an applicant. The professor's recommendation can add credibility to your school's reputation, thereby granting credibility to your entire application. Should you go down this path, however, make sure that the professor is in a position to comment on your leadership capabilities and on your professional goals. If the professor isn't that familiar with you and your story, then it's best to seek out a recommendation from a different source.

Being part of the HBS community is a life-long commitment. This is highlighted by the fact that the alumni network is often one of the first points that is raised when discussing HBS's differentiating factors. It is therefore to your advantage to show ways in which you have been a champion for your alma mater. The admissions committee isn't just concerned about what you will bring to the table during your time in the classroom, but also how you will remain involved with and support the school in the future.

Insider information

The case study method is the lifeblood of the HBS learning model. This cannot be stressed enough. By graduation, students can expect to have conquered more than 500 cases in addition to textbooks, notes, and articles that provide conceptual depth to the case scenarios. Each case addresses a class topic and provides a "real-world" example on how the topic is applicable. New cases are constantly produced by professors and students will often receive a freshly written case hot off the press less than a week before discussing it. Second year students are even granted the opportunity to assist in the case writing process by participating in a field study. Producing cases has become such a core part of HBS that a majority of business schools purchase their case studies from it.

Displaying a grasp of the case method and how it is utilized at HBS is an excellent way to differentiate yourself from other applicants. You should emphasize your ability to engage in open discussions and your desire to learn based on real-world business applications. Both of these components are central to the way in which case studies are taught at HBS. Discussing your learning style and how you would benefit from case studies will also show your understanding of the learning model.

Schools that call for a similar approach

- ☐ INSEAD.
- ☐ University of Virginia (Darden).
- ☐ University of Western Ontario (Ivey).
- ☐ Yale School of Management.

Indiana University (Kelley School of Business)
www.kelley.indiana.edu
Bloomington, IN

Application at a glance
Application due dates (first, second, third, fourth round): Dec. 1, Jan. 15, Mar. 1, Apr. 15.

Requirements
- ❏ Essays: Three essays (two pages each).
- ❏ Interview: Recommended.
- ❏ Recommendations: Two, both should come from people who are familiar with your professional capabilities.
- ❏ Resume.
- ❏ Application fee: $75.

School at a glance
Dean (start of tenure): Dan R. Dalton (1997)
Admissions director: James Holmen
Program size: 520 full-time
Acceptance rate: 22 percent
Yield: 45 percent
Mean GPA: 3.4
Mean GMAT: 651
Middle 80 percent GMAT: 580–710
Average years of work experience: 5.3
International: 30 percent
Women: 25 percent
Minority: 16 percent

Your Kelley application strategy
Curriculum innovation is one of the strongest assets of the Kelley learning model. The curriculum continues to receive accolades for its integrated, cross-functional approach to teaching. The basis of the approach is that real-world business challenges are not discretely segmented into functions and therefore business school should be taught in an integrated manner. The admissions committee is looking for applicants with leadership potential who view business issues in a cross-functional way and are interested in participating in a learning model that is taught in an equally integrated and flexible fashion.

The initial 24 weeks of the first year are split into three sections: Grasping the Foundations of Management and Decision-making, Identifying New Business Opportunities, and Managing an Ongoing Enterprise Profitably. These sections consist of a total of 14 modules, each module building upon the lessons of the previous modules. The goal of the core curriculum is to provide students with tools and intuition that will be invaluable in making management decisions. As a checkpoint, mid-way through the core, students participate in a team-based case competition, which allows them to display the benefits of integrated learning. One way for you to display an appreciation for the Kelley approach is to discuss how the results of actions you've taken in a business environment have been beneficial to multiple functions and not just the one to which you belong.

Outside of the core curriculum, students select majors and minors from a suite of 11 options including: E-Business, Finance, Information Systems, Marketing, Production/ Operations Management, and Strategic Management Consulting. If none of the options suits their needs, students can design their own major that fits with their career interests. To supplement their specialized study, students can apply to participate in an "Academy." Academies are industry-focused and allow students to take part in career-focused course work and professional development activities such as discussions with professionals in the industry, a speaker series, and trips to relevant companies. There are Academies for Consumer Marketing, Entrepreneurship, Global Experience, Health Care, Investment Banking, Investment Management, Sports and Entertainment, and Management Consulting. Discussing these learning opportunities and how they would benefit you in achieving your career goals is a great way to establish fit with Kelley.

Looking into the future, Kelley will continue to focus attention on technology, leadership, and global initiatives. Technology is viewed as a powerful enabler of many of the strategies discussed in the classroom and Kelley strives to be recognized as a front-runner in the usage of technology. Like most other top business schools, Kelley would like to be known as an institution that produces leaders and has established its Leadership Development Institute to help support that objective. From an international perspective, Kelley has gradually increased its international student percentage to 30 percent, and has added several study abroad opportunities. If you have the background or the direction to capitalize on any of these trends, make sure to spell them out in your application.

If the curriculum is the heart of the Kelley learning model, then the faculty is the life-blood. The faculty receives high praise for accessibility, commitment, and expertise. The strong commitment of the faculty has helped create a collegial environment in which teamwork is a strong norm. The admissions committee will be very interested to hear ways in which you can contribute to this environment. Loners and gunners need not apply.

Insider information

While interviewing with Kelley is not required, it is encouraged. Nonetheless, only approximately 50 percent of applicants participate in the interview. The interview is an excellent opportunity for you to establish fit with the program as well as to display a true desire to attend the school. Your initiative will be duly noted by an admissions committee that is looking to increase its yield percentage.

Schools that call for a similar approach

- ❏ Michigan State University (Broad).
- ❏ Purdue University (Krannert).
- ❏ University of Maryland (Smith).
- ❏ University of Texas at Austin (McCombs).

INSEAD

www.insead.edu/mba
Fontainebleau, France, and Singapore

Application at a glance

Application due dates: Feb. 1 for September intake, Jul. 1 for January intake (rolling admissions).

Requirements

- ❏ Essays: Eight (200–500 words each).
- ❏ Interview: By invitation only.
- ❏ Recommendations: Two, both should come from people who are familiar with your professional capabilities.
- ❏ Application fee: • 200.

School at a glance

Dean (start of tenure): Gabriel Hawawini (2000)

Admissions director: Inger Pedersen

Program size: 840 full-time

Acceptance rate: 27 percent

Yield: 80 percent

Mean GPA: N/A

Mean GMAT: 694

Middle 80 percent GMAT: 660–730

Average years of work experience: 5.0

International: 93 percent (foreign nationals)

Women: 24 percent

Minority: N/A

Your INSEAD application strategy

Spanning two continents and with a major presence on a third, INSEAD is making strides toward its goal of being recognized as the preeminent international MBA. The one-year general management program operates on campuses in France and Singapore and maintains an alliance with the Wharton School. Given its goal, INSEAD is in search of applicants who bring significant international exposure, academic excellence, and a solid professional background to the table.

The curriculum itself is general management in nature and lasts for 10 1/2 months. There are two different start dates, one which begins in September and another which begins in January. After receiving admittance into INSEAD, students may state their preference for either the Fontainebleau or Singapore campus. In either case, the program structure is the same and students have opportunities to visit the campus to which they are not assigned. The curriculum is divided into five eight-week periods and calls for students to take 15 required courses and a minimum of seven electives. Electives consist of advanced topics in Finance, Accounting, General Management, Marketing, Entrepreneurship, International Business, Ethics, and Running Family Businesses. Members of the January intake participate in a summer internship between periods three and four.

As far as international diversity goes, you would be hard-pressed to find another business school that rivals INSEAD. No one nationality represents more than 10 percent of the student body and less than half come from Western countries, meaning that the "international student" concept is essentially nonexistent. Students are quick to acknowledge this level of diversity as a differentiating factor, as the learning model gives credence to multiple approaches without showing bias to any. INSEAD also demonstrates its commitment to a global mindset through language requirements. Students must be proficient in at least two languages by matriculation and three by graduation. To establish fit, you should incorporate an international perspective in both your background and in your future goals. The admissions committee will closely evaluate your ability to have an impact on global business, so make sure that your story is not entirely nation-centric.

INSEAD views itself as an academic business institution. This is revealed through the large amount of general research that the school produces in addition to the writing of specific cases. Based on this perspective, INSEAD conducts a thorough assessment of your academic background. Specifically, the admissions committee will look at the reputation of your alma mater(s), your performance in the classroom, and your ability to handle quantitatively rigorous courses. If you don't have a numbers-intensive background or have not fared well in such classes, consider taking a statistics or finance course at a community college.

Due in-part to the abbreviated duration of the program, INSEAD tends to accept applicants with at least several of years work experience (more than 45 percent have more than five years). The school believes that students with more professional experience are better able to adapt to the one-year curriculum and leverage it in their career development. Indeed, INSEAD takes career development very seriously, as each student is matched up with a mentor to assist with the process. The school even has teleconferencing equipment readily available so that students can interview with firms who are unable to make the trip to campus. Your challenge is to present your professional experiences in a way that highlights your success in the workplace and your ability to contribute to the classroom. Despite INSEAD's tendency to accept more experienced applicants, you may still want to consider applying if you are younger, as the school does accept a small number of less-experienced applicants each year (about 15 percent of students have two years or less). If you fall into this category, it is even more important that you emphasize the maturity dimension and discuss an array of experiences that are academic, professional, and personal in nature.

Teamwork is an essential part of the INSEAD learning model. The school's strength in diversity would be pointless if there was no cross-cultural learning involved. As such, students are assigned to study groups of five to seven in order to heighten the learning experience. Groups are diverse across multiple dimensions including: nationality, professional experience, gender, age, and education. Team members work closely together on class assignments and in some cases even exams. Any cross-cultural team-based experiences that you can discuss will go a long way in establishing fit with the INSEAD mission.

Insider information

While INSEAD has won international acclaim for its advances in business education, it is not resting on its laurels. INSEAD is actively seeking to expand the size of its program, especially the Singapore campus, and there are even discussions of establishing an entirely new campus. INSEAD has room to expand its program in part due to its high yield (approx. 80 percent), which should allow for more opportunities among applicants. With expansion on the way, potential applicants should consider INSEAD even if they are not linguistic geniuses. If you have a true desire to pursue a global career and are willing to put in work to develop your foreign language abilities, then INSEAD might be the business school for you.

Schools that call for a similar approach

- ❑ Harvard Business School.
- ❑ University of London (London Business School).

Massachusetts Institute of Technology (Sloan School of Management)
mitsloan.mit.edu
Cambridge, MA

Application at a glance

Application due dates (first, second round): Nov. 13 and Feb. 5.

Requirements

- ❑ Essays: Five (four of 500–800 words each including a cover letter, one of unlimited length).
- ❑ Interview: By invitation only.
- ❑ Recommendations: Two.
- ❑ Resume.
- ❑ Application fee: $175 U.S., $200 international.

School at a glance

Dean (start of tenure): Richard L. Schmalensee (1998)

Admissions director: Rod Garcia

Program size: 638 full-time

Acceptance rate: 13 percent

Yield: 68 percent

Mean undergraduate GPA: 3.5

Mean GMAT: 710

Middle 80 percent GMAT: 650–760

Average years of work experience: 4.9

International: 40 percent

Women: 27 percent

Minority: 18 percent

Your Sloan application strategy

Although not quite as well known as the "other" business school in Boston, MIT's Sloan School of Management has combined the quantitative strengths of its parent school with a focus on entrepreneurship to establish itself as one of the most highly regarded programs in the technology and manufacturing industries. The school is also well-regarded on Wall Street, where Sloan grads are known for their quantitative abilities.

Sloan has traditionally been better known for turning out stronger analysts than business leaders, so the school is making a push to emphasize leadership in its curriculum. The school has appointed a Director of Leadership to create and run leadership programs at the school, as well as to coach Sloan students on their own leadership development. The school even encourages students to fill out a "Leadership Feedback Form" (anonymously, if they want) whenever they observe a fellow student in a leadership role. The school also encourages teamwork, and all first-year students must complete a core project in teams. Sloan's stated goal is to turn out "leaders who innovate."

As expected, the school's curriculum emphasizes the quantitative side of business. Courses such as Finance and Statistics are as quantitative as you would expect, but Sloan also encourages students to apply the skills that they learn in these classes to nearly all of their coursework. Graduates speak highly of the hard skills that they learned at Sloan, so make sure that this is what you want out of your MBA experience. To get in, you will have to demonstrate that you are comfortable utilizing numbers, through your GMAT score, previous coursework, or job experience.

Sloan's curriculum is also notable for its emphasis of "management tracks," instead of traditional majors. The idea behind these tracks is to provide students with a broad study approach to a certain functional area, such as Financial Engineering, Operations Management, and New Product and Venture Development. The tracks' broad approach requires students to complete eight to 10 classes per track. Students can also create their own tracks after their first semester at Sloan. Demonstrating your understanding of Sloan's track system will help you show your enthusiasm for the program.

Entrepreneurship is big at Sloan, as characterized by students' participation in MIT's annual "$50K" entrepreneurship competition. The competition gives Sloan students the chance to develop a business plan and compete against students from other MIT programs for a chance to win the $30,000 grand prize ($10,000 goes to each of the top two runner-up teams). Successful tech companies such as Akamai got their start through the $50K competition, and student teams that get far in the program are often able to attract interest from potential investors and advisors.

One example of Sloan's close ties to the manufacturing sector is its Leaders for Manufacturing (LFM) program, a two-year joint degree program offered in conjunction with MIT's School of Engineering. It offers students courses in engineering, change management, information technology, and operations management through a variety of in-class and on-the-job experiences. Students spend six-and-a-half months on-site as an intern with a sponsor company, culminating in a thesis. The best part of the program is that students receive a scholarship covering the full cost of tuition, thanks to sponsor companies including Boeing, Dell, Harley-Davidson, Intel, and Procter & Gamble. The bad news is that the program is very exclusive—just 50 students participate each year—but give it a look if you are considering working in manufacturing after business school.

Insider information

Sloan has a higher percentage of international students than nearly all of its peer schools—40 percent of the class of 2003 came from abroad. Sloan students therefore tend to be surrounded by international classmates wherever they go. If you are looking to gain international experience, or just want to meet people from new cultures, this is an aspect of the program that may appeal to you. Make sure you demonstrate your enthusiasm for the school's diverse culture in your application, and make your case for why this matters to you, whether you are an American or an international applicant.

Schools that call for a similar approach

- ❏ Carnegie Mellon University.
- ❏ Stanford University.
- ❏ University of Chicago.
- ❏ University of Pennsylvania (Wharton).

Michigan State University (Eli Broad Graduate School of Management)
www.bus.msu.edu/mba
East Lansing, MI

Application at a glance

Application due dates (first, second, third, fourth round): Dec. 16, Jan. 31, Mar. 14, June 2.

Requirements

- ❏ Essays: Two (one page each).
- ❏ Interview: Recommended.
- ❏ Recommendations: Two, with one preferably coming from someone who is familiar with your professional capabilities.
- ❏ Resume.
- ❏ Application fee: $40.

School at a glance

Dean (start of tenure): Robert B. Duncan (2002)
Admissions director: Esmeralda Cardenal
Program size: 210 full-time
Acceptance rate: 22 percent
Yield: 53 percent
Mean GPA: 3.2
Mean GMAT: 639
Middle 80 percent GMAT: 570–710
Average years of work experience: 5.0
International: 30 percent
Women: 23 percent
Minority: 16 percent

Your Broad application strategy

Over the last few years, Broad (rhymes with "road") has expanded its brand beyond "regional MBA" status. This expansion can be attributed to a quick rise in the b-school rankings and Broad's strength in practical specializations. Students can select from four primary specializations (Supply Chain Management, Marketing Technology, Human Resource Management, and Finance). The Supply Chain Management (SCM) specialization has especially helped place Broad on the map. SCM, which focuses on manufacturing operations, logistics, and purchasing, continues to draw recruiters from across the nation that are looking to optimize their product and information flows. Students may supplement these areas of focus with secondary specializations, which include: Business Information Systems, Corporate Accounting, General Management, and Leadership & Change Management. Referencing your specialization interests and explaining how a background in those areas could support your career goals should be key components of your application strategy.

Another large asset of the program is its career services function. Broad's career services group has made extensive efforts to attract a bevy of innovative companies to campus. As a result, Broad students now enjoy an average rate of job offers that is commensurate to or greater than that of other top programs. Some of the major recruiters include: Intel, Cap Gemini Ernst & Young, IBM, Ford, and A.T. Kearney.

You should take note that there is relatively little investment bank presence on campus. Along those lines, make sure that your career goals align well with Broad's strengths.

Broad students rave about the school's small size and the access to professors. They enjoy the intimate environment and the close relationships that are developed within the program. Unlike most other b-school programs, chances are that you will leave Broad knowing all of your classmates' names.

Over the last few years Broad has begun to make a name for itself through case competitions. Held around the globe, case competitions allow teams of three to six students to display their analytical, public speaking, and persuasion skills. Broad actively encourages students to participate in these competitions and assists in students' preparation for them. The results speak for themselves, as Broad students have come away with high placements in a number of these competitions. If you have any interest in participating in case competitions, bring them up as a great discussion point.

Broad's application is fairly compact in comparison to the applications of other top programs. With two short essays, the Broad application makes it more difficult for candidates to differentiate themselves from each other. As such, it is important that your baseline statistics (GMAT and GPA) are close to those of the current MBA class. This importance has been compounded as Broad looks to improve its baseline statistics in order to continue its movement up the rankings. Therefore, you should utilize the optional essay to address weaknesses in baseline statistics that are five percent below the means.

Overall, Broad is looking for bright candidates who aren't afraid to get their hands dirty while working to solve managerial issues. If you can position yourself as such and hit the mark in terms of GMAT and GPA, your application will resonate positively with the admissions committee.

Insider information

A few years ago, Broad grads received criticism for their lack of teamwork capabilities. The Broad administration was quick to react and has made strong efforts to introduce team building exercises into the learning model. Today, a large portion of class assignments are completed in teams. From the moment orientation begins, students are placed on project teams and students' skills are continuously enhanced through team building workshops and activities. As part of the core curriculum, students are required to take the course *Leadership & Teamwork*. This course provides students with an experiential learning opportunity through which they can work in teams under different simulated conditions. The bottom line is that you should present yourself to the admissions committee as a team player who is open to further examination of your team skills.

Schools that call for a similar approach

- ❏ Indiana University (Kelley).
- ❏ Purdue University (Krannert).
- ❏ University of Maryland (Smith).

New York University (Leonard N. Stern School of Business)
www.stern.nyu.edu
New York, NY

Application at a glance

Application due dates (first, second, third round): Dec. 1, Jan. 15, Mar. 15

Requirements

- ❑ Essays: Three (two of two-pages, one "creative" piece involving words, illustrations, etc.).
- ❑ Interview: By invitation only.
- ❑ Recommendations: Two, with at least one preferably coming from a supervisor or coworker.
- ❑ Resume.
- ❑ Application fee: $150.

School at a glance

Dean (start of tenure): Thomas F. Cooley (2002)

Admissions director: Julia Min

Program size: 858 full-time

Acceptance rate: 15 percent

Yield: 52 percent

Mean undergraduate GPA: 3.4

Mean GMAT: 700

Middle 80 percent GMAT: 650–750

Average years of work experience: 4.7

International: 34 percent

Women: 38 percent

Minority: 13 percent

Your Stern application strategy

The fact about NYU's Stern School that comes up most often is its location. Stern sits right in New York City's Greenwich Village, between Manhattan's Midtown and Financial District. Students and grads rave about the school's location, and the administration smartly plays up its ties to New York when promoting Stern.

Given Stern's location, it is not surprising that a large number of grads pursue jobs on Wall Street, where the Stern name and alumni network are the strongest. Eight of the school's top 10 recruiters are investment banks. Although Stern's overall academic reputation is strong, most people consider its finance department to be by far the school's greatest strength. If you are interested in working outside of finance, don't rule out

Stern, but know that finance is where most of the action has historically been. The school is aware of this perceived inequity and has been working hard to balance its strengths across disciplines.

Although many would call Stern a finance school, its approach to management education is mostly a general one. First-year students go through a complete required curriculum of courses in all of the business fundamentals, with the bulk of elective coursework coming in the second year. Most students major in one or two of the school's 12 majors (including Finance, Economics, Marketing, and Operations), and some take a co-major or "program initiative." These latter two programs demonstrate Stern's generalist approach by involving faculty and courses from across the school's academic departments to teach specialized subjects such as Entrepreneurship, Digital Economy, and Law and Business.

Another way in which Stern's New York ties are apparent is in its teaching. The school boasts nearly 100 adjunct professors, many of whom are highly regarded veterans of the New York business community. Some of the bigger names who have taught as visiting professors at Stern include former Federal Reserve Chairman Paul Volcker and Nobel laureate Robert Solow. The school prides itself on giving its students lessons with real-world applications, and part of this is letting students hear lessons straight from these veterans' mouths.

Stern also emphasizes the global orientation of its student body and its curriculum. A third of the class comes from abroad, and Stern offers an International Business co-major option for the many American students there who have some interest in working overseas. You don't need an international angle to your story when you apply to Stern, but at least acknowledging the importance of a globally-focused education should help your cause.

Stern works to cultivate and maintain a spirit of teamwork and cooperation among its students, who do a fair amount of work in groups. Students and grads sometimes comment that they were pleasantly surprised to find that the culture is more cooperative than they expected, especially given the "shark" reputation that bankers tend to have. If you apply to Stern, don't discount the importance of teamwork in your message. The school is less impressed by individual achievers than it is by well-grounded people who have excelled in their past jobs by working with others. Keep this in mind, especially if you are a banker who is looking to distinguish yourself from the pack.

With a yield in the low 50s, Stern gets stiff competition from the likes of Columbia and Wharton for finance-minded students. Showing the admissions committee that Stern really is where you want to be—and having convincing reasons for why this is the case—will greatly help your chances of being admitted.

Insider information

Although Stern's name is best known on Wall Street, the school is also serious about entrepreneurship. The school's Entrepreneurship and Innovation co-major is a popular choice, as is its Entertainment, Media, and Technology program initiative. Stern's annual Maximum Exposure Business Plan Competition gives budding entrepreneurs a chance to compete for cash prizes. Successful business plan teams are matched with experienced entrepreneurs or venture capitalists who serve as mentors. This is an area of the program that the school continues to emphasize. If you consider yourself to be an entrepreneur, or you want to be one, be sure to let the Stern admissions committee know about it.

Schools that call for a similar approach

- ❐ Columbia Business School.
- ❐ University of Pennsylvania (Wharton).

Northwestern University (Kellogg School of Management)
www.kellogg.northwestern.edu
Evanston, IL

Application at a glance

Application due dates (first, second, third round): Nov. 8, Jan. 10, Mar. 14.

Requirements

- ❐ Essays: Six (three of two pages, three short essays).
- ❐ Interview: Required.
- ❐ Recommendations: One "Career Progress Survey" to be completed by the applicant's direct supervisor.
- ❐ Resume.
- ❐ Application fee: $185.

School at a glance

Dean (start of tenure): Dipak Jain (2001)
Admissions director: Beth Flye
Program size: 1,250 full-time
Acceptance rate: 13 percent
Yield: 64 percent
Mean undergraduate GPA: 3.5
Mean GMAT: 700
Middle 80 percent GMAT: 660–750
Average years of work experience: 4.5
International: 33 percent
Women: 31 percent
Minority: 19 percent

Your Kellogg application strategy

The two words you will almost always hear when you mention Kellogg are "teamwork" and "marketing." Donald Jacobs, the school's dean from 1975 to 2001, is responsible for establishing the school as a top-ranked MBA program, and he did it largely on the strength of his philosophy that business managers can't be effective without knowing how to successfully work in teams. Even though Jacobs is no longer involved in the day-to-day running of the school (he's retained the title of Dean Emeritus), his approach is still very apparent in the school's program and culture. Most homework assignments and projects are done in teams, and the school has recently instituted a Web-based peer review system called TeamNet, which students are required to use in some of their classes.

Marketing is the school's other best-known strength, and much of the credit for that goes to Philip Kotler, who has written some of the best-known Marketing textbooks in the world. The rest of the Marketing faculty includes many other heavy-hitters who have distinguished themselves in their own right. All of this leads to heavy recruiting from companies looking for Marketing experts and brand managers.

Lost in the noise about Kellogg's Marketing program is the fact that its other programs are also very strong. In fact, Marketing isn't even the school's most popular major; more Kellogg students study Finance than anything else. Although Kellogg's curriculum is considered to be General Management in nature, students generally specialize in two or three fields.

The school also has noted faculty in areas such as Strategy and Managerial Economics. Just as Finance is a more popular major at Kellogg than Marketing, the biggest recruiters at the other top schools—McKinsey, Boston Consulting Group, Goldman Sachs, etc.—also do more hiring at Kellogg than the biggest marketing-related firms.

As you would expect, Kellogg's admissions office looks for teamwork-oriented applicants. "Sharks" or hot shots need not apply. This doesn't mean that Kellogg looks for 600 touchy-feely people each year, but rather, it looks for applicants who know how to get things done when working with others. Think of the "desert island test"—if you can think of someone whom you'd hate to be stranded with on an island, then Kellogg probably doesn't want that person, either.

Maybe even more importantly, Kellogg looks for people who will get involved at the school. A distinguishing characteristic of Kellogg is that pretty much everything is student-run, from clubs to international study trips ("Global Initiatives in Management") to professional conferences that the school hosts. Chances are that a student will even review your application. It's not uncommon for a student to be involved in five or six different activities or clubs outside of the typical four-class schedule. What this means for you is that you need to demonstrate that you will get involved. The best way to do this is by showing what you've done in the past to get involved in your profession, school, and community. And less can be more: Instead of listing seven clubs that you once participated in while in college, focus on the one or two activities that you're really passionate about and show exactly how you got involved in those activities and made a difference. The grid from Chapter 2 should help strengthen this important part of your application story.

Insider information

Although Kellogg is best known for its teamwork approach, the school is increasingly positioning itself less as a place where students learn to be team leaders, not merely team players. In other words, people who work well with others, but aren't just followers. The administration wants recruiters to come to Kellogg looking for their next generation of leaders, rather than for marketing or finance experts who are easy to get along with. That means that Kellogg is looking for more outstanding leaders in the applicant pool. To this end, think of personal examples of how you've led teams toward a goal in the past. Most applicants will just think about teamwork in terms of how they helped others accomplish a goal, but show the admissions committee how you led a team to success and you'll be in great shape.

Schools that call for a similar approach

- ❐   Duke University (Fuqua).
- ❐   University of Michigan Business School.

Purdue University (Krannert Graduate School of Management)
www.mgmt.purdue.edu
West Lafayette, IN

Application at a glance

U.S. citizen and permanent resident application due dates (first, second, and third round): Nov. 1, Jan. 1, May. 15.

International student application due dates (first and second round): Dec. 1, Feb. 1.

Requirements

- ❐   Essays: Three (two of 500 words, one of 100 words).
- ❐   Interview: By invitation only.
- ❐   Recommendations: Two, with one preferably coming from a direct supervisor.
- ❐   Resume.
- ❐   Application fee: $55.

School at a glance

Dean (start of tenure): Richard A. Cosier (1999)
Admissions director: Ward Snearly
Program size: 400 full-time
Acceptance rate: 30 percent
Yield: 45 percent
Mean GPA: 3.2
Mean GMAT: 651

Middle 80 percent GMAT: 590–730

Average years of work experience: 4.0

International: 36 percent

Women: 23 percent

Minority: 16 percent

Your Krannert application strategy

Originally positioned as a graduate program in operations, Krannert changed its degree title from Masters of Science in Management to MBA in 2001. The new label made official the expansion of the program, which occurred over several years. Today Krannert is recognized as an MBA program with strengths in technology, manufacturing, and other analytical functions. The school is looking for applicants who can thrive within a quantitatively intense environment, support its traditional strengths, and also continue building its brand in other aspects of business. At heart, Krannert is still a quantitatively centered program, so you should display some proficiency in this area through your GMAT score, transcript(s), or professional experiences.

It's not surprising to hear Krannert MBAs refer to their alma mater as "Techno MBA," as the program regularly utilizes technology to support its hands-on learning philosophy. Many students choose to specialize in Information Systems, one of six functional specializations the school offers (the others are: Accounting, Finance, Marketing, Operations Management, and Strategic Management). In addition to functional specializations, the school offers interdisciplinary concentrations in International Management, General Management, and Manufacturing and Technology Management. Discussion of your goals should include a small blurb on where you see one or two of these specializations coming into play.

Technology is used to simulate e-commerce transactions, the power of enterprise application integration, financial trading, and database architecture. In addition to these examples, Krannert provides numerous opportunities for its students to translate theory into application. The Student-Managed Investment Fund (SMIF) provides students with the opportunity to help manage a six-figure financial portfolio and distribute a portion of the gains to Krannert and other graduate programs. During the Digital Information Industry Simulation, students act as the CEO of a large technology company, making decisions that have an impact on the results of the company. Krannert also offers MarkStrat3, another computer simulation that allows student teams to compete against one another, trying to win market share and increase profits in the high-tech industry. Providing an example in which you took an abstract idea and implemented it is a powerful way to highlight your fit with Krannert's philosophy on translating theory into application.

Given Krannert's strong technology focus, it is important that you display familiarity and comfort with technology. This doesn't mean that you have to come across as a techno wiz, but to the extent that you are at ease with discussing the benefits of technology and sharing ideas of technological innovation, you should do so. Keep in mind, however, that Krannert is also trying to expand its brand beyond just technology and operations, so don't shy away from bringing up interests in other aspects of business. Telling a story about how you would like to apply tech-savvy business principles to industries outside of traditional technology can also help your application stand out.

Krannert provides all of the benefits that come along with most small MBA programs, including accessible faculty, a close-knit student community and an emphasis on teamwork. Immediately after beginning the program, you will be assigned to a four- or five-person team. Students within a team come from diverse professional backgrounds and spend time working on group assignments for the first eight weeks of class. Having strong team skills is important to succeeding in these groups, and is therefore something upon which the admission committee will rate you. Use the essays to discuss your ability to contribute to a team.

Insider information

One of the areas that Krannert is actively looking to expand in is its global presence. The program already receives a large number of applications from international candidates (70–80 percent of all applications) and maintains a large number of international students (generally more than 1/3 of students). Krannert is looking to leverage its popularity among international candidates and offer more opportunities abroad. One international program the school is actively promoting is the German International Graduate School of Management and Administration (GISMA) program. This program features an eight-week module in Hannover, Germany, during which students take classes taught by Krannert faculty and visit German companies. To the extent that you have global aspirations, be sure to highlight them in your application. Doing so should benefit your fit with the school.

Schools that call for a similar approach

- ❏ Carnegie Mellon University.
- ❏ Michigan State University (Broad).
- ❏ Indiana University (Kelley).

Stanford University Graduate School of Business
www.gsb.stanford.edu
Stanford, CA

Application at a glance

Application due dates (first, second, and third round): Oct. 30, Jan. 8, Mar. 19.

Requirements

- ❏ Essays: Two (both of unlimited length).
- ❏ Interview: By invitation only.
- ❏ Recommendations: Three—two should come from people who are familiar with your professional capabilities and at least one of which from a

direct supervisor. One letter from a peer with whom you have worked on a team or a project (can be professional, extracurricular, charitable, or otherwise). Academic recommendations are discouraged.

❐ Resume.

❐ Application fee: $200.

School at a glance

Dean (start of tenure): Robert Joss (1999)

Admissions director: Derrick Bolton

Program size: 730 full-time

Acceptance rate: 8 percent

Yield: 80 percent (estimate)

Mean GPA: 3.6 (estimate)

Mean GMAT: 725 (estimate)

Middle 80 percent GMAT: 665–765 (estimate)

Average years of work experience: 4.7

International: 32 percent

Women: 37 percent

Minority: 27 percent (estimate)

Your Stanford application strategy

The instructions to Stanford's application indicate that it evaluates candidates based on three high-level criteria: "demonstrated leadership potential, strong academic aptitude, and contributions to the diversity of the Stanford community." Sounds simple enough, right? The difficulty with navigating the Stanford application is the degree to which these three criteria must be emphasized. In demonstrating your fit with these criteria your emphasis should primarily be on the innovation and leadership dimensions.

The most obvious example of Stanford's alignment with innovation is its strength in entrepreneurship. Closely linked with Silicon Valley, Stanford has achieved an entrepreneurship branding that other b-schools dream of. While Stanford is a general management program to its core (students do not select majors), electives based on entrepreneurship are in abundance. Courses that focus on areas such as venture capital, business model development, private equity, and entrepreneurial strategy are the backbone of Stanford's entrepreneurial strength. Discussing your entrepreneurial inclination can be a great way to unite the innovation and leadership dimensions, but it should not be done to simply appear as though you fit with Stanford's values. Recognize that a large percentage of applicants who apply to Stanford will discuss entrepreneurship in their application. Therefore, should you go down this path, include vivid details about your ideas and also be sure to discuss their potential impact on society. This will help separate you from the pack.

Recommendations should be viewed as an extremely important aspect of your Stanford application. The admission committee will take a close look at your recommendations in evaluating your leadership potential and your teamwork capabilities. If there is one application in which you should avoid submitting generic recommendations at all costs, this is it. Make sure that you follow the instructions closely and submit two professional recommendations and one peer recommendation.

Academic aptitude is a criterion that Stanford evaluates more rigorously than most other top b-schools. Because the curriculum is quantitatively heavy, the admissions committee will look closely for measures that indicate that you will be able to succeed within the learning model. Therefore, your GMAT score will be looked at closely in addition to your transcript(s). If your scores don't reflect a high standard of analytical background, you will need to express it through your professional experiences and/or additional coursework. You should also be aware that while those accepted by Stanford come from a multitude of undergraduate institutions, a large majority attended "high prestige" universities. If you are not among this group, you should discuss your school's strengths and your reasons for attending it.

While Stanford's emphasis on teamwork may not be as strong as it is at Fuqua, Kellogg, or Tuck, it is definitely an important part of the learning model. During their first quarter at Stanford, students are assigned to study groups of four to five people and work together on a daily basis. You can display a penchant for working with others by discussing previous professional and extracurricular team involvement.

The essay portion of the application is your opportunity to demonstrate your ability to contribute to the diversity of the Stanford community. Because the Stanford essays do not have a word limit, you should really focus on telling your unique story, but doing so in a logical, flowing manner. Include headings in your essays so that your readers can follow your framework easily. Consider writing your Stanford essays after you've completed other applications. This will allow your story to be more polished. And don't even bother trying to shoehorn an essay from another application into your Stanford application. Ultimately, your essays should reveal your passions, both professional and personal, and highlight your distinctiveness. You probably haven't scaled Mt. Everest or won a marathon, but don't let that keep you from positioning yourself as unique in some way. One applicant we spoke with, who was denied admission after her interview, mentioned that the alumnus with whom she interviewed suggested that her lack of distinctiveness contributed to her ultimate denial. "He complimented my competitive profile, but stated that I had no point of differentiation in my perspective, which weakened an otherwise strong profile."

You can assert a distinct passion for Stanford by visiting the school, checking out a class, and chatting with current students (yes, this goes for those of you on the East Coast too). Make sure that this visit finds its way into your essays in your discussion of "why Stanford?" Your enthusiasm for Stanford will resonate positively with the admissions committee as it strives to maintain a high yield percentage.

Insider information

The Stanford learning model doesn't offer majors, but it does offer certificates in public management and global management. The Public Management Program (PMP) prepares students for positions in the social sector and the Global Management Program (GMP) prepares students for opportunities at a global level. Both certificates are supported by a large number of electives, programs, and career resources. More than one third of the student body pursues certificates in PMP or GMP, and Stanford is actively looking for ways in which it can augment these programs. Discussing how you would utilize the resources offered by these programs in conjunction with your career objectives is a great way to display fit with Stanford.

Schools that call for a similar approach

- ❏ MIT (Sloan).
- ❏ UCLA (Anderson).

University of California at Berkeley (Haas School of Business)
www.haas.berkeley.edu
Berkeley, CA

Application at a glance

Application due dates (first, second, third, and fourth round): Nov. 1, Dec. 13, Jan. 31, Mar. 14.

Requirements

- ❏ Essays: Eight (seven short essays, one of 500 words).
- ❏ Interview: By invitation only.
- ❏ Recommendations: Two, both should come from people who are familiar with your professional capabilities.
- ❏ Resume.
- ❏ Application fee: $150.

School at a glance

Dean (start of tenure): Tom Campbell (2002)

Admissions director: Ilse Evans

Program size: 480 full-time

Acceptance rate: 11 percent

Yield: 48 percent

Mean GPA: 3.6

Mean GMAT: 703

Middle 80 percent GMAT: 650–760

Average years of work experience: 5.2

International: 34 percent

Women: 30 percent

Minority: 22 percent

Your Haas application strategy

In a world filled with business schools, Haas maintains a high degree of distinction. That distinction can be seen just by reading through the Haas essays, which at times seem more like questions from a psychologist rather than from an admissions committee. Indeed, the essay questions are indicative of a school that is serious about admitting applicants who can maintain almost paradoxical balances—applicants who are committed to traditional business learning, but display a bit of personal panache. Applicants who would be willing to stand alone based on personal conviction, but are willing to unite in the name of teamwork. Applicants who are looking to make waves in the marketplace, but remain cognizant of social and ethical responsibilities. If you can paint a picture of yourself that reflects these traits, in addition to satisfying the more common admissions requirements, then you stand a good chance of being accepted into the Haas family.

The Haas learning model continues to emphasize three main themes: Entrepreneurship and Innovation, Management of Technology, and International Business Management. For the last several years, Haas has benefited from a symbiotic relationship with nearby Silicon Valley. This has resulted, not surprisingly, in an intensified focus on entrepreneurship. Haas now boasts multiple opportunities for students to cultivate and test their business ideas as well as to interact with mentors and experts. The Lester Center for Entrepreneurship and Innovation, founded in 1991, supports a variety of activities such as the Berkeley Business Incubator, UC Berkeley Entrepreneurs Forum, and entrepreneurship fellowships and internships.

Technology has also been a natural outgrowth of Haas' geographical location. The Management of Technology Program offers a number of opportunities including courses such as Strategic Computing and Communication Technology, Information Technology Strategy, and International Trade and Competition in High Technology. The program also features research initiatives, and the annual Leading Edge Technology Conference.

The final theme, International Business Management, is highlighted in Haas' course offerings in addition to its International Business Development (IBD) and International Exchange programs. IBD offers students the opportunity to participate in a global consulting project with a team composed entirely of Haas students. In terms of exchange programs, Haas offers six in locations such as London, Barcelona, and Hong Kong.

Although the Haas learning model is rooted in general management precepts, students can obtain certificates in any one of the three themes in addition to Corporate Environmental Management and Health Management. Displaying an understanding of these themes and how they would benefit you should be a critical part of your application.

Demonstrating the teamwork dimension is also important, as Haas admissions counselors are actively looking for applicants who display team spirit. The learning model promotes a cooperative, intimate environment in which students participate in multiple group assignments and interact closely with faculty. To demonstrate fit with these characteristics, you should display a pattern of getting involved and a sense of community.

The Haas learning model has a strong bent towards applying abstract theories to real-world situations. This approach begins with the faculty, a majority of whom have significant experience within the marketplace, and extends to the students, who boast an average of 5.2 years of work experience. The maturity dimension is highly valued at Haas and gaining acceptance with under three years of work experience can be challenging. As an applicant, you should try to display a diversity of experience and insight into how complex issues such as globalization, ethics, environmentalism, and politics impact business operations.

Insider information

As other business schools scramble to revamp their programs in order to promote a new focus on ethics and social responsibility, Haas will benefit from its reputation as a pioneer in the field. With a required course in ethics, numerous electives, programs, and events focused on the topic, Haas gives full treatment to the interaction of business, ethics, and social responsibility. The National Social Venture Business Plan Competition is a hallmark of that interaction, as business schools across the country compete for a total of $100,000 by presenting plans that outline business propositions that have a societal or environmental component. Although a majority of Haas grads pursue careers in the traditional areas of consulting and finance, they all are all influenced by Haas' incorporation of social issues within the learning model. As you present your profile, make sure that you reflect a cognizance of societal and ethical issues that extend from business issues.

Schools that call for a similar approach

- ❐ Duke University (Fuqua).
- ❐ UCLA (Anderson).
- ❐ USC (Marshall).
- ❐ Yale School of Management.

University of California at Los Angeles (Anderson Graduate School of Management)
www.anderson.ucla.edu
Los Angeles, CA

Application at a glance

Application due dates (first, second, third, and fourth round): Nov. 6, Dec. 27, Jan. 30, Apr. 4.

Requirements

- ❐ Essays: Four (500–1,000 words each).
- ❐ Interview: Recommended.

☐ Recommendations: Two, both should come from people who are familiar with your professional capabilities and one preferably from your direct supervisor.

☐ Resume.

☐ Application fee: $150.

School at a glance

Dean (start of tenure): Bruce Willison (1999)

Admissions director: Linda Baldwin

Program size: 520 full-time

Acceptance rate: 15 percent

Yield: 52 percent

Mean GPA: 3.6

Mean GMAT: 710

Middle 80 percent GMAT: 650–750

Average years of work experience: 4.7

International: 23 percent

Women: 27 percent

Minority: 19 percent

Your Anderson application strategy

Sun, beach, entertainment management program—while Anderson definitely has these assets that few other MBA programs can match, it also excels in the traditional areas that are valued by applicants. The Anderson program offers a general management curriculum that allows students to select from specializations in 11 areas or even create their own specialization. The specializations cover a wide range of topics including Finance, Marketing, Entrepreneurial Studies, Information Systems, Real Estate, and Accounting. In support of its flexible general management learning model, Anderson is in search of candidates who display a unique balance of leadership and teamwork capabilities.

Anderson views leadership in three basic ways. First, it recognizes leaders for their ability to convey strategic direction and vision to others. Vision allows for the unification of the group behind a common goal. Second, Anderson views leaders as problem-solvers who apply their analytical and communication skills to overcome challenges. Finally, Anderson defines leaders as people who cultivate the first two capabilities in others. Anderson does not view leadership and teamwork in separate spheres and therefore notes that the best leaders are also the best team players. The Anderson learning model provides students with opportunities to improve their balance of leadership and teamwork skills through team simulations, team-building exercises, analytical models, and projects. Your challenge is to display fit with Anderson's definition of leadership. One of the best places to do that is in answering the essay questions. Try to provide an example that shows your leadership skills along the lines of the three definitions.

Anderson's entrepreneurship program has served, in many ways, as the model for many other business schools. The program offers a blend of coursework, entrepreneurial resources, and "hands-on" opportunities. At the core of Anderson's entrepreneurship program is the Price Center. The Price Center provides support for the development of course materials, research, and experiential opportunities. One such opportunity, the Knapp Venture Competition, is a traditional business plan contest, through which participants can win venture capital funding. The Venture Fellows Program and the Student Investment Fund—two competitive programs that students must apply for—expose participants to venture capital and investment management activities. Students can also gain exposure to new ventures through the Wolfen Award, which calls for selected students to complete a feasibility study on a start-up as part of an internship. Because of Anderson's strength in entrepreneurship, discussing your own entrepreneurial inclination can be a great way to display fit with the school and to differentiate yourself based on your unique ideas.

Anderson is also often recognized for its leading technology programs. It was one of the first business schools to integrate a wireless network throughout its facilities and often receives praise for its use of technology in the classroom. If you are interested in technology, you will find a number of interesting courses and opportunities in which to participate. Similar in its function to the Price Center, the Center for Management in the Information Economy provides resources to faculty in their research on how technology is impacting the business environment.

Despite Anderson's low acceptance rate and its great reputation, the school has a relatively low yield percentage. The school is looking for improvement in that area and will evaluate applicants closely to see if they are really committed to Anderson or are just applying to diversify risk. Along those lines, establishing fit is extremely important. You are given an explicit opportunity to show that Anderson is your top pick in its essays. Be sure to capitalize on that opportunity by displaying intimate knowledge of the program and then go the extra step by explaining how you would get involved in school activities to further bolster Anderson's reputation.

Insider information

A unique aspect of the Anderson learning model is the Applied Management Research Project. This six month project is the last requirement of the MBA program and follows in line with Anderson's perspective on leadership, teamwork, and applied learning. The projects are completed in teams of three to five and generally consist of a strategic consulting assignment or the development of a business venture idea. In either case, students are able to apply their entire Anderson toolkit in a comprehensive manner. Discussing your interest in this project—and more generally, in the hands-on learning opportunities that Anderson offers—during your interview or in your application is another good way to show fit.

Schools that call for a similar approach

- ❏ Stanford University.
- ❏ University of California at Berkeley (Haas).
- ❏ USC (Marshall).

University of Chicago Graduate School of Business
gsb.uchicago.edu
Chicago, IL

Application at a glance
Application due dates (first, second, third round): Nov. 8, Jan. 8, Mar. 21.

Requirements
- ❏ Essays: Three (two of 750 words, one of 500 words).
- ❏ Interview: Strongly recommended.
- ❏ Recommendations: Two, both should come from people who are familiar with your professional capabilities.
- ❏ Resume.
- ❏ Application fee: $200.

School at a glance
Dean (start of tenure): Edward A. Snyder (2001)
Admissions director: Don Martin
Program size: 1,169 full-time
Acceptance rate: 15 percent
Yield: 67 percent
Mean undergraduate GPA: 3.4
Mean GMAT: 687
Middle 80 percent GMAT: 610–750
Average years of work experience: 4.4
International: 31 percent
Women: 31 percent
Minority: 7 percent

Your University of Chicago application strategy
The University of Chicago Graduate School of Business (GSB) has long had a reputation as a great business school, and it has only grown in stature since Edward Snyder moved into the Dean's office in 2001.

Snyder and his administration have worked hard to promote the GSB's strengths while addressing its perceived weaknesses. Its strengths are impressive, including the school's notable roster of Nobel laureate faculty members—six as of last count, more than any other school—its high number of well-placed alumni, its strong international brand name, and its top-flight reputation with recruiters. As for weaknesses, in addition to its reputation for appealing mainly to quantitative jocks, the school has also faced a perception that GSB students are somewhat less involved in the school than those at other top programs, partly a result of the school having to compete with all that Chicago has to offer.

The school has improved its reputation through a variety of programs. A grade-nondisclosure policy, put in place in 2000, has taken the edge off of grade competition. Leadership Effectiveness and Development (LEAD), a mandatory course for first-year students, helps students develop their leadership, teamwork, and communication skills. The school has also branched out beyond finance, emphasizing the strength of its marketing and general management programs, among others. Additionally, Snyder has made a strong push to augment the Chicago GSB community on campus, which remains an ongoing campaign for the school. Given that, the school will continue to look for applicants who demonstrate a willingness to get involved with meaningful extracurricular activities, maybe even more so than other top business schools. Therefore, be sure that your Chicago GSB application emphasizes your leadership and involvement in past endeavors.

One part of the school's reputation that is unlikely to change is its rigorous academic program. No matter what attributes the school tries to instill in its graduates, it is unlikely that it will lessen its emphases on hard finance and quantitative skills. Finance is still the most popular major, followed by Strategy, Accounting, and Marketing (13 majors are offered). One aspect of the curriculum that students love is its flexibility. LEAD is the only required course in the entire program, with students choosing from a menu of courses to satisfy their core curriculum needs. This level of flexibility truly sets Chicago apart from other business school learning models. Electives include "lab" classes, such as the school's New Product and Strategy Development lab, which gives students an opportunity to take on consulting projects for real companies. Keep this flexibility in mind as you think about how you might fit with the Chicago GSB program. This type of environment suits someone with a strong career focus better than it does a student who is still trying to figure out what he wants to do after business school.

The bottom line is that the school will always take its academics very seriously, and you'll need to communicate that you have the brainpower to keep up, regardless of your academic or professional background. Doing well on the quantitative section of the GMAT will help you a lot here. However, the school is very serious about turning out well-rounded leaders, and this starts by admitting well-rounded applicants who will get involved. If you believe that you can handle the rigorous curriculum, demonstrating that you have polish as well as brains will go a long way toward getting you into Chicago GSB.

Insider information

Chicago GSB's quantitative-heavy reputation has traditionally meant that it attracted a high proportion of people who fit well with the school's learning model. On one hand, the school attracted a less diverse applicant pool than other top schools, but on the other, it knew that a majority of applicants would be a good fit. Now, the school's resurgence in the national rankings means that it may start to attract a broader applicant pool, some of whom may not really be a great fit with the school, or may not even know why they want to attend Chicago GSB other than because it's ranked higher than most other programs. The school's challenge will be to figure out who really belongs at the school. Concentrate on standing out from the pack by emphasizing your fit with the program, ideally by demonstrating some intellectual horsepower as well as the traits of the well-rounded applicant whom the school is looking for.

Schools that call for a similar approach

- ❏ Carnegie Mellon University.
- ❏ Columbia Business School.
- ❏ MIT (Sloan).
- ❏ University of Rochester (Simon).

University of London (London Business School)
www.london.edu
London, UK

Application at a glance

Application due dates (first, second, third, fourth round): Nov. 8, Jan. 3, Feb. 28, May 2.

Requirements

- ❏ Essays: Seven (three of 50–200 words, four of 500 words).
- ❏ Interview: By invitation only.
- ❏ Recommendations: Two, both should come from people who are in a position to comment on your suitability for the LBS program. LBS values both professional and educational references.
- ❏ Resume.
- ❏ Application fee: £120 or U.S. $180.

School at a glance

Dean (start of tenure): Laura D' Andrea Tyson (2002)
Admissions director: David Simpson
Program size: 500 full-time
Acceptance rate: 19 percent
Yield: 58 percent
Mean GPA: N/A
Mean GMAT: 690
Middle 80 percent GMAT: 640–740
Average years of work experience: 5.5
International: 85 percent (foreign nationals)
Women: 26 percent
Minority: N/A

Your University of London application strategy

Looking for a truly international MBA experience? Most other business schools' international immersion claims pale in comparison to what London Business School (LBS) offers. Incoming students can expect that 80–85 percent of their classmates will hail from countries outside of the UK. That representation tallies up to more than 70 nations in total. Combine that with a language proficiency requirement that calls for students to have a reasonable fluency in at least two languages (including English) and exchange programs with 30 business schools abroad, and you have the makings of an environment that encourages a fluid multicultural dialogue. Indeed, "becoming an international citizen" is one of four themes that LBS's program expresses. The admissions committee will be looking closely to see what type of international citizen you will be, so be prepared to discuss your international and cross-cultural experiences. You can expect a good portion of your interview to be dedicated to this subject.

In addition to demonstrating that you have the ability to be an international citizen, you should also make sure to display fit with the other three LBS learning themes: becoming a leader, becoming an independent thinker, and making things happen. These themes should not be viewed in disparate silos, but rather as intertwined objectives. LBS views leadership in three different ways: being competent and confident across a wide range of functions, being creative and flexible in your leadership style, and achieving results. Think of professional and personal examples that display these leadership characteristics and try to integrate as many of them as you can into your essays.

One of the ways that LBS believes your leadership abilities will be enhanced during the MBA program is through team opportunities. Immediately after beginning the program you will be assigned to a study group of six to seven classmates, in which you will tackle a multitude of group assignments. The emphasis on teamwork is so strong that these group projects are worth approximately 50 percent of students' overall first year grade. In addition to participating in a study group there is an expectation that students will also play leading roles in at least one of LBS's 50 club opportunities. In sum, these experiences allow students to enhance the three LBS leadership characteristics, while cultivating their team skills. To show your willingness to get involved, you might want to pick a couple club opportunities that interest you and mention them in your essays.

Becoming an independent thinker highlights LBS's desire to develop not only business leaders, but also to a certain extent, thought leaders. This is underscored by the fact that LBS is one of the only business schools that has its faculty conduct a majority of interviews. Given this type of interview, it is to your advantage to acquaint yourself even more than usual with the curriculum. LBS is also one of the few business schools that values recommendations that are written by professors. The interactive LBS learning model benefits most when students have a high regard for the classroom dynamic and for academic preparation. Discussing your view of academics and how it has played a role in your outlook is a great way to display your stance as an "independent thinker." Ultimately, LBS expects its students to take the academic theories learned in the classroom and "make things happen."

The "making things happen" theme, a mixture of innovation and implementation, is often expressed through entrepreneurial ventures. The combination of the Foundation for Entrepreneurial Management, Sussex Place Investment Management, and the Gavron Business Centre serve as a business incubator and a capital fund from which students can access valuable capital and resources. Students can also opt to participate in the school's Entrepreneurship Summer School, which allows participants to develop and test business plans through their early stages. At the end of the experience, students present the results of feasibility studies to expert panels for feedback. Participants are then encouraged to further hone their business plans throughout their second year. If you have entrepreneurial ambitions, make sure to bring it out in your application.

Insider information

One of the centerpieces of the LBS learning model is its Shadowing Project. As part of the project, first-year students are assigned to a manager for a week and are required to observe that manager's approach to leadership, challenges, and colleague interaction. At the end of the week, students record their observations and reflect on the implications those observations have on their professional development. This reflective nature is something that LBS looks closely for in its applicants; the thought being that reflection produces maturity. Indeed, the LBS learning model suggests that the four themes cannot be achieved without reflection. It is therefore imperative that you demonstrate a thoughtful nature in discussing your past experiences. Describing personal discoveries that you gathered from activities and events is a good way to do so.

Schools that call for a similar approach

- ❏ Columbia Business School.
- ❏ INSEAD.
- ❏ University of Pennsylvania (Wharton).

University of Maryland (Robert H. Smith School of Business)
www.rhsmith.umd.edu
College Park, MD

Application at a glance

Application due dates (International Early, Domestic Early, International Final, Domestic Final): Nov. 15, Dec. 2, Feb. 15, May 1.

Requirements

- ❏ Essays: Three (one of two pages, two of one page).
- ❏ Interview: By invitation only.
- ❏ Recommendations: Three required.
- ❏ Resume.
- ❏ Application fee: $50.

School at a glance

Dean (start of tenure): Howard Frank (1997)

Admissions director: Sabrina White

Program size: 420 full-time

Acceptance rate: 23 percent

Yield: 52 percent

Mean undergraduate GPA: 3.4

Mean GMAT: 655

Middle 80 percent GMAT: 610–710

Average years of work experience: 5.2

International: 33 percent

Women: 34 percent

Minority: 14 percent

Your Smith application strategy

Smith has made a name for itself among business schools for its emphasis on technology. The school's core curriculum works information technology lessons into nearly every one of its classes, and students can tailor their general management education to concentrate in topics including electronic commerce, e-service, information systems, and supply chain management.

One tangible example of the school's technology focus is its Netcentricity Laboratory, or "Net Lab," which Smith has built as a proving ground and learning environment for functions including e-commerce and supply chain management. Students use models and simulations to learn the nuances of these systems in a series of e-business lab courses. The lab is sponsored by industry heavyweights including Oracle, Sun, and Reuters, and features their technologies prominently. The Net Lab also contains a Financial Markets Lab—modeled after a Wall Street trading floor—which gives students a chance to apply what they learn in the classroom to real-time financial decisions. Naturally, the more you can speak with passion about the importance of technology in your career path, the better fit you will demonstrate in your Smith application.

Speaking of Wall Street, the school also has a real-money portfolio called the Mayer Fund, which is run by 10–12 second-year Smith students. Founded in 1993, the fund gives students a chance to manage a portfolio worth more than $1 million. The fund is a great chance for aspiring money managers to get their feet wet and gain exposure to the top executives who make up the fund's external board of directors. If you are interested in finance, consider discussing your interest in the Financial Markets Lab or the Mayer Fund in your application.

Another example of hands-on learning at Smith is its MBA Consulting Project, a required course for all second-year students. Teams of students work to earn credit toward their MBA while consulting for major corporations and government agencies. This is a unique feature of the Smith MBA and one that the school feels sets it apart.

Even if you're not interested in consulting, make sure that you demonstrate enthusiasm for the real-world lessons that this program provides. In fact, if you're not a consultant, emphasizing the appeal of this program may help your application stand out even more, as long as it's consistent with the rest of your story.

Smith students and grads describe the school's culture as being very cooperative. Teamwork figures into a lot of what students do, both in traditional classes and the school's Experiential Learning Modules that augment students' skills in areas such as communications and strategic business analysis. Accordingly, be sure to frame your past successes as instances of team success wherever possible in order to demonstrate fit with the program. And while leadership isn't talked about as much at Smith as at other schools, any examples you can provide to bolster your leadership dimension will help you stand out from the pack.

Like other schools with lower yield percentages, Smith is careful about selecting candidates who are truly interested in its program. Demonstrating your knowledge of the school, and especially your enthusiasm for its focus on technology and entrepreneurship, will help you make your case that Smith is where you want to be.

Insider information

Smith is very committed to entrepreneurship, and its Dingman Center for Entrepreneurship is a major hub for start-up activity in the Washington, D.C., region, giving entrepreneurs access to experienced mentors and potential investors. If you are serious about entrepreneurship, look closely at the school's Dingman and Lamone Scholarships. Students are selected based on their entrepreneurship experience, desire to start a business after business school, and their start-up ideas. They receive personal mentoring and business plan advice from experienced entrepreneurs in the Dingman Center. In exchange, Dingman and Lamone Scholars volunteer at the center, offering their own advice to others and running educational seminars in entrepreneurship and networking. Think about this program if you plan on starting your own business, especially on the East Coast, where Dingman's reputation is strongest.

Schools that call for a similar approach

- ❐ Indiana University (Kelley).
- ❐ Michigan State University (Broad).
- ❐ Vanderbilt University (Owen).

University of Michigan Business School
www.bus.umich.edu
Ann Arbor, MI

Application at a glance

Application due dates (first, second, and third round): Nov. 1, Jan. 7, Mar. 1.

Requirements

- ❏ Essays: Four of two pages each.
- ❏ Interview: Highly recommended.
- ❏ Recommendations: Two—Suggest that both come from a direct supervisor, employer, or someone who is familiar with your professional capabilities.
- ❏ Resume.
- ❏ Application fee: $125.

School at a glance

Dean (start of tenure): Robert Dolan (2001)

Admissions director: Kris Nebel

Program size: 860 full-time

Acceptance rate: 19 percent

Yield: 57 percent

Mean GPA: 3.4

Mean GMAT: 682

Middle 80 percent GMAT: 630–730

Average years of work experience: 5.0

International: 29 percent

Women: 28 percent

Minority: 20 percent

Your University of Michigan application strategy

The key to getting accepted into the University of Michigan Business School (UMBS) is to demonstrate balance across the four dimensions (leadership, innovation, teamwork, maturity) throughout your application. Regardless of the application component(s) in which you emphasize these dimensions, they should each make a couple appearances. It is imperative, therefore, that you take time to analyze your strengths and weaknesses for each of the dimensions before beginning the UMBS application.

UMBS is consistently recognized for its innovation and its focus on applying business principles to real-world scenarios. Both of these attributes are integrated in the learning model along with a solid dose of general management courses. A good example of this combination is UMBS's Multidisciplinary Action Project (MAP). Students are required to work on teams in completing a seven-week project for companies pre-selected by UMBS. The projects are highly analytical and allow students to apply the skills they learned in the classroom to a variety of companies. For those who have inclinations that are more international or entrepreneurial in nature, UMBS offers its IMAP and EMAP programs. The latest example of UMBS's application-based learning is The Tozzi Center. The Tozzi Electronic Business and Finance Center features a trading floor, an elliptical classroom, and a computer laboratory. The trading floor allows for dedicated, real-time access to the global markets. It is used for a multitude of financial class exercises and student projects. Having and displaying knowledge of these types of programs should be a major component of your UMBS application process.

Demonstrating the ability to apply business principles in a rational manner is especially important. Recruiters repeatedly complement UMBS grads on their practical approach, which has been a large reason for UMBS's success in the business school rankings. One applicant, who was recently accepted, displayed a practical approach by explaining how she identified a neglected growth opportunity within her business segment. The applicant took initiative by creating a marketing plan that focused on the opportunity and was able to see her idea through to implementation. These are the types of applicants UMBS seeks.

Given UMBS's focus on professional excellence, it is not surprising to see that accepted students have an average of five years of work experience. This should not discourage applicants with less professional work experience, but recognize that UMBS will especially want to know how you can contribute to the program if you have less than three years of work experience. You should anticipate being questioned on this point during your interview.

Almost all activities at UMBS are team based, so check your ego before beginning the application. Providing one or two examples of your teamwork capabilities should go a long way toward establishing fit with the program.

Overall, if you meet the baseline criteria, express the four dimensions, display knowledge about the learning model and exhibit passion for the school, you should be in a much better position to receive an acceptance letter from UMBS.

Insider information

Over time, entrepreneurship has received greater attention at UMBS and it is now a major aspect of the learning model. The school has vast resources for aspiring entrepreneurs, such as the Samuel Zell-Robert H. Lurie Institute for Entrepreneurial Studies, which supports students as they explore their own business plans and start-up ideas. UMBS will continue to expand its support of entrepreneurial activities because it produces a virtuous cycle. Successful ventures led by students reflect positively on the curriculum, thereby attracting more potential students.

The UMBS application process allows for ample opportunity to discuss innovative entrepreneurial ideas and those opportunities should be capitalized on. That is not to say that all applicants should be aspiring entrepreneurs, but to the extent that you can display entrepreneurial spirit, do so. That spirit can be expressed through an idea for a new business or through an idea for your current company. The admissions committee will certainly take notice of your penchant for entrepreneurship and hopefully recognize your ability to augment the UMBS brand. Being recognized as a potential brand builder is a great way to move your application into the "yes" pile.

Schools that call for a similar approach
- ❏ Cornell University (Johnson).
- ❏ Duke University (Fuqua).

❒ Northwestern University (Kellogg).

❒ USC (Marshall).

University of North Carolina at Chapel Hill (Kenan-Flagler Business School)
www.kenanflagler.unc.edu
Chapel Hill, NC

Application at a glance

Application due dates (first, second, third round): Nov. 22, Jan. 31, Apr. 4.

Requirements

❒ Essays: Three of two pages each.

❒ Interview: Applicant-initiated until mid-December. After mid-December, by invitation only.

❒ Recommendations: Two, at least one should come from a direct supervisor.

❒ Resume.

❒ Application fee: $100.

School at a glance

Dean (start of tenure): Robert S. Sullivan (1998)

Admissions director: Sherry Wallace

Program size: 554 full-time

Acceptance rate: 30 percent

Yield: 46 percent

Mean GPA: 3.2

Mean GMAT: 680

Middle 80 percent GMAT: 640–710

Average years of work experience: 5.2

International: 27 percent

Women: 30 percent

Minority: 16 percent

Your Kenan-Flagler application strategy

Over the last several years, Kenan-Flagler has made great strides in establishing its name among the top business schools. With an intense focus on analytics, leadership and teamwork, and a small-program culture, Kenan-Flagler has grown in popularity among applicants and recruiters. The learning model features an integrated general management curriculum that focuses on four themes: Analyzing Capabilities and Resources, Monitoring the Marketplace and External Environment, Formulating Strategy, and

Implementing Strategy and Assessing Firm Performance. These themes are featured in four corresponding eight-week modules, taken during the first year.

During the second year, students can select from seven "career concentrations" (Corporate Finance, Customer and Product Development, Investment Management, Global Supply-chain Management, Management Consulting, Real Estate, Entrepreneurship, and Venture Development). Students can supplement these career concentrations with "enrichment concentrations" in Sustainable Enterprise, International Business, or Electronic Business and Digital Commerce. As their names indicate, these concentrations are more oriented toward career development than traditional functions. This is indicative of a learning model that prides itself on having close ties to industry development. Those close ties are supported by having a corporate advisory board, comprised of experts from top companies, that provides guidance on the concentrations' curricula. In addition to serving on the board, these experts also provide students with career advice and job opportunities. To fit well with its focus on career development, Kenan-Flagler looks for applicants who are strong in the maturity dimension. The school discourages those with less than two years work experience from applying and takes a close look at applicants' professional records in search of tangible achievements.

Analytics plays a large role in the Kenan-Flagler learning model and therefore in the applicant selection process. The program is known for its quantitative rigor, so if you have a relatively low quantitative GMAT score and a weak quantitative background, you should consider taking a couple extra courses in economics, statistics, or financial accounting. Like many other schools, Kenan-Flagler has an analytical workshop that students can attend before classes start, but taking initiative to shore up your quantitative skills will show the admissions committee that you will be able to succeed in its numbers-driven environment.

The Kenan-Flagler culture strongly emphasizes both leadership and teamwork, but the admissions committee will more actively evaluate your leadership potential. To bolster that potential, first-year students take a two-part course called Leading and Managing. Students begin the course by reviewing leadership evaluations filled out by their former colleagues. These evaluations pinpoint leadership growth opportunities that students focus on throughout the course. Each student ultimately produces a leadership plan which details the areas in which she would like to improve. There should be at least three aspects of your leadership capabilities that you emphasize in your application: Use of analytical skills to assess situations, ability to leverage resources (both people and tools) in developing solutions, and success in implementing solutions. Discussion of these leadership traits will help you establish fit with Kenan-Flagler's mission.

If you are considering an entrepreneurial career path, discussing it in your application is a great way to get your application a second look. We're not talking about merely mentioning that entrepreneurship is an interest, but rather actually discussing the innovation you would like to bring to the market. The latter will get you further because Kenan-Flagler is interested in students who are serious about entrepreneurship. It has spent the last several years augmenting its entrepreneurial program and is hoping to become a household name in the area. Under the direction of the school's Center for Entrepreneurial and Technology Venturing, students can now select from a suite of electives that provide insight into each stage of business model development. The school holds an annual venture capital competition, during which aspiring entrepreneurs put their models to the test and receive feedback from established venture capital firms. It can even be competitive to get into some of the later-stage entrepreneurial classes, which require an application and a business plan.

Despite the accolades Kenan-Flagler has received for making improvements to its program, it still has a relatively low yield percentage. The admissions committee will take a close look at your application to see whether you are serious about attending the school. Naturally, establishing fit with the school's mission and values is a good way to express your interest. An additional, more conventional way to do so is by visiting the campus. The admissions committee looks positively on applicants who visit the campus as a way to get to know the school and the learning model more intimately. Taking this step will express the level of commitment for which the school is looking.

Insider information

In the past, Kenan-Flagler was criticized for its lack of focus on international business. It has since increased its global emphasis by adding an international business concentration, increasing study abroad opportunities, and adding language courses. The school now actively looks for applicants who are interested in pursuing global careers, so if you have any experience or interests along those lines, make sure to bring it out in your application.

Schools that call for a similar approach

- ❑ Cornell University (Johnson).
- ❑ Emory University (Goizueta).
- ❑ Vanderbilt University (Owen).

University of Pennsylvania (The Wharton School)
www.wharton.upenn.edu
Philadelphia, PA

Application at a glance

Application due dates (first, second, third round): Oct. 24, Jan. 9, Mar. 13.

Requirements

- ❑ Essays: Four (two of 1,000 words each, two of 500 words each).
- ❑ Interview: By invitation only.
- ❑ Recommendations: Two, at least one should come from a direct supervisor.
- ❑ Resume.
- ❑ Application fee: $175 (online), $200 (paper).

School at a glance

Dean (start of tenure): Patrick T. Harker (2000)

Admissions director: Rosemaria Martinelli

Program size: 1,600 full-time

Acceptance rate: 13 percent

Yield: 74 percent

Mean GPA: 3.5

Mean GMAT: 711

Middle 80 percent GMAT: 660–760

Average years of work experience: 6.4

International: 36 percent

Women: 34 percent

Minority: 27 percent

Your Wharton application strategy

Wharton sums up its b-school positioning in two words: Wharton Innovates. Indeed, Wharton's stellar reputation and consistent appearance at the top of the rankings can be attributed to the school's ability to transform itself since its establishment in 1881 as the nation's first collegiate business school. Part of your challenge as an applicant is to get the admissions committee to think of your position as *Your Name Here* Innovates.

In support of its Wharton Innovates positioning, Wharton is actively expanding its promotion of entrepreneurial activity. The Small Business Development Center features an opportunity through which students act as consultants to local aspiring entrepreneurs. As consultants, students assist with business model development, raising capital, and conducting feasibility studies. Wharton also hosts an annual business plan competition during which student teams compete for more than $70,000. After completing the business plan, students can utilize the Venture Initiation Program (VIP) to transform their idea into a business. VIP provides Wharton students with the support they need to complete the final part of the entrepreneurial process. If you have any entrepreneurial aspiration, discuss it in detail in your application and it will definitely catch the admission committee's eyes.

There is perhaps no other business school in the United States that is as international minded as Wharton. Incoming classes represent over 65 countries, most students speak a second language, and the learning model encourages students to look at business issues from a global context. The school offers premier global joint programs through Penn's Lauder Institute and Johns Hopkins University's Nitze School of Advanced International Studies. For students who are interested in a more traditional study abroad experience, Wharton offers exchange programs in 11 countries and the Global Immersion Program (GIP). GIP includes six weeks of studying a global region, followed by a four week study abroad to that region. If you have any international experience, make sure to work it into your application, because it will probably be valued by Wharton more so than by other schools. If you haven't worked or studied abroad, demonstrate a global perspective in your professional interests or display an interest in developing one while at Wharton. Overall, Wharton is very serious about its international mission and seeks applicants who aid and or benefit from that mission.

Wharton is often credited for having a top-notch finance curriculum, and its students are widely sought after for their finance capabilities. This means that the admissions committee will be paying close attention to your analytical abilities, as conveyed through your GMAT score, GPA, and professional activities. This doesn't mean that you have to come across as a quantitative guru, but it does mean that you have to show you can "hack it" in the classroom. Wharton has historically been friendly to applicants from non-traditional backgrounds, but that doesn't preclude analytical ability.

While Wharton certainly is a "powerhouse" finance school, its strengths stretch far beyond finance. Wharton offers 19 majors and features approximately 200 electives, more than any other business school in the world. Students can specialize in everything from Real Estate to Health Care Management to Technological Innovation to Strategic Management. Students are also allowed to create their own majors that focus on cross-functional learning paths. The seemingly unending options are like a smorgasbord of delicious treats. It would serve your application well to discuss a Wharton learning path and provide details on how it will aid you in achieving your professional goals.

Over the last several years, Wharton has also placed more emphasis on its students' teamwork capabilities. During their first year, students work on assignments in "learning teams," which are central to the learning model. Members of the Wharton community are quick to emphasize the benefits of learning from students with different professional backgrounds. As such, the school will be extremely interested in your ability to interact in a team-oriented environment. You should expect questions on this to come up during the interview. Additionally, Wharton is genuinely interested in knowing what type of person you are outside of the professional environment. A short discussion of your hobbies or community service activities will show that you are more than a resume.

Insider information

The Wharton admissions committee will look at your application closely to see how you express the maturity dimension. The school really values professional experience, as reflected in its relatively high average years of work experience. Rejected applicants are often told that they could use another year or two of pertinent work experience. That shouldn't dissuade you from applying if your years of experience fall below the Wharton average, but you should be able to answer the "why now?" and "how will you add value to the classroom?" questions. You should especially expect this to come up during the interview if you have less than three years professional experience.

Schools that call for a similar approach

❐ Columbia Business School.

❐ MIT (Sloan).

□ NYU (Stern).

□ University of London (LBS).

University of Rochester (William E. Simon School of Business)
www.simon.rochester.edu
Rochester, NY

Application at a glance
Application due dates (first, second, third, and fourth round): Dec. 15, Feb. 1, Mar. 15, June 1.

Requirements

□ Essays: Four of 350 words each.

□ Interview: Highly recommended.

□ Recommendations: Two, with one preferably coming from a direct supervisor.

□ Resume.

□ Application fee: $125.

School at a glance
Dean (start of tenure): Charles I. Plosser (1993)

Admissions director: Pamela A. Black-Colton

Program size: 429 full-time

Acceptance rate: 32 percent

Yield: 43 percent

Mean undergraduate GPA: 3.2

Mean GMAT: 649

Middle 80 percent GMAT: 590–720

Average years of work experience: 5.3

International: 50 percent

Women: 24 percent

Minority: 25 percent

Your Simon application strategy
Simon offers a heavy dose of quantitative learning within a small school environment. The school's curriculum is unique in that it approaches most of the major academic disciplines from an economics perspective. Simon students study Finance, Marketing, and Organizational Behavior all through the lens of economic theory, and are encouraged to tie these subjects together by using basic economic principles. The school believes strongly in this approach to business training. You won't be expected to

speak intelligently about price elasticity or supply and demand curves in your admissions interview, but be ready to demonstrate an understanding of this learning approach and to explain why it appeals to you.

Simon students are also expected to take a rigorous, analytical approach in nearly every subject, and the school is careful to screen for analytical abilities in the admissions process. In fact, Simon recently raised its minimum requirements for statistics experience among its admitted students. The school will give you every opportunity to get up to speed before you enroll if you haven't already studied statistics or calculus, but be aware that the school will look closely at your quantitative GMAT score and your college transcript for evidence of analytical abilities.

In addition to its emphasis on quantitative skills, Simon's core curriculum gives students an opportunity to develop their leadership and communication skills in a small, team-based environment. Students take their first-year core classes in small cohorts of 40 people each, and also are assigned to five-person study teams in which they participate throughout their entire first year. Simon emphasizes the learning teams in order to expose all students to the diversity of their peers and to try to overcome the competitive pressures that such a rigorous environment can produce. In a small environment like Simon's, the ability to get along with your peers is a must, so think about ways to demonstrate an outgoing personality and knack for teamwork.

Starting in the school's pre-term course and continuing throughout the first year, students also take a series of courses in communication skills, featuring small workshops and one-on-one coaching conducted by second-year students and school staff. This personal coaching is common throughout the school, and is another benefit of its small size. Students are also encouraged to get involved at the school. Part of students' learning outside the classroom—the VISION program, which teaches such skills as negotiation and change management—is run by second-year students. The school looks carefully for evidence that you are truly interested in Simon, and demonstrating your enthusiasm for these unique programs can help convince the admissions committee of your interest.

Simon is best known in finance circles, which is no surprise given its emphases on economic theory and quantitative skills. Students can exercise their finance muscles by managing the student-run Simon Meliora Fund (which is made up of a portion of the university's endowment) or by participating in the school's annual Investment Challenge. While nearly half of each class goes into finance, the school also attracts many consulting and even marketing firms that are interested in students' analytical abilities. Simon recently introduced two new concentrations in Health Sciences Management and E-Commerce to go along with its 12 existing concentrations. Give either of these a look if they complement your background and your career goals.

Insider information

Simon looks for several traits in its applicants, all stemming from the school's definition of what a successful leader can do. It looks for an ability to decipher a murky situation and choose a course of action—an extension of the school's emphasis on analytical abilities. Simon also looks for people who understand how to persuade and motivate people. This is where the school's Organizational Behavior and Communications classes come into play. Finally, the school looks for an ability to recognize talents in other individuals and to encourage their skill development, which is reflected in Simon's emphasis on teamwork. Think about ways in which you can demonstrate these abilities through past experiences, and discuss them in the essays portion of the application.

Schools that call for a similar approach

- ❏ Carnegie Mellon.
- ❏ University of Chicago.

University of Southern California (Marshall School of Business)
www.marshall.usc.edu
Los Angeles, CA

Application at a glance

Application due dates (first, second, third, and fourth round): Dec. 1, Jan. 15, Feb. 15, Apr. 1.

Requirements

- ❏ Essays: Six (four short essays, two of two pages each).
- ❏ Interview: By invitation only.
- ❏ Recommendations: Two, at least one should come from a direct supervisor. Suggest that a written recommendation letter accompany the required evaluation form.
- ❏ Resume.
- ❏ Application fee: $125.

School at a glance

Dean (start of tenure): Randolph W. Westerfield (1993)
Admissions director: Keith Vaughn
Program size: 565 full-time
Acceptance rate: 21 percent
Yield: 51 percent
Mean GPA: 3.4
Mean GMAT: 684
Middle 80 percent GMAT: 640–720
Average years of work experience: 4.5
International: 22 percent
Women: 34 percent
Minority: 41 percent

Your Marshall application strategy

Positioned as more than an MBA program, the Marshall School of Business portrays itself as a life-transforming experience. This experience is referred to as the Marshall Advantage and is highlighted by an application-focused curriculum and special programs in entrepreneurship and international business. The experience is augmented by the Trojan Family culture, which emphasizes teamwork, integrity, and professionalism. Your Marshall application strategy should demonstrate your ability to leverage the Marshall Advantage in addition to displaying fit with the Trojan Family culture.

From the moment students begin the Marshall program, they notice a strong emphasis on career development and putting theory into practice. A majority of the Marshall faculty has significant professional experience. The professors work in teams to discuss ways to highlight the application of theory in the classroom. Not surprisingly, the Marshall Admissions Committee will closely evaluate your maturity dimension. The committee is in search of applicants who can contribute to the classroom based on their success in professional and personal endeavors. Examples that you can provide to impress the committee along these lines include promotions, discussions of passion for your work or community, tangible improvements made to your company, and leadership demonstrated in group settings.

Marshall owns bragging rights to being the first business school with a dedicated entrepreneurship program. That program, supported by the Lloyd Greif Center for Entrepreneurial Studies is now recognized as one of the top in the nation. Students have the opportunity to compete in business plan competitions in addition to developing their own business models. Discussing your entrepreneurial ambitions is a good way to display fit with Marshall's commitment to this subject. Along with Entrepreneurship, Marshall offers almost 20 concentrations in areas such as Business of Entertainment, Corporate Finance, General Marketing, Investments and Financial Markets, Management Consulting, Real Estate Finance, and Technology Development and E-business.

Marshall's commitment to international business is highlighted by the fact that all students are required to travel abroad as part of the Pacific Rim Education Program (PRIME). As part of the first-year curriculum PRIME is a five-week program, during which students become more familiar with the global aspects of business through lectures, casework, and a team project. Students can select from a number a countries including Chile, China, Japan, Singapore, Thailand, Cuba, or Mexico. PRIME has quickly become a favorite among students and a majority of them actually accept internships in the countries that they select for the program. International opportunities outside of PRIME include study abroad programs that come in lengths of three weeks, four weeks, or an entire semester. Marshall will continue to look for ways to make a name for itself in the international arena, and it is therefore important that you display knowledge of or a desire to gain knowledge of global business issues.

Teamwork rests at the core of the Marshall learning model. Students begin the program by participating in a retreat that focuses on developing interpersonal and teamwork skills. When classes begin, students are placed in study groups of four to six classmates who work together during the first term and are then reshuffled in each term thereafter. Additionally, teams of six students participate in a series of case competitions, which call for students to come up with recommendations to real-world business issues and then present to faculty, classmates, and company representatives.

Insider information

Despite the myriad offerings with which Marshall provides its students, it often plays second fiddle to UCLA (Anderson), Berkeley (Haas), and Stanford. Marshall is looking to become more competitive with these area schools by highlighting the quantitative rigor of the program. As such, the admissions committee will take a close look at your quantitative GMAT score in addition to looking at your transcript(s) for evidence of proficiency in numbers-intensive courses. If you don't have a quantitative-heavy background, consider taking an accounting, statistics, or calculus course. The admissions committee will also take a close look and evaluate the probability that you will accept an offer. You can increase your chances by displaying intimate knowledge of the Marshall learning model and passion for the school's mission and values.

Schools that call for a similar approach

- ❐ Emory University (Goizueta).
- ❐ University of California at Berkeley (Haas).
- ❐ UCLA (Anderson).
- ❐ University of Michigan Business School.

University of Texas at Austin (McCombs School of Business)
www.bus.utexas.edu
Austin, TX

Application at a glance

Application due dates (Early, International, Domestic): Nov. 1, Feb. 1, Mar. 15 (rolling admissions).

Requirements

- ❐ Essays: Three of two pages each.
- ❐ Interview: Recommended.
- ❐ Recommendations: Two, with at least one preferably coming from a direct supervisor or coworker.
- ❐ Resume.
- ❐ Application fee: $125.

School at a glance

Dean (start of tenure): George Gau (2002)
Admissions director: Matt Turner

Program size: 805 full-time

Acceptance rate: 29 percent

Yield: 52 percent

Mean undergraduate GPA: 3.4

Mean GMAT: 678

Middle 80 percent GMAT: 640–710

Average years of work experience: 5.0

International: 27 percent

Women: 25 percent

Minority: 10 percent

Your McCombs application strategy

The newly named McCombs School of Business—named after Red McCombs, who gave the school $50 million in 2000—offers a general management program known for innovation in business education. It offers no formal majors, but it does offer concentrations in the traditional business disciplines, such as Marketing and Finance. Students may also choose a "specialization"; a focused set of cross-functional courses designed to address a current business topic such as Entrepreneurship, Market-based Consulting, and Global Business Management. About half of all McCombs students choose one of these concentrations.

Teamwork is a major emphasis at McCombs, with students doing most of their work in project teams. Students also spend their entire first year taking their core classes together in cohorts. Naturally, the school looks for people who will thrive in this environment, so be sure to demonstrate your experience in working with others to make things happen.

One example of McCombs' innovation is its new Plus Program, a two-week mini-term that takes place in the middle of each regular semester. The program is a series of seminars that give students intense, practical training in topics such as sales, communications, and ethics. Students take these courses in one of six "academies," each one having a focus on a particular industry or line of business. Examples of academies are Community Development and Social Enterprise, The Business of Entertainment, and Product Design Innovation. Students apply to these academies in the fall, and are assigned based on their preferences and past experience. Through a series of four two-week Plus Program courses, students work on specific skills and tackle broad business topics within their assigned academies. Much of the work is done in workshops and small teams, and many of these exercises use improvisational exercises and games to help students learn how to think quickly on their feet. These activities exemplify what McCombs is about, so if they appeal to you, make sure to communicate that in your application. Also, as mentioned above, think about ways to demonstrate how you will fit into this environment, particularly by emphasizing your teamwork and maturity dimensions, as described in Chapter 2.

Two programs that demonstrate the school's emphasis on hands-on experience are its MOOT CORP business plan competition and its MBA Investment Fund. Since 1984, the school has hosted MOOT CORP (we wish we knew why it's in all caps), the oldest and largest inter-business school business plan competition in the world. The competition now attracts teams from 30 schools, and winning teams get a chance to start their business in the friendly confines of the Austin Technology Incubator. Be sure to get to know this program better if you plan on applying to McCombs as a prospective entrepreneur.

Each year, 20 students are selected to run the MBA Investment Fund, a $12 million fund that was created in 1994 as the first legally constituted, private investment company to be managed by students. McCombs students have an opportunity to apply growth, value, and fixed-income strategies to several portfolios. The student managers manage a small part of the school's endowment, getting advice from professional money managers along the way. If you have an interest in investment management—or even just like the school's hands-on learning philosophy—be sure to show your enthusiasm for it in your application.

Insider information

Like other highly-ranked schools with relatively low yield percentages, McCombs is careful about selecting people whom it believes have a sincere interest in its program. While most schools hope to see interest and enthusiasm demonstrated throughout your application, McCombs specifically looks for it in its essays questions. Invest considerable time in researching the school and finding out what kind of opportunities interest you (or could be added to the program). Even more importantly, focus less on trying to pick out an obscure activity to impress the admissions committee, and focus more on writing about something that truly interests you and highlighting how you will pursue that interest at McCombs. If your interest isn't currently met by one of the school's activities, then you have a great chance to show your initiative by proposing how you would start an activity around that interest. The key is to write about something for which you truly have passion, and to show how you will bring that same passion to McCombs.

Schools that call for a similar approach

- ❏ Indiana University (Kelley).
- ❏ Vanderbilt University (Owen).

University of Virginia (Darden Graduate School of Business)
www.darden.virginia.edu
Charlottesville, VA

Application at a glance

Application due dates (first, second, third, fourth, and fifth round): Nov. 1, Dec. 3, Jan. 10, Feb. 11, Mar. 25.

Requirements

- ❏ Essays: Four each of unlimited length.
- ❏ Interview: Applicant-initiated until mid-February. After mid-February, by invitation only.
- ❏ Recommendations: Two, work-related recommendations are suggested.
- ❏ Application fee: $140.

School at a glance

Dean (start of tenure): Robert S. Harris (2001)

Admissions director: Dawna Clark

Program size: 600 full-time

Acceptance rate: 18 percent

Yield: 53 percent

Mean GPA: 3.4

Mean GMAT: 683

Middle 80 percent GMAT: 620–740

Average years of work experience: 5.4

International: 27 percent

Women: 30 percent

Minority: 16 percent

Your Darden application strategy

Upon visiting Darden, you will be immediately struck by three traits: the stunning campus, the dynamic classroom interactions, and the academic discipline. Each of these traits is rooted in closely-guarded tradition. While many business schools have changed their models over time to keep up with the latest fads, Darden has remained true to the ideals that have kept its students highly regarded as general managers. Your application should clearly display your fit with the Darden philosophy.

The central tenets of the Darden philosophy are based upon the close-knit feel of the school and the respect among students and faculty. Every weekday morning "First Coffee" is held, during which the Darden community sits down and discusses topics that are pertinent to the school. Students consistently rave about the bonds that are formed throughout their years at Darden, and the alumni are among the most committed to their alma mater. Indeed Darden has the highest endowment per alum of any business school. Although the class size is growing, the small school feeling remains. If you intend to get accepted, you should indicate your desire to become a member of this community and provide examples of how you have and would be a contributing alum. A visit to the Darden campus and classroom is a great way to show commitment to the school; just make sure to mention the visit in your application.

The case study method still remains the major pedagogical tool through which the Darden learning model is taught. Professors select students through cold calls to initiate case analysis and then invite the entire class to participate in the dialogue. Students are placed in the role of the decision maker and must have the ability to articulate and defend their positions in an insightful manner. Your ability to contribute to case conversations will most likely be tested during your Darden interview. The interviewer will be evaluating your ability to provide cogent responses, your confidence level, and your professionalism. Your challenge is to position yourself as a candidate who can play both the student and the teacher roles within the case study framework. It should be noted, however, that while Darden is a case study school at heart, it has added other educational devices to its toolbox such as: video cases, articles, simulations, and experiential activities.

While the cases place you in the role of an individual decision-maker, case preparation is conducted in student learning teams. As a student, you would be placed in a learning team immediately after starting the Darden program. Teams are expected to meet every night, so discussing your ability to interact well with others should be an important piece of your application.

Darden expects its graduates to be leaders in their fields, but it also understands that leadership is learned through a path of progression. Make sure your essays show a progression in leadership and your recommendations highlight your potential to continue growing as a leader.

Darden is also well known for its strong emphasis on ethics. All students are required to take a course on the subject and ethical challenges often arise in cases throughout the rest of the curriculum. The Olsson Center for Applied Ethics supports Darden's continued examination of the ethical aspects of business. Don't be surprised if a question on ethics comes up during your interview. Make sure to review the approach to these types of questions that we outlined in Chapter 4.

Darden is one of the few schools that doesn't impose word limits on its essays. This is nice because of the added flexibility. However, that added flexibility can also lead some applicants to go overboard, writing essays that quickly lose their focus and clarity. It is therefore extra important for you to ensure that your essays answer the stated questions and do so in a powerful and thoughtful manner. Make sure that your essays are segmented using headers and that any background information provided is only given to support your position. Even though the essays have no limit, admissions members certainly have limited patience.

Insider information

While some modifications have been made to the Darden learning model to curb excessive work, the academic experience remains intense. Although students don't take exams on Saturdays, as in the past, the Darden experience is anything but a two year vacation. Perhaps for no other school is the analogy to drinking from a firehose more appropriate. There are no days off at Darden, as students spend more time in the classroom than at any other top business school and conquer 13 cases a week on average. Students are expected to enter the program with a background in statistics, economics, and accounting. The benefit from such a rigorous learning model is that graduates truly feel that they've received value in return for their efforts. The intensity pays off in preparation. Focus on this benefit and your ability to succeed within the parameters of the learning model, and you will be on your way to establishing a good fit with the Darden traditions.

Schools that call for a similar approach

- ❑ Cornell University (Johnson).
- ❑ Dartmouth College (Tuck).
- ❑ Harvard Business School.
- ❑ University of Western Ontario (Ivey).

University of Western Ontario (Richard Ivey School of Business)
www.ivey.uwo.ca
London, Ontario, Canada

Application at a glance

Application due dates (first, second, and third round): Dec. 1, Feb. 1, Apr. 1.

Requirements

- ❑ Essays: Three of 500 words each.
- ❑ Interview: By invitation only.
- ❑ Recommendations: At least one letter of recommendation is encouraged.
- ❑ Application fee: $125 online, $150 paper application (Canadian currency).

School at a glance

Dean (start of tenure): Lawrence G. Tapp (1995)

Admissions director: Joanne Shoveller

Program size: 593 full-time

Acceptance rate: 34 percent

Yield: 57 percent

Mean undergraduate GPA: N/A

Mean GMAT: 661

Middle 80 percent GMAT: 600–720

Average years of work experience: 5.5

International: 43 percent (foreign nationals)

Women: 25 percent

Minority: N/A

Your Ivey application strategy

The Richard Ivey School of Business prides itself on turning out business leaders with well-rounded general management skills. Ivey students don't major in a particular subject, but rather receive a general management degree. All students work through the same core curriculum the first year, and spend their second year taking electives that allow them to focus on a particular discipline, or stay generalists if they so choose. One noteworthy part of the second year is the Ivey Client Field Project (ICFP), the only required course for second-year students. In ICFP, teams of students work with a company to identify business issues and to recommend a course of action. Students spend most of their second year on the project, working with employees from the company and with a faculty advisor along the way. At the end of the project, they present their recommendations to the company's management. ICFP is a great example of the general management approach that Ivey aims to instill in its students. Demonstrating an understanding of the program and the real-world value that it can provide will help show your fit with the school.

More than nearly any other school, Ivey is completely devoted to the case study method of learning. The school estimates that students evaluate and discuss about 600 cases in their two years at Ivey. Students typically spend one to three hours preparing for each case individually and in learning teams, and then discuss their opinions and analysis in class, with the professor directing the discussion. It's a rigorous approach to learning, and one that requires a certain kind of student.

Accordingly, Ivey looks for applicants with strong academic backgrounds, as well as those with a willingness to throw themselves into tough challenges. The school likes applicants who bring a unique point of view to class, in order to encourage consideration of a wide range of perspectives in each discussion. Ivey also looks for applicants with polish who are not afraid to voice their opinions. Any way in which you can demonstrate a time when you had to persuade others to follow you, or when you had to make an unpopular decision, will help greatly. Finally, the school looks for people who will make good citizens in the classroom. The case method works best when everyone involved is willing to consider others' opinions.

Think carefully about how you can demonstrate these kinds of traits in your application, starting with the work you did in Chapter 2. The more easily that the admissions committee can envision you as a thoughtful and active participant in an Ivey case discussion, the better off you will be. Also, remember that Ivey's program is a general management one where a broad perspective is valued over specific quantitative skills. Make sure that a general management education is what you want, and spell out why this is valuable to you in your application.

Finally, Ivey is interested in students with an international perspective. Each year, 50 or so Ivey students take part in programs like the Leader Project, in which students spend three weeks teaching business concepts to students in places such as Russia, Belarus, and Cuba. Students interested in Asia can also spend a month teaching at the School of Economics and Management at Tsinghua University in Beijing. While an international resume isn't required, Ivey will look for an interest in global business issues, and a willingness to stretch outside of your comfort zone. Think about ways in which you can demonstrate these in your essays.

Insider information

As mentioned earlier, Ivey's philosophy and learning style are built around the unique contributions that each student brings to the classroom. While the school places no official minimum on the amount of work experience an applicant needs, Ivey is clear about preferring applicants with at least two years of experience. The admissions committee will not only look at how much experience you have, but also will look for ways in which your experiences make you unique. If you come from an uncommon background, such as entrepreneurship or nonprofit work, then be sure to emphasize what you have learned and how it makes you different than other applicants. At the same time, make clear that you have the business acumen that it takes to succeed in the case study environment. If you come from consulting or banking, then your challenge will be to set yourself apart from similar applicants. Spend a lot of time putting your uniqueness into words, ideally with distinctive work challenges and notable activities outside of the office.

Schools that call for a similar approach

- ❏ Harvard Business School.
- ❏ University of Virginia (Darden).

Vanderbilt University (Owen Graduate School of Management)
www.mba.vanderbilt.edu
Nashville, TN

Application at a glance

Application due dates (first, second, third, and fourth round): Nov. 30, Jan. 31, Mar. 15, Apr. 15.

Requirements

- ❏ Essays: Three of three pages each.
- ❏ Interview: Recommended.
- ❏ Recommendations: Two, both preferably coming from a direct supervisor or coworker.
- ❏ Resume.
- ❏ Application fee: $100.

School at a glance

Dean (start of tenure): William Christie (2000)
Admissions director: Todd Reale
Program size: 577 full-time
Acceptance rate: 47 percent
Yield: 46 percent

Mean undergraduate GPA: 3.3

Mean GMAT: 648

Middle 80 percent GMAT: 588–710

Average years of work experience: 4.7

International: 22 percent

Women: 24 percent

Minority: 12 percent

Your Owen application strategy

Few schools have undergone as much change in the last few years as Owen. After Martin Geisel—who had led the school for 12 years—died in 1999, the school took nearly a year and a half to find a full-time replacement. During that time, it lost nine professors (about 20 percent of its faculty), and students complained that the lack of leadership was hurting the school. Some wondered if the school had peaked.

Enter William Christie, an Owen finance professor who was eventually selected to lead the school in July 2000. Christie is young as far as deans go, but students say that what he might lack in experience is more than made up for by the energy that he displays in the classroom. He has started some innovative new programs to bring the administration closer to the student body, including "The Dean Is In," a regularly scheduled time in which he sets up a table and dispenses advice to any student who has a question. The result is that students now have great things to say about the administration, and they once again feel good about the school's leadership and direction.

Owen is small, and it boasts a faculty-to-student ratio of about 10:1. The school's academic program emphasizes practical application of management knowledge, and that comes through in its Practical Training Internship. This program gives Owen students a look at the issues that most frequently come up in the day-to-day running of a business. Students then apply these lessons during their summer internships, and write in-depth reports of their experiences at the end of the summer.

In addition to completing the core curriculum, Owen students can concentrate in areas such as Finance, Marketing, Operations, or Human and Organizational Performance. The school also offers several "emphases," including Brand Management, Entrepreneurship, and Healthcare. The school is known for maintaining a flexible curriculum, so don't be surprised to see the school add new concentrations or emphases to keep up with the changing times.

As in the case with many small schools, Owen has a collegial, close-knit community where student involvement is high. Students are encouraged to voice their opinions on school-wide matters, and the administration is known to listen to them. Keep this in mind as you think about the aspects of your application that demonstrate your community involvement.

Owen looks for students who really want to attend the school. Owen is likely to sniff out someone who is just looking for a "safety school," so make sure that you demonstrate why you want to spend two years there.

Insider information

Owen made waves with its Electronic Commerce concentration in the late 1990s, as the school made a bold move to establish itself as a leader in the field of e-commerce management training. It was a logical move for a program that was trying to move from having a regional name to a global brand. The tech industry slowdown has meant that Owen's advantage in this arena has been somewhat diminished, but its e-commerce program is still well regarded among recruiters, despite the school's location away from the traditional high tech hotspots. Keep it in mind if you want to build your e-commerce resume and are willing to venture away from the coasts for a couple of years.

Schools that call for a similar approach

- ❏ University of Maryland (Smith).
- ❏ UNC (Kenan-Flagler).
- ❏ University of Texas (McCombs).

Yale School of Management
www.mba.yale.edu
New Haven, CT

Application at a glance

Application due dates (first, second, third, and late round): Nov. 15, Jan. 6, Mar. 14, May 15.

Requirements

- ❏ Essays: Five (one of two pages, four of one page).
- ❏ Interview: Applicant initiated until December, by invitation only thereafter.
- ❏ Recommendations: Three, preferably two from managers and one from an academic instructor.
- ❏ Resume.
- ❏ Application fee: $180.

School at a glance

Dean (start of tenure): Jeffrey E. Garten (1995)

Admissions director: James R. Stevens

Program size: 480 full-time

Acceptance rate: 15 percent

Yield: 63 percent

Mean undergraduate GPA: 3.5

Mean GMAT: 698

Middle 80 percent GMAT: 640–750

Average years of work experience: 5.0
International: 43 percent
Women: 27 percent
Minority: 22 percent

Your Yale application strategy

The Yale School of Management aims to produce leaders who will make a difference both within their organizations and in their communities. The school's stated mission is to educate leaders "for business and society." While over two-thirds of each class go into finance or consulting (like most other business schools), there is a much greater emphasis on nonprofit and public sector lessons and opportunities at Yale than at most other schools. No matter what their career goals are, the candidates who most appeal to the admissions committee are the ones who demonstrate a broad perspective and an understanding of the importance of contributing to society at large.

Yale students spend their first year learning the school's core curriculum. The core includes the usual business school courses (including economics, finance, marketing, and operations), but also covers topics such as Leadership and The Politics of Strategic Management. These courses apply the theory of politics and influence to business management situations, something that is common throughout Yale's curriculum. Think about this approach to learning, how it might appeal to you, and what you may be able to contribute to the classroom. Students take electives in pursuit of one of seven concentrations, including Marketing, Strategy, Finance, Leadership, Public Management, Operations Management, and Nonprofit Management.

Fittingly, Yale's nonprofit program is one of the best-known in the United States. The school offers extensive elective options in nonprofit and public sector management, and also provides students with a variety of opportunities for getting involved in their communities outside of class. Yale's Internship Fund, established in 1979, provides financial assistance to students who take on non- or low-paying jobs in the nonprofit or public sector. Funds are raised from student contributions, and up to one-fifth of the class receives some amount of funding in any given year. Even if you don't plan on pursuing a nonprofit job after school, demonstrating enthusiasm for getting involved in this type of program can help further show your fit with the school.

Entrepreneurship is also a focus at Yale, and students have several opportunities to get involved in building a business. Yale hosts an annual business plan competition, with entries divided into two categories: for profit and social entrepreneurship. The school also hosts a separate National Business Plan Competition for Nonprofit Organizations, blending the school's strengths in community involvement and entrepreneurship. Outside of the nonprofit sector, Yale students also run their own venture capital fund, known as Sachem Ventures. This $1.5 million fund gives students a chance to screen, invest in, and work with startups in the New Haven area.

When thinking about demonstrating fit with Yale, focus especially on the leadership and innovation dimensions of your application. As mentioned previously, the school looks for applicants who contribute to their community, and this is perhaps the most important component of the school's definition of leadership. Additionally, the school stresses the importance of understanding the interaction between the private sector and public sector, so you want to demonstrate a "big picture" view and a willingness to learn about how one affects the other, no matter what your career interest is. As far as innovation goes, Yale looks for applicants who are comfortable with having their thinking challenged and are willing to take intellectual risks. The more you can demonstrate a willingness to "think outside of the box" both on the job and in your extracurricular activities, the better off you will be. Additionally, the school looks for applicants with integrity, so think about how you can demonstrate this as part of your maturity dimension.

Insider information

Yale is looking for business-minded people who are just as comfortable talking about world politics as they are pricing a financial instrument. You can show fit with the program by demonstrating your knowledge of current events and a natural desire to get involved in your community. Note that Yale's essays serve as a great opportunity for you to show that you know what is going on in the world around you, and that you have an opinion that's worth hearing. Don't just try to tell the admissions committee what you think they want to hear. Rather, take a position in which you truly believe and succinctly support it with a real-world example or two.

Schools that call for a similar approach

- ❏ Harvard Business School.
- ❏ University of California at Berkeley (Haas).

11 MBA Trends You Should Be Aware Of

MBA programs are constantly changing. They are as prone to trends as the stock market is to fluctuation. Just a few years ago, cases and courses on e-business dominated the business school scene. While a few schools have kept a strong focus on e-business, most have revamped their curricula to reflect the "new new economy." Being aware of similar trends can be extremely helpful as you develop your application strategy. Here are 11 such trends:

1. **Ethics:** You can thank companies such as Global Crossing, Tyco, and Enron for many of the essay questions on ethics that have been recently added to schools' applications. As discussions of corporate ethics and social responsibility continue to remain prominent in the marketplace, you can expect business schools to place a strong emphasis on them. Many schools are adding or considering adding required courses on ethics and are becoming more aggressive in verifying the accuracy of submitted applications. You should be prepared to answer questions about how you've dealt with ethical dilemmas, both in essay and interview form.

2. **Quantitative rigor:** Success in business school has always required analytical skills, but the level of quantitative rigor that is being introduced into programs is increasing. This is a direct result of recruiters' demands for

graduates who are numbers-oriented. More schools are beginning to require students to have completed a calculus course in addition to other
business courses prior to starting the curriculum. Thankfully, many schools
offer quantitative "boot camps" prior to the first year to get students with
non-quantitative backgrounds up to speed.

3. **Emphasis on leadership:** While the teamwork theme has not lost any
    steam, it seems as though every business school is suddenly referring to its
    students as leaders. The discussion of leadership will continue to gain
    momentum as schools begin to view their students as change agents not
    only within the business realm but also within society as a whole.

4. **Application of theory:** "Our students actually take the knowledge they
    gain in the classroom and apply it in the real world." As you peruse through
    MBA brochures, you will undoubtedly come across messages similar to
    this. Business schools were once criticized heavily for giving students tools
    but not teaching them how those tools are actually used in the business
    environment. Based on that criticism, many schools adopted experiential
    learning methods that allowed students to use principles learned during
    lectures and case discussions in simulations, consulting projects, and busi-
    ness plans. This method of teaching has become exceptionally popular
    and is now used at most schools to varying degrees.

5. **Entrepreneurship:** Courses and activities focused on entrepreneurship
    have become exceedingly popular at business schools. Programs are ac-
    tively pumping millions of dollars into the development of centers that re-
    search and produce research and resources focused on the subject. If you
    have an exciting entrepreneurial idea, you will find that by discussing it in
    your application, you will catch the eye of several admissions committees.

6. **Diversity of experience:** Schools love to brag about the variety of back-
    grounds that their student bodies represent. In fact, at most schools, stu-
    dents that studied business in undergrad are in the minority. Students say
    that having classmates who represent a diversity of experience improves
    the learning process. Schools will continue to actively assemble diverse
    classes, so it's up to you stand out from the pack by presenting a number
    of professional and personal experiences.

7. **Focus on yield:** Yield, the percentage of applicants who accept an offer
    from a school, is becoming more of a focus area among b-schools. Admis-
    sions committees are taking a closer look at applicants to see what their
    level of fit is. It is important that you convince schools that you are serious
    about attending, even prior to receiving an offer.

8. **Widening gap between tiers:** As the popularity of the MBA degree in-
    creased, more schools added it to their graduate offerings. However, with
    the economic downturn, this has allowed recruiters to become more se-
    lective in MBA hiring. The result has been that holding a degree from a
    "top" program has become even more important in terms of salary, posi-
    tion, and more importantly, simply finding a job.

9. **Global opportunities:** The broader trend of globalization has certainly affected business schools. Alongside their investment in entrepreneurship, business schools are developing new exchange, study abroad, and language study opportunities for their students. Many b-schools view increasing their global presence as a good way to build their brand.

10. **Importance of interviewing:** The interview component of the application used to be viewed as relatively unimportant. Now, more schools are placing a greater emphasis on it, and requiring all admitted applicants to go through the interview process. With an increased number of interviews, many schools have moved to a policy of allowing applicants to only interview upon invitation by the school. Look for that trend to continue.

11. **Active communities:** Schools have begun to place a greater emphasis on building vibrant communities. This means searching for applicants who will be active members of the school during their time as students and, just as importantly, after they graduate. For the most part, you can judge how serious a school is about this trend by the amount of student-run activities that are featured on campus. One way you can make a play on this trend is by discussing activities in which you would be interested in participating and showing an overall passion for the school and its community.

FAQs

What is the definition of a safety or stretch school?

A safety school is a business school to which you have greater than a 90 percent chance of being accepted. Generally, safety schools are considered to be those that have 80th percentile of the school's GMAT scores and mean undergraduate GPAs that are lower than your scores. Additionally, you should ensure that you are no more than one year below the school's average number of years of work experience and that you can project a good fit before you assign the safety school moniker. A stretch school is considered to be any school where either your GMAT score or undergraduate GPA is below the 80th percentile of the schools' scores. Of course, because the application process is about much more than just these numbers, you should only use these statistics as a rough guideline. You can also help yourself by meeting students and alumni from the schools in question and seeing how their experiences compare to your own. You will likely be able to get a good feel for whether or not a school is a stretch or a safety this way.

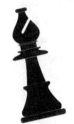
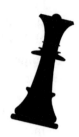

6
ASSEMBLING YOUR
GAME PLAN

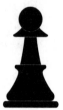

The game plan is the culmination of your research and preparation efforts prior to actually "digging" into the application. The plan includes:

- ❐ A timeline for the application process.
- ❐ Your career goals.
- ❐ Information on your target schools.
- ❐ Professional background.
- ❐ Resume.
- ❐ Academic background.
- ❐ Personal background.

Together, these game plan components will serve as:

- ❐ The formulation of your strategy to get accepted by your target schools.
- ❐ A baseline in writing and reviewing your essays.
- ❐ A reference document for your recommenders.
- ❐ A point of preparation for your interviews.

Putting together a game plan is certainly a time-consuming process, but it's an invaluable tool that is definitely worth the time. Applicants consistently comment that they referenced their plans throughout the application process and that it played a key role in gaining acceptances. Recommenders also find plans to be helpful in crafting recommendations that support the messages that you emphasize in other aspects of your application.

As an example, we'll now step through portions of a game plan that a successful applicant put together in her attempt to gain acceptance to some of the top business schools. As with other sections, we've added our comments to highlight the most important aspects of the document. We will present some sections in their entirety and others in summary form, depending on what we've already covered elsewhere in this book.

The applicant, Lauren, has an engineering background and worked at Hartman Energy for the last four years, assisting customers with their energy needs. She wants to go to business school in order to break into general management, study sustainable development techniques, and eventually assist corporations in pursuing environmentally sustainable business practices.

You'll note that Lauren is a very strong applicant. The purpose of stepping through her game plan is not to emphasize her strengths, but rather to show how useful creating application strategies can be. Keep that in mind as you begin to formulate your own game plan.

Lauren began her plan by addressing her recommenders, who she viewed as the main audience. In addition to supplying the document to her recommenders, she utilized her plan as a launch pad in executing her application strategies.

Lauren's game plan

Introduction

The purpose of this game plan is to provide you with information about me as a professional, student, and individual. Additionally, it will provide you with information on my application timeline and background on the business schools for which you are writing recommendations.

The plan has been written in summary and with detail so that you can glean the information you feel is helpful in completing the recommendation forms. The process of writing this plan has helped me to gain a better sense of my story and to document it as I enter the application process.

The competition to get into the world's top MBA programs is fierce; the average acceptance rate at the top schools ranges from 10 to 20 percent. Top business schools receive thousands of applications from individuals with solid work experience, great GPAs, and outstanding GMAT scores. However, schools are looking for more from candidates than 4.0 GPAs, 700 on the GMAT, and work experience at reputable companies. Top business schools are looking for demonstrated leadership potential, ingenuity, the ability to work in teams, and a genuine interest in making a difference in the world.

Recommendations play an extremely important role in the application process. As Stanford puts it, "We have found that the most useful recommendations provide detailed descriptions, candid anecdotes, and specific evidence that highlights a candidate's potential for leadership. This kind of information helps us to distinguish the very best candidates from a pool of many well-qualified ones."

Thank you for your time and assistance with this process, and in general, for your support! — — — — — — — — — — — —

Many recommenders won't understand how competitive it is to get into top business schools. It's important that they understand the vital role that they play in helping you get accepted.

Why business school and why now?

When I think about my future, I can picture myself moving into a role that is broader and that has a greater impact on society than my current operational position. In the short-term, I definitely see myself returning to the energy industry. I truly enjoy the challenges, the fast pace, the chance to work closely with bright, dynamic individuals, the exposure to a wide variety of customers and business issues, and the constant personal and professional growth that a career of this nature affords. Given this intent, I believe that I am at a natural point in my career to pursue an MBA. While I feel that I am able to add a considerable amount to my joint Hartman/customer teams, I am anxious to contribute a great deal more. An MBA will give me an even stronger general business foundation and understanding of the "big picture," deeper knowledge of the business functions of particular interest to me, the opportunity to master concepts that are difficult or time consuming to master on the job (finance, accounting, statistics), thorough quantitative and leadership training, and added confidence in my abilities—all of which will make me a stronger professional and person. — — —

> Lauren provides good reasoning for why she's at a point in which she wants to make a transition.

In the long-term, I would like to assist companies in coming up with environmentally sustainable business practices that are beneficial to the companies and their constituencies. My background as an environmental engineer gives me some insight into potential steps companies could take, but I need to learn more about the intersection of business and the environment. My current role in operations limits my ability to have a broad impact on the direction of the company or our customers. I believe that the skills and knowledge that I will gain from a MBA program will afford me the career flexibility that I desire. —

> Lauren presents interesting long-term goals that will certainly impact society and leverage her background. She has spent time reflecting on the direction in which she would like to go. Lauren also provided her recommenders with a draft of an essay that contained more details on her career goals.

Given my short- and long-term personal and professional goals, I plan to apply to general management programs that will allow me to develop a background in strategy, finance, and international business. I believe these areas of business will provide me with the tools that I need to analyze sustainable development opportunities and to "sell" companies on how these opportunities can fit in to their long-term visions. I strongly believe that the issues addressed by sustainable development are global in nature and I am therefore interested in how I could introduce solutions at an international level.

Which schools?

I am applying to four schools, all of which have strengths in the areas that I want to study, strong reputations and faculties, and academic environments that appeal to me. In deciding which schools I would apply to, I evaluated the top MBA programs based on: Academic environment/culture, overall fit with my goals and personality, program reputation, international emphasis, teaching quality/style, program features, and location. Although I am equally enthusiastic about each of the four programs, the schools differ slightly in their areas of recognized expertise. I intend to incorporate program-specific messages into each application and hope that you will reflect those program-specific messages in your recommendations. — — — — — — — —

> Lauren demonstrates a good understanding of what she's looking for in a school and provides good reasoning for the selection of her target schools.

The four schools I am applying to are:

- ❏ *The London Business School.*
- ❏ *Kellogg School of Management.*
- ❏ *Stanford Graduate School of Business.*
- ❏ *The Wharton School.* — — — — — — — — — —

> She made the decision not to apply to a safety school, based on her needs.

Academic environment, culture, and fit with my goals and personality

The schools I've targeted have reputations for having "supportive," "team-oriented," and "family-like" cultures. All of the schools emphasize working in teams to enhance learning and developing leadership abilities. I have always enjoyed approaching problems in teams and believe that I am most effective when working within a collaborative culture. The schools I've selected provide the type of environment in which I would flourish.

The collaborative cultures that each of these schools engender supports the introduction of new ideas in the classroom and through extracurricular activities. Although each school has made some strides in terms of supporting the ideas of sustainable development, I would like to further the agenda at the school that I attend. I know that each one of these schools would welcome that and the possibility of establishing a club or volunteer action team would resonate positively with the admissions committee.

In general, I am seeking a relatively relaxed atmosphere (not overly academic or competitive) recognizing that all of the top schools are rigorous and will require my full, best effort.

Overall program reputation and international emphasis

The four schools selected are all widely regarded for their general academic excellence. Additionally, they are known for their particularly strong general management programs. In one case (London Business School) the international emphasis is obvious; the others offer specific programs or exchange opportunities to promote a global view of the business world for its graduates. Ideally, I would like to obtain an internship in France working on a renewable energy project and perhaps spend a semester abroad at one of the MBA programs in France (such as INSEAD or HEC). Each school on my target list would provide ample opportunity for me to achieve these goals.

Teaching quality and program features

The schools also receive praise for the overall quality of their professors. Faculty members at my target schools (for both core and elective courses) are not only accomplished teachers, but also renowned in the academic world for developing theory, authoring enduring textbooks, and advancing management thinking. The schools also have student-to-faculty ratios that allow for a great deal of student/teacher contact. Because professors at my undergraduate school were research-focused and had to deal with large class sizes, outstanding teachers and significant one-on-one time were the exception rather than the rule. I'm looking forward to a more exciting learning experience during b-school.

Each school on my list utilizes a variety of teaching methods; class formats vary to best suit the subject and material covered. Whereas students at a Harvard or Darden use the case study method almost 100 percent of the time, students at my target schools benefit from a range of methods—theoretical, discussion, case study, simulation, role play, team project, and independent study. Based on my undergraduate work and work experience, I believe the varied approach better suits my learning style.

Location

I am generally looking at schools in major economic centers that offer plenty of "real business" opportunities within the local corporate community. These locations are also easy to travel to and from (for me, my friends, and family). Because my (soon to be) husband and I will possibly be living apart for two years, this is of significant importance to me.

I have attached a brief write-up on each of the schools with details about their programs, culture, teaching methods, and criteria for admission (See appendix).

Timeline

The following timeline lays out my plans in terms of the application process. Please note the submission due dates for your recommendations.— — — — — — — — — — — — — —

> The timeline is a great tool for you and your recommenders that helps ensure that all of the required activities get done on time.

Game plan timeline

Date	Action	
December 1–March 1	(GMAT preparation)/initial school selection	**Comment:** Starting early is key! Note, that if you have to take the TOEFL, you'll probably want to get started even earlier.
March 10	Take GMAT exam	
March 15–May 15	Additional GMAT preparation	
May 20	(Retake examination)	**Comment:** Make sure to leave adequate time in case you need to retake the GMAT.
June–July	School research/target school selection	
August 1	Request transcripts	
August–September	Review applications and provide recommenders with forms, game plan, and draft essays	
September 1	(Sign-up for Kellogg interview)	**Comment:** Sign up for your interviews early, because slots go quickly.
September–November	Work on applications/visit schools	
September 20	Kellog interview	
October 1	Submit Kellogg application online	
October 7	(Recommendations are due from recommenders)	**Comment:** Set a due date for your recommenders that is earlier than the actual date by which you need them, so that you have a time buffer.
October 14	Submit Wharton application online	
October 21	Submit Stanford application online	
November 1	(Submit London Business School application online)	**Comment:** Try to submit your applications at least one week before the deadline, to ensure that it receives proper treatment.
December–January	Cross fingers for acceptances	

Summary

My applications will have similar themes interwoven throughout them, but will be tailored for each school's unique set of evaluation criteria. What follows is background information on my work, academic, and personal experience. This background information will be used to support both my general and program-specific messages. Details for each category are included in the appendix.

Work experience

My most meaningful work experience has been my four years with Hartman Energy. In describing my work experience to date, I will try to give details showing:

- ❏ *A wide variety of experience in a relatively short amount of time.*
- ❏ *Performance at a high level (judged by my project managers and peers) in a team environment.*
- ❏ *My determination, intelligence, creativity, and leadership capabilities.*
- ❏ *Recognition (through rapid promotion) and accomplishments.* _ _ _ _ _ _ _ _ _ _ _ _ _ _ _ _

These are all great attributes to express.

Community involvement

I truly enjoy giving back to the various communities to which I belong and have done so for as long as I can remember. In my applications, however, I will emphasize my community involvement since college, as b-schools tend to focus their attention on post-university experience. When discussing my community involvement, I intend to:

- ☐ *Demonstrate my interest in getting involved in my community, when and where possible, despite keeping a busy travel/work schedule.*

- ☐ *Highlight the leadership roles I have taken on (because engineers typically lack significant management experience).*

- ☐ *Show that I am the type of applicant who would take full advantage of the b-school experience and would seek out ways to get involved in the MBA community.*

> Again, great attributes to express. Admissions counselors love applicants who can demonstrate these traits.

Academic history

I have always loved school. Since I was very young, I have been driven (through positive reinforcement and support from my family) to excel academically. I have always worked extremely hard for my grades, and because of this effort, am very proud of what I've accomplished. Schools look at an applicant's academic history as her best predictor of future performance. I will emphasize:

- ☐ *My scholastic strength in a broad array of subjects in order to demonstrate my ability to handle the quantitative rigor of each program, as well as the 'softer' subjects.*

- ☐ *My achievements in the broader context of involvement in undergrad (extracurricular involvement, leadership positions, work experience). By doing so, I hope to demonstrate my energy, time management ability, and enthusiasm for getting the most out of every experience.*

Personal information

I think the biggest challenge in the application process for most applicants is distinguishing themselves—I know this will be the case for me. Where possible, I will look to provide personal information about myself; as Stanford puts it, "the person behind the grades, test scores, job titles, and leadership positions." Through my applications, I hope to:

- ☐ *Describe the unique set of experiences, interests, and perspectives that I would bring to the b-school community.*

- ☐ *Share my influences, motivations, passions, values, interests, and aspirations.*

- ☐ *Paint a picture of a well-rounded, caring, approachable, motivated person who would add to the MBA community.*

Appendix

The appendix to the game plan contains detailed information on the previously covered topics. The appendix serves as a reference for both the applicant and recommenders, so that they can easily provide supporting data in essays, recommendations, data sheets, and interviews.

Work experience

The work experience section allows you to document all of your professional activities, so that you can select the most pertinent experiences for inclusion in your application. You should document your explicit functional or project work in addition to any work-related extracurricular activities in which you're involved. Additionally, try to include positive comments you've received during any of your reviews. These comments can be a great third-party reference that can be included in your essays or recommendations. You should also consider including a section that outlines your strengths and weaknesses. This will give your recommenders a reference point for a question they most certainly will be asked. At the end of the section, you should include a copy of the resume you put together for one of your target schools.

Academic experience

For many applicants, it will have been several years since they thought about their college experiences. This is the section through which you can relive some of the positive ones. Specifically, you'll want to document your accomplishments and activities inside and outside of the classroom. To the extent possible, you want to project yourself as someone who is always willing to get involved and participate. Showing a history of doing so is a great way to display that trait. You'll also want to bring out any special skills that you developed while you were in school. For example, if you studied a foreign language or simply took a broad range of courses that helped improve your perspective on business issues, then be sure to include that here.

Personal experience

The personal experience section is your opportunity to express that you're more than a paper-pusher. You should discuss the hobbies and interests in which you're involved outside of the work environment. This could include community service activities, sports, theatre, or anything else with which you occupy your time. Knowing the personal side of you is always helpful to your recommenders, who might only know the "professional you." Writing this information down will be helpful in preparing for your interviews, as your interviewer will often want to get to know "the person behind the resume."

Which schools?

In this section, you can provide detailed information on your target schools for the purpose of understanding how you will establish fit with each one. There are two types of information that you'll want to include for each target school:

1. Background information about the school, mainline statistics, and your strategy for getting in. The majority of the information can be taken directly from Chapter 5.

2. A discussion of why the school is a good fit for you, which will help you nail down your story for each school before you tackle your essays and interviews.

We've included Lauren's approach to the second component as an example.

The London Business School

LBS's international make-up is one of the main reasons why I'm applying to it. In college, I participated in a study abroad program at the London School of Economics and was the only American in my class. The experience, although brief, was truly life-changing. I learned as much from my team members—about the world and about myself—as I did from the class. I am certain that LBS would offer similar learning and growth experiences.

Another appealing feature is the school's (deliberately) small size, and thus, its sense of intimacy. Students give the school high marks for its culture and friendly atmosphere. According to one second-year MBA, LBS isn't "quite as competitive as some of the U.S. schools. You don't have to get a good grade at the expense of someone else." This is exactly the kind of environment that I am looking for!

Finally, because of its global focus, all LBS students must demonstrate competence in at least one language other than English by the time they graduate. While some students might view this requirement as something to "get over with," I look at is as a golden opportunity to make significant strides towards my goal of becoming fluent in French.

Kellogg School of Management (Northwestern University)

One of the largest b-schools among the Top 30, Kellogg enrolls some 600 students a year in its full-time program. Despite its size, however, Kellogg is able to create a unique, family-like culture through its team learning philosophy—one of the school's biggest draws and differentiators in my opinion. I have always enjoyed a collaborative approach and have never needed a great deal of competition to motivate myself. For these reasons, I believe Kellogg is a perfect fit for me culturally.

Kellogg has an extremely well-balanced program. Although Kellogg is best-known for its marketing program, it actually offers one of the strongest arrays of functional departments available anywhere. Most Kellogg MBAs major in two or three functional areas and can also opt to specialize in an interdisciplinary major. I would most likely major in strategy and finance and specialize in international business. I would also take advantage of the Global Initiatives in Management (GIM) program. Students in this program create specially-designed, two-quarter international independent study courses, and focus on a country of their choice. For each of the geographic areas, students work in groups to create a syllabus, book guest speakers, determine research topics, and identify key issues facing local industries. After coursework is completed during the winter quarter, students travel to the selected country over spring break for a two-week consulting project. Results are then presented to faculty and visiting executives in the spring. I would also take advantage of one of their exchange programs—most likely with HEC in France. Classes at HEC are conducted in both English and French, presenting an ideal opportunity for me to improve my foreign language skills.

Stanford Graduate School of Business

Supporting an entrepreneurial spirit, Stanford's curriculum is very flexible and allows students to select from an array of electives while forming a strong general management foundation. MBA students are not required to major in specific academic disciplines.

Stanford offers a supportive, intimate culture. The business school does not publicly post grades or include overall class rank on academic transcripts. Rather, the collaborative culture frees students to take academic risks and broaden their management and leadership skills. These features are particularly appealing to me. My undergraduate engineering curriculum was extremely grade-focused and, in my opinion, the emphasis only detracted from the learning experience.

Another strength is the school's global management focus. International issues are integrated into the core courses and approximately 25 percent of Stanford electives focus on international topics. Stanford also provides career resources, speakers, student clubs, and conferences to help students connect with global companies.

Many of the global initiatives are provided through the Global Management Program (GMP). The GMP offers an academic certificate in global management for students (like me) who want to focus even more sharply on global issues. To earn the certificate, students complete at least five GSB electives with an international focus. I would definitely take advantage of this option. I would also pursue the Global Management Immersion Experience (GMIX). This program combines a core course in global management, a research project, and a summer internship for students to gain international work experience.

Students can earn up to 16 credits in courses offered outside of the business school. This feature would give me a chance to take advanced French language instruction— something that is nearly impossible to do when working on an out-of-town project.

The Wharton School (University of Pennsylvania)

Wharton is known as a leader and innovator in the b-school arena. It receives praise for its emphasis on international initiatives and creative approaches to teaching. Like Stanford, it has a nondisclosure grading policy which helps to foster a team environment and allows students to concentrate more on their areas of interest.

The first year of the program is divided into four six-week quarters. Students move through their classes as part of a 60 student cohort—a kind of class within a class. Each cluster shares the same team of core professors who work together to integrate the coursework and coordinate student workload. As a member of a cohort, I would be in an intimate environment, without giving up access to resources that larger schools have.

Wharton offers a number of optional programs for its students. One option for first year students that looks particularly appealing to me is the Global Immersion Program (GIP). This program involves six weeks of introductory lectures on a country or region critical to the world economy, with a four-week overseas experience following final exams in which students meet corporate and government officials, tour local businesses, and attend cultural events. Students also submit a written assignment in the Fall. Another enhancement program that fits well with my overall career goals is the Multinational Marketing and Management Program. This program partners Wharton with b-schools in Israel, Canada, and other locations to form multi-school MBA teams that design marketing strategies for companies hoping to enter the North American market. Finally, students can opt to spend a full semester abroad in one of 14 exchange programs with non-U.S. business schools. I am strongly considering a semester at the HEC School of Management in France.

Summary

As you can see, the game plan is a powerful tool that allows you to record and refine your story prior to attacking the applications. This type of preparation will be of great benefit to you and your recommenders as the application process drags on. In fact, you should sit down with your recommenders and step through the plan and perhaps an essay or two that further describes your career goals. This will give them a broader understanding of the plan's purpose and ensure that they use it effectively.

Yes, assembling a game plan is time consuming, but an admittance letter is well worth the additional hours. It's important, therefore, that you not only assemble a dynamic game plan, but that you also execute it.

8 Truths of the Application Process

The one thing that every applicant comes away from the process with is stories. From the applicant whose computer crashed, wiping out all of his freshly written essays, to the applicant who was asked out by her interviewer, we all come away with something. While the unique experiences are probably more interesting, the common ones are probably more useful to you in your application preparation. With that in mind, here are eight experiences that will most probably find their way into your storybook.

1. **Your first interview will be your worst.** Even Michael Jordan looked a little rusty when he first came out of retirement, so you shouldn't expect to be in top-notch condition after not interviewing for several years. This isn't to say that you'll "bomb" your first interview, but generally, applicants need to work through the first one before feeling entirely comfortable with the process again. If you follow the interview advice provided in Chapter 4, then you should be fine, but if possible, set your first interview up with your safety school.

2. **Your last application will be your best.** Many applicants start off working on the application to the school in which they are most interested. More often than not, this is a bad move. By the time you move on to your third or fourth application, you will be in prime application-writing mode. You will have a bunch of base essays from which to start and have already spent tremendous amounts of time revising them. This means that the last application will benefit from all of the knowledge you've gained by working through the first few. If time is not an issue, consider working on your highest priority application last.

3. **Visiting a school is always a good idea.** Would you buy a car that you couldn't see? Probably not, so you should also strongly consider visiting

your target schools. You will be surprised what you pick up, and doing so will help you score big points with the admissions committee.

4. **You will lose perspective and be tempted to make irrational decisions.** A friend of Scott's decided to try and save a couple bucks by sending in her recommendations via the regular mail only a few days before the deadline. As you might have guessed, her documents were lost in the mail and she was denied admittance. If you continue to view b-school as a long-term investment, saving a couple bucks while taking on significant risk becomes an obviously bad tradeoff.

5. **One of your recommenders will not meet the date with which you provide him.** We're busy people and so are our recommenders. Chances are, they'll accept our request to write a recommendation and then put it aside for awhile. It's up to you to ask them early, follow up often, and maybe even more importantly, set a due date that is far in advance of the application deadline.

6. **Your friends and family will get sick of hearing about the process.** Applying to business school can be a consuming process that takes over your life for a whole year. From taking the GMAT, to researching schools, to writing essays, to waiting for responses, the process will seem endless at times. And you will, of course, share your experiences with your friends and family. Unfortunately, they won't be able to understand the trials and tribulations associated with the process unless they've been through it themselves. So, be prepared for their glossy eyes and hollow "uh huh"s as the months drag on.

7. **You will spend more money on the process than you would ever have imagined.** GMAT study guides, exams, and classes; essay consultants; $200 applications; visits to schools; book on application strategy—none of these come for free (although the book on application strategy provides a great ROI). As you get closer to receiving responses from your target schools, you'll notice the expenses piling up. Be prepared to make the necessary investment, because you won't want to go through it again.

8. **Receiving an admittance letter from your dream school will make it all worthwhile.** There are few more satisfying, fulfilling, and overall happy moments than receiving word that you've been admitted to your choice business school. Cartwheels, fist pumps, back flips—it'll all come out. Keep that in mind as your trudging through some of the more mundane aspects of the process.

7
GAME OVER

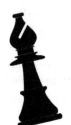
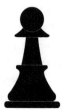
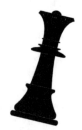

What Happens Once You Submit Your Application?

Like any good business manager, you should design your product (your application) with your customer (the admissions counselor) in mind. To that end, it helps for you to know what will happen to your application once the admissions committee receives it. No two schools are the exact same in how they process admissions applications, but what follows is a general example that will give you an idea of what a "typical" business school application goes through.

Once your application is received, it is usually held until all of your other materials are received (if sent separately), including recommendations or transcripts. Once all of these materials are received and the application is marked as ready for review, a reader will take it in a batch of applications, which can be as few as several applications and as many as dozens. At some schools, the first reader will be a current MBA student, while at other schools only admissions personnel review applications. The first reader will go through your entire application, including a transcript of your interview if you have already had one. The reader will look for evidence of the traits that the school seeks in every applicant (starting with the core dimensions that we outlined in Chapter 2), and will grade you on each of these traits. Based on how your application stacks up, it will receive a simple, high-level grade, such as Yes, Maybe, or No. These grades seem somewhat arbitrary, but for every application a reader fills out an extensive form to back up his decision, citing as many examples as possible or pointing out areas that call for further investigation.

Think about what this reader is faced with: A two-foot stack of applications that mostly look the same, a tight deadline, and the burden of having to decide whether an applicant should be admitted. You can help your cause by putting yourself in the reader's shoes and thinking about how you can make his life easier:

- ❏ **Keep it short.** We cannot emphasize enough how important it is to stick to word limits in essays and data sheets. You are not the most important applicant, nor the one with the most interesting experiences. So make life easy by keeping things concise.

- ❏ **Make it interesting.** Don't use gimmicks, but do remember that your application will be one of dozens that your reader will see. An appropriately humorous paragraph or even whole essay will be appreciated, and will definitely be remembered.

- ❏ **Be organized.** If you don't follow instructions, don't expect a stressed application reader to contact you for missing information. Give yourself extra time to make sure that your application is totally complete.

- ❏ **Be clear about what you have to offer.** Present a focused message, one that your reader will easily understand. Stick only to examples and stories that highlight your core messages.

At most schools a second reader—who also may be a student but is often an admissions officer—will read your application and grade it based on the same exact criteria. The second reader almost never sees what decision the first reader has made on your application, so you can be sure that you will get a fair shake. The second reader will come to a decision and also back up her findings with an in-depth report.

Usually, a third decision-maker then comes into play, someone who is a little more senior in the process. It may be the admissions director, or it may be a somewhat senior admissions officer. If the first two readers agree that you are a Yes or a No, then your fate is quickly sealed, for better or for worse. If they disagree, then the third person will usually read the application herself and come to a final decision. There is sometimes spirited debate about a single application, but remember that everyone involved is trying to get through a huge stack of applications as efficiently as possible. If the third reader still can't decide, or the consensus seems to be "Maybe," then often that is when you will placed on the waitlist.

Contrary to what it often seems, application readers and interviewers are not just looking for reasons to reject you. More than anything, they're looking to find out who you are and how well you embody each of the traits that they look for in an applicant. This sounds simple enough, but it can be especially challenging for a reader when faced with dozens of applications that all look the same. To this end, stay focused on your core messages of who you are and what you can offer to the program. This will make your application readers' jobs much easier, and will greatly improve your chances of admission.

The Five Response Types

Years ago, you could infer a business school's response to your application based on the size of the letter. The traditional belief held that if you received a thick letter in a manila folder then you were in and if you received a thin letter in a business envelope then you were out. Now, b-schools are much more responsive and generally contact applicants via phone, email, or secure Web page before the letter is even sent.

Although the communication vehicle has changed, what hasn't changed is the type of responses you can expect to receive.

There are five types of responses that you could receive:

- ❐ Direct admission.
- ❐ Admission with requirements.
- ❐ Admission with postponement.
- ❐ Waitlist.
- ❐ Denial.

Direct Admission

Hopefully, at least one of your target schools will fall into this category. If this is the case, then pat yourself on the back and celebrate, because you've accomplished what many applicants failed to do. But of course, no sooner than you receive your good news will you have to face a whole new crop of deadlines and decisions. We'll tackle some of the most common ones below.

Deciding Which School to Attend

This is one of the more pleasant decisions that you will ever have to make. Even though you may dread having to actually make the decision, don't forget that this is a dilemma that few others have the luxury of facing.

If you find yourself torn between two or more schools, take an inventory of what mattered most to you when you initially applied. How do you feel about these criteria now? Visit the schools (we highly recommend attending each school's on-campus events for admitted students) and get a feel for your potential future classmates. After all, these are the people with whom you may spend the next two years. Sit in on a class (even if you already did so months ago), and ask yourself if you could see yourself participating in the discussion. Yes, this sounds subjective, but your experience at b-school will largely depend on how well you fit the culture, and vice versa.

Of course, there are more tangible attributes to consider as well, such as each school's reputation in your field of interest, its location, and how much money it offers you in scholarships or grants. First of all, don't become too obsessed with rankings. If two schools are close to one another in rank, then this is a moot question. Don't fool yourself into thinking that two or three notches in a magazine's rankings mean a thing in the real world. However, if you are deciding between a top-five school and a top-30 school, for example, we recommend that you place as little emphasis on scholarship dollars as possible. Even if the lower-ranked school offers you a "free ride," the money shouldn't be your main reason for enrolling there. Yes, mountains of debt can be scary, but you really need to think long-term, and ask yourself which school will help you the most down the road. Greater career opportunities in the future are surely worth more than a few thousand dollars today. The same goes for other factors, such as geography. Remember that business school is just two years, but the benefits that you take away will be with your for the rest of your life. So, don't sell yourself short.

That's not to say that you should always enroll in the higher-ranked school over the lower-ranked one. Far too many applicants make their decision solely on the basis of rankings, and they really aren't being true to themselves. There may very well be a legitimate reason why the top-30 school appeals to you more than the top-five school does, including strength in certain academic fields or unique career opportunities. If that's the case, don't let anyone lead you to believe that you're making the wrong choice. Go where your heart tells you to go. We simply urge that you make your decision for rational reasons, not for the short-term convenience of having less debt or living in a sunnier climate for two years.

Remember, you won't ruin your life by making the "wrong" decision! The b-school you attend won't determine your lot in life. The fact that you were able to gain admission to more than one of these schools is a good indicator that you'll be successful. Where you are 20 years from now will depend much more on your ambition and skills than on whether you choose to attend the number seven- or 10-ranked business school right now. Go where you think you will get the most out of the MBA experience, and the rest will take care of itself.

The deferment question

All schools discourage admitted students from deferring their enrollment, and many explicitly state in their application materials that they don't allow deferment *for any reason*. Still, even those b-schools who purport that they don't allow deferment will generally consider it under certain circumstances. And there are some reasons why you may want to delay the start of your business school experience. The most common reasons for an applicant wanting to defer for a year usually have to do with a professional opportunity or a change in personal circumstances.

If your company offers you a big promotion or a once-in-a-lifetime opportunity to take on a new project, then you may want to think about pushing off b-school for a year. The biggest question to consider is whether it's an opportunity that will come along again anytime in the near future. If you believe that your new role would allow you to gain rare new skills and experiences that will help you down the road, then seriously consider it. If, however, your company is just trying to keep you around for another year by offering you more money or a better title, don't be so quick to defer your enrollment. Yes, the money can look good, but maintain a perspective that extends 20 years into the future. Earning those extra bucks today pales in comparison to the opportunity cost of waiting another year to accelerate your career.

Some people face personal reasons for wanting to defer their enrollment, such as the birth of a child or an illness in the family. If you are faced with a situation that you believe will make it hard to devote 100 percent of your energy to your MBA, then consider deferring. Remember, though, that it's easy to think of *any* time as a bad time to start business school (something always seems to come up). So, only defer if you are sure that your personal circumstances will look significantly different in a year.

If you have decided that you want to defer, and your school will consider letting you do so, then you will have to build a strong case for why it makes sense to wait a year. When it comes to professional reasons, an admissions committee will ask questions along the lines of what we raised previously: What is it about this new opportunity that will make you that much better able to contribute to your class a year from now? Be prepared to argue your case using a framework similar to what you employed in your original application. If you can craft a convincing story that is consistent with your over-all application theme, you will stand a chance of gaining a deferment. Remember, though, that a deferment is never guaranteed.

Schools tend to be a little more willing to listen to personal reasons for deferment because they know that business school will consume your life once you arrive. Honestly let the school know your situation and explain why you are afraid that it may interfere with your business school experience. Schools will usually be very understanding, and will work with you to find a solution. They may not offer you a deferment, but they may at least be able to offer you other options, such as the chance to start during the school's January term.

In any case, be prepared to do some convincing, both via letter and over the phone. Even though many schools tend to be a little more lenient than they let on, many applicants who ask for deferments are not granted them. Also, you will definitely be expected to submit your initial tuition deposit (usually on the order of $1,000 to $2,500) now in order to hold your spot in next year's class. This deposit is non-refundable, so be prepared to kiss it goodbye if you decide next year that business school isn't in your plans after all.

Financial Aid

Once you're admitted and you know which school you will be attending, then you need to worry about how you're going to pay for the whole affair. Most schools will send financial aid information along with your admittance letter, or will send it shortly after admitting you. You will need to submit information about your financial status, both to the school and to the federal government. The latter will receive the information that you enter into your Free Application for Federal Student Aid, or FAFSA (accessible online at *www.fafsa.ed.gov*). Get familiar with these forms as quickly as possible, especially because some schools call for your old tax returns dating back as many as three years. If your jaw just hit the floor when you read that last sentence, don't worry. You can contact the IRS to get these copies (look for IRS Form 4506).

You should submit your financial aid application as early as possible since most schools are doling out a fixed amount of money. Just as applying earlier in the admissions process makes things easier because there are more seats to be had in the class, applying earlier for financial aid gives you a better chance of getting more aid. While being the first one to apply won't necessarily get you a significant amount more, you definitely don't want to be among the last to apply, because the money may already be spoken for by then. In fact, if you're reasonably confident that you will receive admission to at least one of your target schools, then you should consider actually filling out your FASFA forms even before you get your responses. Also, you should still apply if you feel like your situation will make you ineligible for grants given by your business school. Many applicants across all types of situations get a small amount of aid. You'd be crazy to not at least try for this free money, even if the odds seem to be against you.

After you have filled out the requisite forms, your school will get back to you quickly enough to ensure that you have enough time to arrange for other sources of aid, if needed. Some schools offer merit-based aid, some offer need-based aid, and some offer both. Most of this aid will be in the form of grants (money that you don't have to pay back). Whatever the case is for your school, the amount that the school offers is rarely negotiable. Some students have had success negotiating what aid they get, but need-based aid is hard to negotiate (because it tends to go by a formula that takes your assets into consideration), and a majority of merit-based aid decisions will likely have already been made by the time you contact the school. It's worth a shot, but don't expect to get very far in negotiating with the financial aid office.

Assuming that you will need an external source of loans (most students do), there are a few programs in place that make it relatively easy to get money for your education. While your financial situation may not qualify you for grants from the school, you may be eligible for Stafford loans from the federal government. These come in two types: subsidized and unsubsidized. Although you won't have to start paying off either type of Stafford loan while you're in school, subsidized loans are preferable, because interest doesn't accrue until you graduate. Naturally, subsidized loans are harder to qualify for. How much you're eligible to receive and the type of Stafford loan you can get depends on your financial situation (as dictated by your FAFSA results). Who actually services your Stafford loan (who cuts the check) can be anyone from your school to a third party bank such as Sallie Mae. Shopping around can help you save on fees and interest rates.

You'll also have private loan options. Many schools partner with a major bank like Citigroup to offer "preferred" student rates on loans. They are usually fairly competitive, although with some shopping around you can often find a better deal on your own. These loans are usually structured so that you don't start paying them back until you graduate. For American students, these loans tend to be very easy to qualify for, but international students generally have to provide detailed, verifiable proof of assets in order to qualify.

The bottom line is that business school is expensive, but practically no one has to turn down the chance to attend because the costs are too great. Be prepared to fill out lots of forms, patiently research loan options, and take on debt. Just remember: This is a long-term investment!

Scholarships, fellowships, and teaching assistantships

Outside of taking on loans and receiving a b-school grant, graduate business students have it pretty tough in terms of finding sources of income for tuition purposes. The prevailing belief is that we're all going to be rich someday, and therefore aren't in dire need of financial assistance. Although scholarships aren't plentiful for aspiring MBAs, there are definitely some opportunities that exist. Rather than searching for one-off scholarships, check out *www.fastweb.com*. The FastWeb Website will ask you a number of questions in regard to your general background, demographics, and area of study. After completing the detailed questions, you will receive a report that cites the scholarships for which you can apply. Each scholarship has different application requirements and timelines, so you can select those scholarships that suit you best. FastWeb will also continuously send you updates as the year progresses and new scholarships become available.

In addition to these "external" scholarships, there sometimes are additional funding opportunities internal to b-schools to which you may not have access until you actually attend a school. Many b-schools will offer their students the opportunity to apply for additional scholarships, fellowships, or teaching assistantships after they start classes. Keep these additional sources in mind and make sure to ask your b-school about them, so that you can take advantage later down the line.

Admission With Requirements

You may find that you're offered a conditional admission to your target school. Don't worry, this is not an insult. In fact, it speaks pretty favorably of you if the school was willing to admit you despite an obvious weakness. Look at it as an opportunity to get a head start on your MBA experience, or at least to brush up on your weaker subjects.

Most frequently, a school will require you to successfully complete a pre-MBA course in a quantitative subject such as statistics or a business-related course such as accounting. Some schools offer these programs before your first semester begins, but most will ask that you complete this coursework at a local accredited college. Your business school will usually be very willing to work with you to help make this happen.

There are two things to be aware of, though. First, because you don't know what schedule your local college operates on, start researching your options as soon as possible to avoid missing an enrollment deadline. The sooner you can take a class to pass your requirement, the better. Second, you should know that you will have to take these courses on your own dime. So, add these costs into your budget as you plan for business school.

Admission With Postponement

This is a rare decision to receive, and it usually applies to undergraduates and those who have very little business experience. Your school may tell you that it likes what it sees in your application, but that it wants you to work for a year or two more before you enroll. Even though this may be frustrating, it's still much better than a rejection, so take heart. Also know that if the school feels strongly enough about your application to offer you this rare opportunity, then they probably have a point. In the cases with which we're familiar, the applicants have said that the extra work experience helped them get more out of their b-school experience.

Waitlist

Finding out that you've been placed on the waitlist is a melancholy moment. After all of your efforts and patience, you've essentially been asked to wait some more. The immediate question that comes to an applicant's mind at this point is, "What are my chances of getting off the waitlist and into the school?" Generally, your chances of getting off a b-school's waitlist are directly related to that b-school's yield percentage. If, for example, a school has a 90 percent yield, your chances of getting off the waitlist are probably pretty slim. Other factors that will play a role in determining your chances of winning a spot include the total number of applicants accepted, the size of the b-school class, as well as the number of applicants who were placed on the waitlist. While it's nice to know the initial factors that will determine your chances, these numbers differ greatly from school to school and year to year. Regardless of what the chances are, there are a number of steps you can take to greatly increase your chances of turning a waitlist into an admission.

The first step you should take is to understand your target school's policy on the waitlist. Most schools will provide you with a contact within the admissions office who will hopefully be your main advocate in helping you gain admissions. If you haven't already guessed, it's important to get this person to like you, so use tact in your communications. The second step you should take is to review all of your application materials in order to evaluate *why* you weren't directly admitted. The fact that you've been placed on the waitlist means that you're a solid applicant, but there must be at least one aspect of your story that came across as a little weak.

Run down this list of questions when evaluating what your weaknesses might be.

- ❏ Are my career goals defined effectively?
- ❏ What problems will I solve through achieving my career goals?
- ❏ Who will I affect through achieving my career goals?
- ❏ Is it clear how attending b-school will help me achieve my career goals?
- ❏ In what ways do I emphasize fit with the b-school in my application?
- ❏ How do I demonstrate leadership, innovation, maturity, and teamwork abilities?
- ❏ Did I effectively demonstrate my ability to perform well academically at b-school through my GMAT, GPA, transcript, and professional experience?
- ❏ How does my application differentiate me from others with a similar profile?
- ❏ Did I communicate passion for the b-school's mission?
- ❏ Did I do enough in terms of visiting the school, and speaking with current students and alumni?

After running through the list, if you're still not sure what your weakness is, consider having a friend, student, or alum read through your application, asking the same questions. Sometimes having an outside perspective can help you recognize weaknesses of which you were previously unaware. For example, you might think your career goals are crystal clear, while others who read your application are confused about what you're trying to communicate. Naturally, this sort of analysis should be done even before you submit your application, but it can be extremely helpful in crafting your messages when trying to get off the waitlist.

Once you've identified the areas that you would like to strengthen in the eyes of the of the admissions committee, you should select the methods you would like to utilize in your approach. Some of the methods that successful applicants have utilized include:

☐ **Follow-up calls to an admissions officer:** Having semi-frequent conversations with your contact in the admissions committee is a great way to keep your name at the top of his mind. By following up and asking if there are any further developments, you will be able convey your strong interest in gaining admittance. Admissions officers want to make sure that anyone who is admitted from the waitlist will accept, so in these conversations, you can underscore the fact that officer's school is your top choice. Of course, there is a fine line here between sounding interested and becoming annoying. Daily calls or badgering the admissions officer is great way to ensure that you never get off the waitlist. Sometimes the officer will give you guidance in terms of when you should check back in, but in lieu of that guidance we suggest a call every three weeks.

☐ **An additional recommendation:** Sending an additional recommendation can be a great way to emphasize character strengths that the target school values. Coming from a third party, it contains all of the benefits that your initial recommendations contained. Having reviewed your application for potential weaknesses, you can work with the additional recommender in focusing on those perceived weak areas. If, for example, you think that the admissions committee might question your quantitative abilities, your recommender could discuss a rigorous analytical analysis that you recently completed. Ideally, this recommender is an alum of the b-school. Because it's a more targeted recommendation than the originals, it is not a necessity that the recommender know you as well. What you're shooting for is a recommendation that persuades the admissions committee that you have the requisite abilities and that you would be a great addition to the culture. Certainly an alum can speak most effectively to the second objective. Of course, if you don't have access to an alum, a targeted recommendation from someone who can write convincingly about your qualifications is adequate.

☐ **A business course or an improved GMAT score:** Depending on when you hear back from your target school, this method may or may not be option. Given time, however, you might want to consider taking a business course or retaking the GMAT if you get the sense that the school has some reservations about your academic ability. In some cases, a school will actually allude to the fact that you will need to display more academic prowess in order to get off the waitlist. If you go down either or both paths and perform well, this is a great way to push yourself over the top.

☐ **Dialogue with a faculty member:** This method has the least predictable results and therefore is somewhat risky. The goal is to find a faculty member with whom you have similar interests and engage her in regard to those interests. Faculty members tend to like to discuss the topics that they've dedicated their lives to, so they are often open to discussing them. Your hope is that as a result of these brief conversations, the faculty mem-

ber will enjoy the dialogue enough to approach the admission committee and request that you be admitted. Of course, admissions committees
take faculty input very seriously, so if you get that far, a positive result is
more likely than not. The trick is getting that far. Just like contacting the
admissions committee, contacting a faculty member holds the possibility
that you will annoy her. In fact there is a greater possibility of this result,
because the faculty member isn't expecting you to contact her. As such,
you should proceed cautiously when selecting this method. For one thing,
don't go after the world-renowned faculty member. Chances are that
Michael Porter isn't going to freely swap e-mails with you. Rather, go
after a young faculty member who appears open to being engaged in
such a manner. Students can help point you to the professors who fall
into that category. Also, make sure you know what you're talking about.
The point is to find someone with whom you truly share interests, so it's
important that you can speak intelligently about those common interests. Indiscriminately contacting faculty members and blabbering about
how you need to get off the waitlist is a great way to get off that list...and
on to the rejection list.

❏ **A follow-up letter:** The follow-up letter is a great method to use in that it is
the least risky and the method over which you have the most control. As a
result, a well-written letter can be one of the most effective methods to
utilize in getting off the waitlist. Follow-up letters generally provide the
admissions committee with information about your activities since you've
applied. In some cases, you might not find out that you've been placed on
the waitlist until five months after you sent in your application. That means
there are plenty of new experiences to discuss that would improve your
candidacy in the eyes of the admissions committee. Additionally, the follow-up letter is a great method to use to pin-point the weaknesses that
you uncovered in your application evaluation. Finally, the follow-up letter
can highlight your fit with the b-school's culture and your passion for the
b-school's mission.

What follows is an example of a follow-up letter written by a successful applicant
who, after evaluating his application, decided to communicate several messages that
he felt would resonate positively with and admissions. The letter is written to the
applicant's contact in the admissions committee. Although the applicant is very strong
in terms of credentials, he failed to adequately represent himself in his application. In
this follow-up letter, he focuses on demonstrating his abilities, discussing his career
goals, and establishing fit with the target school. This was a very effective combination
and won the applicant a spot in the incoming class.

Sean's follow-up letter

*The purpose of this letter is to further support my candidacy
for admission to Top Business School (TBS). In short, attending TBS would be the perfect "next step" as I progress toward*

my long-term goals. Because fit with any institution is a two-way street, I will focus my comments on my professional progress, business model development, global perspective, community service involvement, and natural affinity with the TBS curriculum. These are all activities and attributes that would allow me to become a dynamic member of the TBS student community and eventually a leading member of the TBS alumni community. — — —

> Nice introduction that lets the admissions officer know exactly what to expect from this communication.

Professional progress

Since submitting my application to TBS, I have played key roles on two additional assignments that have strengthened my professional background. These roles have also provided me with additional experiences that I would bring into the TBS classroom.

As highlighted in my application, I am interested in increasing my knowledge of finance and marketing so that I can develop business cases for technological innovations. The roles that I've played on these assignments have helped start me in that direction. — — — — — — — — — — — — — — — —

> Sean does a nice job of putting his additional professional experiences into perspective in terms of his career goals rather than simply listing what he's done since submitting his application.

I recently completed a project involving an IT value assessment of a large pharmaceutical company. I played an integral part in determining the economic value added (EVA) of the corporation's IT expenditures. In order to determine how to better manage IT costs and enhance value to end-customers, I instituted a process that allowed the team to analyze IT cost drivers and distinguish between non-core and core IT functions. After careful review of the client's current technical solution evaluation processes, I developed a standard technical solution implementation methodology tailored to the demands and requirements of the company. To further enable the client to effectively manage IT expenses while maintaining market share, I created an IT competitive positioning strategy.

Currently, I am working with a core team of employees who recently formed SimTech's pharmaceutical group. In the last few months, my group has released Pharmtek. Pharmtek is a pharmaceutical industry-specific information technology solution package that is expected to experience rapid market growth over the next five years. To maximize our relationships with potential customers who might be interested in the Pharmtek solution, my team is focused on generating sales, recruiting and training skilled resources, developing external marketing campaigns, and generating support materials for sales teams. One of my primary tasks on this project has been to conduct research on major pharmaceutical industry trends. My research has focused on Customer Relationship Management (CRM), supply chain management, and the financing of research and development. Gaining a deeper knowledge of the activities of each functional area has given me a better understanding of our customers' strategic directions and the way in which technology can enable those directions. An added benefit, from a long-term perspective, has been that I have gained further insight into how I can activate a business model in the pharmaceutical industry.

Business model development

In my application to TBS, I stated my long-term ambition is to develop a global electronic exchange through which a select group of pharmaceutical and biotechnology companies can dynamically exchange research techniques and knowledge of various compounds. Through extensive research and a better understanding of the pharmaceutical industry, I have altered my concept to focus on purchasing trends of hospitals. My objective is to create a national exchange that allows hospitals to consolidate their purchasing power, reducing healthcare costs for hospitals and for patients.

Over the past six months, I have spent numerous hours developing a business plan that details the intricacies of my target market, business operations, and financials. The plan's pro forma financial statements indicate that there is a significant opportunity for such offerings both in the United States and in Europe. In the near term, I would like to improve my understanding of finance and marketing, while refining my business model. I also intend to submit my plan to a variety of local investment capital programs, such as the TBS Venture Fund and other lending institutions for financing. — — — — — — —

> Sean mentioned that he felt one of the weaknesses of his application was confusion around his career goals. Certainly this section helps the admissions officer understand the direction in which he's going. Sean actually followed up this letter by submitting an initial draft of his business plan to TBS.

Global perspective

The globalization trend continues to integrate information flow across nations. Having an understanding of globalization is therefore vital to the success of business leaders. A strong global perspective is an attribute that I have been able to impart in both my professional and personal endeavors. On a professional level, a global perspective has allowed me to provide insight in SimTech's analyses of clients who have outsourced operations to East Asian nations. Additionally, being bilingual and maintaining a strong network in Taiwan has been essential to my interactions with our global customers.

Community service involvement

One important component of my personal interests that I was not able to fully convey in my application is my involvement in community service activities. *Upon graduating from Adams University, I decided to participate in the Big Brothers Big Sisters (BBBS) program, which pairs adults with at-risk children from single-parent households. In January of 2000, I was matched with twins. As a Big Brother, it is impossible to count the number of ways that I had an impact on my Littles' lives. Over the course of our relationship, I have tried to instill the value of education and the desire to achieve a college degree. In addition to the impact that I have had on the boys, they have taught me not to always take myself so seriously. I would say that it has been a mutually beneficial relationship.*

The desire to create opportunities for others led me to establish a scholarship program in February 2000 at my alma mater. The scholarship is awarded each year to two entering freshmen who graduate from an inner city high school. The scholarship is given based on academic performance, community involvement, and an essay.

Most recently, I participated in School to Work Day, an annual SimTech team event in which we host local high school students. The day focused on connecting the academic world with the business world. Students were exposed to three different modules: resume building, public speaking, and a business case. As the lead for the public speaking module, I organized the material to be presented and coordinated the session. Each student had the opportunity to practice his or her public speaking skills and learn useful speaking tips that would be useful during presentations under myriad conditions.

Involvement with community outreach will continue to play a large role in my activities. I intend to establish foundations in both the United States and Taiwan that will assist underprivileged children in gaining access to educational opportunities that would otherwise be out of reach. — — — — — — — — — —

Sean made a big mistake in his application by not referencing any of his community service activities even though he's quite active. Certainly this section demonstrates to the admissions committee that he's involved with the community.

Natural affinity with TBS

As stated in my application, I believe that I would learn a great deal from TBS's cross-functional approach and "hands-on" style of teaching. The curriculum is very strong in the areas of finance, marketing, and international business. I have only become more convinced that TBS is the best place for me to pursue an MBA through discussions with current students and alumni, additional visits to campus, and further research on the curriculum and faculty. Moreover, my academic focus in computer science, combined with my professional experiences in high tech have given me a solid background from which my

TBS classmates would benefit and on which I would continue to build. Finally, the team atmosphere that TBS cultivates is inviting, as it reflects the emphasis on teamwork that is inherent within SimTech. — — — — — — — — — — — — — — — — —

> Sean is tactful in the way that he implicitly says that he'd accept an offer from TBS if it was given.

Upon graduating from TBS, I would like to spend a few years further honing my finance and marketing skills by getting on the front lines pitching the added value of technological innovation, all while continuing the development and refinement of my business plan. I am certain that TBS is the best institution for me in terms of preparation for such roles.

Below I have listed additional specific TBS resources from which I could benefit.

Faculty with similar professional interests:

☐ *Professor Ivy E. Lester—Professor of Finance.*

☐ *Professor David Aguliar—Professor of Technological Innovation and Entrepreneurship.*

☐ *Professor Anupam Kumar—Professor of High Technology Marketing.*

Classes of interest:

☐ *Marketing Management.*

☐ *Marketing Technology.*

☐ *Financing Your Start-up.*

☐ *Selling Technical Innovation.*

☐ *Strategic Marketing Planning.*

☐ *Preparing Your Business Plan.*

☐ *Entrepreneurial Management.*

☐ *International Marketing Management.*

☐ *Sources of Venture Capital and Private Equity.*

☐ *Principles of Corporate Finance.*

Activities of interest:

☐ *Asia Business Conference.*

☐ *Global Projects Club.*

☐ *Entrepreneurship Club.*

☐ *Entrepreneurship and Venture Capital Club.* — — — — —

> Simply listing a b-school's resources isn't all that impressive, but after gaining an understanding of Sean's background and goals, having these lists helps show how TBS will help Sean achieve his career goals.

*I am pleased to have been admitted to the waitlist and can
assure you that if I am admitted to TBS, my unique background
and strong spirit in the areas of culture, professional knowledge, academics and community involvement will supplement
the TBS environment and experience. I look forward to joining
you in August.*

   Sincerely,

   Sean

The secret to coming up with a successful strategy for getting off the waitlist is to
put together some combination of the five methods that addresses the weaknesses of
your application. In Sean's case he contacted the admissions committee from time to
time, submitted an additional recommendation from an alum, and of course, sent the
follow-up letter that you just read. Clearly, getting off the waitlist is no easy task, but
for those who are committed to the process and are willing to put together a targeted
strategy, they will be able to greatly increase their chances, just as in the initial application process.

Denial

It feels just like a punch in the stomach. "The Admissions Committee has thoroughly evaluated your application and regretfully cannot offer you a spot in the incoming class." Suddenly you don't want to face any of your friends, family members, or
peers at work. While getting denied by one or more of your target schools can certainly
be a humbling experience, there is a lot to be learned from it.

First, it's important to realize that the world isn't going to come to an end. Applying to top business schools is inherently a competitive process and odds are that you
will receive at least one denial. Second, you should take some time to evaluate your
application using the questions in the section on the waitlist. It's important that you
identify how you went astray in case you decide to reapply. Along those lines, a large
number of schools offer personalized feedback to applicants who are not granted admission. Take advantage of that even you'd prefer never to hear the b-school's name
again. Applicants generally find these feedback sessions to be useful and those that
incorporate the feedback into the following year's application often achieve admittance. In general, rates of admission for reapplicants are higher, but usually not by
more than a few percentage points.

With respect to reapplying, you may face a situation in which you are admitted to
one of your target schools but are still considering reapplying to a school that was higher
on the list. If you are confronted with this situation, then you should ask yourself whether
the b-school to which you've been admitted will provide you with an opportunity to
achieve your career goals. If the answer is no, then you shouldn't have applied to the
school in the first place. Just make sure that you don't pass on an option that would
allow you to achieve your goals so that you can potentially attend a "more prestigious"
business school in the future.

If you do decide to reapply, make sure that you fully understand the weaknesses of your initial applications and that you attack them tirelessly using the techniques we've outlined in previous chapters. With another year to prepare yourself, your application should shine with polish.

Certainly the goal of this book is to help you avoid facing the prospect of receiving denials. We feel strongly that if you closely follow the prescriptions we've outlined, you will be in a much better position to receive a thick letter once decision day comes. All the best!

Closing Thoughts

The one person who controls your application's fate more than anyone is you. Sure, it's difficult sending your application into the abyss not knowing the final outcome, but by the time of submission you'll have spent months maximizing your chances for success. Fit with your target school will be obvious. Your uniqueness will be clear. And your thick letter will be forthcoming. Let us know when you succeed. All the best!

INDEX

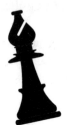
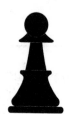
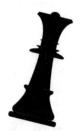

V

W

Y

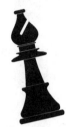
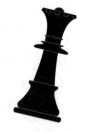

ABOUT THE AUTHORS

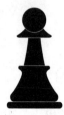

Scott Shrum is a second-year MBA student at the Kellogg School of Management at Northwestern University. His professional experience includes two years of business development for software provider MicroStrategy and several years of product marketing for the financial Website The Motley Fool. Scott used his marketing experience to craft a successful application strategy, gaining admission to both Kellogg and Harvard Business School. His Kellogg application earned him an F.C. Austin Scholarship, one of only 20 handed out by the school each year. In his spare time Scott serves as a professional editor for business school applicants, helping them to apply the principles in this book to their own essays. Scott graduated from the Massachusetts Institute of Technology with a Bachelor of Science degree in Business Administration and a minor in Writing.

Omari Bouknight is a second-year MBA student at Harvard Business School. He studied the business school application process for more than five years in preparation for his own attempt to gain acceptance into a top program. Utilizing application strategy, Omari received admission to Fuqua, Harvard Business School, Kellogg, University of Michigan Business School, and Wharton. Omari's professional experience consists of more than three years with Deloitte Consulting as a management consultant, assisting companies in developing and implementing business strategies. Omari received a Bachelors of Arts from Michigan State University as a triple major in International Relations, German, and Supply Chain Management.